# Assessment and Management of Hepatobiliary Disease

Edited by
L. Okolicsányi, G. Csomós, and G. Crepaldi

With 146 Figures and 110 Tables

Springer-Verlag Berlin Heidelberg New York
London Paris Tokyo

Lajos Okolicsányi, M. D.

Professor, Institute of Internal Medicine,
University of Padova, Via Giustiniani, 2, 35128 Padova/Italy

Géza Csomós, M. D.

Professor, Department of Clinical Research,
Heimhuder Straße 46, 2000 Hamburg/13 FRG

Gaetano Crepaldi, M. D.

Professor, Director, Institute of Internal Medicine,
University of Padova, Via Giustiniani, 2, 35128 Padova/Italy

ISBN-13: 978-3-642-72633-0 e-ISBN-13: 978-3-642-72631-6
DOI: 10.1007/978-3-642-72631-6

Library of Congress Cataloging-in-Publication Data.
Assessment and management of hepatobiliary disease.
Includes index. 1. Liver-Diseases. 2. Gallstones. I. Okolicsanyi, L. II. Csomós, G. (Geza) III. Crepaldi, Caetano. [DNLM: 1. Biliary Tract Diseases-diagnosis. 2. Biliary Tract Diseases-therapy. 3. Liver Diseases-diagnosis. 4. Liver Diseases-therapy. WI 700 A846]
RC845.A86 1987 616.3'6 87-12891


Softcover reprint of the hardcover 1st edition 1987



Typesetting: Appl, Wemding; Printing: Saladruck, Berlin; Bookbinding: Lüderitz & Bauer, Berlin
2121/3020 - 543210

# Preface

Basic and clinical research have in recent years contributed towards clarifying certain aspects of the epidemiology, pathogenesis, prevention, and treatment of liver diseases. New diagnostic techniques have, moreover, facilitated observations on the evolution of such diseases. Nevertheless, a number of questions still remain, especially in the assessment and management of liver patients. The hope that such questions can be answered justifies publications like the present one, which provide experts an opportunity to present the results of their research.

The papers collected in this volume cover all aspects of the assessment and management of hepatobiliary disease. The focal points are three summaries of the state of the art. The first deals with the highly topical problem of liver transplants from the point of view of patient selection. Roger Williams in fact stresses the urgent need to exercise caution in the selection of suitable candidates. This is especially true at the present time when cyclosporin A, a new immunosuppressive drug now available on the market, has significantly changed the natural history of survival after liver transplantation.

In his chapter on drug-induced liver injury, Hans Popper discusses the growing interest in the toxic effects of drugs on the liver, especially in view of the fact that the liver is the main metabolic site for a number of drugs. The final state of the art summary is also by Hans Popper and deals with a highly thought-provoking theme, liver and aging. The basic question Popper poses is, "Does the liver follow the aging process of the host organism?" The conclusion he reaches is that it probably does not, since the liver is an organ with a high regenerative capacity, although, generally speaking, its metabolic capacity does progressively decrease with age. Popper ends this chapter with a glance into the future, confronting the problem of whether the liver of aged liver transplant candidate donors is suitable for grafting.

Apart from these major points, the volume covers the entire range of issues concerning the assessment and management of hepatobiliary disease. First covered are basic research on hepatic transport mechanisms, intrahepatic cholestasis and gallstone disease, which serve as a background for the topics more specifically concerning the assessment of liver function. These topics were chosen in response to the growing need felt by researchers and clinicians for better insight into evaluating quantitative liver function. There is still, in fact, from the practical point of view, some misunderstanding as to whether "liver function tests" should also refer to the common (or routine) biochemical parameters. It was unanimously agreed that in the future the aim should be to have reliable, simple, easy-to-perform tests which provide information on metabolic liver function.

Much of the book is devoted to the management of the commonest forms of liver diseases and their complications, e.g., chronic active hepatitis, liver cirrhosis, portal hypertension, hepatic encephalopathy, hepatorenal syndrome, and ascites. The papers provide confirmation that a lot of progress has been made in this field. It therefore seems worthwhile to say that patients with chronic liver disease and its various complications can be treated with specific drugs, even if prevention remains the essential goal of liver therapy.

We should like to thank all the authors for their great cooperation. Our special thanks go to Niels Tygstrup and John Galambos, and in particular to Hans Popper, for his untiring enthusiasm for the furtherance of science.

We are also grateful to the CNR (National Research Council), the University of Padua, Boehringer Biochemia Robin and Madaus, and all the other pharmaceutical Companies who participated, without whose generous help this publication would not have been possible.

Hamburg, Padua, April 1987

Lajos Okolicsányi
Géza Csomós
Gaetano Crepaldi

# List of Contributors

# Contents

## Hepatic Transport Mechanisms, Intrahepatic Cholestasis and Gallstone Disease

## Assessment of Liver Function

## Management of Liver Disease

# Hepatic Transport Mechanisms, Intrahepatic Cholestasis and Gallstone Disease

# Liver Transplantation: State of the Art

Roger Williams, Rex J. Polson, and John G. O'Grady
Liver Unit, King's College Hospital and School of Medicine and Dentistry, Denmark Hill, London SE5 8RX, United Kingdom

## Introduction

Starzl carried out the first human liver transplant in 1963, and the first liver graft of the Cambridge/King's College Hospital series was performed by Calne in 1968. Two other groups with considerable early experience in this field were led by Pichlmayr in Hannover and Krom in Groningen. The data given by these groups and by the other participants in the National Institutes of Health Consensus Development Conference in 1983 led to the following conclusion: "Liver transplantation is a therapeutic modality for end stage liver disease that deserves broader application" (NIHCDC 1984). This has been followed by a very rapid increase in the number of centres in America and Europe which have either initiated or are planning programmes, as well as marked expansion in the already established transplant programmes. Consequently there has been an exponential increase in the number of patients receiving orthotopic liver transplants in Great Britain, Europe and the United States (Fig. 1). This increase in the number of patients transplanted has been matched by a rapid rise in the number of donor organs offered to our liver transplant co-ordinator between 1982 and 1985 (Fig. 2).

In 1984 and 1985 there has also been a considerable increase in the number of organs offered in the paediatric age-group. This is partly explained by a popular televi-

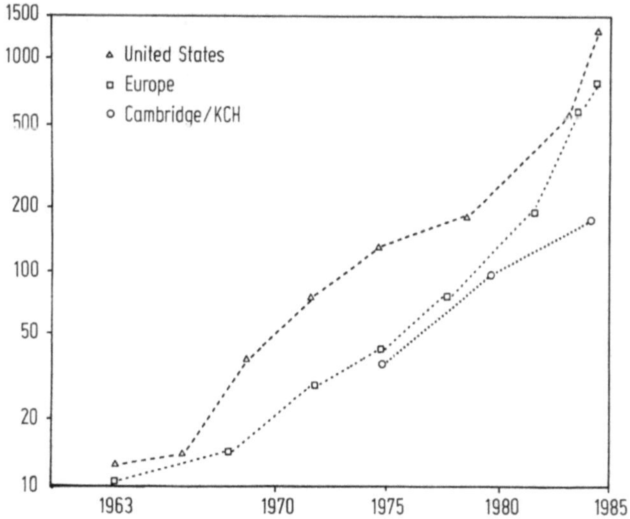


**Fig. 1.** The cumulative number of liver transplants performed in the United States, Europe and in the Cambridge/King's College Hospital series

Assessment and Management of Hepatobiliary Disease
Eds.: L. Okolicsányi, G. Csomós, and G. Crepaldi

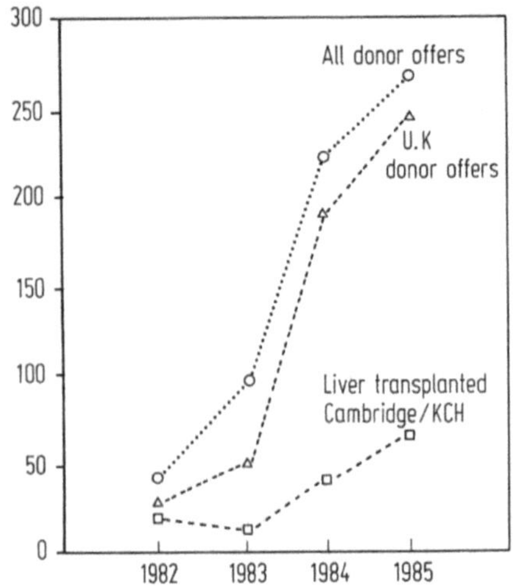


**Fig. 2.** Annual number of donor livers offered to the Cambridge/King's College Hospital programme

sion programme becoming involved in the plight of one of our young children with biliary atresia and the need for transplant facilities for infants and children in the U.K. This has led to an enormous increase in the general public's awareness of liver transplantation and in many instances the request for organs to be used for liver grafting has come from the families of those dying. At the same time doctors in general have been urged to take a more positive attitude to the use of organs from patients dying from accidents or other causes.

## Patient Selection and Pretransplant Assessment

Liver grafting should be considered whenever a patient with a progressive or otherwise fatal liver disorder is no longer able to live a reasonable existence but is still well enough to withstand the considerable trauma of the surgery involved. In practice, the decisions as to which patients should be treated and when can be very difficult. Included in the Cambridge/King's College hospital series, as in most transplant programmes, is almost every type of end-stage liver disease (Fig. 3). The timing of the intervention may be difficult in patients with chronic liver disease, with the exception of primary biliary cirrhosis, where a recently devised prognostic index has proved very useful (Neuberger et al. 1986).

### Malignant Liver Disease

All published experience points to a significant risk of tumour recurrence, and indeed in our programme 45%–100% of patients who survive more than 3 months after transplantation had evidence of recurrence, depending on the tumour type. In spite of the many methods now available for detection of extrahepatic spread, including CT scans, lymphangiography and radionuclide scanning, small tumour deposits, particularly in the porta hepatitis, may still be missed. Thus 20%–47% of various patient groups had macroscopically evident tumour nodules in resected specimens that had been missed on preoperative CT scans (Mittal et al. 1984). Nevertheless some patients with tumours

Orthotopic liver transplantation: Cambridge/King's College Hospital series May 1968-1st April 1986

| | | | | | |
|---|---|---|---|---|---|
| Primary liver tumour | | 66 | Cirrhosis | | 129 |
| Hepatocellular carcinoma | 49 | | Primary biliary | 47 | |
| Intrahepatic cholangiocarcinoma | 13 | | Chronic active hepatitis/cryptogenic | 48 | |
| Sarcoma | 4 | | Alcoholic | 6 | |
| Carcinoma of the hepatic ducts | | 9 | Sclerosing cholangitis/secondary biliary | 16 | |
| Hepatic metastases | | 6 | $\alpha_1$-Antitrypsin deficiency | 6 | |
| | | | Wilsons disease | 3 | |
| | | | Other Metabolic | 3 | |
| | | | Budd-chiari syndrome | | 13 |
| | | | Subacute/fulminant hepatic failure | | 9 |
| | | | Biliary atresia/neonatal hepatitis | | 18 |
| | | | Polycystic liver | | 2 |
| | | Total | 252 | | |

**Fig. 3.** Indications for liver transplantation in the Cambridge/King's College Hospital series (May 1968 to April 1986)

are suitable for treatment by liver transplantation which may even be curative. Our longest survivor remains well 10 years after his transplant, which followed detection of an asymptomatic hepatocellular carcinoma in a liver cirrhotic as a result of familial HBsAg infection. Patients like this in whom hepatoma development is detected at a presymptomatic stage by ultrasound or $\alpha$-fetoprotein screening, are beginning to figure more prominently in transplant series and represent a good group, as do the younger patients whose general condition is good and who have a relatively slow-growing hepatoma, possibly of the fibrolamellar type, which tends to metastasize late.

## Chronic End-Stage Liver Disease

In these patients the presence of ascites, encephalopathy, variceal bleeding or extreme lethargy which are resistant to conventional therapy may be the indication for liver grafting, and the symptomatic relief which follows transplantation is often remarkable.

In several of these conditions there have been reports of recurrence of the disorder in the grafted liver some time after successful transplantation. These include primary biliary cirrhosis (Neuberger et al. 1982); autoimmune chronic active hepatitis (Neuberger et al. 1984); hepatitis B; probably non-A, non-B hepatitis (Wall et al. 1985); and the Budd-Chiari syndrome. Of 13 patients with the latter condition in the Cambridge/King's College Hospital series, five (38%) have developed vascular thromboses after transplantation. In four cases this occurred in spite of treatment with anticoagulants.

## Inborn Errors of Metabolism

Many of these disorders, which would otherwise have proved fatal, have now been successfully treated by liver transplantation. Greater experience with combined organ transplants will also enable more disorders to be treated in which the primary damage is to an organ other than the liver. One example of this is a combined liver and kidney transplant performed recently in our transplant series in a patient with renal failure from primary hyperoxaluria, which led to a correction of abnormal oxalate pools (Watts et al. 1985). Similarly, a combined heart and liver transplant in a 6-year-old girl with familial hypercholesterolaemia provided sufficient low-density lipoprotein receptors in the normal donor liver to restore lipid metabolism to normal (Bilheimer et al. 1984; Starzl et al. 1984). We have recently successfully transplanted a 14-year-old boy with erythropoeitic protoporphyria and severe cholestatic liver disease. He is currently well and has had no further episodes of photosensitive skin rash, suggesting that the transplant has led to a clinically significant improvement in the underlying metabolic defect.

### Severe Hepatic Failure

Many difficulties surround liver transplantation for subacute or fulminant hepatic failure (Williams and Gimson 1984; Van Thiel et al. 1986). These patients usually deteriorate rapidly, and the donor organ has to be available during the short time when it is apparent that all other treatment measures are failing and yet the patient is still able to tolerate surgery. In spite of these difficulties and the marked coagulation deficiencies present in most of these patients, liver grafting has not proved so difficult as might be imagined. Thus, of the 11 patients transplanted for subacute or fulminant hepatic failure in the past 4 years in the Cambridge/King's College hospital series, seven (64%) recovered and left hospital well (O'Grady et al., unpublished observations).

## Operative Details

In children, particularly those aged 2 years or less, there are a greater number of technical difficulties, often related to congenital anomalies. It is also essential that the size of donor organ required by the recipient is matched carefully, so that vascular insufficiency and hepatic infarction are avoided. Older age is, however, less of a barrier than previously, and although cardiopulmonary complications become increasingly common over the age of 40 years, most transplant series, like ours, include occasional patients in their mid-60s.

The postoperative risks are considerably greater if the patients have had previous upper abdominal surgery, as this greatly increases the hazard of dissection and the likely blood loss. Disturbance of coagulation is also of major importance. Bontempo et al. (1985) reported that intraoperative blood usage was closely correlated to the severity of the preoperative coagulation abnormality and, not surprisingly, that blood usage and survival are inversely related. In a further, more recent report from Starzl's group, the survival rate was 70% for adult patients receiving up to 30 units of blood, but only 14% for patients requiring more than 30 units (Van Thiel et al. 1986). Poor nutrition and wasting of patients with chronic parenchymatous liver disease are further adverse factors which often result in reduced resistance to infection postoperatively. Starzl's group have found that the small shrunken liver commonly present in long-standing cirrhosis, instead of being easier, is often technically difficult to replace, and this group has a higher operative and preoperative mortality. Our own experience would support this.

Details of operative techniques differ considerably between centres, particularly with respect to the anastomosis of bile ducts. Calne uses the donor gall bladder as a conduit between donor and recipient ducts, whereas Starzl uses a direct and-to-end anastomosis. Krom et al. (1984) have recently stressed the importance of patency of the hepatic artery anastomosis to provide an adequate blood supply to the extrahepatic bile ducts, essential for their viability. They had a 17% complication rate and only one fatality in 29 patients using a choledocho-choledochostomy. Venoarterial bypass (Shaw et al. 1984) to decompress the splanchnic vein and vena cava is used in nearly all adult patients by Starzl and colleagues, while in the Cambridge/King's College Hospital series bypass is used in only about 10% of cases and venovenous bypass is the method employed (Calne et al. 1984).

## Postoperative Immunosuppression

Most immunosuppresive regimes are now based on Cyclosporin A (CyA). In most centres this is started immediately after the operation, although in our series, because of the drug's nephrotoxicity, we continue to use prednisolone and azathioprine for the first 3-4 days until urine output and electrolytes are satisfactory. Intravenous CyA is then started and continued by mouth when the T-tube is beginning to be clamped and oral intake is satisfactory, usually in the 2nd week after operation. After the first 3 months many patients can be maintained on CyA together with a small dose of prednisolone, and often even this can subsequently be withdrawn.

Work by Starzl's group on the pharmacokinetics of CyA metabolism has shown that when this drug is taken orally with food after an overnight fast, both peak and trough levels are approximately twice those seen when it is taken alone. Food increases bile output which then increases CyA absorption. A similar enhancement of bioavailability is seen when the T-tube is clamped around the time of CyA administration. Awareness of such factors allows reduction of the dose of CyA required to maintain adequate immunosuppression and so results in significant financial savings.

## Long-Term Rehabilitation and Current Results

About 80% of deaths after liver transplantation occur within the first 3 months; in patients who survive beyond this and who leave hospital, rehabilitation is usually excellent. Many return to full-time work, or to school, while of immense satisfaction is the ability to look after family and house again.

It is more relevant to examine the current results in different centres than to look back at overall results of transplant series obtained over a period of years during which there have been major changes in surgical technique, patient selection and immunosuppressive therapy. More patients have been treated in the Cambridge/King's College Hospital programme during the past 2 years than in any similar period previously – 80 patients compared with 147 in the period May 1968 to December 1983. The actuarial 1-year survival for all patients in the past 2 years is currently 45%, with a figure of 56% for patients aged 21 years or under. In Pittsburg, results have also tended to be better in the younger age-group, particularly in the earlier series. Of 47 paediatric patients transplanted over the period 1981-1983, 32 were alive 6-29 months later, including 7 of 15 patients who required retransplantation (Gartner et al. 1984). The latest published actuarial 1-year survival for adult transplants in Pittsburg is 60% (Van Thiel et al. 1986), the same rate as for actuarial 2-year survival in Minneapolis 1983-1985, while the most recent figure given for actuarial 1-year survival in Memphis is 62%. Of the 33 adult patients undergoing liver grafting in the Cambridge/King's College Hospital series in 1985, 24 are currently alive.

Now that a graft can reasonably be offered to patients before they are actually in the terminal phase of the disease, immediate survival results will almost certainly improve. When considering 1-year survival figures it is also important to take into account the frequency of retransplantation. Patients whose grafts do badly for any reason are best treated by early retransplantation. In Starzl's series around 30% of patients are retransplanted, while 5%-10% require a third graft. Such a policy is of course only possible when there is an adequate supply of suitable donor organs.

## References

Bilheimer DW, Goldstein JL, Grundy SM, Starzl TE, Brown MS (1984) Liver transplantation to provide low-density-lipoproteinreceptors and lower plasma cholesterol in a child with homozygous familial hypercholesteraemia. N Engl J Med 311: 1658-1664

Bontempo FA, Lewis JH, van Thiel DH, Spero JA, Ragni MB, Butler P, Isreal L, Starzl TE (1985) The relation of preoperative coagulation finding to diagnosis, blood usage and survival in adult liver transplantation. Transplantation 39: 532-536

Calne RY, Rolles K, Forman JV, Kneeshaw JD, Smith DP, Wheeldon DR (1984) Veno-arterial bypass in orthotopic liver grafting. Lancet 2: 1269

Gartner JC, Zitelli BJ, Malatack JJ, Shaw BW, Iwatsuki S, Starzl TE (1984) Orthotopic liver transplantation in children: two year experience with 47 patients. Paediatrics 74: 140-145

Krom RAF, Kingman LM, Wesenhagen W, Slooff MJH, Haagsma EB, Grips CH (1984) Choledochocholedochostomy is successful in orthotopic liver transplantation. Transplant Proc 16(5): 1228-1229

Mittal R, Kowal C, Starzl T, van Thiel D, Bron K, Iwatsuki S, Schade R, Straub W, Dekker A (1984) Accuracy of computerized tomography in determining hepatic tumour size in patients receiving liver transplantation or resection. J Clin Oncol 2(6): 637-642

National Institutes of Health Consensus Development Conference Statement (1984) Liver transplantation – June 20-23, 1983. Hepatology [Suppl] 4

Neuberger JM, Portmann B, Macdougall B, Calne RY, Williams R (1982). Recurrence of primary biliary cirrhosis after liver transplantation. N Engl J Med 306: 1-4

Neuberger JM, Portmann B, Calne RY, Williams R (1984) Recurrence of autoimmune chronic active hepatitis following orthotopic liver grafting. Transplantation 37: 363-365

Neuberger JM, Altman DG, Christensen E, Tygstrup N, Williams R (1986) Use of a prognostic index in liver transplantation for primary biliary cirrhosis. Transplantation (in press)

Shaw BW, Martin DJ, Marquez JM, Kang YG, Bugbee AC, Iwatsuki S, Griffith BP, Hardesty RL, Bahnson HT, Starzl TE (1984) Venous bypass in clinical liver transplantation. Ann Sug 200: 524-534

Starzl TE (ed) (1969) Experience in liver transplantation. Saunders, Philadelphia

Starzl TE, Bilheimer DW, Bahnson HT, Shaw BW, Hardesty RL, Griffith BP, Iwatsuki S, Zitelli BJ, Gartner JC, Malatack JJ, Urbach AH (1984) Heart-liver transplantation in a patient with familial hypercholesteremia. Lancet 1: 1382-1383

Wall WJ, Duff JH, Ghent CN, Stiller CR, Keown PA, Kutt JL (1985) Liver transplantation: the initial experience of a Canadian centre. 28: 286-289

Watts RWE, Calne RY, Williams R, Mansell MA, Veall N, Purkiss P, Rolles K (1985) Primary hyperoxaluria (Type 1): attempted treatment by combined hepatic and renal transplantation. Q J Med 57: 697-703

Williams R, Gimson AES (1984) An assessment of orthotopic liver transplantation in acute liver failure. Hepatology 4: 225-245

Van Thiel DH, Tarter R, Gavaler JSD, Potanko WM, Schade RR (1986) Liver transplantation in adults. An analysis of costs and benefits at the University of Pittsburg. Gastroenterology 90: 211-216

# Mathematical Models for the Study of Hepatic Metabolism: A New Strategy

N. Dioguardi[1], P. Mussio[2], M. Zuin[1], and A. Lovati[2]

[1] Istituto di Medicina Interna, Via Pace 9, Milano, Italy
[2] Cattedra di Teoria Generale dei Sistemi, Via Viotti, Milano, Italy

The employment of models in the description of reality is a central moment in the scientific method. The employment of mathematical models in medicine has not been very widespread due to the intrinsic complexity of biological phenomena; their formal representation in modeling is made difficult by the unmethodical and often limited availability of in vivo data for simulation.

Disorders and narrowness and restricted application come, first of all, from the measurement modalities adopted (Cobelli et al. 1984). As a matter of fact, the number of variables or parameters which can be obtained from the phenomenon under consideration is often limited; besides this, many of them cannot be directly measured as the construction of the model would require. On the contrary, in those cases in which one is presented with numerous essential variables or parameters, their number may be so high that any formalization achieved by traditionally utilized mathematical tools is impossible. One must add that most measurements are seriously afflicted by "noise" due to experimental error or to uncontrollable physiological perturbations.

Beside these, other difficulties are created by the absence of an actual collaboration between physicians, systemists, mathematicians, and physicists due to the lack of an interface, an essential tool for the construction and application of mathematical models (Cobelli et al. 1984). The systemist is not able to understand thoroughly all details of the physiological phenomena underlying the systems that he has to describe; thence, models and formal representations that he formulates without any collaboration with physicians are in general more directed by the requirements of informatics than by the observed physiologic reality. The mathematician, in fact, is induced to fit reality to formal tools at his disposal. The physician, in contrast, is inclined to consider the mathematical model a useful tool for data analysis rather than an integrant component of an experimental project.

The preferential use of analytical, Cartesian type approaches in the biological field must be added to these motives. Partialization, the fundamental characteristic of this methodology, makes the description of complex phenomena difficult. In fact, while it may enable single components to be identified, an understanding of the individuation of the interrelations and the organization which tie such elements together become very problematic. Models thus obtained are complicated and cannot be expressed through a formalism (Dioguardi 1984).

The analysis of complex phenomena requires, in contrast, an approach with takes into account not only the identification of the single components that constitute reality, but also and above all the interrelations existing between the single components, i.e., the order and the organization which characterizes them.

An approach derived from general systems theory takes into account these method-

Assessment and Management of Hepatobiliary Disease
Eds.: L. Okolicsányi, G. Csomós, and G. Crepaldi

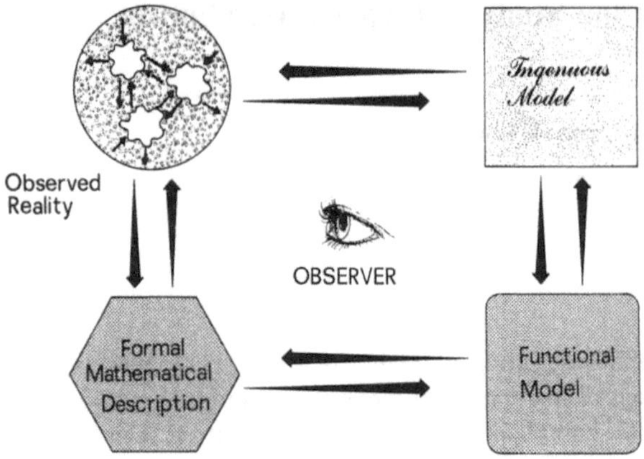


**Fig. 1.** Logical procedure for the construction of a system

ological needs (Miller 1965; von Bertalanffy 1969) and, just because if these characteristics, has already been successfully employed in fields other than biology.

On the basis of these considerations, we have proposed that such a methodology be employed in the study of the liver and its metabolic activities, which are highly complex dynamic realities with regard to both number of components and complexity of mutual interrelations (Dioguardi 1984). In constructing the systemic model we have followed the logical process suggested by Padulo and Arbib (1974) and modified by Dioguardi (1984) (Fig. 1).

According to this approach the observer has, first of all, to identify the components of the complex reality under consideration, including the interrelations among them and between them and the encompassing environment, in relation to the goal for which these entities work.

Since the identification and description of a system is always a multidisciplinary task of groups with different cultures and languages, the reality which one intends to organize in a systemic order must be described by a model which includes all the useful information coming from as wide a range of hypotheses as possible. This first representation is proposed by the physician who describes the reality under examination and its elements on the basis of the theoretical and empirical knowledge at his disposal, oriented around what he has defined to be the system's goal.

Phenomena may be described in an informal, simple, and even coarse way by a natural and/or a graphic language, which must always be comprehensible to the systemist who has to functionalize and formalize the model. This model, proposed by Dioguardi (1984), has been called an "ingenuous model." In constructing the ingenuous model, the physician isolates the operators that effect the modifications of the substance going through the system. The sequence of the operators is the one proposed by Miller (1965b) for a metabolic subsystem (Fig. 2).

A metabolic system, in fact, consists of the following operators:

- An *ingestor,* which regulates the input of matter and energy into the subsystem. It may consist, in turn, of a preselector, a selector, and an introducer. The preselector effects a first selection of the substances which the selector will then sort out in a very rigorous way. Only highly selected matter is introduced by the ingestor.

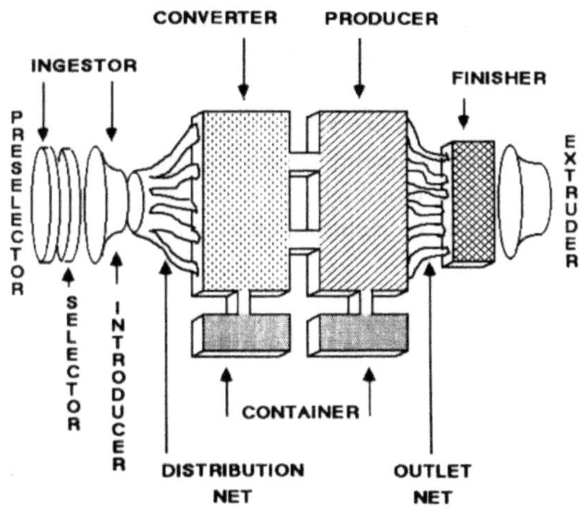


**Fig. 2.** Operators of a metabolic subsystem

- A *distribution net,* which conveys the introduced matter towards the biotransformer.
- The *biotransformer* consists of a converter which transforms input matter in matter recognizable by the producer. The producer works out export material only from matter that it recognizes.
- A *container,* which acts as matter storage for not yet elaborated matter or for matter elaborated for the quick use of the system itself or of the whole organism.
- An *extruder,* which provides the dismissal of the finished product.

In conclusion the ingenuous model may be garded as the "interface" between the physician and the systems engineer. Its insertion in the logical process is particularly important if one considers that incommunicability between physicians and mathematicians is deemed one of the main factors in the limited use of mathematical models in medicine.

The next step consists in the construction of the functional model, in which anatomical structures disappear. The set of functions arranged in a sequence constitutes the metabolic flux line of matter which runs inside the subsystem. From the functional map, one can proceed to the construction of the formal model, applying each time very different mathematical techniques. Each step of this process can be rectified at any moment.

The first experiment on functionalization and formalization of an hepatic subsystem's activity has been carried out on the subsystem for recycling and bile elimination of copper. The choice of this subsystem for our pilot modeling experiment is due to the fact that the liver carries out a central role in the metabolism of this metal. Such metabolism, which has been thoroughly studied under normal and pathological conditions, is relatively simple since it is not integrated very much with the metabolism of other compounds produced in the liver and excreted in bile. In the formal representation of the functional model we have adopted the septuple (Padulo and Arbib, 1974). The septuple is a family of seven sets which describe the evolution in terms of inputs, outputs, and states of the system, according to the preconstituted functional model. The septuple has been translated in a simulation program implemented in APL on PERQ1 ICL workstation under PNX (Unix-Like) operating system.

In this way, it has been possible to obtain a simulation for the behavior of hepatic copper metabolism in normal and pathological conditions (cholestasis, Wilson's disease, Menkes' disease, congenital hypoceruloplasminemia). In our experience the systemic approach thus supplies a model which makes it possible to study, in quantitative and dynamic terms, the activity of the hepatic metabolic subsystems and to predict their behavior in physiological and pathological conditions. It can therefore be regarded as a new strategy for the construction of mathematical models in hepatology.

## References

Bertalanffy L von (1969) General system theory. Braziller, New York
Cobelli G, Carson ER, Finkelstein L, Leaning MS (1984) Validation of simple and complex models in physiology and medicine. Am J Physiol 246: R259-R266
Dioguardi N (1984) Il fegato: un sistema aperto. Masson Italia, Milan
Miller JG (1965a) Living systems: basic concepts. Behav Sci 193-237
Miller JG (1965b) Living systems: structure and process. Behav Sci 337-379
Padulo L, Arbib MA (1974) System and the concept of state. In: System theory. Saunders, Philadelphia

# Mechanism of Hepatic Fatty Acid Uptake*

Wolfgang Stremmel[1] and Paul D. Berk[2]

[1] Medizinische Klinik D der Universität Düsseldorf, Moorenstr. 5, 4000 Düsseldorf, Federal Republic of Germany
[2] The Polly Annenberg Levee Hematology Center and the hepatic Research Group (Department of Medicine), Mount Sinai School of Medicine, New York, NY 10029, U.S.A.

## Background

Long-chain fatty acids are quantitatively the most important substrates for energy production. After absorption by the jejunal mucosa, they are tightly bound to albumin within the circulation and transported to the sites of fatty acid utilization. Cellular fatty acid uptake is rapid and efficient, but little is known about the mechanism by which they permeate the plasma membrane. The lipophilic character of fatty acids suggests that they might diffuse directly through the phospholipid bilayer of the membrane [1-3]. However, cellular influx of other structural components and major energy-yielding substrates, such as glucose and amino acids, has been shown to be a site of metabolic and hormonal control. Therefore it appears plausible that cellular uptake of long-chain fatty acids might also be regulated by a membrane-associated receptor complex. This is supported by the observation that cellular fatty acid influx is modulated by nutritional state, sex hormones, and application of drugs, such as clofibrate [4-6]. Furthermore, a few kinetic studies have suggested that at least a portion of fatty acid uptake might be mediated by a specific transport system. Particularly the observation of saturable fatty acid uptake kinetics in cardiac cells and adipocytes was thought to be compatible with a carrier-mediated transport mechanism [7-10]. However, some investigators have argued that the apparent saturation observed in those studies, as well as the effect on uptake produced by sex hormones, fasting, and clofibrate, reflects intracellular fatty acid metabolism rather than membrane transport [11, 12].

In the following we will review the evidence supporting the concept that the cellular uptake of fatty acids, particularly in rat hepatocytes, represents a carrier-mediated membrane transport process.

## Dissociation of the Fatty Acid - Albumin Complex at the Liver Cell Plasma Membrane

Free fatty acids, as well as other classes of organic anions, are presented to the liver as albumin complexes within the plasma. Since albumin is not taken up by the liver cells, it is clear that albumin-bound ligands are separated from the albumin molecule prior to their hepatocellular uptake. Direct estimation of the in vitro dissociation rates of the

* Supported by grant STR 216/2-3 from the *Deutsche Forschungsgemeinschaft,* grant AM-26438 from the National Institute of Arthritis, Diabetes, Digestive and Kidney Disease, and generous gifts from the Jack Martin Fund and the Polly Annenberg Levee Charitable Trust.

Assessment and Management of Hepatobiliary Disease
Eds.: L. Okolicsányi, G. Csomós, and G. Crepaldi

albumin complexes of ligands such as bilirubin or fatty acids [13–16] indicates that these rates are slow compared to the hepatic uptake rates for the corresponding ligand in vivo [17–19]. Therefore the dissociation rate of ligand-albumin complexes within the space of Disse or at the sinusoidal surface of the liver cell in vivo must appreciably exceed that predicted on the basis of the dissociation rates determined in vitro. It is still controversial whether this accelerated dissociation is due to a specific albumin receptor or, more likely, mediated by high-affinity binding sites for the ligands on the cell surface or by nonspecific interactions with the albumin-ligand complex at or near the hepatocellular plasma membrane [20].

## Kinetics of Cellular Fatty Acid Influx

To evaluate the processes by which fatty acids enter hepatocytes after their dissociation from the albumin molecule, it is essential first to establish whether uptake occurs passively, by simple diffusion through the plasma membrane, or whether the membrane itself participates in some form of facilitated transport. Determination of the cellular uptake rate of a substance as a function of its external concentration can distinguish simple diffusion, which is a linear relationship, from transport, which is a saturable process, provided membrane permeation is the rate-limiting step. Therefore the uptake kinetics of a representative fatty acid, $^{14}$C-oleate, were studied in isolated hepatocytes [21, 22].

First it was shown that uptake of $^{14}$C-oleate into isolated hepatocytes was maximal and linear only over the first 30-s incubation period, and that this initial uptake rate, representing cellular influx, was independent of intracellular fatty acid metabolism, including oxidation and esterification [21]. In the studies illustrated in Fig. 1, $^{14}$C-oleate was added to the incubation mixtures bound to albumin in various molar ratios, which served to modulate the unbound oleate concentration in the medium. At 37 °C, hepatocellular influx of $^{14}$C-oleate increased hyperbolically as a function of its unbound ex-

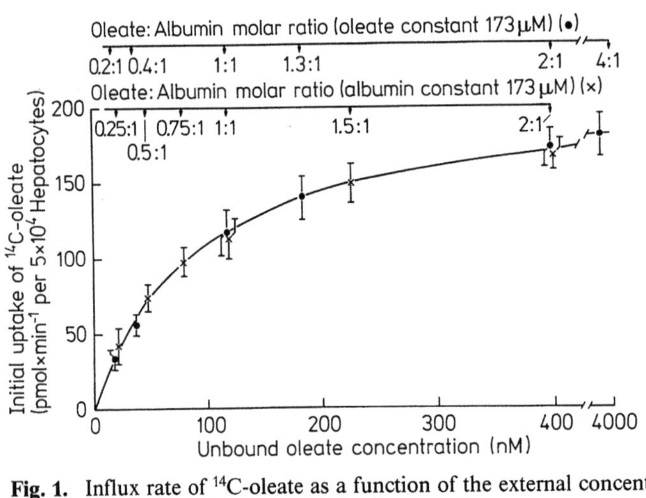


**Fig. 1.** Influx rate of $^{14}$C-oleate as a function of the external concentration of free oleate. Values are means ± SD of β-5 three to five replicate studies

ternal concentration, with the following saturation kinetics: $K_m = 83\ nM$; $V_{max} = 197$ pmol/min/5 × $10^4$ hepatocytes.

Several additional characteristics of hepatocellular fatty acid uptake have now been documented and are suggestive of carrier-mediated transport. In particular, uptake was shown to be specific, since influx of $^{14}C$-oleate was not inhibited by the presence of other organic anions such as BSP, taurocholate, or cholate, but markedly reduced in presence of other long-chain fatty acids. Initial uptake of $^{14}C$-oleate was markedly reduced by preincubation of hepatocytes with trypsin and inhibited by more than 75% in the presence of phloretin, a potent inhibitor of cellular transport processes. Furthermore, $^{14}C$-oleate influx revealed temperature dependency, with an optimum at 37 °C. Collectively these data strongly suggest that hepatocellular uptake of fatty acids is carrier-mediated.

## Binding Characteristics of Fatty Acids to Isolated Rat Liver Plasma Membranes

Since the first step in any carrier-mediated transport process is the binding of ligand to the carrier, binding of $^{14}C$-oleate to isolated rat liver plasma membranes was studied to demonstrate the presence of specific binding sites, presumptively representing the putative carrier (Fig. 2) [23]. Rat liver plasma membranes were incubated with 60 μM $^{14}C$-oleate bound to albumin such that the oleate: albumin molar ratio increased from 0.25:1 to 5:1, thus providing an exponentially increasing concentration of free oleate available in the incubation mixture. With increasing free oleate concentration incubated, total binding to rat liver plasma membranes increased in a nonlinear sigmoidal fashion. In comparison, binding to heat-denatured plasma membranes was much lower and increased linearly with increasing free oleate concentration. It was therefore considered to be a measure of nonspecific binding. When total binding to native plasma membranes was corrected for nonspecific binding, values for specific binding were obtained. Specific binding was shown to be saturable with $10^{15}$ high-affinity binding sites per milligram membrane protein ($K_{av} = 20\ nM$). Furthermore, binding was reversible by postincubation with excess cold oleate, pH- and temperature-dependent, and significantly reduced after trypsin pretreatment [23, 24].

## Identification of a Fatty-Acid-Binding Membrane Protein

The demonstration of saturable, trypsin-inhibitable binding suggested that high-affinity, specific binding is due to an intrinsic membrane protein. This suggestion was pursued by application of solubilized proteins from rat liver plasma membranes to affinity chromatography over oleate-coupled agarose [23]. Figure 3 illustrates SDS rod gels of the original mixture of membrane proteins (column A) and of a single 40000-kd protein recovered from the oleate agarose gel (column B). For comparison the membrane sulfobromophthalein (BSP)/bilirubin-binding protein is shown in column C [25]. The protein isolated from oleate agarose revealed an isoelectric point of 9.0 and lacked lipid or carbohydrate components. On gel filtration, the protein comigrated with various long-chain fatty acids but not with other organic anions such as BSP, bilirubin, and taurocholate or other lipids such as phosphatidylcholine or cholesterol esters.

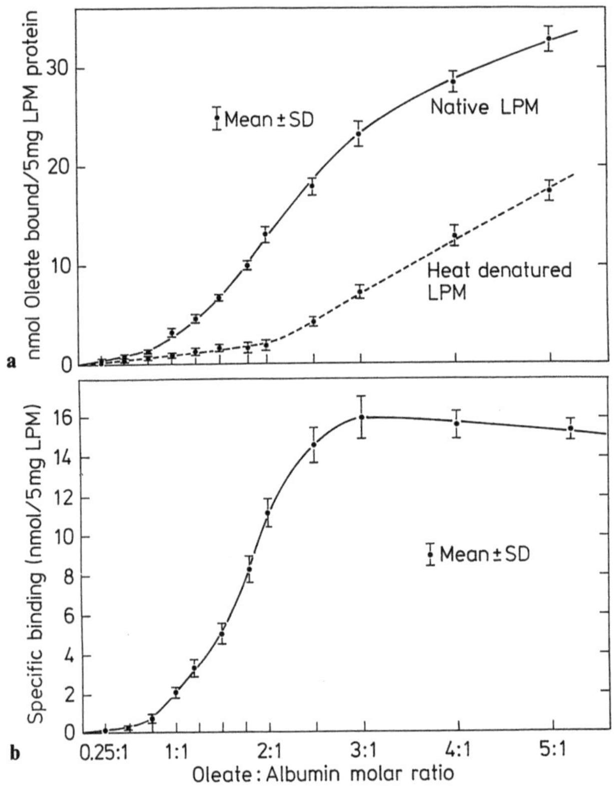


**Fig. 2.** **a** Binding of $^{14}$C-oleate to native and heat-denatured rat liver plasma membranes *(LPM)* (mean ± SD; n = 5). Each incubation contained 5 mg LPM protein and a total oleate concentration of 60 μM. The bovine serum albumin concentration was varied so that the oleate: albumin ratio ranged from 0.25 : 1 to 5 : 1. **b** Specific binding of $^{14}$C-oleate to LPM, calculated from the data in **a** as total binding to native membranes minus binding to heat-denatured LPM

A monospecific antibody against the fatty-acid-binding membrane protein was raised in rabbits, and its effect on binding of selected organic anions to rat liver plasma membranes was tested [23]. In comparison to control incubations containing anti-fibronectin, this antibody inhibited the membrane binding of $^{14}$C-oleate, but not that of BSP or taurocholate, in concentration-dependent fashion (Fig. 4). The fatty-acid-binding membrane protein was localized in rat tissues by a fluorescence antibody technique. In selections of normal rat liver the entire surface membrane appeared to bind the antibody (Fig. 5).

## Biologic Significance of the Fatty-Acid-Binding Membrane Protein in the Hepatocellular Uptake of Fatty Acids

To evaluate the physiologic significance of the isolated fatty-acid-binding membrane protein as a putative carrier in the hepatocellular uptake of fatty acids, the effect of the monospecific antibody to this protein on hepatocellular $^{14}$C-oleate uptake was ex-

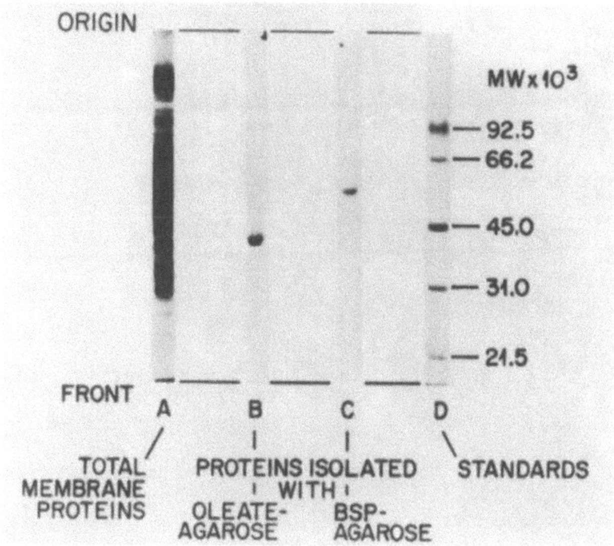


**Fig. 3.** Affinity chromatography of Triton X-100 solubilized proteins from rat liver plasma membrane proteins. Shown are a Coomassie-blue-stained cylindrical gel after SDS PAGE of total solubilized membrane proteins (gel *A*), a 40-kd protein eluted from oleate agarose with 8 *M* urea (gel *B*), a 55-kd protein eluted from BSP agarose with BSP (gel *C*), and standards (gel *D*)

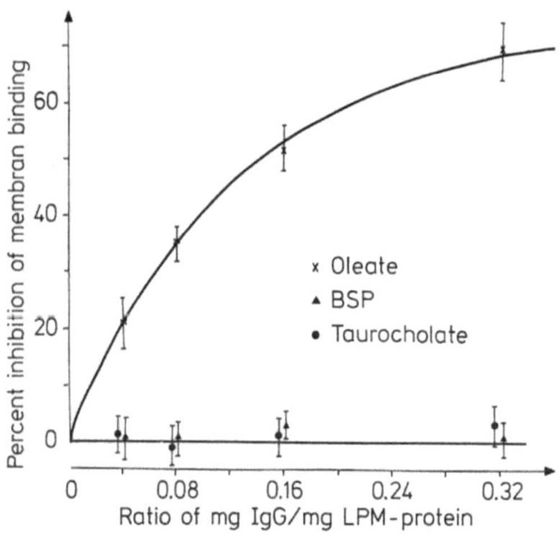


**Fig. 4.** Inhibition of $^{14}$C-oleate binding to rat liver plasma membranes (LPM) by a monospecific antibody to the fatty-acid-binding membrane protein (LPM-FABP). In paired studies, various quantities of LPM (0.625–5 mg protein) were pretreated with 0.2 mg of the IgG fraction of either anti-LPM-FAB P or anti-rat fibronectin (as controls). After addition of $^{14}$C-oleate:albumin (3:1), $^{35}$S-BSP:albumin (1:2), or $^{14}$C-taurocholate, the reaction mixture was incubated for 30 min at 37 °C. Binding of ligand to LPM was determined in the presence of each antibody; results are expressed as percent inhibition by anti-LPM-FABP compared to binding observed in the presence of antifibronectin. Mean values ± SD ($n = 3$)

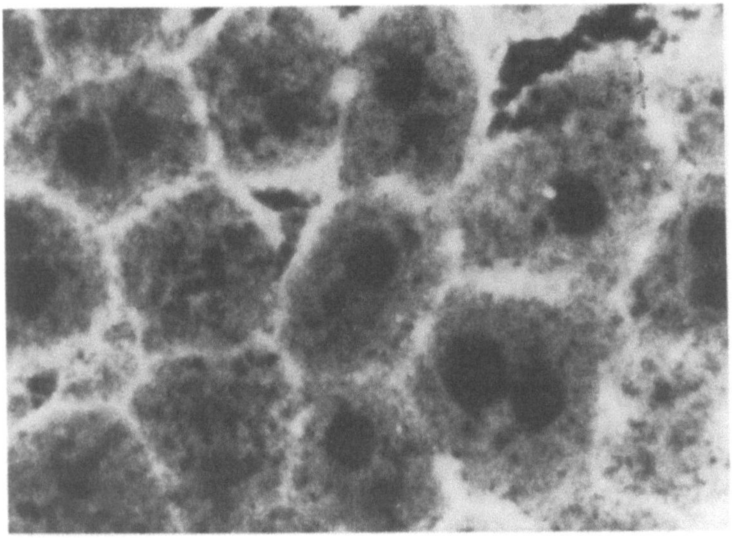

**Fig. 5.** Indirect immunofluorescence staining of the plasma membranes of hepatocytes in normal rat liver sections after incubation with an antibody to the fatty-acid-binding membrane protein

amined (Fig. 6) [22]. When oleate uptake by hepatocytes pretreated with the IgG fraction of this antibody was compared with that of a control preparation pretreated with the IgG fraction of the preimmune serum, a statistically significant ($p < 0.001$) inhibition of the initial uptake velocity by the antibody against the fatty-acid-binding membrane protein was clearly demonstrated. Michaelis-Menten analysis of fatty acid uptake kinetics revealed a predominantly noncompetitive type of inhibition by the antibody.

Similar results were obtained in the experimental model of short-term cultured hepatocytes, where a 70% inhibition of $V_{max}$ but only a 16% reduction of $K_m$ was detected in presence of the antibody against the fatty-acid-binding protein [26]. A similar marked inhibition of the cellular influx of oleic acid, arachidonic acid, palmitic acid, and stearic acid, by 58%–69%, provided evidence that the fatty-acid-binding membrane protein functions as a general carrier protein for long-chain fatty acids (Fig. 7) [26]. In contrast, uptake of representatives of other classes of organic anions, such as BSP, cholic acid, and taurocholic acid were not affected by the antibody to the fatty-acid-binding membrane protein, suggesting that they are transported via a different uptake mechanism. These studies indicate that the liver plasma membrane fatty-acid-binding protein must have a significant role in the hepatocellular uptake of free fatty acids.

## Driving Forces for Hepatic Fatty Acid Uptake

In further studies, the driving forces mediating the hepatocellular uptake of free fatty acids were examined. When uptake was studied in the absence of sodium by means of replacement of sodium chloride in the medium with choline chloride, influx of $^{14}C$-

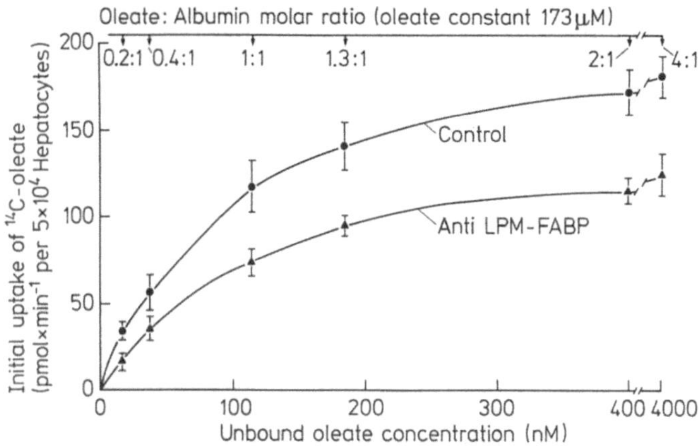


**Fig. 6.** Inhibition of $^{14}$C-oleate uptake into isolated hepatocytes by the antibody to the fatty-acid-binding membrane protein. Cells pretreated with 400 μg of the IgG fraction of the immune serum were compared to a control preparation pretreated with the preimmune serum. 250 μl of the cell suspensions ($2 \times 10^6$ cells/ml) were incubated with 173 μM $^{14}$-oleate bound to albumin in various molar ratios at 37 °C in 1 ml BP S. Illustrated are the initial uptake rates as a function of the calculated unbound oleate concentrations in the incubation media. $^{14}$C-oleate influx is significantly reduced by the antibody to the fatty-acid-binding membrane protein. Values are means ± SD of three replicate experiments

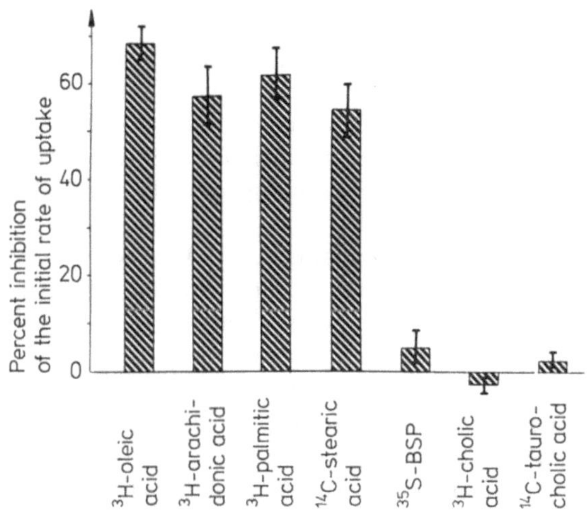


**Fig. 7.** Specificity of the fatty-acid-binding membrane protein on the hepatocellular uptake process of organic anions. Short-term cultured hepatocytes pretreated with the IgG fraction of a monospecific antibody to the fatty-acid-binding membrane protein (LPM-FABP) were compared to a control preparation pretreated with the IgG-fraction of the preimmune serum. The cultures were then incubated with 173 μM $^3$H-oleic acid, $^3$H-arachidonic acid, $^3$H-palmitic acid, $^{14}$C-stearic acid (all bound to albumin in a molar ratio of 1:1), 20 $\mu M$ $^3$H-cholic acid, or 200 $\mu M$ $^{14}$C-taurocholic acid. Initial rate of uptake ($V_o$) was calculated from the linear slopes of the cumulative uptake curves over the first 30-s incubation period. Values are expressed as percent inhibition of $V_o$ by the anti-LPM-FABP compared to the controls and represent means ± SD of three replicate experiments

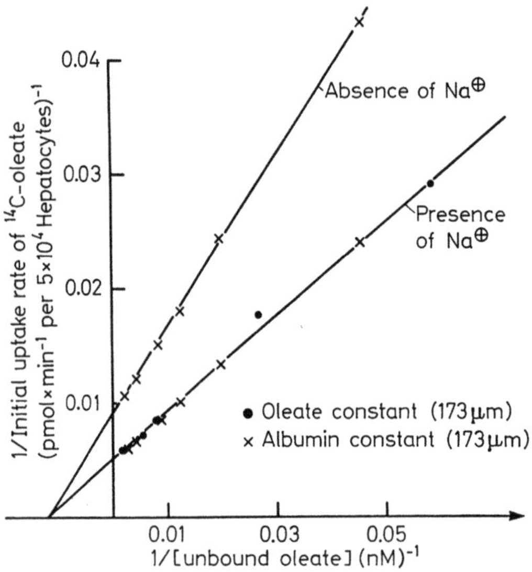


**Fig. 8.** Lineweaver-Burk plot of influx rates of $^{14}$C-oleate as a function of the external concentrations of free oleate. Influx rates of $^{14}$C-oleate were determined in the presence and absence of sodium. Points represent means of three–five replicate studies: coefficient variation averaged 11%

oleate was significantly decreased (Fig. 8) [22]. Calculation of Michaelis-Menten parameters revealed a depression of $V_{max}$ but an unchanged $K_m$ value compared to uptake studies in the presence of sodium. Because similar degrees of inhibition were also observed by replacement of $Na^+$ with sucrose or with various cations such as $K^+$ or $Li^+$ which have different membrane permeabilities and cellular effects, it is likely that these results reflect the specific absence of $Na^+$ and not nonspecific electrochemical alterations.

From these results it was suggested that hepatocellular uptake of fatty acids is coupled to the influx of $Na^+$ down its electrochemical gradient, thus providing the driving force for uptake. The energy for the sodium-coupled uptake of fatty acids is, ultimately, generated by hydrolysis of ATP by the plasma membrane enzyme $Na^+$, $K^+$-ATPase. This inorganic ion pump, maintaining the characteristic low intracellular $Na^+$ and high $K^+$ concentration, establishes an inwardly directed electrochemical $Na^+$ gradient which provides the driving force for fatty acid uptake.

Consistent with this hypothesis, ouabain, a well-known inhibitor of $Na^+$, $K^+$-ATPase reduced initial uptake of $^{14}$C-oleate into isolated hepatocytes, as did metabolic inhibitors such as KCN or dinitrophenol that deplete cellular ATP levels [22]. Collectively, these data suggest that the carrier-mediated transport of free fatty acids is driven by the transmembrane $Na^+$ gradient generated by $Na^+$, $K^+$-ATPase, possibly involving a secondary active $Na^+$-fatty acid symport system which binds $Na^+$ and a fatty acid anion and transports them together into the cell.

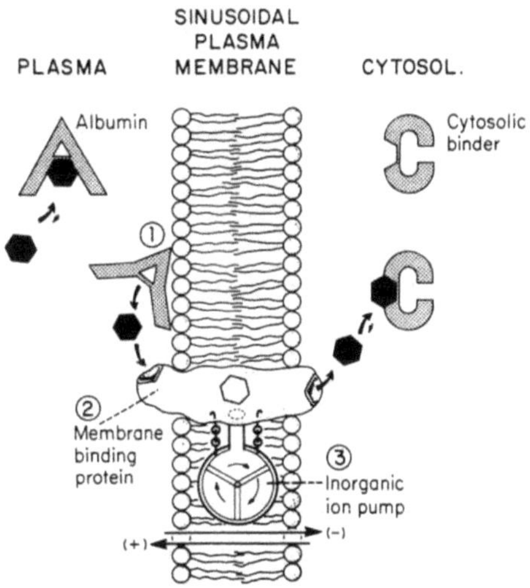


**Fig. 9.** Hepatocellular uptake of albumin-bound organic anions

## Conclusion

The translocation of long-chain fatty acids across the sinusoidal membrane of hepatocytes involves (Fig. 9):

- Accelerated but probably nonspecific dissociation of the albumin-fatty acid complex at the cell surface.
- Binding of fatty acids to a specific membrane protein which functions as carrier for fatty acids across the plasma membrane.
- Movement of fatty acids across the cell membrane coupled to the influx of $Na^+$ down its concentration gradient. After entering the cytoplasm of hepatocytes, fatty acids bind to the low-molecular-weight cytosolic fatty-acid-binding protein which directs fatty acids to the sites of further metabolism.

## References

1. Kuhl W, Spector AA (1970) Uptake of long chain fatty acid methyl esters by mammalian cells. J Lipid Res 11: 458-465
2. Spector AA, Fletcher JE (1978) Transport of fatty acid in the circulation. In: Dietschy, Gotto, Ontko (eds) Disturbances in lipid and lipoprotein metabolism. Williams and Wilkins, Baltimore
3. Heimberg M, Goh EH, Lausner HG, et al. (1978) Regulation of hepatic metabolism of free fatty acids: Interrelationships among secretion of very-low-density lipoproteins, ketogenesis, and cholesterogenesis. In: Dietschy, Gotto, Ontko (eds) Disturbances in lipid and lipoprotein metabolism. Williams and Wilkins, Baltimore
4. Kushlan M, Gollan J, Ma W-L, et al. (1981) Sex differences in hepatic uptake of long chain fatty acids in single-pass perfused rat liver. J Lipid Res 22: 431-436
5. Christiansen RZ (1977) Regulation of palmitate metabolism by carnitine and glucagon in hepatocytes isolated from fasted and carbohydrate re-fed rats. Biochim Biophys Acta 488: 249-262
6. Renaus G, Foliot A, Infante R (1978) Increased uptake of fatty acids by the isolated liver after

raising the fatty acid binding protein concentration with clofibrate. Biochem Biophys Res Commun 80: 327-334

7. Samuel D, Paris S, Ailhaud G (1976) Uptake and metabolism of fatty acids and analogues by cultured cardiac cells from chick embryos. Eur J Biochem 64: 583-595
8. Paris S, Samuel D, Romey G, et al. (1979) Uptake of fatty acids by cultured cardiac cells from chick embryo: evidence for a facilitation process without energy dependence. Biochimie 61: 361-367
9. Abumrad NA, Perkins RC, Park JH, et al. (1981) Mechanism of long chain fatty acid permeation in the isolated adipocyte. J Biol Chem 256: 9183-9191
10. Abumrad NA, Park JH, Park CR (1984) Permeation of long chain fatty acid into adipocytes. J Biol Chem 259: 8945-8953
11. DeGrella RF, Light RH (1980) Uptake and metabolism of fatty acids by dispersed rat heart myocytes. I. Kinetics of homologous fatty acids. J Biol Chem 255: 9731-9738
12. DeGrella RF, Light RJ (1980) Uptake and metabolism of fatty acids by dispersed rat heart myocytes. II. Inhibition by albumin and homologous fatty acids, and the effect of temperature and metabolic reagents. J Biol Chem 255: 9739-9745
13. Faerch T, Jacobsen J (1975) Determination of association and dissociation rate constants for bilirubin-bovine serum albumin. Arch Biochem Biophys 168: 351-357
14. Gray RD, Stroupe S (1978) Kinetics and mechanism of bilirubin binding to human serum albumin. Arch Biochem Biophys 168: 351-357
15. Scheider W (1978) Dissociation rate of serum albumin-fatty acid complex from stop-flow dielectric study of ligand exchange. Biophys J 24: 260-262
16. Svenson A, Holmer E, Andersson L (1974) A new method for the measurement of dissociation rates for complexes between small ligands and proteins applied to the palmitate and bilirubin complexes with serum albumin. Biochim Biophys Acta 342: 54-59
17. Goresky CA (1977) Hepatic membrane carrier transport processes: their involvement in bilirubin uptake. In: Berk. Berlin (eds) The chemistry and physiology of bile pigments. US Government Printing Office, Washington
18. Goresky CA (1964) Initial distribution and rate of uptake of sulfobromophthalein in the liver. Am J Physiol 207: 13-26
19. Wolkoff AW, Goresky CA, Sellin J, et al. (1979) Role of ligandin in transfer of bilirubin from plasma into liver. Am J Physiol 236: E638-E648
20. Berk PD, Stremmel W (1986) Hepatocellular uptake of organic anions. Prog Liver Dis 8: 125-144
21. Stremmel W, Berk PD (1986) Hepatocellular influx of $^{14}$C-oleate reflects membrane transport rather than intracellular metabolism or binding. Proc Natl Acad Sci USA, 83: 3086-3090
22. Stremmel W, Strohmeyer G, Berk PD (1986) Hepatocellular uptake of oleate is energy dependent, sodium linked, and inhibited by an antibody to a hepatocyte plasma membrane fatty acid binding protein. Proc Natl Acad Sci USA, 83: 3584-3588
23. Stremmel W, Strohmeyer G, Borchard F, et al. (1985) Isolation and partial characterization of fatty acid binding protein in rat liver plasma membranes. Proc Natl Acad Sci USA 82: 4-8
24. Stremmel W, Kochwa S, Berk PD (1983) Studies of oleate binding to rat liver plasma membranes. Biochem Biophys Res Commun 112: 88-95
25. Stremmel W, Gerber MA, Glezerov V, et al. (1983) Physicochemical and immunohistological studies of a sulfobromophthalein- and bilirubin-binding protein from rat liver plasma membranes. J Clin Invest 711: 796-805
26. Stremmel W, Theilmann L (1986) Selective inhibition of long chain fatty acid uptake in short-term cultured rat hepatocytes by an antibody to the rat liver plasma membrane fatty acid binding protein. Biochim Biophys Acta 877: 191-197

# Vesicular Transport of Fluid Phase Markers by Hepatocytes*

Bruce F. Scharschmidt, John R. Lake, Eberhard L. Renner, Vojtech Licko, and Rebecca Van Dyke

Department of Medicine and Liver Center, University of California, San Francisco, CA, U.S.A.

## Introduction

Endocytosis is a general term which refers to the internalization of extracellular material via invagination of a portion of the plasma membrane, which then pinches off to form a vesicle. The ability to internalize extracellular material is a property shared by most, if not all, animal cells. Hepatocytes are actively endocytic and internalize a variety of specific ligands, including asialoglycoproteins, low-density lipoproteins, and IgA, via a process called receptor-mediated endocytosis (Ashwell and Harford 1982; Goldstein et al. 1979; Renston et al. 1980). Certain ligands, such as asialoglycoproteins and low-density lipoproteins, are transported predominantly to lysosomes via receptors which recycle to and from plasma membrane and participate in many rounds of endocytosis before ultimately being degraded. Other receptors, such as the receptor for IgA, do not recycle, but instead escort their ligands to bile. A third pathway involves the recycling of intact receptor-ligand complexes back to the cell surface. This appears to occur to a variable degree for a variety of receptors and ligands and is characteristic of the interaction between transferrin and its receptor. Despite this considerable body of information regarding the endocytosis of ligands, relatively little is known regarding the role of transcellular vesiclar transport in canalicular bile formation, the rate at which hepatocytes endocytose extracellular fluid, or the mechanism by which fluid phase markers commonly used in studies of bile formation (e.g., erythritol, sucrose) are transported into the canaliculus. We therefore undertook a series of studies in both perfused rat liver and cultured hepatocytes with the overall objective of characterizing and quantitating rates and pathways of hepatic fluid phase endocytosis.

## Role of Transcellular Vesicular Transport in the Biliary Secretion of Fluid Phase Markers

Our initial studies were undertaken to assess the contribution of transcellular vesicular transport to the biliary secretion of fluid phase markers (Lake et al. 1985a). We used the isolated rat liver perfused with a 20% fluorocarbon solution, and studied the movement from perfusate to bile of several solutes specifically selected to cover a wide range of molecular weights (m.w.). These solutes are all commonly used as markers of

* Supported in part by NIH, grants AM-26270, AM-07453, and AM-01254, UCSF Liver Core Center grant AM-26743, grants from the American Liver Foundation, and a fellowship from the Swiss National Science Foundation.

Assessment and Management of Hepatobiliary Disease
Eds.: L. Okolicsányi, G. Csomós, and G. Crepaldi

fluid phase transport, as they are known not to bind to specific receptors or carriers. Their movement therefore reflects the movement of bulk fluid. Erythritol (m.w. = 120), sucrose (m.w. = 342), methoxyinulin (m.w. = 5000), and dextran (m.w. = 70000) were used in radiolabeled form, and methoxyinulin and dextran were chromatographically purified prior to use to eliminate low-molecular-weight radiolabeled contaminants. Microperoxidase (m.w. = 1879) and horseradish peroxidase (m.w. = 40000) were measured by bioassay.

### Biliary Secretion of Markers Under Steady-State Conditions

Under steady-state conditions, the perfused rat liver secreted even large markers in appreciable amounts. The bile-to-plasma ratio of these different markers ranged from 0.04 to 1.0 (erythritol = 1.0; sucrose = 0.21; microperoxidase = 0.06; methoxyinulin = 0.09; horseradish peroxidase = 0.04; dextran = 0.09), and the bile-to-perfusate ratio for the four largest markers exhibited no apparent ordering based on size. Infusion of taurocholate (2.5-μmol bolus + 90 nmol/g liver/min) produced a 71% increase in bile flow and a commensurate drop in the bile-to-perfusate ratio of these markers, with little or no increase in their biliary output.

### Biliary Secretion of Markers Under Non-Steady-State Conditions

The appearance in or disappearance from bile of erythritol, sucrose, and dextran was then studied under non-steady-state conditions following the abrupt addition to or removal from perfusate of these markers. Following its addition to perfusate, erythritol achieved a bile-to-perfusate ratio of about 1 within 2 min. Dextran, in contrast, appeared in bile in significant quantities only after a lag of about 12 min and then slowly approached a maximal bile-to-perfusate ratio of 0.10. Sucrose exhibited an intermediate type of behavior and achieved a maximum ratio of 0.24. Following their abrupt removal from perfusate, erythritol concentration in bile fell abruptly and again achieved a bile-to-perfusate ratio of 1 within minutes. Dextran, by contrast, fell only after a lag of about 12 min, and the absolute bile-to-perfusate concentration ratio exceeded 5 for greater than 15 min after its removal from perfusate. Sucrose again exhibited an intermediate pattern.

When these data were subjected to kinetic analysis (Fig. 1), the behavior of erythritol was compatible with rapid movement from perfusate to bile via a pathway described by a single rate constant. Dextran's behavior was strikingly different, and the initial lag phase was satisfactorily described only as movement from perfusate to bile via several interposed delay compartments, which are presumably cellular in nature. Sucrose movement was adequately described as a combination of these two routes, as well as a third route with a single interposed delay compartment, with up to 35% of sucrose movement estimated to occur via the dextran, or multiple-delay pathway (Fig. 1).

### Subcellular Localization of Internalized Markers

Several approaches were used to explore the subcellular localization of these markers. First, following perfusion with radiolabeled markers, liver tissue was homogenized and centrifuged at low speed to remove intact cells. The supernatant was then recentrifuged

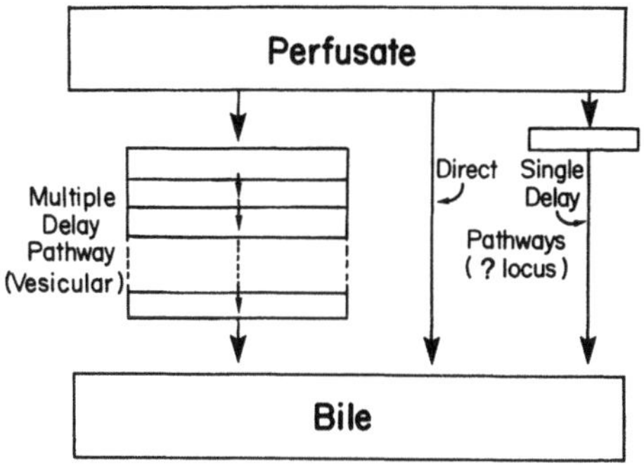


**Fig. 1.** Proposed model for movement of fluid phase markers from perfusate to bile based upon analysis of non-steady-state data. Dextran movement to bile, which is characterized by a 12-min lag period, occurs almost exclusively via the multiple-delay pathway, which is tentatively identified as transcytosis. Erythritol movement to bile is very rapid and is satisfactorily described by a single rate constant; further characterization is precluded by a lack of detailed data during the first 60 s. Sucrose movement to bile is kinetically intermediate between that of dextran and erythritol and occurs via a combination of these two pathways as well as via a third pathway represented by a single delay compartment. The anatomic identities of the zero-delay (erythritol) and single-delay pathways are unknown

at 100000 *g* to pellet subcellular organelles. Forty to sixty percent of sucrose, inulin, and dextran was recovered in the pelleted subcellular structures, compared with only 8% of erythritol. Much of the pelleted marker was relased into the supernatant by addition of the detergent Triton X-100, which would be expected to disrupt vesicles. Second, electron micrographs of perfused liver tissue demonstrated the presence of horseradish peroxidase in intracellular vesicle, and, third, fluoresceinated dextran was localized to subcellular vesicular-like structures in primary cultures of adult rat hepatocytes by fluorescence microscopy.

### Conclusions

Collectively, these observations demonstrate the existence of a perfusate-to-bile transport pathway which is able to accommodate very large fluid phase markers and exhibits little discrimination based on size. This pathway appears to be minimally affected by taurocholate and is kinetically distinct from that traversed by erythritol. These findings, in conjunction with the localization of markers to subcellular vesicles, suggest that the pathway traveled by dextran and other large fluid phase markers represents transcellular vesicular transport or transcytosis.

## Comparative Effects of Colchicine and Chloroquine on the Vesicular Transport of Fluid Phase Markers Vs Ligands in Perfused Rat Liver

In order to further explore the vesicular nature of this pathway and examine the possible role in this process of microtubules and vesicle acidification (Lake et al. 1985b), we studied the effects of colchicine (1.2 mg/kg body weight to donor rat 3 h prior to hepatectomy and 10 μmol added to perfusate, with lumicolchicine used as a control) and chloroquine (50 mg/kg to donor rat 1 h prior to hepatectomy and added to perfusate in concentration of 1 m*M*). We again used erythritol, sucrose, and dextrân as fluid phase markers and employed both steady-state and non-steady-state protocols. Asialofetuin (ASF), which is known to be taken up by hepatocytes via receptor-mediated endocytosis (Ashwell and Harford 1982), was radiolabeled with 125-I and studied simultaneously to serve as a frame of reference. ASF was added to the perfusate as a bolus, and intact (precipitable with 20% tricholoroacetic acid/4% phosphotungstic acid) and degraded (nonprecipitable) ASF (100 μg) were measured in perfusate and bile. Under control conditions, intact ASF disappeared rapidly from perfusate and was replaced almost quantitatively by degraded ASF in perfusate in a period of 1 h. Less than 1.0% of the total ASF added appeared intact in bile during this same period.

### Effects of Chloroquine

Chloroquine decreased ASF degradation by 70% and increased the biliary output of intact ASF by about 50%, but had no effect whatsoever on the absolute amounts of fluid phase marker secreted in bile or the rates of secretion.

### Effects of Colchicine

Colchicine reduced ASF degradation by 50% compared with lumicolchicine and decreased the cumulative biliary secretion of intact ASF in bile by about 80%, but had little effect on initial ASF disappearance from perfusate. Cholchicine had no effect on the biliary secretion of erythritol, but decreased the biliary secretion of dextran by about 80% without altering the time course of appearance in bile, kinetically consistent with inhibition of the multiple-delay or transcytosis pathway. The output of sucrose, by contrast, was actually increased by about 60%, and sucrose appeared in bile at an accelerated rate, consistent with enhanced transport via the zero- or single-delay pathway.

### Conclusions

These observations indicate that intact microtubular function is necessary for the biliary secretion of fluid phase markers such as dextran, strongly supporting the hypothesis that such markers move from blood to bile by vesicular transport. They further indicate that changes in the steady-state, bile-to-perfusate ratio of commonly used fluid phase markers such as sucrose may result from changes in vesicular as well as nonvesicular transport. Thus, the use of such markers as indices of tight-junction permeability is unreliable.

## Fluid Phase Endocytosis by Cultured Rat Hepatocytes

While providing rather compelling evidence for the role of transcytosis in the blood-to-bile transport of fluid phase markers, these studies provided limited insight into the overall handling of such markers by hepatocytes. For example, they permitted no estimate of either the total rate of fluid internalization by hepatocytes or the pathways taken by internalized markers. In order to address these general questions, we extended our studies to measurements of fluid phase endocytosis in rat hepatocytes in 2-day-old primary culture (Scharschmidt et al. 1986). Inulin (5000 m.w., chromatographically purified) was employed as the fluid phase marker. Its appropriateness in this regard was supported by the observations that (a) inulin uptake was concentration-independent, (b) inulin was not degraded intracellularly, as determined by chromatographic analysis of inulin extracted from cells at 1 h, (c) inulin uptake was decreased at 4 °C, and (d) identical rates of fluid phase endocytosis were measured with dextran, which was demonstrated earlier (see above) to be present in intracellular vesicles.

## Uptake and Efflux of Inulin in Cultured Hepatocytes Under Control Conditions

Inulin uptake by cultured hepatocytes at 37 °C was most rapid during the first 1–2 min. This initially rapid uptake was followed by a slower, apparently steady rate of inulin accumulation to 120 min. This biphasic pattern was not the result of cell exhaustion during prolonged incubation or inulin exposure, since it was unaltered by varying periods of preincubation with unlabeled inulin. Uptake was decreased by at least 75% at all time points when cells were incubated at 4 °C. Kinetic analysis of these findings required a two-component function and indicated the present of two intracellular compartments (Fig. 2). The initially rapid rate of inulin uptake was postulated to correspond to endocytosis of inulin into a small pool which rapidly exchanged with plasma and exhibited a half-life of about 1 min. The slower, steady rate of uptake was postulated to correspond to transfer of inulin to storage compartments which turned over slowly in relation to the time course of the study.

To determine whether movement of inulin between medium and cells was in fact bidirectional, cells were incubated in radiolabeled inulin for either 5 or 60 min and then transferred to inulin-free medium. Inulin efflux did occur, and a kinetic analysis of inulin efflux data also required a two-compartment model in which both compartments exchanged, either directly or indirectly, with the extracellular space (Fig. 2). The rate and absolute amount of efflux corresponded closely to that predicted from the uptake curve. The estimated half-life of the early compartment was again about 1–2 min,

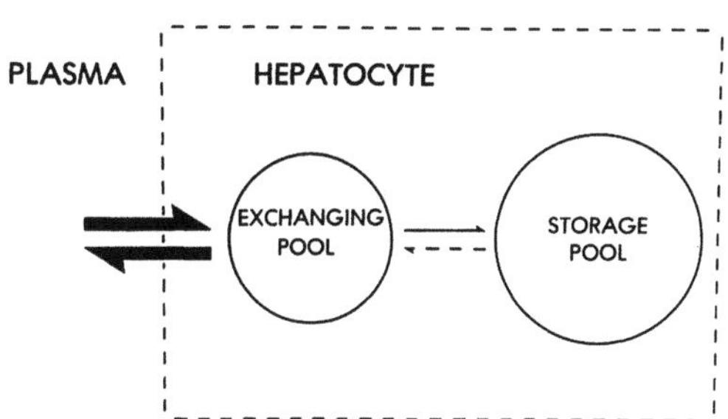


**Fig. 2.** A minimal model which adequately describes the uptake and efflux of inulin in cultured hepatocytes. Kinetic analysis of these data requires the presence of two intracellular compartments, including a smaller, rapid-turnover (half-life 1–2 min) compartment, which presumably represents the endosomal compartment, and a slow-turnover (half life much greater than 1 h) storage compartment

and the apparent half-life of the storage compartment(s) was considerably greater than 1 h. More precise estimates of the half-life of the storage compartment would have required considerably longer periods of observation than were employed in our study.

### Effects of Experimental Agents on Inulin Uptake

Neither taurocholate (200 μ*M*) nor chloroquine (1 m*M*) had any effect on inulin handling by the cultured cells. Colchicine (10 μ*M*), in contrast inhibited the apparent transfer of inulin to storage compartments by more than 50% compared with lumicolchicine.

### Inulin Uptake by Perfused Rat Liver

To determine the relevance of these observations in cultured cells to intact liver, livers were perfused in the presence of radiolabeled inulin and uptake into liver tissue was measured by sequential biopsies taken from the periphery of the liver lobes over a period of 90 min. Inulin uptake into perfused liver tissue was linear with time to 90 min, and in four perfusions inulin uptake, expressed as the apparent rate of fluid internalization, averaged 65%–75% of that observed in the cultured cells.

## Discussion

Collectively, these observations in intact perfused rat liver and cultured rat hepatocytes permit a quantitative overview of the vesicular trafficking of fluid phase markers in hepatocytes, as illustrated in Fig. 3. The present studies suggest that inulin is first internalized into a compartment, presumably an "endosomal" compartment, which has an apparent volume based upon kinetic analysis of uptake and efflux curves of about 3% of hepatocyte volume. This endosomal compartment exchanges with the extracellular space and turns over with a half-life of 1–2 min. This estimated half-life is considerably shorter than previous estimates of 5–20 min in other cell types, including macrophages, fibroblasts, and adipocytes, based on comparatively few early time points (Besterman et al. 1981; Gibbs and Lienhard 1984; Morrill et al. 1984). Our observations regarding the rate of endocytic vesicle recycling underscore the potential rapidity with which hepatocytes or other cells can regulate transport via vesicular insertion into or removal from the plasma membrane of receptors or carriers (Gluck et al. 1982; Schwartz et al. 1984; Stanton 1984). The present studies also provide new information regarding the rate of internalization and hence turnover of the hepatocyte plasma membrane via endocytosis. Based upon the known dimensions of the hepatocytes in culture, and assuming a mean endocytic vesicle diameter of 50–200 nm, the present findings indicate that an area of membrane equivalent to about 5–20 times the total surface of the hepatocyte is endocytosed every hour.

Integration of the present observations in cultured hepatocytes and perfused liver, which appears justified based upon the quantitative and qualitative similarities in the results obtained in the two systems, also permits an overview of the pathways of fluid phase marker transport by liver cells. Of total inulin internalized via endocytosis, about 80% is rapidly regurgitated back into the extracellular space across the basolateral

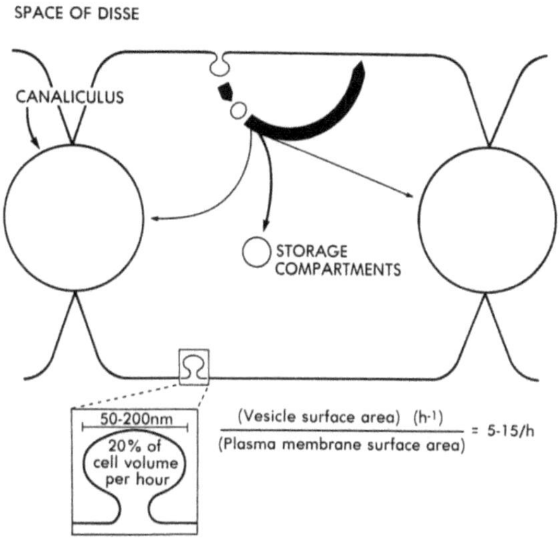


**Fig. 3.** An overview of fluid phase marker transport by hepatocytes. Based on analysis of all data in perfused liver and cultured hepatocytes, inulin appears to be endocytosed initially into a rapid-turnover compartment which comprises about 3% of hepatocyte volume. Of total inulin internalized, most (about 80%) is regurgitated rapidly back into the extracellular space, with smaller amounts transported to storage compartments (about 18%) and bile (about 2%). Every hour, hepatocytes appear to endocytose the equivalent of 20% or more of their cell volume. Based upon the known dimensions of hepatocytes in culture and assuming a mean endocytic vesicle diameter of 50–200 nm, the findings suggest that hepatocytes internalize the equivalent of 5–20 times their plasma membrane surface area each hour

membrane. Of the remainder, most (18% of total internalized) is transported to storage compartments. In contrast to the plausible estimates of apparent endosomal volume noted above, which are in remarkably good agreement with estimates in fibroblasts using stereologic techniques (Steinman et al. 1976), the unrealistically large volume of the storage compartment (>50% of cell volume) indicates that marker is progressively concentrated *en route* to these intracellular sites. Finally, about 2% of marker internalized is transported to bile via a vesicular pathway exhibiting a transit time between the basolateral and canalicular membranes of about 12 min. The participation of this pathway in the blood-to-bile transport of fluid phase markers such as sucrose makes it difficult to use the bile/blood ratio of these markers as an index of tight-junction permeability (Elias et al. 1980) and further indicates that the current conceptualization of marker movement as occurring via diffusion and convection requires reevaluation (Strasberg et al. 1979).

Finally, the observations in both cultured hepatocytes and in perfused rat liver indicate that the cellular mechanisms responsible for fluid phase marker movement via these pathways are unaffected by taurocholate and do not require vesicle acidification. In contrast, intact microtubular function is essential both for the transfer of internalized marker to lysosomes and for their secretion into bile.

## References

Ashwell G, Harford J (1982) Carbohydrate-specific receptors of the liver. Annu Rev Biochem 51: 531-554

Besterman JM, Airhard JA, Woodworth RC, Low RB (1981) Exocytosis of pinocytosed fluid in cultured cells: kinetic evidence for rapid turnover and compartmentalization. J Cell Biol 91: 716-727

Gibbs EM, Lienhard GE (1984) Fluid phase endocytosis by isolated rat adipocytes. J Cell Physiol 121: 569-575

Gluck S, Cannon C, Al-Awqati Q (1982) Exocytosis regulates urinary acidification in turtle bladder by rapid insertion of H+ pumps into the luminal membrane. Proc Natl Acad Sci USA 79: 4327-4331

Goldstein JL, Anderson RGW, Brown MS (1979) Coated pits, coated vesicles, and receptor-mediated endocytosis. Nature 279: 679-685

Lake JR, Licko V, van Dyke RW, Scharschmidt BF (1985a) Biliary secretion of fluid-phase markers by the isolated perfused rat liver: role of transcellular vesicular transport. J Clin Invest 76: 676-684

Lake JR, George CP, Licko V, Scharschmidt BF (1985b) Vesicular transport of fluid phase markers (FPM) and ligands by liver: Effects of colchicine and chloroquine. Clin Res 33: 322A

Morrill GA, Kostellow AB, Weinstein SP (1984) Endocytosis in the amphibian oocyte: Effect of insulin and progesterone on membrane and fluid internalization during the meitoic division. Biochim Biophys Acta 803: 71-77

Renston RH, Jones AL, Christiansen WD, Hradek GT (1980) Evidence for a vesicular transport mechanism in hepatocytes for biliary secretion of immunoglobulin A. Science 208: 1276-1278

Scharschmidt BF, Lake JR, Renner EL, Licko V, van Dyke RW (1986) Fluid phase endocytosis by cultured rat hepatocytes and perfused rat liver: Implications for plasma membrane turnover and vesicular trafficking of fluid phase markers. Proc. Natl. Acad. Sci. USA 83: 9488-9492

Schwartz AL, Bilognesi A, Fridovich SE (1984) Recycling of the asialoglycoprotein receptor and the effect of lysosomotropic amines in hepatoma cells. J Cell Biol 98: 732-738

Stanton BA (1984) Regulation of ion transport in epithelia: role of membrane recruitment from cytoplasmic vesicles Lab Invest 51: 255-257

Steinman RM, Brodie SE, Cohn ZA (1976) Membrane flow during pinocytosis. J Cell Biol 68: 665-687

Strasberg SM, Petrunka CN, Ilson RG, Paloheimo JE (1979) Characteristics of inert solute clearance by the monkey liver. Gastroenterology 67: 259-266

# The Hepatic Uptake of Organic Anions: An Overview*

Claudio Tiribelli[1], Gian Carlo Lunazzi[2], Marcello Persico[2], Nicoletta Orzes[1], Maddalena Miccio[2], Bruno Gazzin[2], Giulia Baldini[2], and Gian Luigi Sottocasa[2]

[1]Istituto Patologia Medica and [2]Dipartimento Biochimica, Biofisica e Chimica delle Macromolecole, Universita' di Trieste, 34100 Trieste, Italy

## Introduction

The complex process by which organic anions are efficiently taken up, stored, metabolically modified, and eventually excreted into the bile has been the subject of intensive investigation.

The liver plays a major role in removing exogenous and endogenous compounds from plasma and excreting them into the bile after possible, but not obligatory, metabolic transformation. The compounds taken up by the liver are usually grouped under the name of xenobiotics. They are a composite class of substances having in common a more or less pronounced hydrophobic character and one or more negative charges on their molecules. They include: bile pigments, bile acids, fatty acids, bilirubin, dyes (di- and tetrasulfobromophthalein, indocyanine green) and many drugs (nicotinic acid, rifamycins, etc.). Of particular interest is sulfobromophthalein (BSP) which was introduced as a diagnostic probe of liver function as early as 1925. Since then, BSP has been extensively applied as a reference substance in studies of the hepatic uptake of organic anions.

Many mechanisms operating in series and/or in parallel have been shown at the level of the sinusoidal and canalicular plasma membrane. In general they are involved in mantaining ionic fluxes across the membrane and are closely linked to intracellular events. A schematic drawing of these mechanisms is shown in Fig. 1.

The most extensively studied factors influencing the hepatic removal of substances from the plasma include the following: total blood flow to the liver, binding of the substrate to blood constituents (mainly albumin), binding and translocation across the sinusoidal plasma membrane, intracellular binding to specific proteins, metabolic transformation, and biliary excretion.

In this paper we will briefly review the steps accounting for the hepatic uptake of organic anions, mainly in relation to their translocation across sinusoidal and basolateral plasma membranes. The possible clinical implication of the new concepts emerging in this area will also be discussed.

* Supported by grants from the Ministero Pubblica Istruzione, Rome, Italy. Drs. M. Persico, N. Orzes and M. Miccio were partially supported by career development awards from the *Fondo per lo Studio e la Ricerca Scientifica delle Malattie del Fegato, FVG.*

Assessment and Management of Hepatobiliary Disease
Eds.: L. Okolicsányi, G. Csomós, and G. Crepaldi

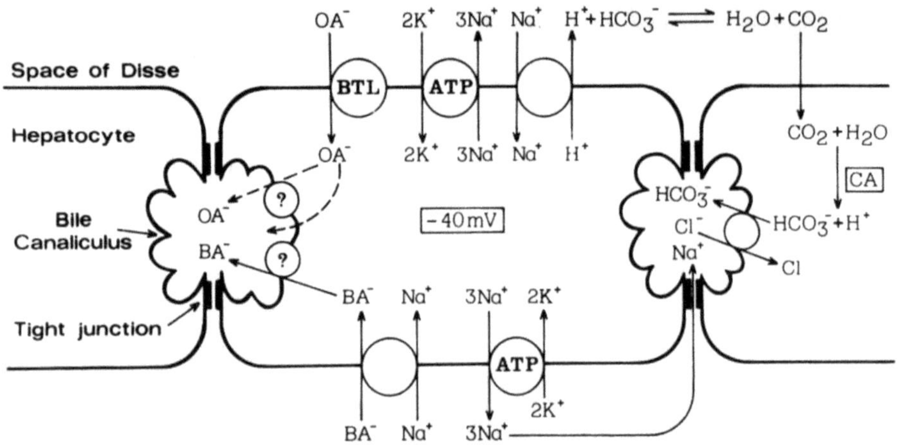


**Fig. 1.** Diagram of some mechanisms involved in the hepatic uptake of organic anions operating at the level of the sinusoidal-basolateral and the canalicular plasma membrane of the liver cell. *OA*, organic anions; *BA*, bile acids/salts; *CA*, carbonic anhydrase; *BTL*, bilitranslocase

## Factors Governing Hepatic Clearance

The clearance of a compound mostly depends on the blood flow *(Q)* and its intrinsic clearance *(Cli)*, defined as the capacity of the liver to remove the substrate extrapolated at an infinite value. Accordingly, hepatic clearance *(ClH)* may be represented as:

$$ClH = Q \times [(Cli/(Q + Cli)]$$

where $(Cli/Q + Cli)$ is the extraction ratio *(E)* of a given substance. When $E$ is high ($>0.7$), the *ClH* will be mostly determined by the hepatic blood flow, whereas when $E$ is low ($<0.3$), the clearance will reflect the velocity at which the compound crosses the hepatocyte plasma membrane [1, 2]. Intermediate situations exist with $E$ values between 0.3 and 0.7.

## Factors Governing Transport Mechanisms

It is accepted nowadays that the transport of organic anions across the sinusoidal plasma membrane occurs via a carrier-mediated process. Saturable uptake kinetics have been shown in vivo for BSP, bilirubin, and indocyanine green [3-5], long chain fatty acids [6], rose bengal [7], and bile acids [8]. All these substances have in common the property of being avidly bound to albumin in serum in view of their amphipathic characteristics. Based on the very low dissociation rate of these compounds from albumin and the consequent low concentration of free ligand available for uptake (10 n*M* in the case of bilirubin [9]), the hypothesis has been developed that a specific albumin receptor might exist at the level of the sinusoidal plasma membrane [6]. This receptor was thought to interfere with the albumin-ligand complex and thus facilitate the uptake by increasing the dissociation rate of the ligand from the complex. This stimulating hypothesis was subsequently challenged on the basis of experimental evidence such as the lack of specific binding of albumin to rat liver plasma membrane [10]. In addition, in vivo experiments showed that the plasma disappearance and biliary excretion of BSP was found to be comparable in normal and mutant Nagase analbuminemic rats, indicating that BSP binding to serum albumin was not critical to the hepatic uptake of this organic anion in vivo [11]. However, albumin is involved in the zonal distribution of the dye, as shown by the finding that its omission resulted in a much greater BSP accumulation in zone 1 (periportal), whereas in its presence the dye was evenly distributed along the sinusoid [12]. An interesting alternative to the so-called albumin receptor hypothesis has recently been presented by Weisiger [13], who has developed a mathematical model in which the rate of dissociation of the ligand-albumin complex is also considered. Conditions are described in which this rate may become limiting, in addition to flow and intrinsic limitations.

## Driving Forces for Hepatic Uptake

It is important to mention that the uptake of cholephylic anions occurs via two independent pathways, one specific for bile acids [14-17] and the other for bilirubin and related substances [3-5]. Data reported in the literature suggest that an additional common pathway may also exist [18, 19]. The bile acid uptake pathway is well defined in terms of energy requirements, being essentially and specifically dependent on the existence of a sodium ion gradient across the plasma membrane. The process has been described as an electroneutral cotransport of sodium and bile acids [20, 21]. The subject of the electroneutrality of this transport is somewhat controversial in the literature, for other authors have described bile acid hepatic uptake as an electrogenic process [17, 22, 23]. Hepatic uptake of bilirubin and related anions does not depend specifically on the presence of sodium in the medium [24-26], and much experimental evidence is accumulating indicating that it occurs elecrogenically. The data have been obtained under various experimental conditions, for example, with plasma membrane vesicles [27-29] or proteoliposomes containing purified bilitranslocase (see below) [30]. In the case of BSP, the movement of the dye was promoted by the creation of a potassium diffusion potential induced by valinomycin. This finding suggests that negatively charged species are carried across the sinusoidal membrane against a negative-inside (around $-30$ mV) membrane potential [31]. It is expected, therefore, that this energy barrier is overcome by a downhill chemical potential which is somehow maintained across the membrane. A number of mechanisms are operating in the cytoplasm to lower the free ligand concentration, e.g., ligandin [32], metabolic transformation, and biliary excretion.

## Isolation of Putative Plasma Membrane Carriers for Organic Anions

Liver plasma membrane contains specific binding sites for BSP [33, 34], which may be shown to compete with bilirubin [35]. More direct evidence in favor of the existence of a specific carrier molecule came from the isolation, in 1978 [36], of a protein from rat liver plasma membrane showing binding properties very similar to those displayed by isolated membranes. In the presence of deoxycholate (0.4%) this protein showed a molecular weight (mol.wt.) of 170000 daltons. The protein could bind up to 15 mol BSP/mol protein with a dissociation constant (Kd) for the complex in the order of 5 μmol/l. Interestingly, this Kd was identical to that found in plasma membrane preparations [35]. Further studies on this protein, named bilitranslocase, showed that the native molecule prepared in the absence of deoxycholate can be resolved, by treatment with reducing agents (2-mercaptoethanol) in the presence of SDS and BSP, into two distinct subunits $\alpha$ and $\beta$ of 37000 and 35500 daltons respectively [37]. Native bilitranslocase showed a lower Kd (1.2 μmol/l), with a ratio of 3 mol BSP/mol protein [38].

Immunological studies provided evidence for a physiological function of bilitranslocase. Injection into the portal vein of the rat of specific, affinity-chromatography-purified rabbit anti-bilitranslocase antibodies resulted in a significant increase of serum unconjugated bilirubin [39, 40]. The same effect was also present after administration of specific Fab fragments of the antibodies. These data suggested that the specific blockade of the receptor resulted in an impairment of bilirubin uptake by the liver. Similar results were obtained in isolated and perfused liver. In his system, anti-bilitranslocase antibodies significantly reduced the uptake of dibromosulphonphthalein (DBSP), whereas the biliary excretion was not affected by the treatment [41]. The specificity of the effect was supported by the observation that treated livers removed taurocholate from the perfusate at a normal rate, thus confirming that the hepatic uptake of bile acids and other organic anions operate mainly via two independent pathways [3, 5, 14, 42].

At a functional level, the insertion of purified preparations of bilitranslocase into liposomes reconstituted BSP transport. The transport was shown to be electrogenic, being highly accelerated by the creation of a negative-inside potential after addition of valinomycin in potassium-preloaded artificial vesicles [30]. These data strongly support the view that bilitranslocase may act as a specific permeabilizer of the lipid bilayer. This makes bilitranslocase a good candidate for being the carrier molecule operating in translocation, at least of BSP, across the hepatic plasma membrane. Similar results have been obtained in rat liver membrane vesicles. Also in this case, the BSP transport was shown to be electrogenic as greatly enhanced by the creation of a positive-inside membrane potential by valynomicin. Moreover, the bilitranslocase-mediated transport is paralleled by the enzymatic distribution of $Na^{+}$-$K^{+}$ATPase indicating that it occurs almost exclusively at the sinusoidal domain of the liver plasma membrane [29].

Other putative membrane receptors for organic anions have been described in the literature.

Reichen and Berk [39] described the isolation of a Sudan black- and PAS-negative organic-anion-binding protein from rat liver plasma membrane fractions with a mol.wt. of 60000 daltons, a Kd in the order of 0.1 $\mu M$, and a valence of 2.

Wolkoff and Chung [40] reported on the isolation, by affinity chromatography on a glutathione BSP-agarose column, of a protein with a mol.wt. of 55000 daltons that bound bilirubin with a Kd of 20 μmol/l. It was immunologically distinct from rat albumin and ligandin. The protein also showed high affinity binding for BSP (Kd 4 μmol/l, a value very close to that described for bilitranslocase) [36].

Stremmel et al. [41] also isolated, by affinity chromatography on BSP- agarose and bilirubin-agarose columns, one electrophoretically homogeneous protein with a mol.wt. of 55000 daltons under dissociative conditions. When the detergent was omitted, the estimated mol.wt. was in the order of 100000 daltons. Both the 55000- and 100000-dalton peaks cochromatographed with [$^{35}$S]BSP. Immunohistochemical studies revealed the presence of the antigen on all surface domains of rat hepatocytes, but its absence from other cell populations of normal rat liver and of other organs.

Any possible relation between these putative organic anion receptors and bilitranslocase remains to be established.

Other organic anions undergoing rapid hepatic uptake are fatty acids. In the past, the process of hepatic removal of these compounds has been regarded as passive diffusion [46]. However, kinetic studies have revealed that at least at low plasma concentrations, this phenomenon might take place via a carrier-mediated mechanism [47-49]. A putative oleate-binding protein was reported to be present in rat liver plasma membranes [50]. This protein showed a mol.wt. of 40000 daltons and did not stain with either Sudan black or PAS reagent. On the other hand, bilitranslocase was previously demonstrated also to be involved in fatty acid hepatic transport, with the observation that in the rat, anti-bilitranslocase antibodies was able to reduce the hepatic uptake of palmitate both in isolated and perfused liver and in isolated hepatocytes [51]. The Km of the carrier-mediated part of the process was 13 μmol/l, a value very close to that described in cardiac cells of chick embryo [47]. Immunofluorescence studies showed, in addition, that bilitranslocase was present in a number of tissues oxidizing fatty acids but lacking in organs devoid of this metabolism. Here also, no relationship between the plasma membrane protein described by Stremmel et al. [50] and bilitranslocase has yet been established.

## Sex Influence in Hepatic Uptake

Sex seems to play an important role in modulating the hepatic uptake of various organic anions, since in general, females show more efficient hepatic handling of these compounds than males. In humans, the plasma disappearance rate of low doses of indocyanine green is faster in females [52], and the plasma clearance of bilirubin, when calculated per kilogram body wt., is more rapid in normal women than in men [53]. Similarly, female rats were reported to excrete higher amounts of indocyanine green into the bile than males at low doses [54]; this sex-related difference disappeared with higher doses [55]. All these experimental findings are in line with the recent finding that in the case of BSP, the apparent Km for transport was lower in the female rat liver, whereas comparable Vmax values were observed in the two sexes [56].

Other organic anions, such as long-chain fatty acids, have been demonstrated to be better utilized in female rat hepatocytes. This finding correlated with a higher cytosol content of fatty-acid-binding protein [57]. In keeping with this was the observation that first-pass extraction by perfused female rat livers is more efficient than that seen in males [58]. Sex differences have also been described to occur inside the hepatocyte. In the case of bilirubin, the activity of the conjugating enzyme (UDP-glucuronyltransferase) and the maximal biliary excretion rate of the pigment were found to be higher in female rats [59].

## Clinical Aspects

Gilbert's syndrome (GS), first described in 1901 [60], is characterized by a chronic, low-grade, fluctuating unconjugated hyperbilirubinemia in the absence of overt hyperhemolysis and in the presence of normal liver function. GS has been considered as a good human model in the study of bilirubin metabolism. The molecular defect(s) underlying GS are still considered an open question. In addition to the well-known reduction in hepatic UDP-glucuronyltransferase activity [61-64], a defect in the hepatic uptake of various organic anions has been described in this condition. The plasma clearance of bilirubin was found to be constantly reduced [65-67] owing mainly to a reduction in the uptake step of the process as assessed by multicompartmental analysis of the plasma disappearance curve [68, 69]. On the other hand, the plasma clearance of other organic anions, such as BSP and indocyanine green, is reported to be impaired in only some subjects [70, 71].

Recent data suggest that a defective bilitranslocase function may be one of the metabolic defects in GS. The demonstration of a specific binding to the protein of both nicotinic acid [27] and rifamycin-SV [28] is consistent with the reduction in their plasma clearance observed in GS [72, 73]. In the case of nicotinic acid, the impaired clearance and the consistently higher hyperbilirubinemic effect were demonstrated not to be related to a higher degree of nicotinate-induced hemolysis [74]. Altogether, these data are in line with the view that a defective carrier molecule function is associated with GS and that this defect is sex-linked, being more evident in males than in females. The demonstration that bilitranslocase-mediated activity is lower in male than in female rats is in line with these results [56]. It is also tempting to speculate that this experimental evidence could account for the higher incidence of GS in men than in women.

## Concluding Remarks and Prospects

The process of hepatic organic anion uptake is far from being fully understood. In spite of the relevant and rapid progress achieved in the last few years, many aspects remain to be elucidated. In particular, the driving forces governing the process, the interaction between the ligand and the sinusoidal membrane receptor(s), the translocation mechanism(s) across the lipid bilayer, the possible physiochemical transformation upon entry into the liver cell, and the binding to intracellular "storage" proteins will certainly attract the attention of investigators in coming years. It is expected that progress in the understanding of this basic function of the liver will also shed further light on congenital and acquired liver disorders involving the metabolism of bilirubin and related compounds.

## References

1. Roberts RK, Schenker S (1983) Clearly there is intrinsic value in intrinsic clearance. Hepatology 3: 1036-1038
2. Branch RA (1982) Drugs as indicators of hepatic function. Hepatology 2: 97-105
3. Scharschmidt BF, Waggoner JG, Berk PD (1975) Hepatic organic anion uptake in the rat. J Clin Invest 56: 1280-1292

4. Goresky CA (1964) Initial distribution and rate of sulfobromophthalein in the liver. Am J Physiol 207: 13-26
5. Paumgartner G, Reichen J (1975) Kinetics of hepatic uptake of unconjugated bilirubin. Clin Sci Mol Med 51: 169-176
6. Weisiger RA, Gollan JL, Ockner RK (1981) Receptor for albumin on the liver cell surface may mediate uptake of fatty acids and other albumin-bound substrates. Science 211: 1048-1051
7. Forker EL, Luxon BA, Snell M, Shurmantine WO (1982) Effect of albumin binding on the hepatic transport of rose bengal: surface-mediated dissociation of limited capacity. J Pharmacol Exp Ther 223: 342-347
8. Forker EL, Luxon BA (1981) Albumin helps mediate removal of taurocholate by rat liver. J Clin Invest 67: 1517-1522
9. Faerch T, Jacobsen J (1975) Determination of association and dissociation rate constants for bilirubin-bovine serum albumin. Arch Biochem Biophys 168: 351-357
10. Stremmel W, Potter BJ, Berk PD (1983) Studies of albumin binding to rat liver plasma membrane: implications of the albumin receptor hypothesis. Biochim Biophys Acta 756: 20-27
11. Inoue M, Ohajiama K, Nagase S, Morino J (1983) Plasma clearance of sulfobromophthalein and its interaction with hepatic binding proteins in normal and analbuminemic rats: is plasma albumin essential for vectorial transport of organic anions in the liver? Proc Natl Acad Sci USA 80: 7654-7658
12. Gumucio DL, Gumucio JJ, Wilson JAP, Cutter C, Krauss M, Caldwell R, Chen E (1984) Albumin influences sulfobromophthalein transport by hepatocytes of each acinar zone. Am J Physiol 246: G86-G95
13. Weisiger RA (1985) Dissociation from albumin: a potentially rate-limiting step in the clearance of substances by the liver. Proc Natl Acad Sci USA 82: 1563-1567
14. Reichen J, Paumgartner G (1976) Uptake of bile acids by perfused rat liver. Am J Physiol 231: 734-742
15. Glasinovich JC, Dumont M, Duval M, Erlinger S (1975) Hepatocellular uptake of taurocholate in the dog. J Clin Invest 55: 419-426
16. Inoue M, Kinne R, Tran T, Arias IM (1982) Taurocholate transport by rat liver sinusoidal membrane vesicles: evidence of sodium cotransport. Hepatology 2: 572-579
17. Ruifrok PG, Meijer DKF (1982) Sodium ion-coupled uptake of taurocholate by rat liver plasma membrane vesicles. Liver 2: 28-34
18. Laperche Y, Preaux AM, Berthelot P (1981) Two systems are involved in the sulfobromophthalein uptake by rat liver cell: one is shared with bile salts. Biochem Pharmacol 30: 1333-1336
19. Laperche Y, Preaux AM, Feldman G, Mahu JL, Berthelot P (1981) Effect of fasting on organic anion uptake by isolated rat liver cells. Hepatology 1: 617-621
20. Duffy MC, Blitzer BL, Boyer JL (1983) Direct determination of the driving forces for taurocholate uptake into rat liver plasma membrane vesicles. J Clin Invest 72: 1470-1481
21. Rouse DJ, Lack L (1979) Ion requirements for taurocholate transport by ileal brush border membrane vesicles. Life Sci 25: 45-52
22. Scharschmidt BF, Stephens JE (1981) Transport of sodium chloride and taurocholate by cultured rat hepatocytes. Proc Natl Acad Sci USA 78: 986-990
23. Edmonson JW, Miller BA, Lumeng L (1985) Effect of glucagon on hepatic taurocholate uptake: relationship to membrane potential. Am J Physiol 249: G427-G433
24. Schwenk M, Burr R, Schwarz L, Pfaff E (1976) Uptake of sulfobromophthalein by isolated liver cells. Eur J Biochem 64: 189-197
25. Schwarz LR, Gotz R, Klassen CD (1980) Uptake of sulfobromophthalein-glutathione conjugate by isolated hepatocytes. Am J Physiol 239: C118-C123
26. Blom A, Keulemans K, Meijer DKF (1981) Transport of dibromosulphthalein by isolated rat hepatocytes. Biochem Pharmacol 30: 1809-1816
27. Gentile S, Tiribelli C, Baldini G, Lunazzi GC, Sottocasa GL (1985) Sex differences of nicotinate-induced hyperbilirubinemia in Gilbert's syndrome: implication of bilitranslocase function. J Hepatol 1: 417-429
28. Gentile S, Persico M, Baldini G, Lunazzi GC, Tiribelli C, Sottocasa GL (1985) The implication of bilitranslocase function in the impaired rifamycin-SV metabolism in Gilbert's syndrome. Clin Sci 68: 675-680

29. Baldini G, Passamonti S, Lunazzi GC, Tiribelli C, Sottocasa GL (1986) Cellular localization of sulfobromophthalein transport activity in rat liver. Biochim Biophys Acta 865: 1-10
30. Sottocasa GL, Baldini G, Sandri G, Lunazzi GC, Tiribelli C (1982) Reconstitution in vitro of sulfobromophthalein transport by bilitranslocase. Biochim Biophys Acta 685: 123-128
31. Claret M, Mazet JL (1972) Ionic fluxes and permeabilities of cell membranes in rat liver. J Physiol (Lond) 233: 279-295
32. Levy AJ, Gatmaitan Z, Arias IM (1969) Two hepatic cytoplasmic proteins, Y and Z, and their possible role in the hepatic uptake of bilirubin, sulfobromophthalein and other anions. J Clin Invest 48: 2156-2167
33. Frezza M, Tiribelli C, Panfili E, Sandri G (1974) Evidence for the existence of a carrier for bromosulphonphthalein in the liver cell plasma membrane. FEBS Lett 38: 125-128
34. Cornelius CE, Ben-Ezzer J, Arias IM (1967) Binding of sulfobromophthalein sodium (BSP) and other organic anions by isolated hepatic cell plasma membranes in vitro. Proc Soc Exp Biol Med 124: 665-667
35. Tiribelli C, Panfili E, Sandri G, Frezza M, Sottocasa GL (1976) In: Leevy CM (ed) Diseases of the liver and biliary tract. Karger, Basel, p 55
36. Tiribelli C, Lunazzi GC, Luciani M, Panfili E, Gazzin B, Liut G, Sandri G, Sottocasa GL (1978) Isolation of a sulfobromophthalein-binding protein from hepatocyte plasma membrane. Biochim Biophys Acta 532: 105-112
37. Lunazzi GC, Tiribelli C, Gazzin B, Sottocasa GL (1982) Further studies on bilitranslocase, a plasma membrane protein involved in hepatic organic anion uptake. Biochim Biophys Acta 685: 117-122
38. Gentile S, Bajema BL, Baldini G, Lunazzi GC, Groothuis GMM, Tiribelli C, Meijer DKF, Sottocasa GL (1985) Measurement of the association of cholephylic organic anions with different binding proteins. Biochem Pharmacol 34: 2439-2444
39. Reichen J, Berk PD (1979) Isolation of an organic anion binding protein from rat liver plasma membrane fractions by affinity chromatography. Biochem Biophys Res Commun 28: 484-489
40. Wolkoff AW, Chung CT (1980) Identification, purification and partial characterization of an organic anion binding protein from rat liver cell plasma membrane. J Clin Invest 65: 1152-1161
41. Stremmel W, Gerber MA, Glezerov V, Thung SN, Kochwa S, Berk PD (1983) Physicochemical and immunohistological studies of a sulfobromophthalein- and bilirubin- binding protein from rat liver plasma membranes. J Clin Invest 71: 1796-1805
42. Tiribelli C, Kunazzi GC, Luciani M, Gazzin B, Sottocasa GL (1978) Carriers and specific hepatocellular receptors for endogenous and exogenous anions. In: Gentilini P, Popper H, Sherlock S, Teodori U (eds) Problems in intrahepatic cholestasis. Karger, Basel, p 111
43. Sottocasa GL, Tiribelli C, Luciani M, Lunazzi GC, Gazzin B (1979) Isolation and some properties of a protein molecule involved in hepatic uptake of bilirubin – and other anion – transport. In: Quagliariello E, Palmieri F, Papa S, Klingenberg M (eds) Function and molecular aspects of biomembrane transport. Elsevier/North-Holland Biochemical, Amsterdam, p 451
44. Tiribelli C, Meijer DKF, Lunazzi GC, Hardonk MJ, Sottocasa GL (1982) Specific inhibition of the hepatic uptake of dibromosulfonphthalein (DBSP) by anti-bilitranslocase antibody. Hepatology 2: 749
45. Paumgartner G, Reichen J (1975) Different pathways for hepatic uptake of taurocholate and indocyanine green. Experientia 31: 306-307
46. Heimberg M, Goh EM, Klausner HA, Soler-Argilaga C, Weinstein I, Wilcox HG (1978) Regulation of hepatic metabolism of free fatty acids. Interrelationships among secretion of very low density lipoproteins, ketogenesis and cholesterogenesis. In: Dietschy JM, Gotto AM Jr, Onthro JA (eds) Disturbances in lipid and lipoprotein metabolism. American Physiologic Society, Washington, p 251 (Clinical physiology series)
47. Samuel D, Paris S, Ailhaud G (1976) Uptake and metabolism of fatty acids and analogues by cultured cardiac cells from chick embryo. Eur J Biochem 64: 583-595
48. Abumrad MA, Perkins RC, Park JH, Park CR (1981) Mechanism of long chain fatty acid permeation in the isolated adipocyte. J Biol Chem 256: 9183-9191
49. Mahadevan S, Saver F (1979) Effect of trypsin, phospholipases and membrane-impermeable reagents on the uptake of palmitic acid by isolated rat liver cells. Arch Biochem Biophys 164: 185-193

50. Stremmel W, Strohmeyer G, Borchard F, Kochwa S, Berk PD (1985) Isolation and partial characterization of a fatty acid binding protein in rat liver plasma membranes. Proc Natl Acad Sci USA 82: 4-8
51. Tiribelli C, Luciani M, Lunazzi GC, Gazzin B, Renaud G, Infante R, Sottocasa GL (1981) The possible role of bilitranslocase in fatty acid transport. In: Okolicsanyi L (ed) Familial hyperbilirubinemia. Wiley, Chichester, p 43
52. Martin JF, Mikulecky N, Blaschke TF, Waggoner JG, Vergalla J, Berk PD (1975) Differences between plasma indocyanine disappearance rate of normal men and women. Proc Soc Exper Biol Med 150: 612-617
53. Berk PD, Howe RB, Bloomer JR, Berlin NI (1969) Studies of bilirubin kinetics in normal adults. J Clin Invest 48: 2176-2190
54. Hart LG, Guarino AM, Adamson RH (1969) Effects of phenobarbital on biliary excretion of organic acids in male and female rat. Am J Physiol 217: 46-52
55. Klassen CD, Strom SC (1978) Comparison of biliary excretory function and bile composition in male, female and lactating rats. Drug Metab Disp 6: 120-124
56. Orzes N, Bellentani S, Aldini R, Simoni P, Ferretti I, Lunazzi GC, Sottocasa GL, Tiribelli C (1985) Sex differences in the hepatic uptake of sulfobromophthalein in the rat. Clin Sci 69: 587-593
57. Ockner RK, Burnett DA, Lysenko N, Manning JA (1979) Sex differences in long chain fatty acids utilization and fatty acid binding protein concentration in rat. J Clin Invest 64: 172-181
58. Ockner RK, Weisiger RA, Gollan JL (1983) Hepatic uptake of albumin bound substances: albumin receptor concept. Am J Physiol 245: 413-418
59. Muraca M, De Groote J, Fevery J (1983) Sex differences of the hepatic conjugation of bilirubin determine its maximal biliary excretion in non-anaesthetized male and female rats. Clin Sci 64: 85-90
60. Gilbert A, Leboullet P (1901) La cholemie simple familiale. Sem Medic 21: 241-245
61. Arias IM (1962) Chronic uncojugated hyperbilirubinemia without overt signs of hemolysis in adolescents and adults. J Clin Invest 41: 2233-2242
62. Arias IM, Gartner LN, Cohen N, Ben-Ezzer J, Levi AJ (1969) Chronic non hemolytic unconjugated hyperbilirubinemia with glucuronyltransferase deficiency: clinical, biochemical, pharmacologic and genetic evidence for heterogeneity. Amer J Med 47: 395-409
63. Black M, Billing BH (1969) Hepatic bilirubin UDP glucuronyltransferase activity in liver disease and Gilbert's syndrome. N Engl J Med 280: 1266-1271
64. Felsher BF, Craig JR, Carpio N (1973) Hepatic bilirubin glucuronidation in Gilbert's syndrome. J Lab Clin Med 81: 829-837
65. Billing BH, Williams R, Richards TC (1964) Defect in hepatic transport of bilirubin in congenital hyperbilirubinaemia: an analysis of plasma bilirubin disappearance curves. Clin Sci 27: 245-251
66. Berk PD, Bloomer JR, Howe RB, Berlin NI (1970) Constitutional hepatic dysfunction (Gilbert's syndrome): a new definition based on kinetic studies with unconjugated radiobulirubin. Am J Med 49: 296-305
67. Frezza M, Perona G, Corrocher R, Cellerino R, Bassetto MA, de Sandre G (1973) Bilirubin H3 kinetic studies: pattern of normals, Gilbert's syndrome and hemolytic state. Acta Hepato-gastroenterol (Stuttg) 20: 363-371
68. Cobelli C, Frezza M, Tiribelli C (1975) Modeling, identification and parameter estimation of bilirubin kinetics in normal, hemolytic and Gilbert's state. Comp. Biomed Res 8: 522-537
69. Okolicsanyi L, Ghidini O, Orlando R, Cortellazzo S, Benedetti G, Naccarato R, Mannitto P (1978) An evaluation of bilirubin kinetics with respect of the diagnosis of Gilbert's syndrome. Clin Sci Mol Med 54: 539-547
70. Berk PD, Blaschke PF, Waggoner JC (1972) Defective BSP clearance in patients with constitutional hepatic dysfunction (Gilbert's syndrome). Gastroenterology 63: 472-481
71. Cobelli C, Ruggieri A, Toffolo G, Okolicsanyi L, Venuti M, Orlando R (1981) BSP vs bilirubin kinetics in Gilbert's Syndrome. In: Okolicsanyi L (ed) Familial hyperbilirubinemia. Wiley, Chichester, p 121
72. Frezza M, Pozzato G, Quaranta C, Tiribelli C, Piccinini C (1980) Abnormality in the hepatic transport of rifamycin-SV in Gilbert's syndrome. Ital J Gastroenterol 12: 1-5
73. Gentile S, Saponara A, Foglia F, Grigni N, Garofano ML, Porcellini M, Coltori M (1981) Im-

paired plasma disappearance of nicotinic acid and interference with rifamycin-SV in Gilbert's syndrome. A defect in hepatic uptake of organic anions? Ital J Gastroenterol 13: 94-99
74. Gentile S, Tiribelli C, Persico M, Bronzino P, Marmo R, Orzes N, Orlando C, Rubba P, Coltorti M (1986) Dose dependence of nicotinic acid-induced hyperbilirubinemia and its dissociation from hemolysis in Gilbert's syndrome. J Lab Clin Med 107: 166-171

# Mechanisms of Transport of Tauroconjugated Bile Acids in the Hepatocyte: Functional Significance

S. Bellentani[1], F. Manenti[1], and W. G. M. Hardison[2]

[1] Cattedra di Gastroenterologia, Policlinico, Via Del Pozzo 71, 41100 Modena, Italy
and Cattedra di Gastroenterologia, Policlinico Via Del Pozzo 71, 41100 Modena Italy
[2] VAMC-GI Section 111D, 3350 La Jolla Village Drive, San Diego, CA 92161, U.S.A.

New techniques such as these employing isolated perfused liver, isolated hepatocytes, and, more recently, membrane vesicles and hepatocyte couplets have increased our understanding of hepatic transport processes. The isolated perfused liver is the most complicated model used to study liver transport, because all aspects of hepatic architecture participate in the process. Highly purified canalicular and/or basolateral rat liver membrane vesicle preparations are very useful for exploring transport function in various domains of the plasma membrane and for identifying and isolating putative membrane carriers. Isolated hepatocytes are simple to prepare and are useful especially in studying uptake function of the hepatocyte. One limitation of this model is that isolated liver cells in suspension lose their polarity; thus, it is impossible to examine canalicular excretion processes. This problem has been partially solved by the use of hepatocyte couplets [12, 31]. However, this technique is technically demanding and does not lend itself to quantification of water or solute flux.

In this review we shall summarize current knowledge concerning bile acid uptake by the hepatocyte, focusing particularly on our studies performed during the last 3 years. Because our early attempts at identifying a specific bile-acid-binding protein in liver plasma membranes were not successful [1, 4], we turned to the freshly isolated hepatocyte preparation as a tool. Many studies [2, 10, 14, 15, 23-26, 28] have demonstrated that hepatic uptake of proteinated bile acid, especially taurocholate (TC) is mostly a secondary active transport process. The "uphill" movement of TC into hepatocytes is coupled to the inwardly directed sodium gradient generated by the $Na^+$-$K^+$-ATPase activity. This is the main symport for TC, but, as schematically illustrated in Fig. 1, other ion-coupled transport systems may be coupled with it [21, 22]. Unconjugated bile acids, however, are transported primarily via a nonsaturable sodium-independent process [8, 14, 18, 22, 24].

## Active Sodium-Coupled Transport of Taurocholate

Because TC is the major endogenous bile acid in both man and the rat, we chose the uptake site responsible for the transport of this bile acid to study hepatocyte transport. To assess the structural requirements of this uptake site, we measured the ability of a series of bile acid analogs to inhibit the sodium-dependent uptake of TC. Both single-concentration and kinetic studies of TC uptake were performed. Hepatocytes were isolated by perfusion with collagenase [5, 13, 25] and uptake studies were completed within 2 h of isolation. The single-concentration TC uptake experiments were carried out by incubating the isolated liver cells with 5 $\mu M$ $^{14}C$-taurocholic acid in the presence or

Assessment and Management of Hepatobiliary Disease
Eds.: L. Okolicsânyi, G. Csomós, and G. Crepaldi

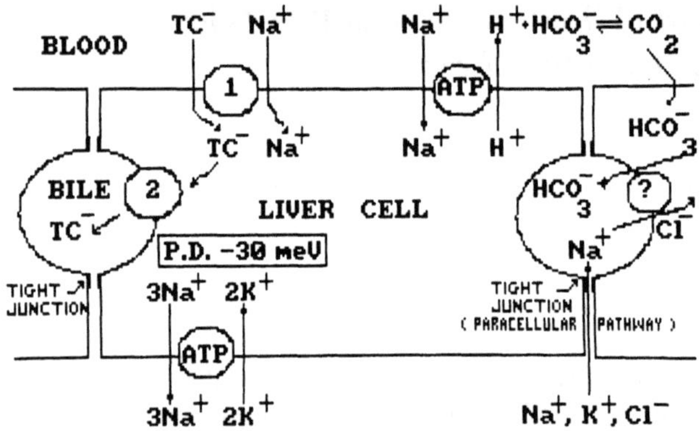


**Fig. 1.** Model for the proposed mechanisms of taurocholate transport at the basolateral and canalicular level of the hepatocyte and their coupled ion antiports. Hypothetical taurocholate translocators are also indicated (① and ②)

absence of a fixed concentration (100 μ*M*) of a bile acid analog. $^3$H-Inulin was used to correct for extracellular fluid space included in the cell pellet. A previously determined TC diffusion constant was used to correct TC uptake for passive diffusion. In this way, the active portion of the TC uptake process was calculated. The kinetic studies were carried out only with tauroconjugated bile acid inhibitors. Isolated hepatocytes were incubated with five different concentrations of TC (2.5, 8, 20, 50, and 100 μ*M*) in the presence or absence of a single concentration (5 or 25 μ*M*) of the bile acid inhibitor. All experiments were performed with 140 m*M* sodium and at 37 °C. Cells were sampled after 15, 30, 45, and 60 s incubation at a time when uptake was linear. They were immediately centrifuged through a silicon-oil layer into 50 μl 3 *N* KOH [5, 13]. Samples were then processed as described in our earlier work [13]. By plotting time (seconds) vs TC cell uptake (nmol/mg protein) a linear function was obtained, and from the slope of this line the velocity of TC uptake could be calculated. From the data for TC concentration vs uptake velocity, kinetic parameters (Km and Vmax) of TC uptake could be calculated with a nonlinear least-squares program [19]. By comparing these parameters obtained with or without the bile acid inhibitor, the type of inhibition could be defined. Thus, competitive inhibitors will not change Vmax but will increase Km (Fig. 2), while noncompetitive inhibitors will lower Vmax but will not change Km (Fig. 3). By applying a simple mathematical formula, the inhibition constant (Ki) for the competitive inhibitors could also be computed. The Ki is inversely related to inhibitory potency. In this way, we were able to characterize the effect of bile acid molecular structure upon inhibitory potency for TC uptake and thereby gain insight into molecular conformations which provided the "best fit" for the TC uptake site.

## Structural Specificity of $Na^+$-Dependent taurocholate Transport

We found the $Na^+$-dependent transport site of TC to be structurally specific for bile acid. Other $Na^+$-dependent uptake processes have been demonstrated in rat liver basolateral membrane vesicles, such as the $Na^+$-dependent amino acids system [7, 9].

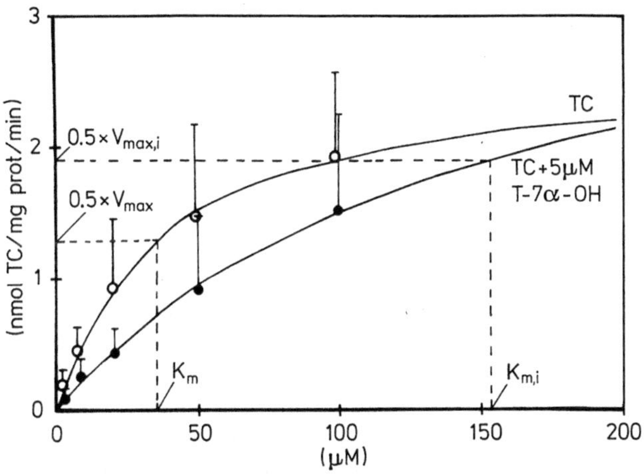


**Fig. 2.** Taurocholate uptake velocity in the absence *(TC)* presence *(TC+ T-7α-OH)* of a typical competitive inhibitor (T-7α-OH). Kinetic parameters are also indicated (Km, $Km_i$ and Vmax, $Vmax_i$ are the affinity constants and the maximal velocities of taurocholate uptake in the absence and presence, respectively, of the inhibitor). Note that the Vmax values are almost identical, while the Km values are significantly different ($p < 0.05$)

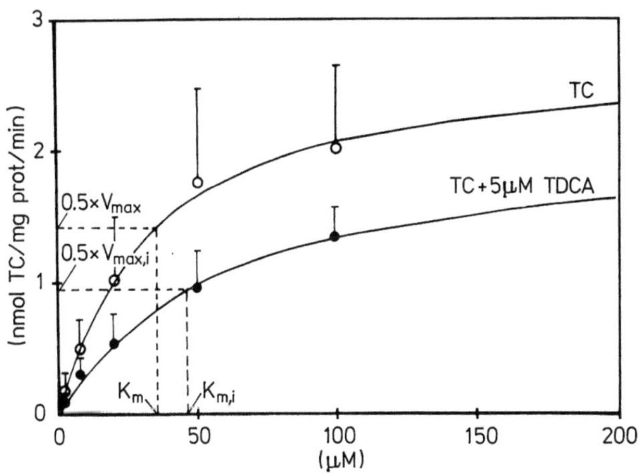


**Fig. 3.** Taurocholate uptake velocity in the absence *(TC)* and presence *(TC+ TDCA)* of a typical noncompetitive inhibitor (taurodeoxycholate). Kinetic parameters are also indicated (see Fig. 2 for details). Note that the Km values are almost identical while the Vmax values are significantly different ($p < 0.05$)

These systems, however, are separate from those for bile acids, sharing only a common requirement for an inwardly-directed sodium gradient [7]. We also demonstrated, by single-concentration experiments, that the most potent inhibitors of TC uptake (the tauro-3-α-OH, tauro-7-α-OH, and tauro-7-β-OH derivatives of 5-β-cholanic acid) did not inhibit the $Na^+$-dependent uptake of L-alanine [5]. These and other studies [7, 9, 13] support the view that amino acids and bile acids do not share the same transport systems in the hepatocyte.

We also found other evidence that the transport system for tauroconjugated bile acids recognizes a specific chemical structure, and either the steroid ring structure or the number, the position, and the orientation of the hydroxyl groups in the steroid moiety of the molecule is important in determining the fit of the bile acid in the $Na^+$-dependent TC transport site [13].

## Role of Structure of Steroid Ring

The TC uptake site is not only specific for excluding non-bile acid compounds, but also shows some degree of specificity even within the bile acid class. By means of single-concentration inhibition studies, we were able to demonstrate that progressive replacement of at least two of three hydroxyl groups by keto groups, which increases polarity and alters carbon-carbon bond angles to distort ring structure, diminishes the inhibitory capacity of the compound. The 3,7,12-triketo derivative bile acid, which has a planar steroid ring, did not inhibit the uptake of TC at all. These studies suggest that when a molecular distortion of the ring occurs or polarity increases, the bile acid is no longer recognized by the TC uptake site and does not compete.

## Role of Charge and Length of Side Chain

Both the charge and the length of the nonsteroid moiety of the bile acid molecule can influence the inhibitory potency of the acid for TC uptake. We found that positively charged compounds, such as cholylamine, inhibited weakly, while both neutral and negatively charged compounds were more potent inhibitors [13]. These findings are supported by those of Anwer et al. [3], who demonstrated, in isolated and perfused rat liver, that a single negative charge on the bile acid side chain gave optimal overall transport. This is similar to the situation in the intestine [22].

The length of the nonsteroid moiety is also important for recognition by the TC uptake site. We found that inhibitory potency increased as chain length increased from 0.5 to 1.2 nm. The only compound we studied with a longer chain (1.8 nm) was CHAPS. Although this compound did not inhibit TC uptake, its side chain is zwitterionic, so that definite conclusions about chain length vs. charge cannot be made. Compounds with a long negatively charged side chain need to be studied.

## Role of Number, Position, and Orientation of Hydroxyl Group in Steroid Moiety

The most interesting findings we obtained during our recent studies concern the importance of the OH groups in determining the inhibitory mechanism of tauroconjugated bile acids for TC uptake by the hepatocyte. The number of OH groups is important in determining the potency of inhibition of TC uptake: the fewer the hydroxyl substituents, the stronger the inhibition (and the lower the Ki) (Fig. 4). Also, orientation of the OH group at position 3 seems to be particularly critical: compounds with a 3-$\beta$-OH group are less inhibitory than those with a 3-$\alpha$-OH group [5, 13]. The orientation of the

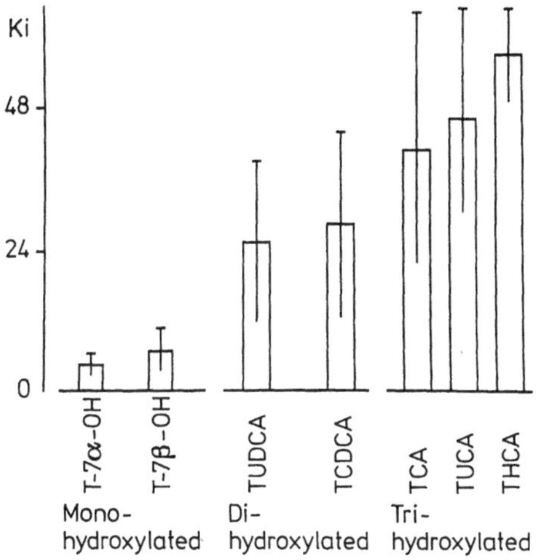


**Fig. 4.** Inhibition constant (Ki) of the competitive inhibitors of taurocholate uptake. The Ki is inversely correlated with inhibitory potency. *TUDCA*, tauroursodeoxycholic acid; *TCDCA*, taurochenodeoxycholic acid; *TCA*, taurocholic acid; *TUCA*, tauroursocholic acid; *THCA*, taurohyocholic acid

OH group in position 7 seems to be less important, while the presence of an OH group in position 6 or 7, no matter what the orientation, is necessary for a bile acid to compete with TC for uptake. Compounds without a 6- or a 7-OH group exhibited behavior most compatible with noncompetitive rather than competitive inhibition. Examples of both competitive and noncompetitive inhibition are illustrated in Figs. 2 and 3. In spite of the fact that compounds lacking a 6- or 7-OH group are noncompetitive inhibitors, they still probably utilize the $Na^+$-dependent TC uptake site for transport into the cell. This is suggested by the fact that taurolithocholic acid (TLCA) and TC, at the same concentration, show mutual inhibition of uptake.

In summary, we believe that all the tauroconjugated bile acids share the same mechanisms of uptake. The presence or absence of a 6- or a 7-OH group dictates the mechanism of inhibition, while the number of OH substituents determines the potency of competitive inhibition. How these noncompetitive inhibitors work is unknown. They do not dissipate the sodium gradient (unpublished observations) and do not inhibit $Na^+$-dependent alanine uptake [13]. Nor do they alter membrane potential (unpublished observations). At present we have no data to address this question. These structure-activity relationships support the view that all tauroconjugated bile acids are transported via the TC uptake site by the same carrier protein. Various candidates for the TC translocator at the sinusoidal level have recently been described. Kramer et al. [17] described three peptides of 52, 48, and 43 kd that could be involved in the transport of conjugated bile acids during their passage across the hepatocyte membrane. Von Dippe and Levy [29, 30] using a photoreactive derivative of TC, namely 7,7-azo-3alpha,-12-alpha-dihydroxy-5-beta-cholan-24-oyl)-2-aminoethansulfonic acid (7-ADTC), isolated another 54-kd membrane protein which was present in the normal hepatocyte but not in non-bile-acid-transporting hepatoma cells, suggesting that this could be the bile acid plasma membrane receptor. They also suggested that the 54-kd membrane protein was the receptor for both conjugated and unconjugated bile acids, but other evidence [22, 24, 27] suggests that the transport systems for the two species of bile acid are different. However, none of these authors reported clear evidence that the bile acid transporter could be reconstituted within proteoliposomes.

## Transport of Bile Acid at Canalicular Pole

Transport processes at the canalicular pole of the hepatocyte are less well understood, because they are more difficult to study. Recently, authors using isolated canalicular membrane vesicles [10, 16, 20, 22] and isolated rat hepatocyte couplets [12] have suggested that the TC transport system at the canalicular level is sodium-independent, carrier-mediated, and driven by an inward-directed intravesicular potential (Fig. 1). Another group, using a bile acid photoprobe, suggested that a 100-kd protein is the transport carrier [21]. An $HCO_3/Cl^-$ exchanger has also been identified in canalicular membrane vesicles [21, 22]. However, further investigations are necessary in order to establish a definitive role for these pumps.

Other unexplained and unidentified transport systems and driving forces could contribute to both the uptake and the secretion of bile acid. All the evidence already discussed indicates that the mechanism of conjugated bile acid uptake, which is the major driving force for bile secretion, is mainly an $Na^+$-dependent secondary active transport mechanism at the sinusoidal pole, whereas the mechanism of bile acid excretion is a $Na^+$-independent carrier-mediated process at the canalicular pole. The $Na^+$-$K^+$-ATPase pump, which was considered the unique driving force of both the bile-acid-dependent (BADBF) and the bile-acid-independent (BAIBF) components of bile secretion, remains the major mechanism for maintenance of the sodium gradient, but is not the only one. The recent finding of a basolateral $Na^+/H^+$ and a canalicular $Cl^-/HCO_3^-$ exchanger (Fig. 1) now permit a unifying hypothesis for bile flow. The basic mechanisms of hepatic bile formation are as follows:

1. Sodium-coupled transport of bile acids at the sinusoidal membrane ($Na^+$-$K^+$-ATPase antiport)
2. Transcellular transport of bile acids toward the canalicular pole
3. Transport of bile acids across the canalicular membrane into the canalicular lumen
4. Osmotic equilibration of bile acids inside the canaliculi (the paracellular pathway)
5. Bile-acid-independent secretory mechanisms ($Cl^-/HCO_3^-$ and $Na^+/H^+$ antiport)
6. Cytoskeletal elements (microfilaments and microtubules) driving the movements of canaliculi and pushing the bile forward

These mechanisms closely resemble the anion transport systems demonstrated in intestinal and renal epithelial cells [22], with the peculiar addition that the most important anions transported by the hepatocyte and driving bile secretion are the conjugated bile acids.

## References

1. Accattino L, Simon FR (1976) Identification and characterization of a bile acid receptor in isolated liver surface membranes. J Clin Invest 57: 496-508
2. Anwer MS, Hegner D (1978) Effect of $Na^+$ on bile acid uptake by isolated rat hepatocytes. Hoppe Seylers Z Physiol Chem 359: 181-192
3. Anwer MS, O'Maille ERL, Hofmann AF, Di Pietro RA, Michelotti E (1985) Influence of side-chain charge on hepatic transport of bile acids and bile acid analogues. Am J Physiol 249: G479-G488
4. Bellentani S, Hardison WGM, Grisendi A, Barbieri I, Manenti F (1984) Bile acid binding to isolated liver plasma membranes: failure to find a specific binding site. Hoppe Seylers Z Physiol Chem 365: 357-363

5. Bellentani S, Hardison WGM, Marchegiano P, Zanasi G, Manenti F (1986) Bile acid inhibition of taurocholate uptake by rat hepatocyte: role of OH-groups. Am J Physiol, (in press)
6. Blitzer BL, Boyer JL (1982) Cellular mechanisms of bile formation. Gastroenterology 82: 346-357
7. Blitzer BL, Bueler RL (1985) Kinetic and energetic aspects of the inhibition of taurocholate uptake by $Na^+$-dependent amino acids: studies in rat liver plasma membrane vesicles. Am J Physiol 249: G120-G124
8. Blitzer BL, Terzakis C, Carolan MA (1984) Hydroxyl-bile acid exchange: a new mechanism for the uphill transport of cholate by basolateral liver plasma membrane vesicles (Abstr). Hepatology 4: 1037
9. Bucuvalas JC, Goodrich A, Blitzer BL, Suchy FJ (1985) Amino acids are potent inhibitors of bile acid uptake by liver plasma membrane vesicles isolated from suckling rats. Pediatr Res 19: 1298-1304
10. Duffy MC, Blitzer BL, Boyer JL (1983) Direct determination of the driving forces for taurocholate uptake into rat liver plasma membrane vesicles. J Clin Invest 72: 1470-1481
11. Edmondson JW, Miller BA, Lumeng L (1985) Effect of glucagon on hepatic taurocholate uptake: relationship to membrane potential. Am J Physiol 249: G427-G433
12. Graf J, Gautam A, Boyer JL (1984) Isolated rat hepatocyte couplets: a primary secretory unit for electrophysiologic studies of bile secretory function. Proc Natl Acad Sci USA 81: 6516-6520
13. Hardison WGM, Bellentani S, Heasley V, Shellhamer S (1984) Specificity of a $Na^+$-dependent transport site in isolated rat hepatocytes. Am J Physiol 246: G477-G483
14. Iga T, Klaassen CD (1982) Uptake of bile acids by isolated rat hepatocytes. Biochem Pharmacol 31: 211-216
15. Inoue M, Kinne R, Tran T, Arias IM (1982) Taurocholate transport by rat liver sinusoidal membrane vesicles: evidence of sodium cotransport. Hepatology 2: 572-579
16. Inoue , Kinne R, Tran T, Arias IM (1983) The mechanisms of biliary secretion of reduced glutathione. Analysis of transport process in isolated rat-liver canalicular membrane vesicles. Eur J Biochem 134: 467-471
17. Kramer W, Bickel U, Buscher HP, Gerok W, Kurz G (1982) Bile-salt-binding polypeptides in plasma membranes of hepatocytes revealed by photoaffinity labelling. Eur J Biochem 129: 13-24
18. Klaassen CD, Watkins JB III (1984) Mechanisms of bile formation, hepatic uptake, and biliary excretion. Pharmacol Rev 36: 1-67
19. Marquardt DW (1963) An algorithm for least-squares estimation of non-linear parameters. J SIAM Soc 11: 431-436
20. Meier PJ, Meier-Abt AS, Barrett C, Boyer JL (1984) Mechanisms of taurocholate transport in canalicular and basolateral rat liver plasma membrane vesicles: evidence for an electrogenic canalicular organic anion carrier. J Biol Chem 259: 10614-10622
21. Meier PJ, Knickelbein R, Moseley RH, Dobbins JW, Boyer JL (1985) Evidence for carrier-mediated chloride/bicarbonate exchange in canalicular rat liver plasma membrane vesicles. J Clin Invest 75: 1256-1263
22. Moseley RH, Boyer JL (1985) Mechanisms of electrolyte transport in the liver and their functional significance. Semin Liver Dis 5: 122-135
23. Reichen J, Paumgartner G (1976) Uptake of bile acids by perfused rat liver. Am J Physiol 231: 734-742
24. Scharschmidt BF, Stephens JE (1981) Transport of sodium, chloride, and taurocholate by cultured rat hepatocyte. Proc Natl Acad Sci USA 78: 986-990
25. Schwartz LR, Barth CA (1979) Taurocholate uptake by adult rat hepatocytes in primary culture. Hoppe Seylers Z Physiol Chem 360: 1117-1120
26. Schwartz LR, Burr R, Schwenk M, Pfaff E, Greim H (1975) Uptake of taurocholate into isolated rat liver cells. Eur J Biochem 55: 617-623
27. Strange RC (1984) Hepatic bile flow. Physiol Rev 64: 1055-1103
28. Van Dyke RW, Stephens JE, Scharschmidt BF (1982) Bile acid transport in cultured rat hepatocytes. Am J Physiol 243: G484-G492
29. Von Dippe P, Levy D (1983) Characterization of the bile acid transport system in normal and transformed hepatocytes. Photoaffinity labeling of the taurocholate carrier protein. J Biol Chem 258: 8896-8901

30. Von Dippe P, Drain P, Levy D (1983) Synthesis and transport characteristics of photoaffinity probes for the hepatocyte bile acid transport system. J Biol Chem 258: 8890–8895
31. Watanabe S, Phillips MJ (1984) $Ca^{++}$ causes active contraction of bile canaliculi: direct evidence from microinjection studies. Proc Natl Acad Sci USA 81: 6164–6168

# Determinants of Biliary Cholesterol Secretion

Nicola Carulli, Paola Loria, Marco Bertolotti, and Alberto Tripodi
Istituto di Clinica Medica 1, Università di Modena

## Introduction

The major route by which the body eliminates cholesterol is biliary excretion, either as intact molecule or after degradation to bile acids. Thus biliary output of cholesterol could contribute to maintaining body cholesterol balance in equilibrium; however, an excess of cholesterol into the bile is considered a prerequisite for gallstone formation. Despite intensive research in this field, regulation of cholesterol secretion into the bile is not as yet well defined.

In many animal species, including man, biliary secretion of cholesterol and phospholipids is linked to that of bile acids. In kinetic terms, the relation is usually described by a curvilinear function where the ratio of cholesterol to bile acids is higher at low bile acid output than at high bile acid output [1]. The absolute value of this function, i.e., moles of cholesterol secreted per mole of bile acid, varies from animal to animal and in man among different subjects [2].

This would suggest that although the output of bile acids is a necessary event for cholesterol secretion into the bile, other factors play a role in determining how much cholesterol is to be secreted. Definition of these factors would require a sound knowledge of *where* biliary cholesterol comes from and *how* cholesterol enters the bile.

Broadly speaking, some determinants might regulate the availability of cholesterol for biliary excretion and others might affect the very process of cholesterol transport into the bile. In this brief review we will summarize the aspects of cholesterol secretion with emphasis given to human physiology.

## Availability of Cholesterol for Biliary Secretion

In Fig. 1 is shown schematically the cholesterol traffic through the liver cell. Input of cholesterol to the liver is provided by two sources: circulating cholesterol and local neosynthesis. Cholesterol derived from both exogenous (diet) and endogenous (other tissues) sources is delivered to the liver as lipoprotein of varying composition and most of it is taken up by means of a receptor-mediated mechanism. Local neosynthesis constitutes an important, though variable from animal to animal, proportion of liver cholesterol [2].

From the available evidence it can be assumed that cholesterol entering the liver cell, by whatever means, and the neosynthesized cholesterol feed into a metabolically active pool which the liver uses for bile acid synthesis, VLDL secretion, biliary secretion, and storage as esters. However, the possibility exists that cholesterol coming from

Assessment and Management of Hepatobiliary Disease
Eds.: L. Okolicsányi, G. Csomós, and G. Crepaldi

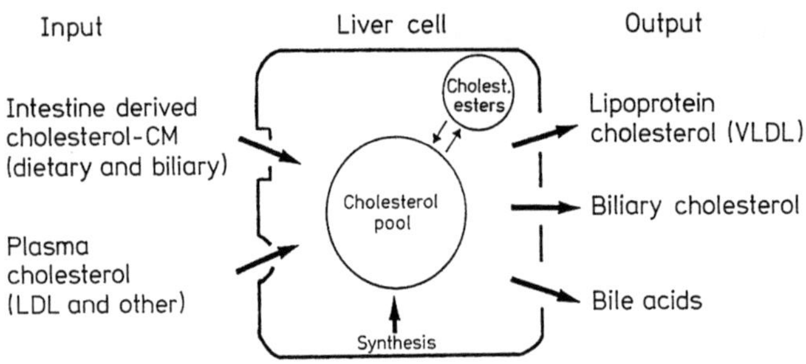


**Fig. 1.** Cholesterol balance across the liver

one source is channeled to a specific excretory pathway. Thus, isotopic kinetic studies have suggested that cholesterol delivered to the liver as HDL might be preferentially used for biliary excretion [3, 4]. At variance with these findings, recently it has been reported that newly synthesized cholesterol is a preferred source of biliary cholesterol [5]. In addition, the pathway for biliary secretion seems to be different for newly synthesized and preformed cholesterol. The latter, delivered by circulating lipoproteins, could be incorporated into plasma membrane and from there be secreted into the bile without being internalized and without being mixed with intracellular cholesterol [5].

Complex though the traffic of cholesterol through the liver may be, it is possible that biliary excretion is influenced by the balance between input of cholesterol on one hand and degradation of cholesterol to bile acids, secretion into VLDL, or storage as esters on the other hand. However, attempts to relate changes of biliary output to changes of the different processes of cholesterol metabolism have not always produced clear-cut results.

## Cholesterol Synthesis

A strong relation between total body synthesis of cholesterol and its biliary excretion was established by studies in obesity. Obese subjects show a linear relationship between degree of overweight, body synthesis of cholesterol, and its biliary secretion [6].

Another line of evidence linking synthesis to biliary secretion of cholesterol was the finding that patients with cholesterol gallstones and supersaturated bile displayed, at least in some studies, an increased HMG-CoA reductase activity in the liver [7, 8, 9] thus suggesting an increased hepatic synthesis of cholesterol. This latter finding is controversial, for some other studies have reported no difference between gallstone and control subjects [10, 11]. Moreover, extensive studies in experimental animals have produced evidence that newly synthesized cholesterol contributes to biliary cholesterol [12]; however, dramatic changes of the rate of synthesis, induced by various means, are not paralleled by similar changes in the excretory rate [13].

## Dietary Cholesterol

Of practical significance could be the possibility that biliary cholesterol output is influenced by dietary intake of the sterol. In theory an increased load of cholesterol, delivered to the liver with chilomicrons, could increase the cholesterol available for secre-

**Table 1.** Effect of cholesterol feeding on bile and plasma cholesterol

| Cholesterol (g) (feeding period) | Bile | | | Plasma cholesterol | Authors, year |
|---|---|---|---|---|---|
| | Bile acids | Cholesterol | Saturation | | |
| 1.5 (1 week) | → | → | → | n.d. | Sarles et al. 1970 [14] |
| 0.5–4 (5–12 weeks) | →[a] | ↑[a,b] | ↑ | ↑→ | Quintao et al. 1971 [16] |
| 1.5–3 (6 weeks) | → | → | → | ↑ | Dam et al. 1971 [15] |
| 0.75 (3 weeks) | ↑[a] | ↑[a] | ↑ | ↑ | Den Besten et al. 1973 [17] |
| 1.5 (2 weeks) | | | → | ↑ | Andersen and Hellstrom 1979 [18] |
| 0.5–1 (3 weeks) | | | ↑ | n.d. | Lee et al. 1983 [19] |

[a] Balance studies
[b] Secretion data

tion into the bile. However, reports from several studies on cholesterol feeding in man indicate that no such relation is evident. In addition, it seems that in most cases of increased dietary cholesterol, humans respond by increasing plasma cholesterol concentration rather than increasing biliary output [14–19] (Table 1).

In addition to the cholesterol absorbed in the intestine and that newly synthesized in the liver, circulating lipoprotein cholesterol also contributes to biliary output. A definite relationship in quantitative terms is, however, difficult to establish, and the critical issue remains whether cholesterol arriving in the liver mixes in a common pool or is directly utilized for one or the other pathway.

Availability of cholesterol for biliary secretion may also be dictated by the amount used for other excretory processes.

## Synthesis of Bile Acids

Synthesis of bile acids is quantitatively the most important mechanism for reducing the liver's load of cholesterol, and an increased degradation to bile acids would be expected to reduce the biliary output of cholesterol. In man, however, the administration of cholestyramine, a bile-acid-binding resin which interrupts the enterohepatic circulation, does not seem to change biliary output of cholesterol [20] whereas it is effective in reducing plasma concentration [21].

## Lipoprotein Secretion

Lipoprotein secretion could, in theory, be a way for the liver to remove cholesterol. However, VLDL, the only quantitatively important lipoprotein secreted by the liver, carries little cholesterol. Furthermore, cholesterol removed by lipoprotein secretion is returned to the liver by various mechanisms.

### Cholesterol Esterification

Recently attention has been focused on the balance between hepatocyte free and esterified cholesterol as a possible determinant of cholesterol output into the bile. Nervi and colleagues [22] investigated the relationship between the activity of acylcoenzyme A: cholesterolacyltransferase (ACAT), and hence cholesterol esterification rate, and biliary secretion of cholesterol in rats. They observed that chronic administration of progesterone, a compound that decreases ACAT activity, is associated with an increased biliary cholesterol content. Subsequently Stone et al. [23] addressed this problem in more detail by inducing, in rats, changes of both HMG-CoA reductase and ACAT activities, in different combinations. From the obtained results they suggested that the size of a free cholesterol pool, determined in part by the rates of synthesis and of esterification of cholesterol, is a key determinant of biliary cholesterol output. In this context Andersen and Cook [24] have reported that liver free cholesterol content correlates with biliary cholesterol concentration.

In summary, biliary cholesterol could be derived from the different sources of preformed cholesterol as well as from newly synthesized cholesterol. The rate at which cholesterol is delivered to or synthesized in the liver would influence only the relative contribution of these sources to biliary cholesterol, not the total output [25]. In fact, availability for biliary excretion most likely depends on the balance between cholesterol input to and disposition by the liver. In addition, the actual balance between the free and esterified forms of the sterol could be an immediate determinant of biliary secretion.

## Transport of Cholesterol into the Bile

The precise mechanism by which cholesterol is coupled to bile acids and enters the bile is not well defined. Bile acids could stimulate the formation of cholesterol-phospholipid complex inside the hepatocyte [26, 27] or on the canalicular membrane [28] or alternatively bile acids, once having entered the canalicular lumen, could leech away complexed phospholipid and cholesterol from the membrane [29]. Lipids could be secreted as vesicles which are transformed into mixed micelles as bile acids approach and exceed the micellar concentration [30, 31]. Canalicular cholesterol and phospholipids lost into the bile would be replaced from a microsomal pool [32, 33].

Whatever the exact physical mode of cholesterol transport, there is no doubt that the secretory process is made possible by the amphipathic properties of the bile acids. Micelle-forming capacity seems to be a prerequisite for bile acid to stimulate phospholipid and cholesterol secretion [34–36].

### Bile Acid Structure and Bile Lipid Secretion

A great deal of information on the regulation of biliary cholesterol secretion has come from the use of some bile acids as cholesterol-gallstone-dissolving agents. Administration of chenodeoxycholic (CDCA) or ursodeoxycholic (UDCA) acid to humans leads to a predominance of the administered bile acid in the pool and to a marked reduction of biliary cholesterol [37, 38]. The time sequence of these two events strongly suggests a cause-effect relationship. The mechanism linking changes of bile cholesterol to changes of bile acid pool composition was thought to be attributable to changes of cholesterol metabolism, including the rate of hepatic synthesis and/or the extent of intestinal absorption of cholesterol.

However, it was seen that CDCA and UDCA, while both decreasing bile cholesterol secretion, have disparate and controversial effects on HMG-CoA reductase, in that CDCA seems in all reported studies to decrease the enzyme activity [8-11], whereas for UDCA some authors have reported a decrease [9, 39], others no change [40] or even an increase [11], in HMG-CoA reductase activity.

Intestinal absorption of cholesterol is depressed by UDCA [41-43] and probably also by CDCA [44], and this has suggested that changes of absorption could have a direct influence on biliary secretion of cholesterol. This view was somewhat limited by the observation that the administration of deoxycholic acid (DCA), while depressing both the hepatic synthesis [45] and the absorption [46], of cholesterol, is nevertheless associated with no change [45, 47, 48] or even with an increase [46, 49] of biliary cholesterol content. Altogether, these findings would suggest that the effect of bile acids on biliary cholesterol secretion is not mediated by changes of cholesterol metabolism.

A possibility which has been considered is that the various bile acids, due to their different structure, may alter the coupling of cholesterol to bile acids, thus leading to changes of biliary secretion. Some studies have been performed, in patients with T-tubes, in which the endogenous bile acid pool was drained off and replaced by individual bile acids infused through the duodenum. In these acute experiments infusion of UDCA was associated with a biliary cholesterol output lower than that observed when CDCA or cholic acid (CA) were infused [50-52]. These results provide evidence that CDCA- or, even better, UDCA-induced bile desaturation is due to a direct effect of these bile acids on the secretory process.

A more systematic approach to the definition of the effect of bile acid structure on biliary cholesterol secretion was employed in our laboratory. Due to the number, the reciprocal position, the orientation of the hydroxyl group, and the conjugation with glycine or taurine, bile acid molecules possess a different hydrophilic-hydrophobic balance, which dictates their detergent strength: the more hydrophobic the bile acid, the greater its detergency and its ability to solubilize lipids in vitro [53]. Physiological bile acids of man could be ranked in order of decreasing detergency as follows: DCA, CDCA, CA, UDCA. We postulated that bile acid capacity to stimulate bile lipid secretion is a direct correlate of their detergent strength. Using a T-tube model, we investigated in cholecystectomized patients the effect on bile lipid secretion of DCA, CDCA, CA, and UDCA [54] and of ursocholic acid (UCA), the 7 $\beta$-epimer of cholic acid [55]. It was seen that when the endogenous pool was replaced by the individual bile acid, the biliary output of cholesterol and phospholipid was linearly related to the detergency of the infused bile acid, the highest being observed during DCA and the lowest during UCA secretion. Regarding the nature of the experiment, i.e., acute replacement of the bile acid pool, it could reasonably be assumed that changes of intracellular metabolism of cholesterol and phospholipids that might have occurred as a consequence of bile acid infusion had little, if any, relevance for their biliary secretion. In our study the biliary output of alkaline phosphatase, a canalicular membrane-bound enzmye, paralleled that of cholesterol in that it was directly related to the detergent strength of the secreted bile acid. This finding supports the view that biliary secretion involves solubilization of membrane constituents.

Acute studies performed on different experimental animals and using bile acids with different structures have, in general, produced results consistent with the view that biliary output of cholesterol and phospholipid is related to the detergency of the secreted bile acids [56–63].

Though obtained in nonphysiological conditions, the results of acute experiments are relevant to the interpretation of the results observed with chronic bile acid feeding, and in addition they furnish the basis for a generalized and physiological concept that physicochemical properties of the bile acid molecule, namely its solubilizing capacity, are the key determinant of bile lipid secretion.

## Bile Acid Pool Composition and Bile Cholesterol Saturation

In fact the bile acid pool, taken as a mixture of bile acids, possesses a detergent strength that can be regarded as the resultant of the solubilizing capacity of the bile acids present within the pool. From what has been said above, we can assume that in physiological conditions the pool will stimulate an output of cholesterol and phospholipid into the bile somewhat proportional to its detergency. It follows that changing the composition, e.g., by means of chronic bile acid feeding, would lead to a decrease or increase of bile cholesterol secretion and saturation, depending on the change of detergency of the pool. This view is supported by several observations.

Studies on dose-response relationship in patients receiving CDCA or UDCA for gallstone dissolution have shown that chronic administration leads to a cholesterol desaturation of the bile provided that the administered bile acid reaches a certain proportion in the pool. It could be presumed that the proportion of bile acid at which bile desaturates is the one effective in reducing the detergency of the pool. If so, the more hydrophilic the bile acid, the lower its proportion in the pool that would be necessary to reduce detergency. Administration of UDCA, the least detergent of the physiological bile acids in man, produces a fall of bile cholesterol content greater than that associated with the feeding of the more detergent CDCA, in spite of the fact that the proportion of UDCA in the pool never exceeds 60%, in contrast with the 80%–90% levels of CDCA observed after CDCA administration [64].

One may find it intriguing that two bile acids such as CDCA and UDCA, which have different detergent strengths, produce the same effect, i.e., bile desaturation, in man. The mechanism by which the detergency of the physiological bile acid pool is reduced as a consequence of the administration of one or the other of the two bile acids may be dual: the pool becomes enriched in a weak detergent such as UDCA, while the proportion of a very strong detergent such as DCA is reduced during CDCA administration.

Following this line of reasoning, the administration of CA, a weak detergent, should also reduce the detergency of the pool and decrease bile saturation. However, attempts to desaturate bile by feeding CA to man have not produced consistent results. The most likely explanation for this failure, in our opinion, is that feeding CA leads to an increase in the proportion of DCA which may overcome the effect of CA. If the increase of DCA is prevented, e.g., by reducing its intestinal production, the CA pool expands and bile cholesterol saturation falls [65]. It is tempting to speculate that a relation might exist between the detergency of the bile acid pool and the degree of saturation even in physiological conditions. The bile acid pool in men is constituted two-thirds by dihydroxy bile acids such as CDCA and DCA, the latter being the most hydrophobic of all and having the strongest detergency, and human bile is saturated or supersaturated [66]. Such an interpretation would make the abundance of DCA in the bile of man an important factor for bile supersaturation with cholesterol. This view was first put forward by Low-Beer and Pomare [49], who suggested that an increased proportion of DCA in the pool might cause cholesterol supersaturation by depressing the proportion of CDCA. Regardless of the mechanism responsible, support for the role of DCA in supersaturating the bile is provided by the results of several investigations. Some authors have found that the fraction of DCA is greater in the bile of patients with gallstones than in normal controls [67-71]. A relationship between DCA fraction and bile cholesterol saturation was observed by van der Linden and Bergman [72], Bennion et al. [73], Thornton et al. [74], and Hofmann et al. [75]. When the proportion of DCA into the pool is increased by feeding physiological doses of DCA, the relative content of biliary cholesterol increases both in normal controls [49] and in cirrhotic subjects [76]. Moreover, drug treatments which, by whatever mechanism, lead to changes of DCA fraction produce parallel changes in bile cholesterol saturation [77-81]. These findings stress the role of physicochemical determinants of bile cholesterol secretion.

Undoubtedly the actual secretion of cholesterol into the bile is the net result of the complex interplay between the metabolic factors which govern the availability of hepatocyte cholesterol and the physicochemical characteristics of the bile acid pool which influence the transport of the sterol into the bile.

## References


1. Wagner CI, Trotman BW, Soloway RD (1976) Kinetic analysis of biliary lipid excretion in man and dog. J Clin Invest 57: 473-477
2. Turley SD, Dietschy JM (1982) Cholesterol metabolism and excretion. In: Arias, Popper, Schachter, Shafritz (eds) The Liver: biology and pathobiology. Raven, New York, pp 467-492
3. Schwartz CC, Berman M, Vlahcevic ZR, Halloran LG, Gregory DH, Swell L (1978) Multicompartmental analysis of cholesterol metabolism in man. Characterization of the hepatic bile acid and biliary cholesterol precursor sites. J Clin Invest 61: 408-423
4. Schwartz CC, Halloran LG, Vlahcevic ZR, Gregory DH, Swell L (1978) Preferential utilization of free cholesterol from high-density lipoprotein for biliary cholesterol secretion in man. Science 200: 62-64
5. Robins SJ, Fasulo JM, Collins MA, Patton GM (1985) Evidence for separate pathways of transport of newly synthesized and preformed cholesterol into bile. J Biol Chem 260: 6511-6513
6. Grundy SM, Mok HYL, von Bergmann K (1976) Regulation of biliary cholesterol secretion in man. In: Preisig, Bircher, Paumgartner (eds) The liver. Quantitative aspects of structure and function. Editio Cantor, Aulendorf, pp 393-403
7. Salen G, Nicolau G, Shefer S, Mosbach EH (1975) Hepatic cholesterol metabolism in patients with gallstones. Gastroenterology 69: 676-684
8. Coyne MJ, Bonorris GG, Goldstein LI, Shoenfield LJ (1976) Effect of chenodeoxycholic acid and phenobarbital on the rate-limiting enzymes of hepatic cholesterol and bile acid synthesis in patients with gallstones. J Lab Clin Med 87: 281-291
9. Maton PN, Ellis HJ, Higgins MJP, Dowling RH (1980) Hepatic HMG-CoA reductase in human cholelithiasis: effects of chenodeoxycholic and ursodeoxycholic acids. Eur J Clin Invest 10: 325-332
10. Ahlberg J, Angelin B, Einarsson K (1981) Hepatic 3-hydroxy-3-methyl glutaryl coenzyme A

reductase activity and biliary lipid composition in man: relation to gallstone disease and effects of cholic and chenodeoxycholic acid treatment. J Lipid Res 22: 410-422
11. Carulli N, Ponz de Leon M, Zironi F (1983) Evaluation of hepatic cholesterol synthesis in man: results with the HMG-CoA reductase activity assay. In: Barbara, Dowling, Hofmann, Roda (eds) Bile acids in gastroenterology. MTP Press, Lancaster, pp 69-74
12. Turley SD, Dietschy JM (1981) The contribution of newly synthesized cholesterol to biliary cholesterol in the rat. J Biol Chem 256: 2438-2446
13. Turley SD, Dietschy JM (1979) Regulation of biliary cholesterol output in the rat: dissociation from the rate of hepatic cholesterol synthesis, the size of the hepatic cholesteryl ester pool and the hepatic uptake of chylomicron cholesterol. J Lipid Res 20: 923-934
14. Sarles H, Crotte C, Gerolami A, Mulè A, Domingo N, Hauton J (1970) Influence of cholestyramine, bile salt and cholesterol feeding on the lipid composition of hepatic bile in man. Scand J Gastroenterol 5: 603-608
15. Dam H, Prange I, Jensen MK, Kallehauge HE, Fenger HJ (1981) Studies in human bile. IV. Influence of ingestion of cholesterol in the form of eggs on the composition of bile in healthy subjects. Z Ernährungswiss 10: 178-187
16. Quintao E, Grundy SM, Ahrens EH (1971) Effects of dietary cholesterol on the regulation of total body cholesterol in man. J Lipid Res 12: 233-247
17. Den Besten L, Connor WE, Bell S (1973) The effect of dietary cholesterol on the composition of human bile. Surgery 73: 266-273
18. Andersen E, Hellstrom K (1979) The effect of cholesterol feeding on bile acid kinetics and biliary lipids in normolipidemic and hypertriglyceridemic subjects. J Lipid Res 20: 1020-1027
19. Lee DW, Gilmore CJ, Bonorris GG, Cohen H, Marks JW, Meiselman MS, Schoenfield LJ (1983) Effect of dietary cholesterol on biliary lipids in women with and without gallstones. In: Paumgartner, Stiehl, Gerok (eds) Bile acids and cholesterol in health and disease. MTP Press, Lancaster, pp 237-238
20. Grundy SM, Mok HMY (1979) Effects of diets and drugs on biliary cholesterol secretion. In: Fisher, Goresky, Shaffer, Strasberg (eds) Gallstones. Phenum, New York, pp 283-298
21. Levy RI (1980) Drugs used in the treatment of hyperlipoproteinemia. In: Goodman, Goodman, Gilman (eds) The pharmacological basis of therapeutics. MacMillan, New York, pp 834-847
22. Nervi FO, Del Pozo R, Covarrubias CF, Ronco BO (1983) The effect of progesterone on the regulatory mechanisms of biliary cholesterol secretion in the rat. Hepatology 3: 360-367
23. Stone BG, Erickson SK, Craig WY, Cooper AD (1985) Regulation of rat biliary cholesterol secretion by agents that alter intrahepatic cholesterol metabolism. Evidence for a distinct biliary precursor pool. J Clin Invest 76: 1773-1781
24. Andersen JM, Cook LR (1986) Regulation of gallbladder cholesterol concentration in the hamster. Role of hepatic cholesterol level. Biochim Biophys Acta 875: 582-592
25. Turley SD, Spady DK, Dietschy JM (1983) Alteration of the degree of biliary cholesterol saturation in the hamster and rat by manipulation of the pools of preformed and newly synthesized cholesterol. Gastroenterology 84: 253-264
26. Gregory DH, Vlahcevic ZR, Prugh MF, Swell L (1978) Mechanism of secretion of biliary lipids: role of a microtubular system in hepatocellular transport of biliary lipids in the rat. Gastroenterology 74: 93-100
27. Reuben A, Allen RM (1986) Intrahepatic sources of biliary-like micelles. Biochim Biophys Acta 876: 1-12
28. Small DM (1970) The formation of gallstones. Adv Intern Med 16: 243-264
29. Coleman R, Holdsworth G, Vyvoda OS (1977) Hepatocyte surface enzymes and their appearance in the bile. In: Popper, Bianchi, Reutter (eds) Membrane alterations as basis of liver injury. MTP Press, Lancaster, pp 143-156
30. Sömjen GJ, Gilat T (1985) Contribution of vesicular and micellar carriers to cholesterol transport in human bile. J Lipid Res 26: 699-704
31. Cohen DE, Angelico M, Carey MC (1986) Evidence for vesicular secretion of biliary lipids and their transformation into mixed micelles in native bile. Gastroenterology 90: 1786
32. Gregory DH, Vlahcevic ZR, Schatzki P, Swell L (1975) Mechanism of secretion of biliary lipids. I. Role of bile canalicular and microsomal membranes in the synthesis and transport of biliary lecithin and cholesterol. J Clin Invest 105-114
33. Barnwell S, Yousef I, Tuchweber B (1986) The extent of biliary phospholid secretion and can-

alicular membrane solubilization may be common determinates for the secretory rate maximum (SRm) of bile acids. Gastroenterology 90: 1710
34. Hardison WGM (1971) Metabolism of sodium dehydrocholate by the rat liver: its effect on micelle formation in bile. J Lab Clin Med 77: 811-820
35. Hardison WGM, Apter JT (1972) Micellar theory of biliary cholesterol excretion. Am J Physiol 222: 61-67
36. Wheeler HO, King KK (1972) Biliary excretion of lecithin and cholesterol in the dog. J Clin Invest 51: 1337-1350
37. Northfield TC, La Russo NF, Hofmann AF, Thistle JL (1975) Effect of chenodeoxycholic acid treatment in gallstone subjects. Gut 16: 12-17
38. Makino I, Nakagawa S (1978) Changes in biliary lipid and biliary bile acid composition in patients after administration of ursodeoxycholic acid. J Lipid Res 19: 723-728
39. Salen G, Colalillo A, Verga D, Bagan E, Tint GS, Shefer S (1980) Effect of high and low doses of ursodeoxycholic acid on gallstone dissolution in humans. Gastroenterology 78: 1412-1418
40. Einarsson K, Ahlberg J, Angelin B, Ewerth S (1981) Bile acids and hepatic HMG-CoA reductase in man. In: Paumgartner, Stiehl, Gerok (eds) Bile acids and lipids. MTP Press, Lancaster, pp 67-71
41. Ponz de Leon M, Carulli N, Loria P, Iori R, Zironi F (1980) Cholesterol absorption during bile acid feeding. Effect of ursodeoxycholic acid (UDCA) administration. Gastroenterology 78: 214-219
42. von Bergmann K, Leiss O, Streicher U, Strotkoetter H (1983) Effect of various bile acids on cholesterol absorption in man. In: Paumgartner, Stiehl, Gerok (eds) Bile acids and cholesterol in health and disease. MTP Press, Lancaster, pp 203-212
43. Hardison WGM, Grundy SM (1984) Effect of ursodeoxycholate and its taurine conjugate on bile acid synthesis and cholesterol absorption. Gastroenterology 87: 130-135
44. Ponz de Leon M, Carulli N, Loria P, Iori R, Zironi F (1979) The effect of chenodeoxycholic acid (CDCA) on cholesterol absorption. Gastroenterology 77: 223-230
45. Carulli N, Ponz de Leon M, Zironi F, Iori R, Loria P (1980) Bile acid feeding and hepatic sterol metabolism: effect of deoxycholic acid. Gastroenterology 79: 637-641
46. Ponz de Leon M, Carulli N, Iori R, Loria P, Romani M (1983) Regulation of cholesterol absorption by bile acids: role of deoxycholic and cholic acid pool expansion on dietary cholesterol absorption. Ital J Gastroenterol 15: 86-93
47. La Russo NF, Sczepanik PA, Hofmann AF (1977) Effect of deoxycholic acid ingestion on bile acid metabolism and biliary lipid secretion in normal subjects. Gastroenterology 72: 132-140
48. Ahlberg J, Angelin B, Einarsson K, Hellström K, Leijd B (1977) Influence of deoxycholic acid on biliary lipids in man. Clin Sci Mol Med 53: 249-256
49. Low-Beer TS, Pomare EW (1975) Can colonic bacterial metabolites predispose to cholesterol gallstones? Br Med J 1: 438-440
50. Lindblad L, Lundholm K, Scherstén T (1977) Influence of cholic and chenodeoxycholic acid on biliary cholesterol secretion in man. Eur J Clin Invest 7: 383-388
51. Scherstén T, Lindblad L (1979) Biliary cholesterol output during ursodeoxycholic acid secretion in man. In: Paumgartner, Stiehl, Gerok (eds) Biological effects of bile acids. MTP Press, Lancaster, pp 53-60
52. Sama C, La Russo NF, Lopez del Pino V, Thistle JL (1982) Effect of acute bile acid administration on biliary lipid secretion in healthy volunteers. Gastroenterology 82: 515-525
53. Armstrong MJ, Carey MC (1982) The hydrophobic-hydrophilic balance of bile salts. Inverse correlation between reverse-phase high performance liquid chromatographic mobilities and micellar cholesterol-solubilizing capacities. J Lipid Res 23: 70-80
54. Carulli N, Loria P, Bertolotti M, Ponz de Leon M, Menozzi D, Medici G, Piccagli I (1984) Effects of acute changes of bile acid pool composition on biliary lipid secretion. J Clin Invest 74: 614-624
55. Loria P, Carulli N, Medici G, Menozzi D, Salvioli G, Bertolotti M, Montanari M (1986) Effect of ursocholic acid on bile lipid secretion and composition. Gastroenterology 90: 865-874
56. Bilhartz LE, Dietschy JM (1984) Bile salt hydrophobicity dictates biliary cholesterol output. Gastroenterology 86: 1028
57. Gilmore IT, Barnhart JL, Hofmann AF, Erlinger S (1982) Effect of individual taurine-conjugated bile acids on biliary lipid secretion and sucrose clearance in the unanesthetized dog. Am J Physiol 242: G40-G46

58. Gilmore IT, Stokes K, Hofmann AF, Gurantz D, Lorenzo D (1980) Differing effects of chenodeoxycholyl conjugates and ursodeoxycholyl conjugates on biliary phospholipid and cholesterol secretion in gallstone patients. Gastroenterology 79: 1020
59. Gurantz D, Gilmore IT, Hofmann AF, Kozmary SV (1981) Biliary lipid secretion in the hamster: greater cholesterol secretion induced by unconjugated bile acids. Hepatology 1: 513
60. Hoffman NE, Sewell RB, Smallwood RA (1978) Bile acid structure and biliary lipid secretion. A comparison of three hydroxy and two keto bile acids. Am J Physiol 234: E637-E640
61. O'Maille ERL, Kozmary SV, Hofmann AF, Gurantz D (1984) Differing effects of norcholate and cholate on bile flow and biliary lipid secretion in the rat. Am J Physiol 246: G67-G71
62. Sewell RB, Hoffman NE, Smallwood RA, Cockbain S (1980) Bile acid structure and bile formation: a comparison of hydroxy and keto bile acids. Am J Physiol 238: G10-G17
63. Smallwood RA, Hoffman NE (1976) Bile acid structure and biliary secretion of cholesterol and phospholipid in the cat. Gastroenterology 71: 1064-1066
64. Stiehl A, Czygan P, Kommerell B, Weis HJ, Holtermueller KH (1978) Ursodeoxycholic acid versus chenodeoxycholic acid. Comparison of their effects on bile acid and bile lipid composition in patients with cholesterol gallstones. Gastroenterology 75: 1016-1020
65. Carulli N, Ponz de Leon M, Loria P, Iori R, Rosi A, Romani M (1981) Effect of the selective expansion of cholic acid pool on bile lipid composition: possible mechanism of bile acid induced biliary cholesterol desaturation. Gastroenterology 81: 539-546
66. Holzbach RT, March M, Olzewski M, Holan K (1973) Cholesterol solubility in bile. Evidence that supersaturated bile is frequent in healthy man. J Clin Invest 52: 1467-1479
67. Pomare EW, Heaton KW (1973) Bile salt metabolism in patients with gallstones in functioning gallbladders. Gut 14: 885-890
68. Fisher MM, Youssef IM (1973) Sex differences in the bile acid composition of human bile: studies in patients with and without gallstones. Can Med Assoc J 109: 190-193
69. Hepner GW, Hofmann AF, Malagelada JR, Szczepanik PA, Klein PD (1974) Increased bacterial degradation of bile acids in cholecystectomized patients. Gastroenterology 66: 556-564
70. Arnesjö B, Bodvall B, Stahl E (1975) Bile acid patterns of gallbladder and hepatic bile in patients with and without cholesterol gallstones. Acta Chir Scand 141: 135-138
71. McDougall RM, Walker K, Thurston OG (1976) Bile acid alterations in patients with cholesterol gallstones. J Surg Res 21: 233-237
72. van der Linden W, Bergman F (1977) An analysis of data on human hepatic bile. Relationship between main bile components, serum cholesterol and serum triglycerides. Scand J Clin Lab Invest 37: 741-747
73. Bennion LJ, Mott DM, Howard BV (1980) Oral contraceptives raise the cholesterol saturation of bile by increasing biliary cholesterol secretion. Metabolism 29: 18-22
74. Thornton JR, Emmett PM, Heaton KW (1983) Diet and gallstones: effects of refined and unrefined carbohydrate diets on bile cholesterol saturation and bile acid metabolism. Gut 24: 2-6
75. Hofmann AF, Grundy SM, Lachin JM, Lan S-P, Baum RA, Hanson RF, Hersh T, Hightower NC Jr, Marks JW, Mekhjian H, Shaefer RA, Soloway RD, Thistle JL, Thomas FB, Tyor MP, and the National Cooperative Gallstone Study Group (1982) Pretreatment biliary lipid composition in white patients with radiolucent gallstones in the National Cooperative Gallstone Study. Gastroenterology 83: 738-752
76. Di Donato P, Carubbi F, Ponz de Leon M, Carulli N (1986) Effect of small doses of deoxycholic acid on bile cholesterol saturation in patients with liver cirrhosis. Gut 27: 23-28
77. Low-Beer TS, Nutter S (1978) Colonic bacterial activity, biliary cholesterol saturation, and pathogenesis of gallstones. Lancet 2: 1063-1065
78. Thornton JR, Heaton KW (1981) Do colonic bacteria contribute to cholesterol gallstone formation? Effects of lactulose on bile. Br Med J 282: 1018-1020
79. Salvioli G, Salati R, Bondi M, Fratalocchi A, Sala BM, Gibertini A (1982) Bile acid transformation by the intestinal flora and cholesterol saturation in bile. Effects of *Streptococcus faecium* administration. Digestion 23: 80-88
80. Angelin B, Einarsson K, Leijd B (1983) Bile acid metabolism in hypothyroid subjects: response to substitution therapy. Eur J Clin Invest 13: 99-106
81. Marcus SN, Heaton KW (1986) Intestinal transit, deoxycholic acid and the cholesterol saturation of bile – three inter-related factors. Gut 27: 550-558

# The Enterohepatic Circulation of Sulfated and Nonsulfated Bile Acids*

Folkert Kuipers, Charles M. A. Bijleveld, Rick Havinga, John Fernandes, and Roel J. Vonk

Department of Pediatrics, University of Groningen, Bloemsingel 10, 9712 KZ Groningen, The Netherlands

## Introduction

Bile acids are synthesized in the liver from cholesterol and after conjugation with taurine or glycine are excreted into bile. After release in the intestine, the greater part of the bile acids is reabsorbed and returns to the liver via the portal blood stream. In this way bile acids are conserved in an enterohepatic circulation. One of the components of the bile acid pool in man is lithocholate (3$\alpha$hydroxy-5$\beta$cholanoic acid). This secondary bile acid posesses cholestatic properties which have been well established in experimental animals. Intravenous administration of lithocholate and its taurine or glycine conjugate to rats or hamsters causes a dose-dependent reduction in bile flow (Javitt 1966; Kakis and Yousef 1978; King and Schoenfield 1971). Little is known about the significance of lithocholic acid in the pathogenesis of cholestasis in man. It has been claimed that the human liver is protected from lithocholic acid hepatotoxicity by efficient sulfation of the 3$\alpha$hydroxy group, which increases the bile acids' polarity (Cowen et al. 1975; Marks et al. 1981). Sulfated bile acids are poorly absorbed from the intestine (De Witt and Lack 1980; Low-Beer et al. 1969) and their renal clearance is relatively high (Makino et al. 1975). The hypothesis that sulfation per se might be a protecting factor against hepatotoxic bile acids will be discussed in this chapter.

In recent years some reports have been published in which cholestatic effects of sulfated monohydroxy bile acids were described. The first study, by Yousef et al. (1981), reported hepatotoxic effects of sulfated glycolithocholate in anesthetized rats. Intravenous injection of 240 µmol/kg body weight induced cholestatis, and effect which turned out to be dose-dependent. Similar experiments with sulfated taurolithocholate showed that the toxic effect of this particular compound was much less pronounced. These studies suggest that taurine could protect the liver against cholestasis, because excess taurine leads to the formation of sulfated taurolithocholate rather than the toxic sulfated glycolithocholate. Two other studies reported on the cholestatic effects of sulfated monohydroxy bile acids: Vonk et al. (1981) demonstrated a high cholestatic potency of sulfated allomonohydroxy bile acids (3$\beta$hydroxy-5$\alpha$cholanoic acid). It is not known whether these bile acids are present in man. Mathis et al. (1983) published data on the cholestatic effect of sulfated cholenoic acid (3$\alpha$hydroxy-5cholenoic acid), which is present in man under certain circumstances.

* This work was supported by grant 13-53-44 from the Dutch Health Organization (TNO)

Assessment and Management of Hepatobiliary Disease
Eds.: L. Okolicsányi, G. Csomós, and G. Crepaldi

## Clinical Studies

We studied the prevalence and origin of sulfated lithocholic acid conjugates (SGLC) in children. A group of 268 pediatric patients with various hepatic and gastrointestinal disorders were screened for the presence of SGLC in serum (Kuipers et al. 1985a). SGLC concentrations were measured by radioimmunoassay (Abbott Laboratories, Chicago). In a group of 42 patients without distinct cholestasis and with a moderately increased serum bile acid concentration, an increased SGLC level was found. This group included patients with intestinal dysfunctions such as Crohn's disease, celiac disease and gastroenteritis, acute lymphatic leukemia treated with methotrexate, contaminated small bowel syndrome, and three patients with benign recurrent intrahepatic cholestasis (BRIC), measured during the anicteric period. In two patients with BRIC, brothers born in 1969 and 1972, we studied the prevalence and origin of the elevated SGLC levels in more detail. BRIC is a syndrome that has been described in a familial form (Tygstrup and Jensen 1969; de Pagter et al. 1976) and in a nonfamilial form (Summerskill and Walshe 1959). The clinical features include episodes of jaundice with biochemical signs of cholestasis alternating with symptom-free intervals of several months or years. The etiology remains obscure; although Van Berge Henegouwen et al.

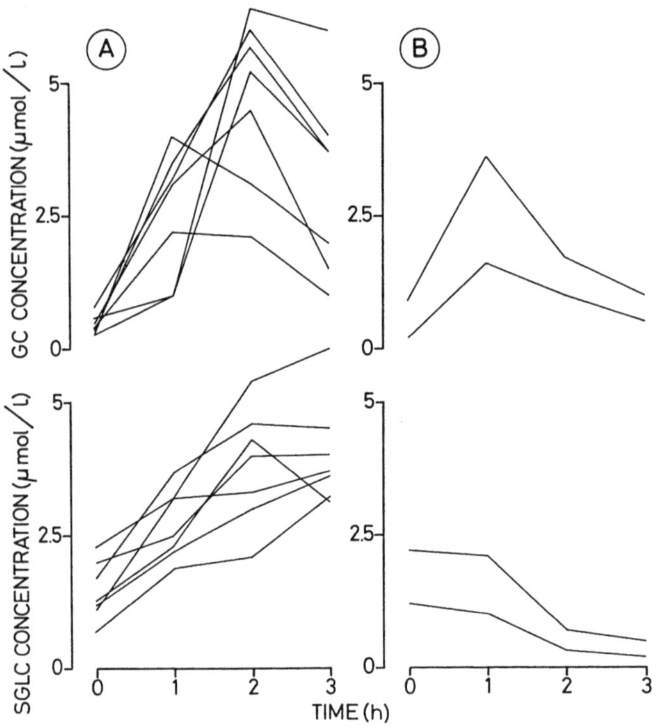


**Fig. 1 a, b.** Serum concentrations of SGLC (lower panels) and GC (upper panels) after a test meal at t=0 in nine tests performed in two patients with intermittent intrahepatic cholestasis. **a** Test performed during symptom-free periods, $n=7$. $\Delta SGLC = 2.8 \pm 0.2$ μmol/l, $\Delta GC = 4.2 \pm 0.5$ μmol/l, (mean ± SEM). **b** Test performed during symptom-free periods, 4 g of cholestyramine added to the test meal. (With permission of Scand J Gastroenterol)

(1974) suggested that a selective defect in bile acid transport might be responsible, no factor initiating a cholestatic attack has ever been described. The older of the two brothers had recurrent cholestatic attacks characterized by very high serum bile acid concentrations (>400 μmol/l) preceding the rise in serum bilirubin levels. The same pattern was reported by other groups (Van Berge Henegouwen et al. 1974; Summerfield et al. 1981). During symptom-free intervals, in which neither clinically nor biochemically abnormalities could be detected, the serum concentrations of SGLC were elevated (Vonk et al. 1982).

To investigate the origin of the elevated serum levels of SGLC in these two BRIC patients, the postprandial response of serum SGLC was measured after a test meal of 1.0 g fat/kg body weight. Serum SGLC concentrations were determined at 0, 60, 120, and 180 min after the test meal. In addition, serum concentrations of glycocholate (GC; radioimmunoassay, Abbott) were measured to ascertain gallbladder contraction. The response was expressed as maximal increase toward fasting values ($\Delta$, μmol/l). In the patient group with basal SGLC levels below 1.2 μmol/l, the SGLC response was small or absent (0.2±0.1, mean±SEM, $n=26$). In contrast, when the test was performed in the pediatric BRIC patients during anicteric intervals, the mean $\Delta$SGLC was 2.8±0.2, ($n=7$) (Fig. 1 A). In these tests, the mean $\Delta$GC was 4.2±0.5, higher than in the control group ($\Delta$GC=2.1±0.32, $n=26$) but much lower than in patients with cholestatic liver disease ($\Delta$GC=18.4±2.8, $n=6$). No correlation was found between $\Delta$SGLC and $\Delta$GC in the total group of patients studied, which indicates that the observed $\Delta$SGLC is not caused by a decreased hepatic clearance of bile acids. When cholestyramine (4 g) was added to the test meal, a postprandial decrease in SGLC levels was found and the GC response was strongly reduced (Fig. 1 B).

## Animal Studies

The results presented suggest that the elevated serum levels of SGLC found in BRIC patients might be caused by an increased influx of these sulfated bile acids from the intestine. The postprandial rise in serum SGLC is possibly a reflection of an altered net intestinal transport in these patients. We therefore studied some factors influencing the intestinal absorption of these potentially hepatotoxic bile acids in vivo in rats. The animals were equipped with permanent catheters in bile duct and duodenum as described elsewhere (Kuipers et al. 1985b). Radiolabelled bile acids were introduced via the duodenal catheter during a 4-h infusion. Intestinal absorption was calculated from the recovery of radioactivity in bile and urine. When SGLC or GLC were administered at an infusion rate of 125 nmol/min, equivalent to 7% of the total biliary bile acid excretion in rats with an intact enterohepatic circulation (Kuipers et al. 1985b), it could be shown that sulfation markedly delayed the biliary appearance, but only slightly reduced the 24-h absorption: 90.0%±3.6% and 94.4%±1.1% for SGLC and GLC respectively (Fig. 2). Urinary excretion was less than 2% of the infused dose for both bile acids studied. Absorption of a tracer dose of $^{3}$H-taurocholate (TC), which was added to the infusate in all experiments as an "internal control," was 99.9%±0.5%. These data clearly indicate that SGLC can be efficiently absorbed from the intestine. Because we are dealing with hepatotoxic bile acids, it is of practical importance to study factors which could be involved in protection.

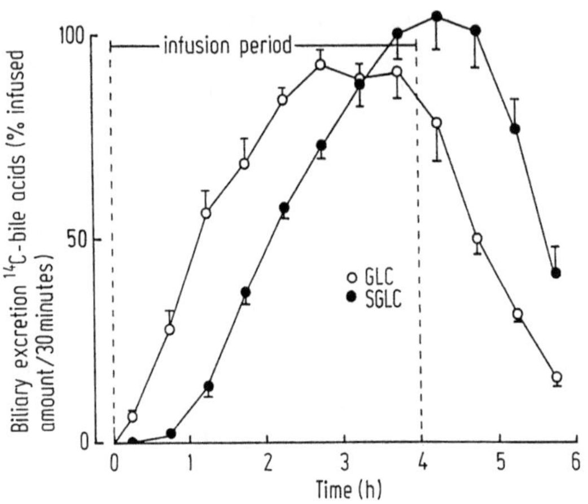


**Fig. 2.** Biliary excretion of $^{14}$C-labelled bile acids during and after a 4-h intraduodenal infusion of $^{14}$C-glycolithocholic acid or its 3-sulfate ester at a rate of 125 nmol/min. Mean values ± SEM, $n=4$–6

## Protecting Factors

One possible protective mechanism is binding of the bile acids in the intestine followed by enhanced fecal excretion, and a second is interactions at the hepatic level. One of the agents which binds SGLC with high affinity is cholestyramine (Kuipers et al., unpublished data). Cholestyramine is able to prevent a postprandial rise in serum SGLC levels, as mentioned before, and therefore cholestyramine treatment might be useful in preventing cholestasis in BRIC patients. Experiments in rats have also releaved that calcium salts interfere with the intestinal absorption of sulfated monohydroxy bile acids (Kuipers et al. 1986). Figure 3 shows that in the presence of excess calcium the absorption of lithocholate conjugates was dramatically reduced, and that this inhibitory effect was most pronounced for the sulfate ester. The absorption of SGLC decreased from 90.9% ± 3.6% to 33.2% ± 2.0%. GLC absorption was reduced to 76.3 ± 0.4%, but that of a tracer amount of TC only to 94.5% ± 0.6%. The therapeutic possibilities of these observations are not clear.

Protective interactions against SGLC-induced cholestasis at hepatic level may be twofold:

1. *Taurine Administration.* Dorvil et al. (1983) suggested that taurine might have protective effects on cholestasis induced by monohydroxy bile acids, because taurine administration would favor the formation of sulfated taurolithocholate instead of the more toxic SGLC. In the two BRIC patients described above, administration of 800 mg taurine/day in the anicteric period did not prevent a rise in serum bile acids and increased urinary bile acid excretion in one patient after treatment for 7 weeks. Consecutive cholestyramine administration suppressed the cholestatic attack in this patient.
2. *Endogenous bile acids.* Kuipers et al. (1985b) have shown that rats with an intact endogenous bile acid pool are less susceptible to cholestatic effects of sulfated monohydroxy bile acids than rats with a biliary drain and no endogenous bile acid pool. Whether patients with a diminished bile acid pool size are also more susceptible to cholestatic agents is not clear at the moment. If this is the case, enlargement of the

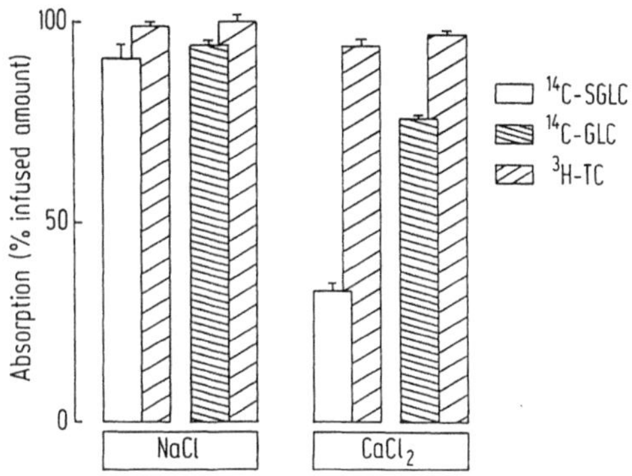


**Fig. 3.** Absorption efficiency of $^{14}$C-labeled SGLC and GLC and of $^{3}$H-labeled TC after intraduodenal administration of the $^{14}$C bile acids at a rate of 125 nmol/min, in the presence of either 154 m*M* NaCl *(left)* or 154 m*M* $CaCl_2$ *(right)*. $^{3}$H-TC was added to all bile acid solutions in a tracer amount

bile acid pool by administration of exogenous bile acids would have beneficial effects in certain situations.

## Methodological Approach

The question of whether sulfated monohydroxy bile acids play a direct role in the etiology of cholestasis in man remains difficult to answer because of the relative inaccessibility of the enterohepatic circulation. We have recently developed two new approaches to tackle this problem. A *computer simulation* of transport processes in the enterohepatic circulation has been made (Fig. 4). With this ten-compartment model one can calculate the concentration changes vs time in plasma, liver, intestinal compartments, etc. The relative contribution of the various transport constants on whole body kinetics can be studied with such a model. Furthermore, we have developed a *string test* to facilitate sampling of duodenal bile acids in man. For this purpose we employ ENTERO-TEST, an encapsulated nylon thread originally used for diagnosis of enteral parasites. The capsule is swallowed in the fasting state. The proximal end of the thread is taped at one corner of the mouth, the distal end is propelled into the duodenum by peristaltics. Four hours after swallowing, the thread is withdrawn and bile acids are eluted with buffer. The solution is applied to a Sep-Pak C-18 cartridge to extract bile acids, which are subsequently analyzed by capillary gas chromatography or liquid chromatography. In vitro analyses showed that there was no preferential binding to the thread of any bile acid and that binding was pH-independent. A high correlation ($r=0.98$) was found between direct analyses of bile and analyses by ENTERO-TEST after in vitro incubation. The values obtained using ENTERO-TEST were similar to those of duodenal bile simultaneously collected using the normal intubation technique ($r=0.99$) (Vonk et al. 1986). In 19 healthy volunteers the following bile acid composition of unstimulated duodenal juice was found (mean ± SD; %): cholate 56 ± 13 (glycine/taurine ratio 1.7 ± 0.9); chenodeoxycholate 29 ± 8 (G/T ratio 2.0 ± 1.2); deoxycholate 15 ± 9 (G/T ratio 5.9 ± 4.3); lithocholate < 1; ursodeoxycholate < 1. The technique described proved to be easily applicable for determination of duodenal bile acids in man. This enables longitudinal studies concerning the factors that determine the bile acid pool composition and its relevance to various diseases.

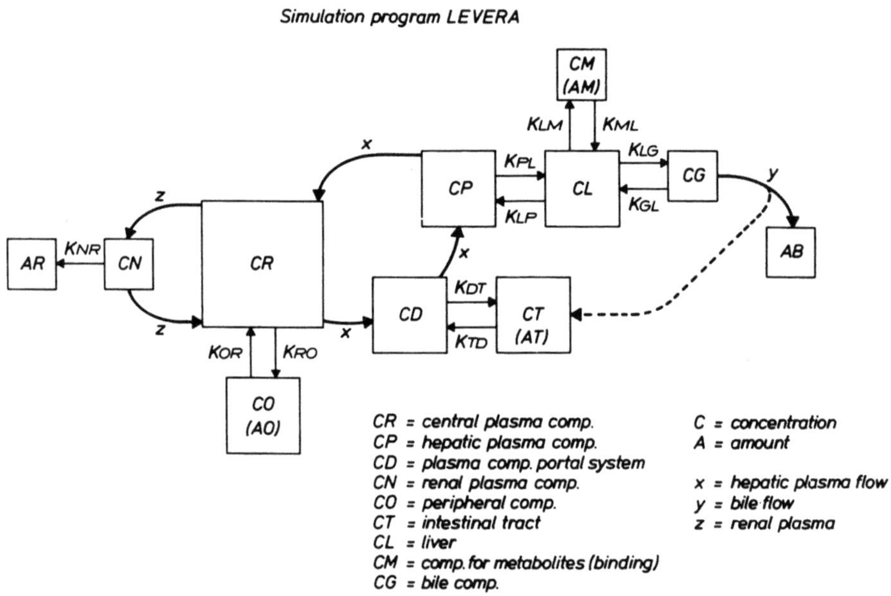


**Fig. 4.** Schematic diagram of the 10-compartment computer simulation of transport processes in the enterohepatic circulation


## Summary

Sulfated monohydroxy bile acids can be absorbed from the intestine and can therefore travel around the enterohepatic circulation. This process presumably has little physiological importance under normal conditions because of the presence of intestinal binding agents (food components) which have a high affinity for these bile acids. However, in certain circumstances, when these binding agents are absent (for instance during total parenteral nutrition) or during increased formation of these particular bile acids, reabsorption of sulfated monohydroxy bile acids might become of importance. The new techniques presented here can be used to investigate the enterohepatic circulation of sulfated bile acids in man in more detail.


## References


Cowen AE, Korman MG, Hofmann AF, Cass OW, Coffin SB (1975) Metabolism of lithocholate in healthy man. II. Enterohepatic circulation. Gastroenterology 69: 67-76

De Witt EH, Lack L (1980) Effects of sulfation patterns on intestinal transport of bile salt sulfate esters. Am J Physiol 238: 34-39

Dorvil NP, Yousef IM, Tuchweber B, Roy CC (1983) Taurine prevents cholestasis induced by lithocholic acid sulfate in guinea pigs. Am J Clin Nutr 37: 221-232

Javitt NB (1966) Cholestasis in rats induced by taurolithocholate. Nature 210: 1262-1263

Kakis G, Yousef IM (1978) Pathogenesis of lithocholate- and taurolithocholate induced intrahepatic cholestasis in rats. Gastroenterology 75: 595-607

King JE, Schoenfield L (1971) Cholestasis induced by sodium taurolithocholate in isolated hamster liver. J Clin Invest 50: 2305-2312

Kuipers F, Bijleveld CMA, Kneepkens CMF, van Zanten A, Fernandes J, Vonk RJ (1985a) Sulphated lithocholic acid conjugates in serum of children with hepatic and intestinal diseases. Scand J Gastroenterol 20: 1255-1261

Kuipers F, Havinga R, Bosschieter H, Toorop GP, Hindriks FR, Vonk RJ (1985b) Enterohepatic circulation in the rat. Gastroenterology 88: 403-411

Kuipers F, Heslinga H, Havinga R, Vonk RJ (1986) Intestinal absorption of lithocholic acid sulfates in the rat: inhibitory effects of calcium. Am J Physiol, (in press)

Low-Beer TS, Tyor MP, Lack L (1969) Effects of sulfation of taurolithocholic and glycolithocholic acids on their intestinal transport. Gastroenterology 56: 721-726

Makino I, Hashimoto H, Shinozaki K, Yoshino K, Nakagawa S (1975) Sulfated and nonsulfated bile acids in urine, serum, and bile of patients with hepatobiliary diseases. Gastroenterology 68: 545-553

Marks JW, Sue SO, Pearlman BJ, Bonorris GG, Varady P, Lachin JM, Schoenfield LJ (1981) Sulfation of lithocholate as possible modifier of chenodeoxycholic acid-induced elevations of serum transaminase in patients with gallstones. J Clin Invest 68: 1190-1196

Mathis U, Karlaganis G, Preisig R (1983) Monohydroxy bile salt sulfates: tauro-3$\beta$-hydroxy-5-cholenoate-3-sulfate induced intrahepatic cholestasis in rats. Gastroenterology 85: 674-681

Pagter de AGF, van Berge Henegouwen GP, Ten Bokkel Huinink JA, Brandt KH (1976) Familial benign recurrent intrahepatic cholestasis: interrelation with intrahepatic cholestasis of pregnancy and from oral contraceptives. Gastroenterology 71: 202-207

Summerfield JA, Kirk AP, Chitranukroh A, Billing BH (1981) A distinctive pattern of serum bile acid and bilirubin concentrations in benign recurrent intrahepatic cholestasis. Hepatogastroenterology 28: 139-145

Summerskill WHJ, Walshe JM (1959) Benign recurrent intrahepatic 'obstructive' jaundice. Lancet 2: 686-690

Tygstrup N, Jensen B (1969) Intermittent intrahepatic cholestasis of unknown etiology in five young males from the Faroe Islands. Acta Med Scand 185: 523-530

Van Berge Henegouwen GP, Brandt KH, de Pagter AGF (1974) Is an acute disturbance in hepatic transport of bile acids the primary cause of cholestasis in benign recurrent cholestasis? Lancet 1: 1249-1251

Vonk RJ, Tuchweber B, Massé D, Perea A, Audet M, Roy CC, Yousef IM (1981) Intrahepatic cholestasis induced by allomonohydroxy bile acids in rats. Gastroenterology 80: 242-249

Vonk RJ, Bijleveld CMA, Jousma C, Havinga R, Fernandes J, van Zanten A (1982) Cholestatic effects of sulfated bile acids. In: Mulder GJ, Caldwell J, van Kempen GMJ, Vonk RJ (eds) Sulfate metabolism and sulfate conjugation. Taylor and Francis, London, pp 231-237

Vonk RJ, Kneepkens CM, Havinga R, Kuipers F, Bijleveld CMA (1986) The enterohepatic circulation in man. A simple method for the determination of duodenal bile acids. J Lipid Res, 27: 901-904

Yousef IM, Tuchweber B, Vonk RJ, Massé D, Audet M, Roy CC (1981) Lithocholate cholestasis-sulfated glycolithocholate induced intrahepatic cholestasis in rats. Gastroenterology 80: 233-241

# Estrogens and Bile Secretion

M. Frezza[1], G. Pozzato[1], and C. Di Padova[2]

[1]Institute of Medical Pathology, University of Trieste, Trieste, Italy
[2]Third Medical Clinic, University of Milan School of Medicine, Milan, Italy

The purpose of this report is to present an overview of the influence of natural and synthetic estrogen on the bile-secreting apparatus. Estrogen-induced alterations of hepatobiliary function range from modifications of bile lipid composition, so that bile becomes supersaturated with cholesterol, to bile flow impairment, i.e., intrahepatic cholestasis (Kern et al. 1978). Most of the knowledge regarding estrogen-induced liver dysfunction has been obtained from experiments focusing on estrogen treatment of animals as well as from clinical experience of estrogen hepatotoxicity in pregnant women and in subjects receiving drugs containing these hormones (Stricker and Spoelstra 1985). The mechanism(s) whereby estrogens interfere with bile secretion is still unknown.

Recent investigations have indicated that both liver and gallbladder can be regarded as target organs for these hormones, as they have receptors of high affinity and low capacity for estrogens (Porter et al. 1983; Frezza et al. 1986) (Fig. 1). A major implication of these findings is that the response of the hepatobiliary system to estrogens may be mediated by the number and/or the affinity of estrogen receptors for their substrates. By means of the irreversible binding to microsomal proteins, estrogen metabolites such as catecholestrogens may also interfere with the liver microsomal mixed-function oxidase system, which is involved in steroid hydroxylation and, therefore, in bile salt synthesis (Stramentinoli et al. 1979; Tritapepe et al. 1980).

In rats, ethinyl estradiol, the steroid widely used in oral contraceptives, causes cholestasis, i.e., bile flow impairment, mainly due to an inhibitory effect on bile salt independent fraction (BSIF) (Schreiber and Simon 1983) (Fig. 2). This phenomenon seems to be mediated by changes of liver plasma membrane composition and fluidity with ensuing alterations of $Na^+/K^+$-ATPase-dependent pump. In addition, ethinyl estradiol may exert marked effects on bile lipid composition, reducing the bile salt/cholesterol ratio (Davis and Kern 1976). Also, in humans estrogens alone or combined with progestins are able to induce changes in biliary lipid composition, as reported by

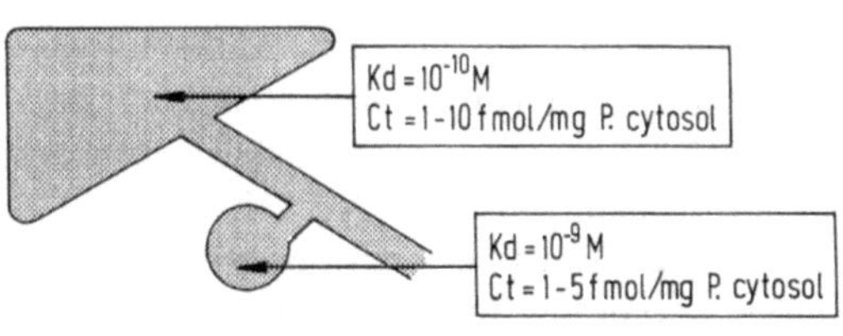


**Fig. 1.** Presence of specific and saturable bindings of high affinity *(Kd)* and low capacity *(Ct)* in human liver and gallbladder. [Data from Frezza et al. (1986) and Porter et al. (1983)]

Assessment and Management of Hepatobiliary Disease
Eds.: L. Okolicsányi, G. Csomós, and G. Crepaldi

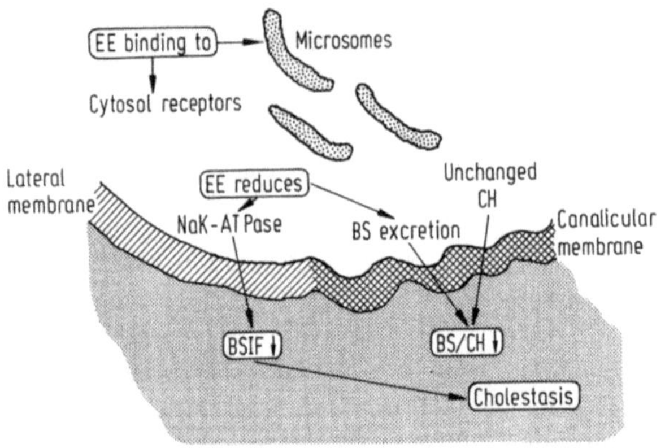


**Fig. 2.** Interactions of ethynil estradiol (EE) with the hepatic bile-secreting apparatus. [Data from Kern et al. (1978) and Schreiber and Simon (1983)]

Tritapepe et al. (1976), Anderson et al. (1980), Nakagaki and Nakayama (1982), and Podda et al. (1985). These authors have indicated that estrogen, and not progestin, is reponsible for the increase of bile lithogenicity which accompanies the use of oral contraceptives. Bile cholesterol supersaturation after estrogen administration is due to the increase in the molar percentage of cholesterol and phospholipids and the concomitant decrease in the molar percentage of bile salts. These findings are in agreement with epidemiological studies which have shown clearly that women treated with oral contraceptives or synthetic estrogens have an increased incidence of cholesterol gallstones (Scragg et al. 1984).

In subjects who exhibit a high susceptibility to estrogens, e.g., women with a past history of intrahepatic cholestasis of pregnancy (ICP) (Reyes 1982), a constant production of lithogenic bile may persist even in basal conditions. In seven of nine women with previous ICP, we found cholesterol supersaturation of gallbladder bile at least 6 months after delivery. The cholesterol saturation index was significantly higher than in the control group ($1.34 \pm 0.08$ vs $0.76 \pm 0.09$, mean $\pm$ SE, $p < 0.05$ by Student's t test). All subjects were neither obese nor pregnant and had cholecystograms negative for gallstones. Frezza et al. (1985) recently documented functional biliary alterations in the same women (Fig. 3). The gallbladder fasting volume and the residual volume after a standard meal were significantly greater in these subjects than in pair-matched controls. Both findings are in agreement with epidemiological reports which have underlined that the prevalence of gallstones in patients with history of ICP is 2–3 times that in controls matched for age and parity (Reyes 1982).

Some years ago, we showed that *S*-adenosylmethionine (SAMe) prevents the negative effects of ethinyl estradiol on bile flow, BSIF, and bile salt/cholesterol ratio (Figs. 4, 5) (Stramentinoli et al. 1979, 1981). Other authors (Schreiber et al. 1982; Boelsterli et al. 1983; Arias et al. 1983; Arias and Kine 1984) have confirmed these observations and have also demonstrated that SAMe maintains liver $NA^+/K^+$-ATPase to control values. The mechanism by which SAMe affords hepatocytoprotection against estrogen toxicity has not yet been clarified. According to a first hypothesis, SAMe, whose capability to enter hepatocytes has been clearly shown (Giulidori et al. 1984), may act as a methyl donor in the presence of the enzyme catechol-*O*-methyltransfer-

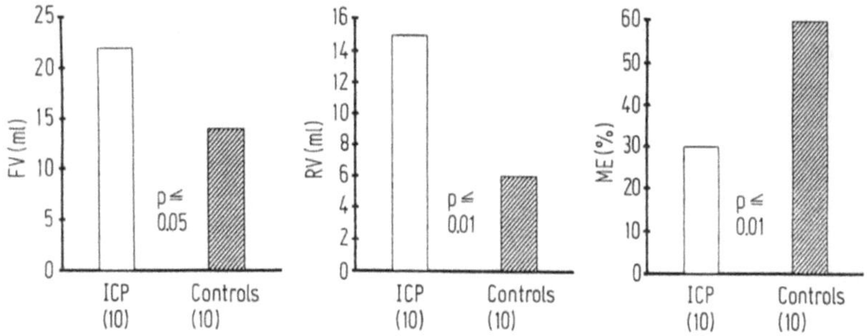


**Fig. 3.** The fasting *(FV)* and residual *(RV)* gallbladder volume and maximum percentage emptying *(ME)* of women with previous ICP were significantly different from those of pair-matched controls. [Data from Frezza et al. (1985)]

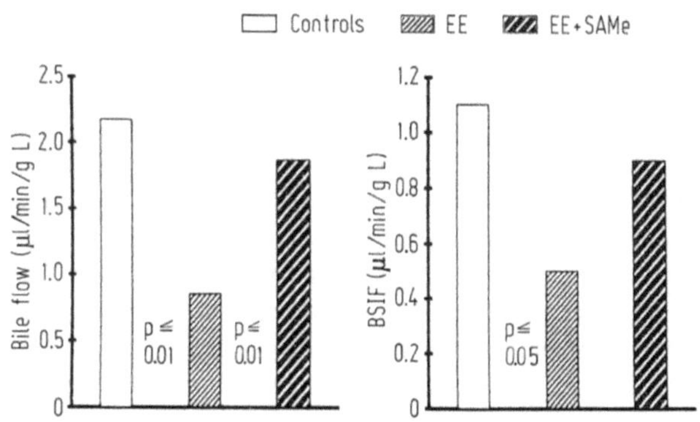


**Fig. 4.** Mean values of bile flow and bile salt independent fraction *(BSIF)* in control rats and in rats treated with ethinyl estradiol *(EE)* alone (5 mg/kg body weight orally for 3 days) or with the same dosage of EE plus SAMe (25 mg/kg body weight i.m. tid for 3 days). SAMe exerts a preventive action on the effects of EE. [Data from Stromentinoli et al. (1979, 1981)]

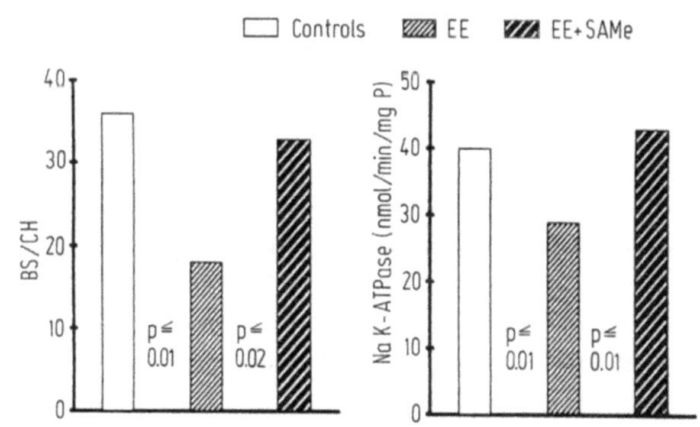


**Fig. 5.** Mean values of bile salt/cholesterol ratio *(BS/CH)* and $Na^+/K^+$-ATPase in control rats and in rats treated with ethinyl estradiol *(EE)* alone (5 mg/kg body weight orally for 3 days) or with the same dosage of EE plus SAMe (25 mg/kg body weight i.m. tid for 3 days). SAMe has a preventive action on the effects of EE. [Data from Schreiber et al. (1982) and Stramentinoli et al. (1981)]

ase. Methylation at position 2 of catecholestrogens could antagonize the binding of the highly reactive estrogen metabolites to liver microsomes, preventing the hepatotoxicity of these derivatives, which are metabolically inert (Bolt 1979). In this regard, Stramentinoli et al. (1981) have shown that rats treated with ethinyl estradiol plus SAMe excrete into bile an amount of methoxy derivatives of the estrogen significantly higher than that secreted by animals receiving ethinyl estradiol alone. An alternative hypothesis is that SAMe-dependent methylation of membrane phospholipids could influence liver membrane fluidity, which has been shown to decrease after estrogen administration (Schachter 1984). Arias (1986) has stressed the concept that ethinyl estradiol interferes with liver membrane viscosity, and reduces bile secretion mainly by altering the sodium pump and its symports and antiports in the sinusoidal membrane. According to Arias, through membrane phospholipid methylation SAMe prevents these effects and restores membrane fluidity as well as sodium pump and $Na^+/H^+$ antiporter activities to control values.

On the basis of these encouraging experimental observations, we carried out a clinical trial aimed at evaluating whether SAMe could reverse ICP, a syndrome whose pathogenesis has been attributed to an abnormal reaction of maternal liver to endogenous estrogens (Frezza et al. 1984). Eighteen women with ICP were randomly divided into three groups of six and treated for 20 days. The first group received 200 mg/day SAMe i.v., the second group received 800 mg/day SAMe i.v., and the third group served as control. After 10 and 20 days of treatment with the higher dose of SAMe, the mean values of serum transaminases, conjugated bilirubin, and total bile salts had fallen significantly in respect to initial levels, in contrast to the other two groups. Moreover, the final values of these laboratory parameters were lower in the group of subjects treated with 800 mg/day SAMe than in the other two groups of women. Pruritus evaluated according to a scoring system was significantly reduced in patients treated with the higher dose of SAMe. We concluded that SAMe may ameliorate pruritus and abnormal biochemical parameters referable to cholestasis in pregnant women who have an exaggerated response to estrogens.

The purpose of a further investigation was to verify whether SAMe could also prevent the hepatotoxic effects induced by ethinyl estradiol (given as a small oral dose for a few days) in women with a past history of ICP. Four nonobese fertile women (29 ± 7 years) volunteered for this study, which was performed at least 1 year after the episode of ICP. Before receiving the estrogen, the women underwent complete medical examination, venous blood collection for liver function tests, and ultrasound examination of the gallbladder, with normal results in all cases. The absence of pregnancy was indicated by negative urine tests for human chorionic gonadotropin. All subjects denied the intake of drugs or hormones during the previous 3 months with the exception of occasional analgesics for minor ailments. In the second half of a normal menstrual cycle, the subjects received ethinyl estradiol 0.1 mg/day orally for 7 days (Reyes et al. 1981). After one week of hormone intake, the individuals underwent another complete medical and biochemical assessment. A 3-month interval was observed before the women were given the same ethinyl estradiol dose plus SAMe 800 mg/day orally for 7 days. SAMe was administered as follows: one tablet containing 200 mg in the morning, two similar tablets at noon, and a fourth tablet at bedtime. At the end of this rechallenge phase of the study, the patients underwent a final clinical evaluation, including laboratory parameters.

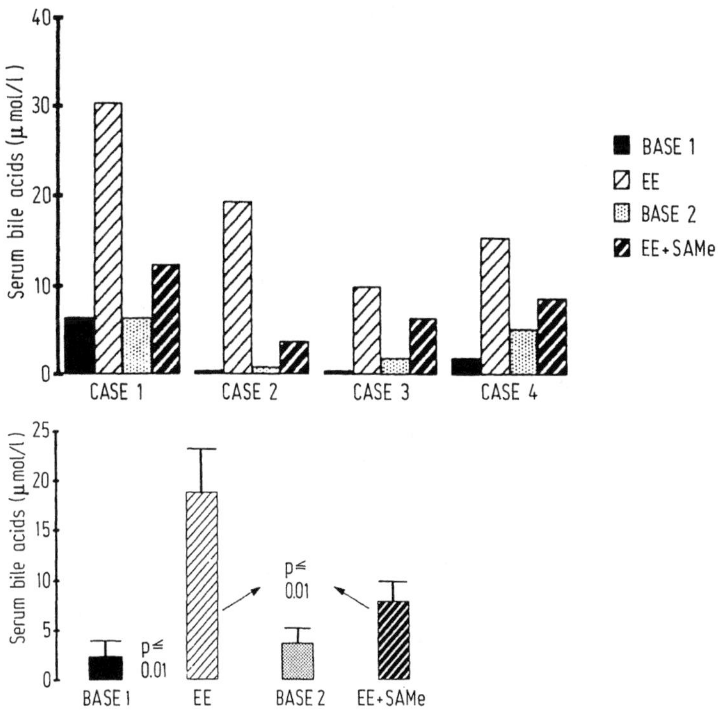


**Fig. 6.** Serum total bile acids in basal conditions, after 1 week of oral ethinyl estradiol (*EE;* 0.1 mg/day), and after 1 week of the same dosage of oral EE plus oral SAMe (800 mg/day) in four women with a past history of ICP. Individual cases are reported in the *upper panel,* while the *lower panel* shows the mean values ± SE. EE induced a significant increase of serum bile acid concentration in respect to both basal assessments and the value obtained after EE plus SAMe

To maintain the double-blind status of the study, during the challenge with the steroid the women received placebo tablets which were similar to SAMe tablets. The data were analyzed according to a one-way within-subjects analysis of variance (randomized block design). The Tukey test was used for comparisons between and within groups. Ethinyl estradiol significantly ($p < 0.05$) increased serum transaminases and total bile acids in respect to basal values (GOT 112 ± 44 vs 17 ± 1 IU/l, GPT 59 ± 15 vs 18 ± 2 IU/l, bile acids 18 ± 4 vs 2 ± 1 μmol/l; mean ± SE).

In the rechallenge with ethinyl estradiol plus SAMe, serum transaminases did not differ from basal levels and bile acids (7 ± 1 μmol/l) were significantly lower than the value obtained after ethinyl estradiol alone (Fig. 6). These results give evidence of the ability of SAMe to afford effective protection against estrogen-related side effects in a high-risk population. The data are in agreement with previous reports showing that SAMe counteracts estrogen-induced cholestasis in animals (Stramentinoli et al. 1981; Boelsterli et al. 1983; Arias 1986) and in pregnant women (Frezza et al. 1984), and support the belief that SAMe acts as an antidote to estrogen hepatotoxicity. This concept is also consistent with other studies showing that SAMe prevents bile cholesterol supersaturation induced by estrogens (Di Padova et al. 1982, 1984). We propose further investigations to clarify whether this methyl-donor compound might represent an innovative approach to the therapeutic management of liver dysfunction induced by estrogens in humans.

## References


Anderson A, James OFW, MacDonald HS, Snowball S, Taylor W (1980) The effect of ethynyl oestradiol on biliary lipid composition in young men. Eur J Clin Invest 10: 77-80

Arias IM (1986) Mechanisms and consequences of ion transport in the liver. In: Popper H, Schaffner F (eds) Progress in liver disease, 8th edn. Grune and Stratton, New York, pp 145-159

Arias IM, Kinne R (1984) On the pathophysiology and reversibility of intrahepatic cholestasis. Clin Res 32: 548

Arias IM, Adachi Y, Tran T (1983) Ethynyl estradiol cholestasis: a disease of the sinusoidal domain of hepatocyte plasma membrane. Hepatology 3: 872

Boelsterli UA, Rakhit G, Balazs T (1983) Modulation by *S*-adenosyl-L-methionine of hepatic $Na^+,K^+$-ATPase, membrane fluidity, and bile flow in rats with ethinyl estradiol-induced cholestasis. Hepatology 3: 12-17

Bolt HM (1979) Metabolism of estrogen – natural and synthetic. Pharmacol Ther 4: 155-181

Davis RA, Kern F (1976) Effect of ethynyl estradiol and phenobarbital on bile acid synthesis and biliary bile acid and cholesterol excretion. Gastroenterology 70: 1130-1135

Di Padova C, Tritapepe R, Cammareri G, Humpel M, Stramentinoli G (1982) *S*-Adenosyl-L-methionine antagonizes ethynylestradiol-induced bile cholesterol supersaturation in humans without modifying the estrogen plasma kinetics. Gastroenterology 82: 223-227

Di Padova C, Tritapepe R, Di Padova F, Frezza M, Stramentinoli G (1984) *S*-Adenosyl-L-methionine antagonizes oral contraceptive-induced bile cholesterol supersaturation in healthy women: preliminary report of a controlled randomized trial. Am J Gastroenterol 79: 941-944

Frezza M, Pozzato G, Chiesa L, Stramentinoli G, Di Padova C (1984) Reversal of intrahepatic cholestasis of pregnancy in women after high dose *S*-adenosyl-L-methionine administration. Hepatology 4: 274-278

Frezza M, Chiesa L, Ricci C, Pozzato G, Bazzocchi M, Pison G, Gallegari P (1985) Gallbladder volume and contraction in non-pregnant women previously affected with intrahepatic cholestasis of pregnancy. Ital J Gastroenterol 17: 311-313

Frezza M, Borean M, Pozzato G, Pison G, Rinaldi C, Terpin M, Santini G (1986) Estrogen and progesterone receptors on human gallbladder: the first description. Ital J Gastroenterol, (in press)

Giulidori P, Galli-Kienle M, Catto E, Stramentinoli G (1984) Transmethylation, transsulfuration, and aminopropylation reactions of *S*-adenosyl-L-methionine in vivo. J Biol Chem 259: 4205-4211

Kern F, Erfling W, Simon FR, Dahl R, Mallory A, Starzl TE (1978) Effect of estrogens of the liver. Gastroenterology 75: 512-522

Nakagaki M, Nakayama F (1982) Effect of female sex hormones on lithogenicity of bile. Jpn J Surg 12: 13-18

Podda M, Ghezzi C, Battezzati PM, Zuin M (1985) Steroidi sessuali femminili e secrezione biliare. In: Roda A, Roda E, d'Ascenzo G, Barbara L (eds) La bile: aspetti chimici, farmacologici e fisiopatologici. Atti del Seminario Interdisciplinare di Studio, Bologna, 18-19 January, pp 201-205

Porter LE, Els MS, van Thiel DH, Dugas MC, Eagon PK (1983) Characterization and quantitation of human hepatic estrogen receptor. Gastroenterology 84: 704-712

Reyes H (1982) The enigma of intrahepatic cholestasis of pregnancy: lessons from Chile. Hepatology 2: 87-96

Reyes H, Ribalta J, Gonzalez MC, Segovia N, Oberhauser E (1981) Sulfobromophthalein clearance tests before and after ethynyl estradiol administration, in women and men with familial history of intrahepatic cholestasis of pregnancy. Gastroenterology 81: 226-231

Schachter D (1984) Fluidity and function of hepatocyte plasma membranes. Hepatology 4: 140-151

Schreiber AJ, Simon FR (1983) Estrogen-induced cholestasis: clues to pathogenesis and treatment. Hepatology 3: 607-613

Schreiber AJ, Sutherland E, Simon FR (1982) Prevention of ethynyl estradiol cholestasis by *S*-adenosylmethionine: possible role of phosphotidylcholine. Hepatology 2: 697

Scragg RKR, McMichael AJ, Seamark RF (1984) Oral contraceptives, pregnancy, and endogenous oestrogen in gall stone disease – a case-control study. Br Med J 288: 1795-1799

Stramentinoli G, Gualano M, Rovagnati P, Di Padova C (1979) Influence of *S*-adenosyl-L-methionine on irreversible binding of ethynylestradiol to rat liver microsomes, and its implication in bile secretion. Biochem Pharmac 28: 981-984

Stramentinoli G, Di Padova C, Gualano M, Rovagnati P, Galli-Kienle M (1981) Ethynylestradiol-induced impairment of bile secretion in the rat: protective effects of *S*-adenosyl-L-methionine and its implication in estrogen metabolism. Gastroenterology 80: 154-158

Stricker BHC, Spoelstra P (1985) Drug-induced hepatic injury. Elsevier, Amsterdam, pp 237-245

Tritapepe P, Di Padova C, Zuin M, Bellomi M, Podda M (1976) Lithogenic bile after conjugated estrogens. N Engl J Med 295: 961-962

Tritapepe R, Di Padova C, Chiesara E, Cova D (1980) Effects of ethynyl estradiol on bile secretion and liver microsomal mixed function oxidase system in the mouse. Biochem Pharmacol 29: 677-680

# Transport of UDPG in Vitro and Reversal of Ethanol-Induced Effects

M. Earl Balis[1] and Paul J. Higgins[2]

[1]Memorial Sloan-Kettering Cancer Center, 1275 York Avenue New York, NY 10021 U.S.A.
[2]Veterans Administration Medical Center, 113 Holland Avenue Albany, NY, 12208 U.S.A.

5-Phosphoribosyl pyrophosphate (PRPP) is a necessary metabolic intermediate in the synthesis of purine and pyrimidine nucleotides as well as other important molecules. Perturbation of the intracellular level of PRPP has been found to be relevant to the origin of certain metabolic diseases [1, 2]. Too little PRPP leads to a condition that to a limited degree mimics Lesch-Nyhan disease. Too much leads to overproduction of purines and the catabolic end product uric acid, and hence gout.

PRPP is synthesized by the enzyme PRPP synthetase. Part of each cell's component of PRPP is membrane-bound. A number of compounds, both natural and synthetic, have been shown in our laboratory to affect the concentration of PRPP, probably by action on the synthetase. Under normal physiologic conditions the enzyme catalyzes the forward (synthetic) reaction at a rate roughly comparable to the rate at which it catalyzes the reverse (degradative) reaction. Among other interesting properties, PRPP synthetase changes in catalytic activity with the age of certain cells. As a result the equilibrium between PRPP and its precursors is altered.

Much of the cellular component of PRPP is found associated with the cell membrane (Table 1). Thus, upon exposure of lymphocytes to mitogens it is not surprising that one of the first responses should be an increase in PRPP. Nor should it be unexpected that a variety of metabolic inhibitors whose site of action appears to be far distant from PRPP homeostasis should be found upon closer analysis to be acting through changes in PRPP level or availability.

Because many earlier investigations had demonstrated that a variety of sugar derivatives alter the action of enzymes involved in the synthesis and utilization of PRPP, we undertook a study of the effects of uridine diphosphoglucose (UDPG) on PRPP metabolism. UDPG has been shown to have tissue-specific effects that have proved to be

**Table 1.** Purine-metabolizing enzymes of erythrocyte membranes

| | APRT | | HPRT | | PRPP SYN | |
|---|---|---|---|---|---|---|
| Hemolysates | | | | | | |
| Normal control | 333 | | 1335 | | 831 | |
| $HPRT^-$-patient | 640 | | 0 | | 739 | |
| Membrane PREP | | | | | | |
| Triton | – | + | – | + | – | + |
| Normal control | 15 | 21 | 23 | 42 | 173 | 222 |
| $HPRT^-$-patient | 9.6 | 13 | 0 | 23 | 439 | 745 |

APRT, adenine phosphoribosyltransferase; HPRT, hypoxanthine phosphoribosyltransferase; PRPP SYN, phosphoribosyl pyrophosphate synthetase

Assessment and Management of Hepatobiliary Disease
Eds.: L. Okolicsányi, G. Csomós, and G. Crepaldi

of clinical value in the treatment of some liver ailments. In an effort to determine something about the mechanism of action, we investigated the effect of UDPG on the levels of PRPP and PRPP synthetase in mouse liver, spleen, and transplanted tumors. Three strains of mice were studied with and without tumors under various experimental conditions. The PRPP level in the liver was found to increase threefold. A slight increase was noted in the activity of PRPP synthetase.

## Experimental Studies

### Determination of PRPP Concentration

The concentration of PRPP was determined through the reaction of $^{14}$C-orotic acid with PRPP to form $^{14}$C-carboxyl orotidine-5′-phosphate (OMP) in the presence of orotate phosphoribosyltransferase followed by the liberation of $^{14}CO_2$ under the catalysis by OMP decarboxylase [3].

### Studies on the In Vitro Incorporation of UDPG into Hepatocytes

We studied the transport of tritiated UDPG at 10, 30, and 40 min. The cells were prepared as single-cell suspensions under conditions that left them viable in terms of several biochemical parameters and vital dye exclusion. The plot (Fig. 1) shows the fraction of the material in each of the three compounds that were derived from the glucose moiety of the UDPG.

There is an uptake of intact UDPG which is maximal at 30 min. By 40 min the cells have begun to die in this medium and the UDPG has broken down. At 3 min about one-sixth of the label is in the form of UDPG. A major proportion of the UDPG enters the cells intact. The data further show that the initial product is glucose phosphate, which in time is dephosphorylated to glucose. It is obvious that the UDPG does not

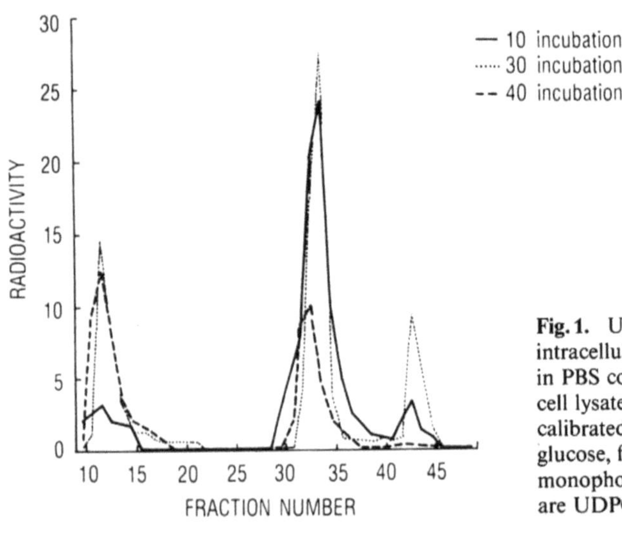


**Fig. 1.** UDPG uptake: distribution of intracellular label. Cells were incubated in PBS containing 0.5 m*M* UDPG, and cell lysates were analyzed by HPLC on calibrated columns. Fractions 11-15 are glucose, fractions 32-36 are glucose monophosphate, and fractions 41-46 are UDPG

break down before entering the cell, not only from its presence intact, but also from the fact that the breakdown products to not cause the same metabolic response that UDPG does.

Other preliminary studies show the presence of some intact UDPG in the cell membranes. This suggests that there may be an active transport mechanism responsible for the entry of UDPG into the hepatic cell.

Our data on the permeability of cell membranes to UDPG indicate that a significant amount (ca. 20%) of the UDPG, even though it is a highly polar compound, does pass through the membrane unchanged. A large fraction of the UDPG added to incubation media, however, is found in the cell as glucose phosphate, indicating cleavage after penetration of the cell. Eventually, all the UDPG to enter the cells is degraded to glucose phosphate and glucose. The in vitro studies show that glucose-6-phosphate is not the active form, and several tests show that uridine does not lead to changes like those seen with UDPG [4–6]. Thus, the most likely mechanism of action involves the membrane. The effects of UDPG on cell metabolism do not appear to be limited to enzyme induction.

### Determination of $^3$H-UDPG Incorporation

Isolated mouse hepatocytes were incubated at 37° in MEM with 0.21 m*M* $^3$H-UDPG. After 30 min the cells were layered on top of 1.0 ml dibenzylamine and centrifuged at 4 *g* immediately to separate the cells from the incubation medium. The cells were lysed in 0.2 ml KPB (pH 7.4) by vigorous vortexing. The solution was clarified by centrifugation at 30000 *g* for 15 min, and 25 µl of 10% TCA was added to 0.1 ml of supernatant solution. The initial pellet (containing cell membranes) was solubilized in 2% Triton X-100 in 10 m*M* Tris (pH 7.4) buffer and deproteinized. Solubilized membrane and cytoplasm were analyzed for $^3$H-containing components by HPLC fractionation through a PXS-102SAX column with a linear gradient from 0.007 *M* $KH_2PO_4$ to 0.25 *M* $KH_2PO_4$, 0.5 *M* KCl (pH 4.5). The flow rate was 0.8 ml/min and fractions were 0.4 ml each. The UV absorption and the radioactivity profiles were compared to values of known standards, and radioactivity levels were determined by liquid scintillation.

## Reversal of Ethanol Effects by UDPG

Appropriate ethanol-sensitive cells exhibit marked proliferative restrictions with associated entrance into a quiescent substrate [7] following acute exposure to ethanol in vitro [8]. This proliferative restriction is characterized by a gradual withdrawal of cells from the S and $G_2+M$ compartments of the cell cycle, an increase in the fraction of cells in the $G_1$ phase and an accumulation (also in the $G_1$ phase) of cells with a very low mean RNA content (designated "$G_1$e" cells, i.e., ethanol-induced cells of the $G_1$ substrate) [8]. Cells of both rat and mouse are susceptible to this proliferative restriction, although mouse cells appear to be particularly sensitive. In addition, mouse cells tend to aggregate into tight colonies of closely juxtaposed cells during the period of ethanol treatment, thereby affording an additional parameter for rapid assessment of the potential effects of ethanol in a given cell population. The cell line used in the

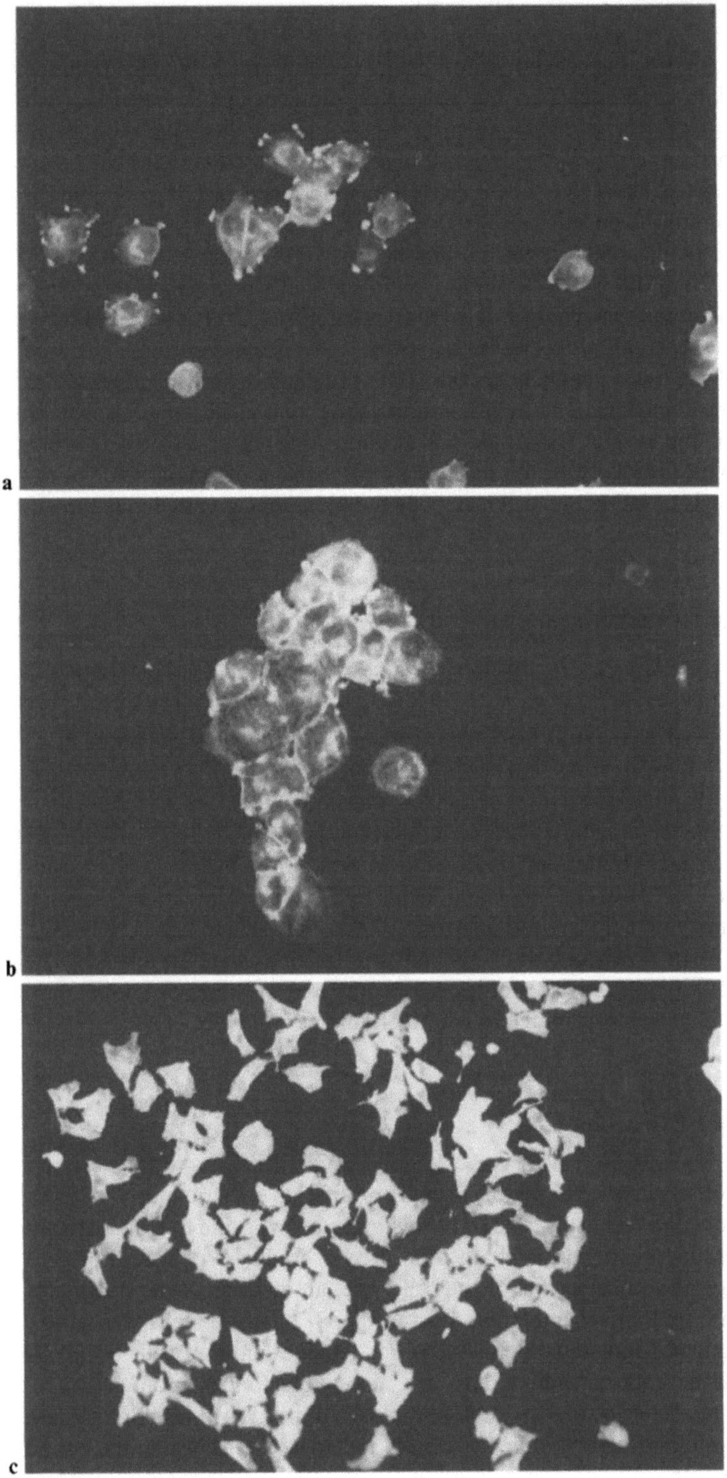

**Fig. 2 a–c.** Exposure of cells to ethanol and UDPG. **a** Cells at start of experiment; **b** cells exposed to ethanol; **c** cells exposed to both ethanol and UDPG

**Table 2.** Effect of UDPG on cell division

| Ethanol concentration (m*M*) | UDPG concentration (m*M*) | Time of onset of division (h) |
|---|---|---|
| 10 | 0 | 8.6 ± 5 |
| 10 | 0.1 | 2.2 ± 1 |
| 50 | 0 | 17.9 ± 9 |
| 50 | 0.1 | 5.4 ± 2 |
| 100 | 0 | 22.7 ± 7 |
| 100 | 0.1 | 6.9 ± 4 |

Ethanol and UDPG were added simultaneously to 25% confluent MH cell cultures. After 3 days the culture fluid was replaced with fresh medium containing neither ethanol nor UDPG. The values reported are those reported at the time of initial onset of cell division (> 10% dividing cells)

studies to be described is an established line of albumin-secreting murine epithelial liver cells derived from the BW 7756 hepatoma and is referred to as MH [9, 10].

Addition of UDPG (0.1-1 m*M*) simultaneously with the change-over to chemically defined medium containing ethanol was sufficient to inhibit the formation of cell clusters (Fig. 2). This was obvious in cells stained with Giemsa and fixed with 10% formalin in phosphate buffered saline (PBS), permeabilized in 1% nonidet-P40, and then stained with 1 g/ml rhodamine-labelled phalloidin for visualization of actin cables. Analysis of a great many actin-stained cells suggested that UDPG did not significantly alter cell morphology, but clearly inhibited the ballooning or enlargement of the hepatocytes that was typically observed in ethanol-containing media (Fig. 2). We feel that inhibition of clustering is a major factor in the shortening of the time to mitosis seen in Table 2 since MH cells forced to cluster or to grow in dense aggregates by culture in semisolid medium or on the surface of microbeads have a prolonged entrance into mitosis, compared to cells grown in sparse monolayer cultures, when released into liquid media culture.

## Morphologic Alterations

Addition of ethanol (50-100 *M*) to log-phase MH cells resulted in a dose-dependent reduction in cell proliferation, as seen in Table 3 as well as the marked development of cell clumping. Since this clumping was most evident in cultures treated with 100 *M* ethanol, which have a greatly reduced rate of cell proliferation, it is likely that growth of cells in cluster formations was not the only factor in the development of such aggregates. The marked change in size has been attributed inter alia to accumulation of protein, and it seemed likely that UDPG might interfere with this phenomenon. As can be seen in Table 4, there is a considerable accumulation of protein in the ethanol-treated cells, and this is blocked by the presence of m*M* UDPG. The morphologic and biochemical changes induced by ethanol in these cultured liver cells have some at least superficial similarities to changes induced by alcohol in humans, there is obvious reason to investigate these actions of UDPG in depth.

**Table 3.** Effect of ethanol on MH cell population density

| Medium | Cells per culture ($\times 10^{-5}$) |
|---|---|
| CD | 16.3 ± 2.1 |
| CD + 50 m*M* ethanol | 12.7 ± 3.1 |
| CD + 100 m*M* ethanol | 6.2 ± 1.7 |

MH cells were seeded to a low population density ($2.1 \times 10^{-5}$). After 24 h the medium was changed to chemically defined (CD) medium or ethanol-containing CD. Four days later the cells were harvested and counted

**Table 4.** Effects of UDPG on protein accumulation in ethanol-treated cells

| Culture conditions | Protein/$10^9$ cells (mg) |
|---|---|
| No additive | 501 ± 55 |
| UDPG 1 m*M* | 529 ± 68 |
| Ethanol 50 m*M* | 619 ± 47 |
| Ethanol 100 m*M* | 771 ± 89 |
| Ethanol 50 m*M* + UDPG 1 m*M* | 554 ± 43 |
| Ethanol 100 m*M* + UDPG 1 m*M* | 574 ± 29 |

Cells were seeded in RPMJ 1640 containing 10% FBS. After 24 h the growth medium was changed to CD. Cells were cultured for an additional 3 days, at which time they were lysed by sonication. Protein determinations were made on defined numbers of cells using the Bio-Rad assay

Another interesting effect of UDPG on cell development, as expressed morphologically, is shown in Fig. 3. Figure 3 A shows cells with typical Mallory body formation and distorted nuclei that have been induced by ethylnitrosamine. Although these are rat cells, the appearance and structure of the hepatocytes closely resembles the abnormality seen in the liver of human alcoholics. Figure 3 B shows a similar culture grown for 5 days in the presence of 1 m*M* UDPG: The Mallory body is reduced, absent, or redistributed. Note also the inhibition of aggregation and the more centrally located and more clearly defined nuclei. It is too early to attempt to explain these preliminary findings biochemically, but it is quite evident that the presence of UDPG greatly alters cell metabolism, apparently for the better. These studies were carried out in serum-free chemically defined media. Some of the changes might not have been the same had fetal calf serum been present.

Using gel electrophoresis, no evidence could be obtained for the induction of new proteins by UDPG, nor did UDPG influence the release of secretory proteins, including transferin, albumin, and alpha-fetoprotein. There was no evidence of specific deletion or diminishment of any protein. The intracellular concentrations of the major structural proteins of MH cells (actin, cytokeratin A, C, and D) were apparently unchanged by exposure to UDPG.

At the present time we have only limited biochemical leads as to the mechanisms of action. Perhaps the two compounds, UDPG and ethanol, act by altering membrane

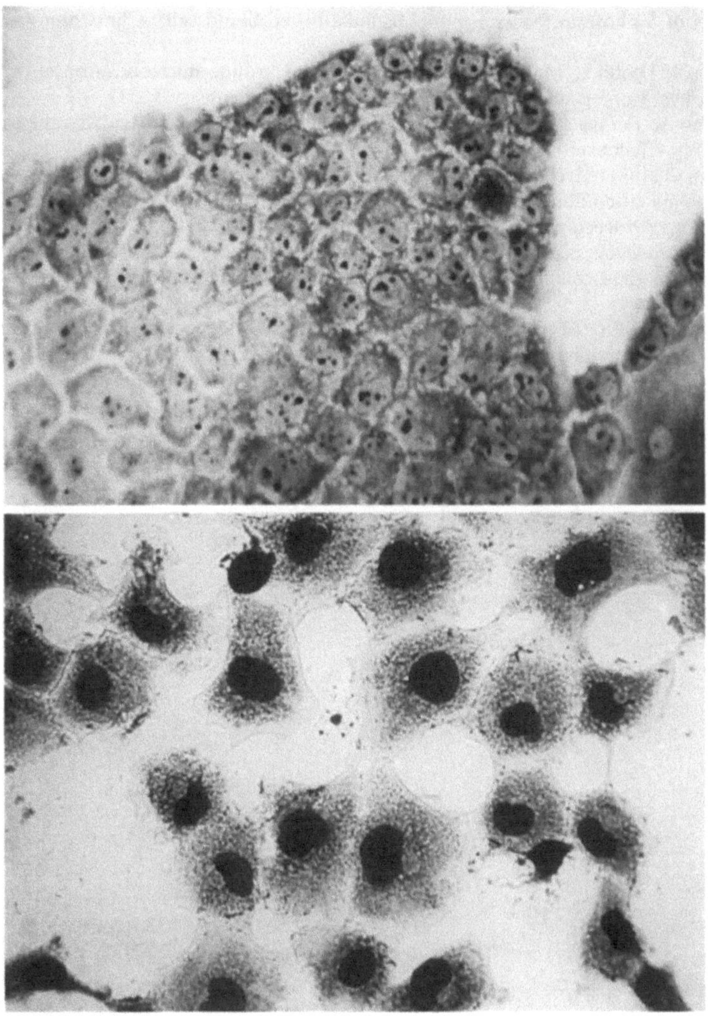

a b

**Fig. 3 a, b.** Effect of UDPG on Mallory bodies. **a** Control cells showing Mallory bodies; **b** cells grown in the presence of 1 m*M* UDPG

transport or other membrane functions and do so in opposing directions. Perhaps PRPP plays a role in the toxic manifestations of ethanol. Whatever the mechanisms, the unusual effects of UDPG on liver may provide a useful biochemical probe for investigation of both normal and abnormal liver function.

## References


1. Balis ME (1976) Uric acid metabolism in man. Adv Clin Chem 18: 213
2. Kelley WN, Wyngaarden JB (1974) Enzymology of gout. Adv Enzymol 14: 1
3. Tax WJM, Veerkamp JH (1977) A simple and sensitive method for estimating the concentra-

tion and synthesis of 5-phosphoribosyl 1-pyrophosphate in red blood cells. Clin Chim Acta 78: 209
4. Bossa R, Galatulas I, Leotta L, Mantovani E (1975) Effect of uridine nucleotides on energy metabolism in rat liver homogenates IRCS Medical Science. Biochemistry 3: 531
5. Pinelli A, Colombo A, Fumagalli D, Tofanetti O (1976) 5-Amino-Levulinic-Acid Synthetase inauction; inhibitory effect exerted by administration of UDPG. Biochem Pharmacol 25: 623
6. Pinelli A, Tofanetti O (1981) Livelli di acidi grassi liberi plasmatici e trigliceridi epatici in ratti trattati con adrenalina o teofillina. In: Some physiopathological, diagnostic and therapeutic aspects in hepatology (Proceedings of symposium), Pacini, Padua, p 121
7. Higgins PJ (1985) Cell cycle compartments of adult mouse hepatocytes identified by flow cytometric analysis of total cellular and nuclear RNA content: Effect of aging on $G_1$ substrates. Age 8: 122
8. Higgins PJ, Borenfreund E (1986) Alterations in growth rate and cell cycle kinetics of rat liver tumor cells in ethanol-containing medium. Biochem Pharmacol 35: 3857
9. Higgins PJ, Tong C, Borenfreund E, Bendich A (1979) Differential association of fetal antigen with hepatoma tissue grown in vivo and in vitro. Eur J Cancer 15: 423
10. Higgins PJ, Darzynkiewicz Z, Melamed MR (1983) Secretion of albumin and alpha-foetoprotein by dimethyl sulphoxide-stimulated hepatocellular carcinoma cells. Br J Cancer 48: 485

# Associated Factors in Gallstone Disease

L. Barbara, C. Sama, A. M. Morselli Labate, and A. G. Rusticali

Clinica Medica 3, Universita' degli Studi di Bologna, Ospedale Policlinico S. Orsola, via G. Massarenti 9, 40138 Bologna, Italy

## Introduction

Prevention of cholelithiasis, still at a very early stage of development, depends largely on a clear understanding of events concerning pathogenesis and risk factors. There has been a tremendous surge of new knowledge concerning the pathogenesis of cholesterol gallstones in recent years, particularly in the last decade, but there is much less information available on the risk factors of gallstone disease.

Although many factors have been considered, (Table 1), the current literature about the epidemiology of gallstone disease makes it very difficult to support clinical impressions with statistics. Most of the studies proposing the relationship of gallstone disease to possible pathogenetic factors concern mainly data from clinical observations, necroscopy series, or surgical records (Newman and Northrup 1949; Torvick and Hoivik 1960; Holland and Heaton 1972).

The major problem concerning an epidemiological approach in large population groups was related to the fact that no simple and noninvasive diagnostic technique for detecting gallstones had been available. In the last few years, ultrasound scanning has been introduced and fulfills the fundamental prerequisites for use in epidemiological studies: besides its high sensitivity and specificity compared with X-ray procedures, this technique is simple, safe, and noninvasive. In the pre-echographic era two major studies on epidemiology of gallstones were published: the Framingham (Friedman et al. 1966) and the Bainton (Bainton et al. 1976) studies. The Framingham study reported

**Table 1.** Factors associated with the presence of gallstones

| | |
|---|---|
| Ethnic | - American Indians |
| | - Northern Europe |
| | - West > Orient |
| Age | |
| Sex | - Women |
| | - Pregnancy |
| Familial | |
| Weight | - Obesity |
| | - Rapid weight loss |
| Bile acid malabsorption | - Distal ileal disease, resection or bypass, cystic fibrosis |
| Drugs | - Clofibrate |
| | - Oral contraceptives |
| Diabetes | |
| Hyperlipidemias | |
| Diet | |

Assessment and Management of Hepatobiliary Disease
Eds.: L. Okolicsányi, G. Csomós, and G. Crepaldi

"clinical prevalence," i.e., cases obtained from clinical practice. In this study, possible risk factors for gallstone disease were also discussed. Bainton and colleagues performed oral cholecystography on a weighted sample of the population of an industrial town in South Wales.

Two studies on the epidemiology of gallstone disease on free-living populations have been recently initiated in Italy using ultrasound: the GREPCO (GREPCO 1984) and the Sirmione (Barbara and Progetto Sirmione 1984) studies. The first cross-sectional part of these studies has been completed and gives us the opportunity of evaluating the factors associated with gallstone disease. Only some of the proposed factors have proved to be associated. They are: age, sex, parity, obesity, hypertriglyceridemia, and hypocholesterolemia.

We will now examine the results of the two studies in detail.

## Age

Both prevalence and incidence of gallstone disease seems to increase with age. These findings have been reported in the past based on autopsy studies (Newman and Northrup 1949; Torvick and Hoivik 1960) and hospital studies (Holland and Heaton 1972) and have been confirmed by the Framingham study (Friedman et al. 1966).

The Bainton study failed to find a positive correlation between gallstones and age. This is probably due to the fact that the considered age span (about 20 years) did not allow a wide distribution of subjects in different age groups (Bainton et al. 1976).

Both the GREPCO and the Sirmione studies show that the prevalence of gallstone disease increases steadily with age in both sexes (Table 2). This does not necessarily mean that the risk of developing gallstones is really much higher in the elderly than in other age groups. It is well known, in fact, that prevalence is about equal to incidence times duration of disease; therefore, because cholelithiasis is a long-standing disease with negligible recession or mortality, this factor may account for a higher prevalence in older subjects, even without an increase in incidence.

**Table 2.** Prevalence of gallstone disease

| Age group (years) | Total no. of subjects | Chole-lithiasis | Chole-cystectomy | Gallstone disease | |
|---|---|---|---|---|---|
| | | | | no. | % |
| Females | 1033 | 92 | 59 | 151 | 14.6 |
| 18-29 | 241 | 6 | 1 | 7 | 2.9 |
| 30-39 | 232 | 11 | 11 | 22 | 9.5 |
| 40-49 | 267 | 27 | 16 | 43 | 16.1 |
| 50-65 | 293 | 48 | 31 | 79 | 27.0 |
| Males | 878 | 40 | 19 | 59 | 6.7 |
| 18-29 | 188 | 2 | 0 | 2 | 1.1 |
| 30-39 | 226 | 8 | 2 | 10 | 4.4 |
| 40-49 | 228 | 13 | 8 | 21 | 9.2 |
| 50-65 | 236 | 17 | 9 | 26 | 11.0 |
| Total | 1911 | 132 | 78 | 210 | 11.0 |

**Table 3.** Female/male ratio of prevalence of gallstone disease

| Age (years) | F/M ratio |
|---|---|
| 18-29 | 2.6 |
| 30-39 | 2.2 |
| 40-49 | 1.8 |
| 50-65 | 2.5 |
| Overall | 2.2 |

## Sex

The old, well-known aphorism by which the typical gallstone patient is "female, fat, fair, and forty" has been confirmed by epidemiological studies. Autopsy studies (Torvick and Hoivik 1960) have shown in the past that in the western world females have a higher frequency of gallstones.

However the male/female ratio seems to have changed since the very first reports, which reported a figure of 1:4-6, to the present value of 1:2 (Holland and Heaton 1972; Friedman et al. 1966; Bainton et al. 1976).

This trend has been confirmed by the Sirmione study (Barbara and Progetto Sirmione 1984), where a significantly higher prevalence of gallstone disease was observed in all age groups, with a female/male ratio of 2:1 (Table 3).

The causes of this difference are not fully understood at present. Pregnancy does not seem to play a fundamental role; in fact, in the Sirmione study the risk of developing gallstones is higher than in males even in women who have never been pregnant. Sex hormones could be involved by altering biliary secretion and/or gallbladder motility.

## Pregnancy

Pregnancy is thought by many investigators to promote gallstone formation. In both the GREPCO (Angelico and GREPCO 1984) and the Sirmione (Roda and Progetto Sirmione 1984) studies the relative risk of gallstones increased with the number of pregnancies. Furthermore both studies demonstrated that the increase in the relative risk due to pregnancy is higher among younger than among older women.

Pregnancy could influence gallstone formation in several ways. Composition of bile may be altered adversely by hormonal changes during pregnancy.

Recent studies (Braverman et al. 1980) have shown sluggish gallbladder emptying during the third trimester; this could induce gallstone formation by altering bile acid enterohepatic circulation and promoting retention of cholesterol crystals, a prerequisite for gallstone formation. In addition, rapid weight variation during and after pregnancy can influence biliary lipid secretion.

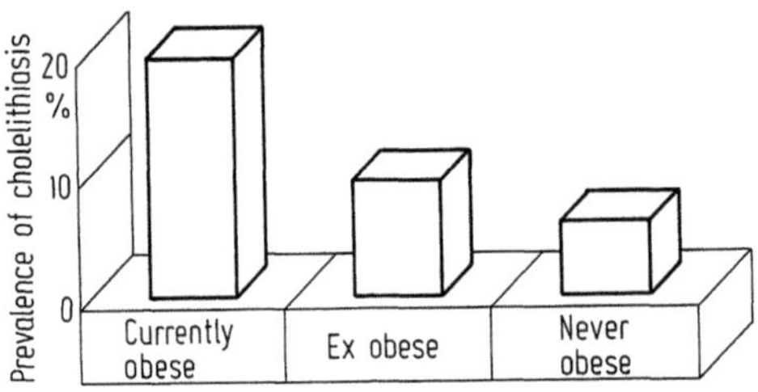


**Fig. 1.** Prevalence of cholelithiasis and obesity

**Table 4.** Prevalence of cholelithiasis and current obesity

| Age (years) | RRMH[a] | 95% confidence limits |
|---|---|---|
| 18-39 | 9.04 | 4.24-19.3 |
| 40-49 | 1.94 | 0.94-4.04 |
| 50-65 | 1.83 | 1.08-3.09 |
| Overall[b] | 2.32 | 1.60-3.36 |

[a] Age-specific relative risk standardized for sex (Mantel-Haenszel)
[b] Standardized for sex and age

## Obesity

Many clinical and epidemiological studies indicate that cholesterol gallstones are more common in obese subjects than in the nonobese. For instance, the Framingham study (Friedman et al. 1966) has shown a positive correlation between gallstones and obesity. In agreement with previous reports, obesity is associated with a higher frequency of gallstones in both the GREPCO (Angelico and GREPCO 1984) and the Sirmione study (Roda and Progetto Sirmione 1984).

In the Sirmione study, we have also evaluated the effect of present or previous obesity on the prevalence of gallstones, which turned out to be higher in those subjects who were obese at the time of the study (Fig. 1). Moreover, the Sirmione study showed that the risk of developing gallstones for currently obese subjects is higher in the lower age groups (Table 4).

The link between obesity and gallstones is supersaturated bile. Obesity raises the saturation of bile by increasing hepatic secretion of cholesterol. The high output of cholesterol in bile is secondary to a heightened synthesis of cholesterol in obese people.

## Serum Lipids

In the Western World serum cholesterol levels do not seem to be higher in gallstone sufferers than in normal subjects. This has been confirmed by both the Framingham (Friedman et al. 1966) and the Sirmione (Roda and Progetto Sirmione 1984) studies.

**Table 5.** Prevalence of cholelithiasis and serum triglyceride levels

| Age (years) | RRMH[a] | 95% confidence limits |
|---|---|---|
| 18-39 | 0.73 | 0.31-1.72 |
| 40-49 | 1.76 | 0.89-3.50 |
| 50-65 | 1.65 | 1.01-2.75 |
| Overall[b] | 1.43 | 1.01-2.06 |

[a] Age-specific relative risk standardized for sex and obesity (Mantel-Haenszel);
[b] Standardized for sex, age, and obesity

Moreover, in the GREPCO study cholesterol serum levels were found to be inversely correlated with the prevalence of gallstones (Angelico and GREPCO 1984), confirming the observations on Pima Indians (Sampliner et al. 1970), where a high prevalence of gallstones is associated with low cholesterol serum levels.

However, hypertriglyceridemia was found to be associated with a higher frequency of gallstones in both studies. The Sirmione study also showed that the higher relative risk of gallstones observed in hypertriglyceridemic subjects is independent of other factors like obesity (Table 5).

## Conclusions

Knowledge of the risk factors is fundamental to any program of prevention of cholesterol gallstone disease.

Many factors have been considered (Table 1), but most are based on clinical impressions, experimental studies, or studies on selected series of patients, which in no way represent the general population. Only studies actively investigating general populations will give us real insight into the problem.

The two Italian studies on the epidemiology of gallstone disease, the GREPCO and the Sirmione studies, have indicated some factors associated with the disease: age, sex, parity, obesity,hypertriglyceridemia, and hypocholesterolemia. These results come from cross-sectional studies, and therefore only at the end of the longitudinal study will we have more information on the true risk factors.

## References

Angelico F, Grepco (1984) Factors associated in the gallstone disease: observations in the GREPCO study. In: Capocaccia L, Ricci G, Angelico F, Angelico M, Attili AF (eds) Epidemiology and prevention of gallstone disease. MTP Press, Lancaster, pp 185-192

Bainton D, Davies GT, Evans KT et al. (1976) Gallbaldder disease. Prevalence in a South Wales industrial town. New Engl J Med 294: 1147-1149

Barbara L and Progetto Sirmione (1984) Epidemiology of gallstone disease: the Sirmione study. In: Capocaccia L, Ricci G, Angelico F, Angelico M, Attili AF (eds) Epidemiology and prevention of gallstone disease. MTP Press, Lancaster, pp 23-25

Bennion LJ, Grundy SM (1978) Risk factors for the development of cholelithiasis in man. N Engl J Med 299: 1161-1167, 1221-1227
Braverman DZ, Johnson ML, Kern F Jr (1980) Effect of pregnancy and contraceptive steroids on gallbladder function. N Engl J Med 302: 362-364
Friedman GD, Kamel WB, Dawber TR (1966) The epidemiology of gallbladder disease: observations in the Framingham study. J Chronic Dis 19: 273-292
GREPCO (1984) Prevalence of gallstone disease in a Italian adult female population. Am J Epidemiol 119: 796-805
Holland C, Heaton KW (1972) Increasing frequency of gallbladder operations in the Bristol area. Br Med J 3: 672-675
Newman HF, Northrup JD (1949) The autopsy incidence of gallstones. Int Abstr Surg 109: 1-13
Roda E (1984) Progetto Sirmione. Factors associated with gallstone disease: observations in the Sirmione study. In: Capocaccia L, Ricci G, Angelico F, Angelico M, Attili AF (eds) Epidemiology and prevention of gallstone disease. MTP Press, Lancaster, pp 207-209
Sampliner RE, Bennet PH, Courres LJ et al. (1970) Gallbladder disease in Pima Indians: demonstration of high prevalence and early onset by cholecystography. N Engl J Med 283: 1358-1364
Torvick A, Hoivik B (1960) Gallstones in an autopsy series. Acta Chir Scand 120: 168-174

# Epidemiology of Gallstone Disease in Hungary

A. Gógl[1], T. Szabó[1], Lenke Molnár[2], Z. Than[1]
[1]County Hospital, Székesfehérvár, Hungary
[2]Medical University, Pécs, Hungary

It must be said at the outset that one cannot disagree with Professor Heaton in saying the study of epidemiology of gallstones is both exciting and frustrating. Despite the latter, I have become an enthusiastic researcher of this topic. As you will probably have noticed, there were no data for Hungary accompanying the AMG map. At that time, only experienced clinicians estimates were available, according to which the occurrence of gallstones in Hungary was between 5% and 15%, similar to that in the USA.

The problem is almost insoluble from the financial and surgical viewpoints. However, something had to be done and therefore we began to collect data about gallstone disease. We wanted to determine the exact frequency and the actual number of patients suffering from gallstones and to clarify the factors influencing the development of the disease, in the hope that we would find ways of preventing it. Our clinical studies aimed at more reliable diagnosis with simultaneous cost reduction.

First of all – like everybody else – we went through autopsy records of 2 separate years. In each case the number of adults was near 1000 and the sex distribution almost equal (Table 1).

Table 2 shows the frequency of the disease among autopsy subjects. In 1970 gallstones were found in 9% of men and 24% of women, while in 1975 the corresponding

**Table 1.** Autopsy records from 1970 and 1975 (Institute of Pathology, Medical University, Pécs)

| | 1970 | 1975 |
|---|---|---|
| Men | 466 | 586 |
| Women | 436 | 543 |
| Under 14 years | 216 | 277 |
| Total | 1115 | 1406 |

**Table 2.** Frequency of gallstones in autopsy records

| | 1970 | | 1975 | |
|---|---|---|---|---|
| | Number | % | Number | % |
| Men | 43 | 9.2 | 68 | 11.6 |
| Women | 106 | 24.3 | 137 | 25.2 |
| Total | 149[a] | 16.5 | 205[b] | 18.0 |

[a] Includes 30 operated on for gallstones
[b] Includes 35 operated on for gallstones

Assessment and Management of Hepatobiliary Disease
Eds.: L. Okolicsányi, G. Csomós, and G. Crepaldi

**Table 3.** Obesity and diabetes in gallstone patients

| | 1970 | | 1975 | |
|---|---|---|---|---|
| | Obese | Diabetic | Obese | Diabetic |
| Men | 13.9% | 6.9% | 17.6% | 5.8% |
| Women | 23.6% | 14.1% | 37.8% | 16.7% |

**Table 4.** Complications in the gallstones patients

| | 1970 | | 1975 | |
|---|---|---|---|---|
| | Women | Men | Women | Men |
| Carcinoma | 8 | 2 | 4 | 2 |
| Perforation | 2 | 2 | – | – |
| Acute cholecystitis | 2 | 1 | 2 | 1 |
| Chronic cholecystitis | 10 | 3 | 10 | 11 |
| Cholangitis | 1 | 2 | 3 | 1 |
| Occluded icterus | 5 | 4 | 6 | 4 |
| Pancreatitis | 2 | 2 | 3 | 1 |
| Fistula | – | – | 1 | – |
| Total | 30 | 16 | 29 | 20 |

figures were 11.6% and 25.2%. In both years the overall figure remained under 20%. The material included some people who had been operated on for gallstones (30 in 1970 and 35 in 1975).

In both years and in both sexes, a striking number of obese and diabetic patients are found among the studied records (Table 3). In the women, diabetes is five times more frequent than in the general population.

According to pathologists, among the studied material in 1970, 20.3% of complications somehow connected with the possible cause of death represented gallstone disease. Even where no such connection could be demonstrated, some kind of sign could be noticed in 26.5% of gallstone cases.

In 1975 the data were similar. The distribution of complications connected with death can be seen in Table 4. I believe it is clear that most of these fatal outcomes could have been prevented if operations had been carried out in time. Since the majority of the patients had such diseases as cholecystitis and cholangitis, it is obvious that with optimal medical management of the disease – at the appropriate stage – the possibility of fatal outcome could be decreased.

Recently, it has become possible to dissolve some types of stones, so we analyzed the stones in our material in this light (Table 5). Unfortunately, our material does not contain the stone analysis of those who had been operated on, and the stones or records of some of the others got lost somehow. About half of the analyzed stones seemed to be soluble. In our opinion this is the very group whose development of stones could have been avoided with suitable lifestyle and diet.

Figure 1 shows the frequency of gallstones according to age in the 2 years' autopsy records (excluding operated subjects). The only possible conclusion – surely common knowledge – is that men have significantly lower values in every age group than wom-

**Table 5.** Gallstones according to type

| | 1970 | | 1975 | |
|---|---|---|---|---|
| | Women | Men | Women | Men |
| Cholecystectomy | 21 | 9 | 11 | 24 |
| Unknown | 20 | 6 | 22 | 44 |
| Mixed | 35 | 13 | 26 | 46 |
| Cholesterol | 21 | 11 | 4 | 14 |
| Bilirubin | 5 | 2 | 5 | 9 |

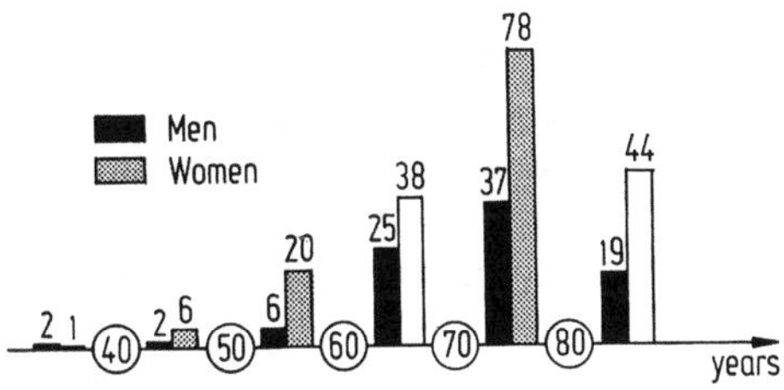


**Fig. 1.** Gallstones according to age (1970–1975). Patients operated on for gallstones are excluded

en. These findings generally correspond with those reported in literature, although the ratio of cholesterol stones may be lower than in the American data.

Knowing the high occurrence of gallstones, we started to study all the patients admitted to the internal medicine department of Szekesfehérvár county hospital in 1982 (Table 6). We wanted to ascertain the workload the gallstone patients represented for the department and whether the strategy for treatment was up to standard.

In 13 patients we found gallstones with family history. These families are in our follow-up study. We feel it is of interest that 58 of our patients had been taking diuretics for 2 years or more before diagnosis was made. In 83 cases – one-quarter of the patients – we diagnosed diabetes mellitus or impaired glucose tolerance.

The first step of our diagnostic strategy – after suitable anamnesis and physical examination – was ultrasound, which permitted definite diagnosis in 225 cases. In 63 cases, we needed intravenous cholegraphy, in four cases ERCP. In ten cases gallstone disease was verified on autopsy. In 37 cases the diagnosis was not clear but the existence of gallstones was judged probable and the patients were referred to surgical intervention, where the disease was substantiated. I shall show the age and distribution of all our gallstone patients. In contrast to many literature data, in our material there is an uneven distribution of men and women even after the age of 60 (Fig. 2).

**Table 6.** Data from Department of Internal Medicine, County Hospital, Székesfehérvár 1982

| | |
|---|---|
| Population | 270000 |
| Patients admitted | 6165 |
| Gallstone disease admissions | 354[a] |
| Average hospitalization | 12.4 days |
| Recommended for operation | 158[b] |

[a] One patient 4 times, seven 3 times, 57 twice
[b] Mortality 1.4%

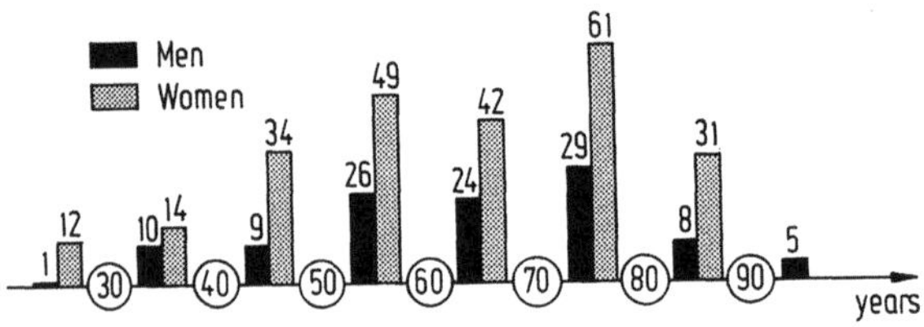


**Fig. 2.** Gallstones according to age and sex (hospital 1982)

The ultrasound examination seems to be reliable, is noninvasive and relatively inexpensive, and has the potential to become a basic method of screening.

Although we recommended half of our patients for operation, some of those who did not undergo surgery had to be admitted to the hospital several times. This suggests that however good our diagnostic skill, if the patient with gallstone diagnosis is not recommended for operation, the diagnosis is in vain. It is imperative to have the patient operated on. Naturally, this does not include those who for some reason just cannot be operated on, those in whom operation is contraindicated.

Of course, we are well aware of the importance and usefulness of the follow-up study.

To determine the exact occurrence and clarify the etiopathogenesis, a prospective study was carried out on 1700 residents of the catchment area of the hospital. Using first questionnaires and then examinations (physical, laboratory, ultrasound, X-ray) the subjects' complaints, eating habits, and relevant laboratory data were evaluated in order to establish the existence of gallstones. The sample was only partly representative.

The occurrence of gallstone disease in men was 13.7%, while in women – to our surprise – it was 31.6%. In the total population, the frequency of gallstones is 24.5% (50% silent). Naturally, we included cases where cholecystectomy had been carried out (one-quarter of the total gallstone patients). 6.5% of our sample underwent surgical intervention (Table 7).

**Table 7.** Gallstone disease frequency in our sample

| | *n* | Gallstone | Operated |
|---|---|---|---|
| Men | 680 | 13.7% | 27% |
| Women | 1020 | 31.6% | 26% |
| Total | 1700 | 24.5 | |

Figure 3 shows the absolute and relative frequency of gallstone disease in respect to age in our prospective study. One thing is certain: above the age of so the frequency increases sharply. It is also noticeable that in contrast to the autopsy records, the incidence at advanced age was similar in men and women.

Gallstone patients' body weight is significantly higher than normal, as their food includes an excess of carbohydrates and calories (Table 8).

The frequency of diabetes is several times higher among gallstone patients than that in the general population, which in Hungary is around 3%. More than one-quarter of the gallstone patients have contents of cholesterol and triglyceride so high as to be considered abnormal. This contrasts with the figure of 3% in those without gallstone disease at the time of examination (Table 9).

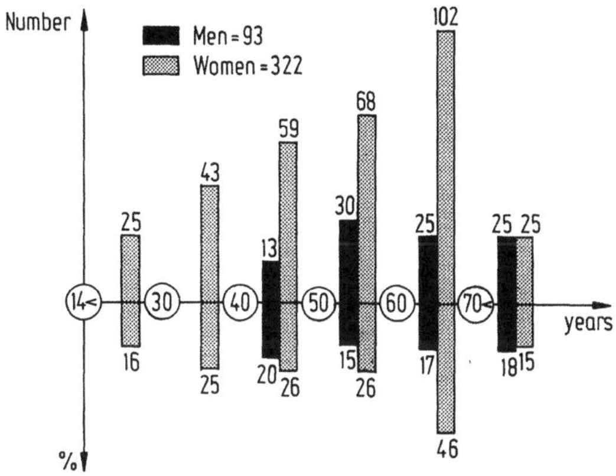


**Fig. 3.** Absolute and relative frequency of gallstone disease according to age and sex

**Table 8.** Relative body weight, eating habits, and diabetes in gallstone patients

| | Rel. B.W. | Diet[a] | Diabetes |
|---|---|---|---|
| Men | 113 | 91% | 18% |
| Women | 118 | 87% | 15.7% |

[a] Excessive carbohydrates and calories

**Table 9.** Abnormal cholesterol and triglyceride levels in gallstone patients (cholesterol >6.0 mmol/l, triglyceride >2.0 mmol/l)

| | Gallstone | Without stone |
|---|---|---|
| Men | 36% | 3.7% |
| Women | 26% | 2.5% |
| Men | 36% | 3.0% |
| Women | 26% | 2.5% |

We were disappointed with our questionnaire, mainly because it did not make it possible to separate people with and without gallstones. The answers of the silent gallstone subjects did not differ significantly from those of gallstone disease sufferers. The questionnaire is not suitable, in our opinion, for the screening of gallstone patients who are free of symptoms. Neither did the laboratory examinations fulfill our expectations - pathological signs were only obtained in patients already known to have gallstones.

We think direct examination of the bile is indispensable for the establishment of the inclination to form stones. For correct diagnosis, ultrasound is highly useful.

The following conclusions can be drawn:

- For more effective prevention of gallstone disease, people's eating habits must be changed. The diet should contain fiber-rich food and be poor in carbohydrates.
- The screening and exploration of the disease must not be impersonally "computerized."
- Ultrasound is the most suitable method of screening and verification.

– The diagnosed gallstone patients must be recommended for surgery as soon as possible.

Finally, I would propose the elaboration of an effective method for detecting the inclination to form gallstones in order to improve our preventative work in this rather common disease.

## References

1. Ingelfinger FJ (1968) Gastroenterology 55: 102
2. Newman-Northrup (1959) Internat. Abstr. Surg. 109: 1
3. Holzbach R Thomas (1983) Raven Press, New York

# The Role of the Gallbladder in Cholesterol Gallstone Pathogenesis

Gianfranco Salvioli[1], Ruggero Lugli[2], and Maurizio Pulvirenti[2]

[1] Cattedra di Geriatria e Gerontologia dell'Università di Modena
[2] USL n° 16 di Modena,
Ospedale Estense, Viale Vittorio Veneto 9, 41100 Modena, Italy

## Introduction

Normal human bile is a nonechogenic fluid containing mixed micelles, commonly supersaturated in cholesterol (Ch), plus proteins and electrolytes. Interestingly, formation of cholesterol gallstones (CG) is limited to the gallbladder (GB), despite the fact that bile in other compartments of the biliary tree is more saturated in cholesterol. The importance of the GB in the pathogenesis of CG was suggested more than a century ago: biliary stasis or alteration of GB mucosa were considered the primary cause of CG. Virchow (1857) noted that GB epithelium accumulated lipids. More recently, other studies have demonstrated that the GB wall, which has the same embryological origin as the intestine, has the capacity to both synthesize and absorb lipids, such as Ch, lecithin, triglycerides, and long-chain fatty acids (Niederhiser et al. 1976; Tilvis et al. 1982), and can metabolize Ch to Ch esters. The absorption and transport rates of Ch increase with increasing Ch saturation, reaching a maximum of 3-5 $nmol/cm^2/min$ (Jacyna et al. 1985): this slow process induces little variation of bile composition. Of greater importance seems to be fast absorption of water and electrolytes, regulated by gastrointestinal hormones and other secretagogues: as in the intestine, these can reverse the direction of the transport processes, so that a net absorption becomes a net secretion (Wood and Svanvik 1983), with consequent dilution of GB content.

A layer of mucus adheres to the epithelial surface of the GB; it is produced by the tubular alveolar glands in the neck region and has important rheological functions which can influence the flow of bile (Lee et al. 1981[b]).

The question is whether these metabolic functions of the GB can influence the rate of Ch crystal formation. Other physiological properties of the GB can also influence CG formation, such as its motility, the viscosity and pH of its content, and the secretion of nucleating and antinucleating agents into the bile (Salvioli et al. 1984). These factors help to explain why not all subjects with Ch-supersaturated bile develop Ch gallstones.

## Concentration of Lipid Components

Hepatic bile contains 100-nm particles (vesicles) which solubilize large quantities of Ch in stable form (Mazer and Carey 1983). Therefore the increase of total lipid concentration during stagnation of bile in the GB reduces the metastable zone: consequently, the possibility of forming a solid Ch phase is increased. GB motility and the sphincter of Oddi directly influence some parameters of the enterohepatic circulation of bile acids,

Assessment and Management of Hepatobiliary Disease
Eds.: L. Okolicsányi, G. Csomós, and G. Crepaldi

and also residence time, lipid composition, and lithogenicity of bile. Therefore it has primary importance in CG pathogenesis. But even after cholecystectomy, a diurnal rhythm of biliary lithogenicity suggests the presence of a complex chronobiological regulation of lipid secretion in bile (Kurtz et al. 1985).

Nuclear magnetic resonance (NMR) provides anatomic and chemical information: a strong NMR signal is recorded in the GB because of the absorption of water and inorganic ions, whereas hepatic bile emits a weak signal (Hricak et al. 1983; Demas et al. 1985): low specific gravity hepatic bile settles above the higher specific gravity GB bile (Hricak et al. 1983; Demas et al. 1985).

## Motility of the Gallbladder

The main functions of the GB are storage of bile during fasting and mobilization of the bile acid pool during digestion. Around 60% of the bile acid pool is contained in the GB during fasting. Cycling frequency of the bile acid pool in the enterohepatic circulation is the main regulator of the quantity and quality of biliary lipid secretion. It especially affects the Ch/lecithin (Lec) ratio: GB storage of the bile acid (BA) pool reduces lipid secretion and increases the Ch/Lec molar ratio of bile.

Regulation of GB motility is complex: neural control prevails during fasting, but is replaced by humoral control when cholecystokinin (CCK) is released after a meal (Ryan 1981). This hormone is a powerful stimulant of GB contraction and its production is increased by the ingestion of food, water and $MgSO_4$ (Ryan 1981; Svenberg et al. 1984; Hopman et al. 1985). During fasting, cyclic motor activities of the GB and the sphincter of Oddi are present and related to those of the lower esophageal sphincter and stomach (Peeters et al. 1980): these periodic contractions, observed at 80-min intervals, are not suppressed by vagotomy (Pellegrini et al. 1985) and occur in connection with phase II fasting motor pattern complexes of the proximal digestive tract (Kraglund et al. 1984). After a meal, cyclic motor activity is altered by the release of gastrointestinal hormones such as CCK, motilin, gastrin, secretin, pancreatic polypeptides, insulin, and VIP, which have contrasting effects on GB motility (Ryan 1981).

CCK is the most important contracting hormone and has a very short half-life. The role of motilin is less clear: even though GB emptying and motilin release in man are casually related events (Svenberg et al. 1985), intravenous motilin administration does not induce GB contraction (Svenberg et al. 1985). The role of high plasma levels of pancreatic polypeptide – an inhibitor of GB emptying – during CCK infusion is not clear (Hopman et al. 1985). VIP and somatostatin antagonize the contractile effect of CCK; gallstones are frequently present in somatostatinoma (Krejs et al. 1979). Gallbladder contraction induced by CCK or acetylcholine requires the presence of extracellular calcium (Ryan 1985).

### Gallbladder Motility in Gallstone Patients

Gallstone patients have normal meal-stimulated plasma CCK profiles, but reduced GB contraction. Thus GB motility, rather than CCK release, is abnormal in gallstone patients (Forgacs et al. 1984). Fisher et al. (1982) clearly demonstrated that GB emptying is abnormal in CG subjects after a standard liquid meal, but not after CCK-OP octopeptide administration. Pomeranz and Shaffer (1985) have recently shown that GB contraction induced by low doses of CCK is reduced in a group of CG subjects and that this occurs irrespective of clinical features, stone size, and number of stones. Animal models of cholelithiasis have shown that early stages of stone formation are characterized by defective GB contractility in vitro, as if GB muscle functions were affected by changes in bile composition. Moreover, GB emptying in response to exogenous CCK is altered early during gallstone formation in the prairie dog (Pellegrini et al. 1986). The absence of abnormal GB filling under these conditions would seem to exclude the possibility of diminished cystic duct flow as a cause of GB stasis. It has been mentioned that development of lithogenic bile in the prairie dog is associated with increased flow resistance (Pitt et al. 1982), and sphincterotomy prevents gallstone formation in this experiment (Hutton et al. 1981).

### Bile Stratification During Stasis

Prolonged GB retention of bile increases the probability that retained Ch crystals can grow. During stasis, stratification of GB content occurs (Thureborn 1966; Nakayama and van der Linden 1975; Holzbach 1984). This has been further evaluated with NMR (Hricak et al. 1983). When low-weight vesicles enter a GB filled with concentrated bile, rich in dense mixed micelles, the buoyant material tends to float (Holzbach 1984) and is responsible for layering of the GB content. The upper layer has a lower lipid concentration and a higher Ch/Lec molar ratio (Nakayama and van der Linden 1975). Stratification of bile phases also occurs experimentally in tubes containing samples of abnormal GB bile. The lighter layer may form a nidus for Ch crystallization, even though vesicles dissolve large quantities of Ch.

Two compartments having different flow behaviors have been hypothesized in the GB (Howard et al. 1986). The infundibulum has rapid washout, and entering bile remains only for a short time, not mixing with the stored bile; the corpus region has slow washout. These hydraulic properties, influencing the residence time in the two GB compartments, could play a role in the retention of Ch crystals.

### Sludge Formation

Roslyn et al. (1983) found a high incidence of sludge formation in the GB of patients receiving total parenteral nutrition (TPN). Moreover, 33% of patients undergoing prolonged fasting for gastrointestinal surgery have sludge (Bolondi et al. 1985). It is noteworthy that TPN does not increase bile saturation in Ch, but induces GB stasis; in fact, CCK administration prevents sludge formation in these patients (Doty et al. 1985). These observations underline the importance of bile stasis in the formation of a solid phase in the GB (calcium bilirubinate in the case of TPN).

Cholesterol monohydrate crystals and bilirubin granules embedded in a matrix of mucus gel make up the sludge (Lee and Nicholls 1986). When sludge is present, the GB wall shows mucus hypersecretion and glandular metaplasia. Therefore mucus hypersecretion in the GB is associated with sludge, which may represent a step in the development of gallstones (Lee and Nicholls 1986).

### Influence of Vagotomy

Animal studies show that vagotomy is associated with increased incidence of gallstones (Ihasz and Griffith 1981; Stempel and Duane 1978) and with increased resistance of bile to flow through the Oddi sphincter. Other studies report that vagotomy increases the lithogenicity of bile in some species but not in humans (Stempel and Duane 1978). Augmented GB emptying after exogenous CCK has been observed in vagotomized subjects, who show reduced GB emptying after a liquid meal (Fisher et al. 1985). Pellegrini et al. (1985) have shown that CCK activity is not affected by vagotomy.

### Gallbladder Motility and Pregnancy

Pregnancy seems to be a risk for Ch cholelithiasis. Pregnant women have a slow rate of emptying; the fasting volume and the residual and average hourly volume are increased in all trimesters of pregnancy (Everson et al. 1982). GB contraction induced by acetylcholine and CCK requires the presence of calcium, and pregnancy reduces intracellular calcium release (Ryan 1985).

### Gallbladder Motility in Diabetes

Besides Ch supersaturation of bile, diabetics frequently have an enlarged GB, in some cases resembling postvagotomy cholecystomegaly (Gitelson et al. 1969). Onodera et al. (1983) studied the diurnal profile of GB size in diabetic patients and found that emptying is especially reduced in subjects with symptoms of autonomic neuropathy.

### Gallbladder Motility and Aging

It is well known that gallstone prevalence increases with age, as shown by epidemiological studies and autopsy. Apart from progressively increasing cholesterol saturation of bile during life (Einarsson et al. 1985), gastrointestinal motility is also reduced in old people. But volumes of the fasting and maximally contracted GB are the same in old and young subjects alike, even though plasma CCK levels after fasting or fat stimulation increase with age (Khalil et al. 1985). The sensitivity of GB muscle is seemingly reduced with age, and increased concentrations of CCK could compensate for the reduced responsiveness of GB muscle and also explain the slow gastric emptying observed in old people (Khalil et al. 1985).

In conclusion, GB emptying is frequently reduced in gallstone patients. The problem is whether the observed variations are cause or consequence of anatomical changes in the GB wall due to the presence of gallstones. Another point is that the method used for studying GB motility and the type of stimulus inducing GB contraction could influence the results.

## Altered Nonlipid Bile Content: Importance of Proteins

The metabolic activities of the GB wall and their influence on bile composition have already been described. The influences of neuropeptides and autonomic innervation on fluid transport of the GB wall are not well known, but these factors do affect the dilution of bile components and their residence time in the GB. The inflamed GB secretes fluid into the lumen; the same effect is obtained after administering secretin, VIP, and prostaglandins (Wood and Svanvik 1983; Jivegård et al. 1985). These variations probably become important when the GB wall displays abnormalities consequent to cholelithiasis.

## Bile pH

Past studies have reported pH values of 5.6-8.0 for GB bile and 6.2-8.5 for hepatic bile (Sutor and Wilkie 1976). The GB mucosa reduces $[HCO_3^-]$ and $[CO_3^{--}]$, and this change depends on the secretion of $H^+$ions (Rege and Moore 1986). Lower pH of the GB reduces calcium carbonate lithogenicity in dogs (Rege and Moore 1986). Free fatty acids, insoluble at low pH, are present in bile and can precipitate, as can unconjugated bilirubin. Low pH activates endogenous $\beta$-glucuronidase: the activity at pH 7 is only 23% of its maximum, which occurs at pH 5.2 (Ho 1985).

## Merocrine Secretion of Mucous Glycoproteins

Glycoproteins are found as complexes in the core of gallstones (Smith and LaMont 1985). Their concentration in bile is 20-40 mg%. Total proteins amount to 400-600 mg%, about 5% of total biliary solids (Reuben 1984). Holan et al. (1979) found a lower amount of solid and proteins in GB bile of gallstone patients. Others have reported a reduced concentration of nondialyzable hexoses (372 vs 643 mg/dl) (Pearson et al. 1982). The vagus is involved in the regulation of glycoprotein synthesis, which increases after meals. The molecular weight (MW) of biliary proteins ranges from $10^4$ to $10^8$, and mucus is represented by high-MW polymerized glycoproteins (Pearson et al. 1982) released by exocytosis of granules of the apical portion of epithelial cells (LaMont et al. 1983). Mucus has a pH-dependent affinity for calcium and bilirubin (Allen et al. 1981; Forstner and Forstner 1975): increased concentration of mucus induces high bile viscosity and sludge formation under certain conditions (Lee and Nicholls 1986). High-MW mucus is produced in increased concentrations in patients with lithogenic bile (Bouchier et al. 1965) and in experimental Ch-fed prairie dogs (Ho 1985).

Endogenous prostaglandin levels raise mucus secretion. They increase consequent to high levels of both Ch and arachidonic acid in bile (LaMont et al. 1983). In man, hydrophobic and detergent bile acids (DCA and CDCA) have been shown to promote the preferential secretion into bile of Lec species rich in arachidonic acid (Salvioli et al. 1985).

Administration of aspirin (an inhibitor of glycoprotein synthesis) prevents gallstone formation in the prairie dog, in spite of persistent Ch supersaturation of bile (Lee et al. 1981a). The increased viscosity of bile containing higher concentrations of mucus is an underestimated pathogenetic factor (LaMont et al. 1984): development of lithogenic bile in the prairie dog is associated with increased production of glycoproteins and with a high resistance of bile flow through the cystic duct (Doty et al. 1985), with altered GB compliance in addition to defective GB contractility (Fridhandler et al. 1983).

The depletion of mucous glycoproteins could be an effect of the more detergent bile salts, as hypothesized for the gastric mucosa (Slomiany et al. 1984); in this regard, the proportion of deoxycholate (the most detergent bile acid) has been found to be higher in the lower layers of GB bile (Nakayama and van der Linden 1975).

### Nucleating and Antinucleating Factors

Normal bile is frequently supersaturated in Ch (Holzbach et al. 1973); the process of Ch precipitating out of metastable bile is termed nucleation. The rate of this process is influenced by the balance between nucleating and anti-nucleating factors (Holan et al. 1979; Holzbach et al. 1984). Values of Ch saturation of bile do not clearly discriminate between normal and gallstone bile. Nucleation times provide a better distinction between the two groups (Holan et al. 1979). Desquamated cells, bacteria, proteins, and glycoproteins can induce or accelerate the heterogeneous nucleation rate. Inflamed GB epithelium produces phospholipases which can cleave fatty acids from biliary lecithin, precipitating as calcium salts.

Mucous glycoproteins have been considered good candidates for nucleating factors because their biliary concentration increases before Ch crystal formation (Lee et al. 1981b). Available data favor this hypothesis (LaMont et al. 1984), but some studies failed to find any quantitative or qualitative changes of mucous glycoproteins in normal and Ch gallstone subjects (Gollish et al. 1983; Harvey et al. 1986). Complete removal of mucous glycoproteins from bile does not slow the nucleation time of abnormal bile (Harvey et al. 1986; Gallinger et al. 1985). A specific heat-labile nucleating factor has been identified in the proteins of abnormal bile (Gallinger et al. 1985). Since the nucleation time of artificial bile is faster than that of human bile having the same composition, the presence and identification of antinucleating factors seems more important than that of nucleating factors (Holzbach et al. 1984). These have been identified as apolipoproteins AI (Kibe et al. 1984), originating from the catabolism of hepatic lipoproteins. Holzbach et al. (1984) separated two protein fractions having different MW: the lighter fraction has a great degree of lipid association and inhibits Ch nucleation. It is possible that these low-MW proteins characterize bile samples supersaturated in Ch, but without gallstones.

However measurements of nucleation time may be incorrect. For example, calcium oxalate crystallization is slower in a urothelium-lined system than in glass containers (Gill et al. 1980); the metastable limit of oxalate is also higher in the former. No data are available on the influence of the materials used to incubate bile samples on Ch nucleation time (Gill et al. 1980).

The effect of sludge on nucleation requires more in-depth study. In fact, a retained precipitated phase induces nucleation at comparatively lower supersaturation levels, and secondary nucleation mechanism (due to the presence of a solid interface) could become important in such cases (Garside 1982).

The evaluation of both Ch nucleation and crystal growth remains a problem requiring further study. The formation of crystals is probably a very common event, but they usually only remain in the GB for a short time. When they are retained, secondary nucleation becomes relevant and crystals rapidly increase in number (Salvioli et al. 1984). The importance of standing and stirring on the nucleation of Ch should also be evaluated using appropriate methods in a system where heterogeneous and secondary nucleations predominate.

## References

Allen B, Bernhoft R, Blanckaert N, Svanvik J, Filly R, Gooding G, Way L (1981) Sludge is calcium bilirubinate associated with bile stasis. Am J Surg 141: 51-54
Bolondi L, Gaiani S, Casanova P, Ferrentino M, Santi V, Bazzocchi R, Amenta E, Labò G (1985) Early detection of biliary sludge and gallstones after surgery of the G. I. tract. In: Barbara L, et al. (eds) Recent advances in bile acid research. Raven, New York, pp281-285
Bouchier IAD, Copperband SR, El Kidsl BM (1965) Mucous substances and viscosity of normal and pathological human bile. Gastroenterology 49: 343-352
Demas BE, Hricak H, Moseley M, Wall SD, Moon K, Goldberg HI, Margulis AR (1985) Gallbladder bile: an experimental study in dogs using MR imaging and proton MR spectroscopy. Radiology 157: 453-455
Doty JE, Pitt HA, Porter-Fink V, DenBesten L (1985) Cholecystokinin prophylaxis of parenteral nutrition-induced gallbladder disease. Ann Surg 201: 76-80
Einarsson K, Nilsell K, Leijd B, Angelin B (1985) Influende of age on secretion of cholesterol and synthesis of bile acids by liver. N Engl J Med 313: 277-282
Everson GT, McKinley C, Lawson M, Johnson M, Kern F Jr (1982) Gallbladder function in the human female; effect of the ovulatory cycle, pregnancy, and contraceptive steroids. Gastroenterology 82: 711-719
Fisher RS, Stelzer F, Rock E, Malmud LS (1982) Abnormal gallbladder emptying in patients with gallstones. Dig Dis 27: 1019-1024
Fisher RS, Rock E, Malmud LS (1985) Cholinergic effects on gallbladder emptying in humans. Gastroenterology 89: 716-722
Forgacs IC, Maisey MN, Murphy GM, Dowling RH (1984) Influence of gallstones and ursodeoxycholic acid therapy on gallbladder emptying. Gastroenterology 87: 299-307
Forstner JF, Forstner GG (1975) Calcium binding to intestinal goblet cell mucin. Biochim Biophys Acta 1386: 283-292
Fridhandler TM, Davison JS, Shaffer EA (1983) Defective gallbladder contractility in the ground squirrel and prairie dog during the early stages of cholesterol gallstone formation. Gastroenterology 85: 830-836
Gallinger S, Harvey PRC, Petrunka CN, Strasberg SM (1985) The effect of mucous glycoprotein on nucleation time of human bile. Gastroenterology 89: 648-658
Garside J (1982) Nucleation. In: Nancollas GH (ed) Biological mineralization and demineralization. Springer, Berlin Heidelberg New York, pp23-33
Gill WB, Ruggiero KJ, Fromes MC (1980) Elevation of the metastable limits and absence of container surface nucleation for calcium oxalate crystallization in a urotheliallined system as compared to glass containers. Invest Urol 18: 158-161
Gitelson S, Oppenheim D, Schwartz A (1969) Size of the gallbladder in patients with diabetes mellitus. Diabetes 18: 493-498
Gollish SH, Burnstein MJ, Ilson RG, Petrunka CN, Strasberg SM (1983) Nucleation of cholesterol monohydrate crystals from hepatic and gall-bladder bile of patients with cholesterol gallstones. Gut 24: 836-844
Harvey P, Rupar CA, Gallinger S, Petrunka CN, Strasberg SM (1986) Quantitative and qualitative composition of gall bladder mucus glycoprotein from patients with and without gallstones. Gut 27: 374-381
Ho KJ (1985) Human $\beta$-glucuronidase. Studies on the effects of pH and bile acids in regard to its role in the pathogenesis of cholelithiasis. Biochim Biophys Acta 827: 197-206
Holan KR, Holzbach RT, Hermann RE, Cooperman AM, Claffey WJ (1979) Nucleation time: a key factor in the pathogenesis of cholesterol gallstone disease. Gastroenterology 77: 611-617
Holzbach RT (1984) Effects of gallbladder function on human bile: compositional and structural changes. Hepatology 4: 57S-60S
Holzbach RT, Marsh M, Olszewski M, Holan K (1973) Cholesterol solubility in bile. Evidence that supersaturated bile is frequent in healthy man. J Clin Invest 52: 1467-1479
Holzbach RT, Kibe A, Thiel E, Howell JH, Marsh M, Hermann RE (1984) Biliary proteins. Unique inhibitors of cholesterol crystal nucleation in human gallbladder bile. J Clin Invest 73: 35-43
Hopman WPM, Rosenbusch G, Jansen JBM, de Jong AJL, Lamers CBHW (1985) Gallbladder contraction: effect of fatty meals and cholecystokinin. Radiology 157: 37-39

Howard P, Murphy GM, Dowling RH (1986) Impaired gallbladder motor function in gallstone disease (Abstr) International Bile Acid Meeting, Cortina

Hricak H, Filly RA, Margulis AR, Moon KL, Crooks LE, Komfman L (1983) Nuclear magnetic resonance imaging of the gallbladder. Radiology 147: 481-484

Hutton SW, Sievert CE Jr, Vennes JA, Duane WC (1981) The effect of sphincterotomy on gallstone formation in the prairie dog. Gastroenterology 81: 663-667

Ihasz M, Griffith CA (1981) Gallstones after vagotomy. Am J Surg 141: 48-50

Jacyna MR, Ross PE, Hopwood D, Bouchier AD (1985) Cholesterol absorption by the human gallbladder. Gut 26: A 1132

Jivegård L, Thornell E, Björk S, Svanvik J (1985) The effects of morphine and enkephaline on gallbladder function in experimental cholecystitis. Inhibition of inflammatory gallbladder secretion. Scand J Gastroenterol 20: 1049-1059

Khalil T, Walter JP, Wiener I, Fagan CJ, Townsend CM, Greeley GH Jr, Thompson JC (1985) Effect of aging on gallbladder contraction and release of cholecystokinin-33 in humans. Surgery 98: 423-429

Kibe A, Holzbach RT, LaRusso NF, Mao SJT (1984) Inhibition of cholesterol crystal formation by apolipoproteins in supersaturated model bile. Science 225: 514-516

Kraglund K, Hjermind J, Jensen FT, Stødkilde-Jørgensen H, Øster-Jørgensen E, Pedersen SA (1984) Gallbladder emptying and gastrointestinal cyclic motor activity in humans. Scand J Gastroenterol 19: 990-994

Krejs GJ, Orci L, Conlon JM, Ravazzola M, Davis GR, Raskin P, Collins SM, McCarthy BM, Baetens D, Rubinstein A, Aldor TAM, Unger RH (1979) Somatostatinoma syndrome. Biochemical, morphologic and clinical features. N Engl J Med 301: 285-292

Kurtz W, Leuschner U, Schneider S, Classen M (1985) Diurnal rhythm of bile lipid composition after cholecystectomy and papillotomy, Postpapillotomy biliary lithogenicity. Scand J Gastroenterol 20: 1001-1006

LaMont JT, Bradley BS, Di Benedetto D, Haudin R, Schafer AI (1983) Arachidonic acid stimulates mucin secretion in prairie dog gallbladder. Am J Physiol 245: G92-G98

LaMont JT, Smith BF, Moon JRL (1984) Role of gallbladder mucin in pathophysiology of gallstones. Hepatology 4: 51S-56S

Lee SP, Nicholls JF (1986) Nature and composition of biliary sludge. Gastroenterology 90: 677-686

Lee SP, Carey MC, LaMont JT (1981[a]) Aspirin prevention of cholesterol gallstone formation in prairie dog. Science 211: 1429-1431

Lee SP, LaMont JT, Carey MC (1981[b]) Role of gallbladder mucus hypersecretion in the evolution of cholesterol gallstones. J Clin Invest 67: 1712-1723

Mazer NA, Carey MC (1983) Quasielastic light scattering studies of aqueous biliary liquid systems. Cholesterol solubilization and precipitation in model bile solutions. Biochemistry 22: 425-442

Nakayama F, van der Linden W (1975) Stratification of bile in the gallstone and gallstone formation. Surg Gynecol Obstet 141: 587-590

Niederhiser DH, Harmon CK, Roth HP (1976) Absorption of cholesterol by the gallbladder. J Lipid Res 17: 117-124

Onodera H, Sugawara H, Hirata T, Imai N, Nagasaki A, Yoda B, Toyota T, Soto Y (1983) Diurnal profile of gallbladder size in diabetic patients: ultrasonographic evaluation of diabetic neurogenic gallbladder. Tohoku J Exp Med 139: 179-186

Pearson JP, Kaura R, Taylor W, Allen A (1982) The composition of polymeric structure of mucus glycoprotein from human gallbladder bile. Biochim Biophys Acta 706: 221-228

Peeters TL, Vantrappen G, Janssens J (1980) Bile acid output and interdigestive migrating motor complex in normals and in cholecystectomy patients. Gastroenterology 79: 678-681

Pellegrini CA, Lewin M, Patti MG, Thomas MJ, Ryan T, Way LW (1985) Gallbladder filling and response to cholecystokinin are not affected by vagotomy. Surgery 98: 452-458

Pellegrini CA, Ryan T, Broderick W, Way LW (1986) Gallbladder filling and emptying during cholesterol gallstone formation in the prairie dog. A cholescintigraphic study. Gastroenterology 90: 143-149

Pitt HA, Doty JE, DenBesten L, Kuchenbecker SL (1982) Stasis before gallstone formation: altered gallbladder compliance or cystic duct resistance? Am J Surg 143: 144-149

Pomeranz J, Shaffer EA (1985) Abnormal gallbladder emptying in a subgroup of patients with gallstones. Gastroenterology 88: 787-791
Rege RV, Moore EW (1986) Pathogenesis of calcium-containing gallstones. Canine ductular bile, but not gallbladder bile, is supersaturated with calcium carbonate. J Clin Invest 77: 21-26
Reuben A (1984) Biliary proteins. Hepatology 4: 46S-50S
Roslyn JJ, Pitt HA, Mann LL, Arvent ME, DenBesten L (1983) Gallbladder disease in patients on long-term parenteral nutrition. Gastroenterology 84: 148-154
Ryan JP (1981) Motility of the gallbladder and biliary tree. In: Johnson LR (ed) Physiology of the gastrointestinal tract. Raven, New York, pp 473-494
Ryan JP (1985) Calcium and gallbladder smooth muscle contraction in the guinea pig: effect of pregnancy. Gastroenterology 89: 1279-1285
Salvioli G, Lugli R, Pradelli JM (1984) Physicochemical aspects of cholesterol gallstone formation. In: Capocaccia L, Ricci G, Angelico F, Angelico M, Attili AF (eds) Epidemiology and prevention of gallstone disease. MTP Press, Lancaster, pp 37-48
Salvioli G, Romani M, Loria P, Carulli N, Pradelli JM (1985) Effect of acute administration of bile acids on fatty acid composition of biliary phosphatidylcholine in man. J Hepatol 1: 291-300
Slomiany BL, Aono M, Murthy LN, Piasek A, Slomiany A (1984) Effect of bile acids on the glycoprotein constituent of gastric mucus. J Appl Biochem 6: 308-313
Smith BF, LaMont JT (1985) Identification of gallbladder mucin-bilirubin complex in human cholesterol gallstone matrix. Effects of reducing agents on in vitro dissolution of matrix and intact gallstones. J Clin Invest 76: 439-445
Stempel JM, Duane WC (1978) Biliary lipids and bile acid pool size after vagotomy in man. Evidence against a predisposition to gallstones. Gastroenterology 89: 716-722
Sutor DJ, Wilkie LI (1976) Diurnal variations of the pH of pathological gallbladder bile. Gut 17: 971-974
Svenberg T, Nilsson I, Samuelson K, Welbourn RD (1984) Studies on the causal relationship between gall-bladder emptying and motilin release in man. Acta Chir Scand [Suppl] 520: 59-61
Svenberg T, Christofides ND, Fitzpatrick ML, Bloom SR, Welbourn RB (1985) Oral water causes emptying of the human gallbladder through action of vagal stimuli rather than motilin. Scand J Gastroenterol 20: 775-778
Thureborn E (1966) On the stratification of human bile and its importance for the solubility cholesterol. Gastroenterology 50: 775-780
Tilvis RS, Strandberg TE, Lempinen M, Miettinen TA (1982) In vitro synthesis of triglycerides and cholesterol in human gallbladder mucosa. Scand J Gastroenterol 17: 335-340
Virchow R (1857) Über das Epithel der Gallenblase und über einen intermediären Stoffwechsel des Fettes. Virchows Arch Pathol Anat 2: 374-578
Wood JR, Svanvik J (1983) Gall-bladder water and electrolyte transport and its regulation. Gut 24: 579-593

# Mechanism of Gallstone Formation in Obese Subjects

E. Roda, M. Malavolti, P. Simoni, G. Mazzella, N. Villanova, and M. Ronchi

Istituto di Clinica Medica e Gastroenterologia, Universita' degli Studi di Bologna, Ospedale S. Orsola, v. G. Massarenti 9, 40138 Bologna, Italy

The connection between cholesterol gallstones and obesity has been known for some time (Mabee et al. 1976; Burnett 1971; Gross 1929). Recent epidemiological studies carried out in Italy have confirmed this clinical knowledge by showing that there is a prevalence of gallstones in obese subjects. Obesity is a factor in the formation of gallstones (Roda 1983).

The aim of this work is to outline the possible mechanisms leading to the formation of gallstones in obese subjects. Several studies on obese subjects have demonstrated the following:

a) The majority of obese subjects have supersaturated bile.

b) Examination of daily biliary lipid secretion has shown that the excess of cholesterol in the bile of an obese subject is due not so much to decreased bile acid secretion but rather to increased cholesterol secretion.

c) The synthesis of cholesterol measured using the "sterol balance" method is particularly high in obese subjects (Bennion and Grundy 1975; Mabee et al. 1976; Miettinen 1971).

A close relationship between the synthesis of cholesterol and its bile secretion has not yet been shown. The mechanism which leads to the increased synthesis and secretion of cholesterol in obese subjects remains obscure.

We have studied groups of obese subjects during weight maintenance and weight reduction, evaluating the following factors:

- The bile acid pool size
- The composition of the bile acids in the gallbladder bile
- The degree of exposure of the bile acid pool to the intestinal bacterial flora, using the cholyl glycine breath test
- The bile lipid secretion

The metabolic characteristics of biliary lipid secretion in obese patients can be summarized in this way: the total bile acid pool size is significantly higher. Analysis of the biliary lipids shows a significant percentage increase of deoxycholic acid in bile. The breath-test with cholyl-glycine shows a marked increase in the elimination of $CO_2$ in breath.

Principally, our data confirm that the fundamental mechanism leading to the formation of lithogenic bile is an overproduction of cholesterol (Bennion and Grundy 1975). This study demonstrates that there is an increase in the bile acid pool with a normal secretion of bile acids in obese subjects. The biotransformation of hepatic cholesterol to bile acids is increased and efficient, but not to the point of compensating for the oversecretion of cholesterol; there is a relative increase in cholesterol secretion in obese patients. A new aspect that has emerged from this study is the enlargement of

Assessment and Management of Hepatobiliary Disease
Eds.: L. Okolicsányi, G. Csomós, and G. Crepaldi

the deoxycholic acid pool, which is probably due to greater exposure of the cholic acid pool to the intestinal bacterial flora because of an increased number of cycles of the bile acid molecules in the enterohepatic circulation. This is probably related to the frequency and the quantity of the meals consumed, which are significantly higher in obese subjects (Miettinen 1971).

The enrichment of deoxycholic acid in the enterohepatic circulation probably contributes greatly to substaining the oversecretion of cholesterol in obese subjects.

The effect of caloric restriction (1080 Kcal/day) was evaluated on the same biochemical parameters. During rapid weight loss, bile acid secretion decreased and cholesterol secretion slightly decreased, leading to an increase of the saturation of bile; therefore obese subjects continue to risk developing gallstones even during weight loss. At the same time, we found normalization of deoxycholic pool size and of the turnover of cholyl glycine.

We have also examined the effect of chronic administration of chenodeoxycholic acid (CDCA) and ursodeoxycholic acid (UDCA), two bile acids widely used in the treatment of cholesterol cholelithiasis, on biliary lipid secretion in obese patients during a period of weight maintenance and during a period of weight reduction (Fromm et al. 1983). During weight maintenance only UDCA induced a significant decrease in cholesterol saturation in bile by reducing cholesterol secretion. This data confirms previous reports showing a resistance to CDCA treatment in obese patients with gallstones (Iser et al. 1978). In contrast during weight loss both bile acids are able to decrease cholesterol saturation and secretion in bile.

These biochemical results suggest that UDCA is the ideal drug for preventing the formation of gallstones in obese people.

## References


Bennion LJ, Grundy SM (1975) Effects of obesity and caloric intake on biliary lipid metabolism in man. J Clin Invest 56: 996-1011

Burnett W (1971) The epidemiology of gallstones. Tijdschr Gastroenterol 14: 79-89

Fromm H, Roat JW, Gonzales V, Sarva RP, Farivar S (1983) Comparative efficacy and side effects of ursodeoxycholic and chenodeoxycholic acid in dissolving gallstones: a double blind controlled study. Gastroenterology 85: 1257-1264

Gross DMB (1929) A statistical study of cholelithiasis. J Pathol Bacteriol 32: 503-526

Iser JH, Maton PN, Murphy GM, Dowling RH (1978) Resistance to chenodeoxycholic acid (CDCA) treatment in obese patients with gallstones. Br Med J 1509-1512

Mabee TM, Mayer P, DenBest L et al. (1976) The mechanism of increased gallstone formation in obese human subjects. Surgery 79: 460-468

Miettinen TA (1971) Cholesterol production in obesity. Circulation 44: 842-850

Roda E (1983) Sirmione study. In: Capocaccia L, Ricci G, Angelico F, Angelico M, Attili AF (eds) Epidemiology and prevention of gallstone disease. MTP Press, Lancaster, pp 207-209

# Medical Treatment of Cholesterol Gallstones: Present and Future

U. Leuschner, H. Baumgärtel, W. Kurtz, M. Leuschner, and W. D. Strohm

Zentrum der Inneren Medizin der Johann Wolfgang Goethe-Universität Frankfurt am Main, Abteilung für Gastroenterologie, Theodor-Stern-Kai 7, 6000 Frankfurt/M 70, Federal Republic of Germany

For 15 years it has been possible to dissolve cholesterol gallstones with chenodeoxycholic acid or ursodeoxycholic acid. There are now about 30 different chenodeoxycholic and ursodeoxycholic acid preparations available worldwide [10].

Applying strict criteria of eligibility, a mean rate of 60% of cholesterol stones can be dissolved. This is shown, for example, in studies by Dowling et al. [4] and Barbara et al. [2] (Table 1), who used chenodeoxycholic acid and ursodeoxycholic acid to treat large and small stones with varying dosages and treatment times, and in our own investigations in 45 patients treated with CDCA and 145 patients treated with UDCA.

In the CDCA group, 17 patients (37.8%) refused therapy within a couple of weeks after onset of the treatment, i. e., were never treated regularly. Of the remaining 28 patients, 17 (60.7%) were treated successfully, 11 (39.3%) not. Of the 145 UDCA patients, six patients (4.1%) were lost to follow-up because they moved away and further data were not available. Four patients (2.8%) underwent surgery on the advice of their family physicians, although there were no contraindications against medical treatment and no complications. The success rate in regularly treated UDCA patients was 62.2% (Tables 2, 3).

**Table 1.** Response rate and dissolution rate (%)

| | Small stones | | | | Large stones | | | |
|---|---|---|---|---|---|---|---|---|
| | UDCA | | CDCA | | UDCA | | CDCA | |
| | Low* dose | High** dose | Low dose | High dose | Low dose | High dose | Low dose | High dose |
| | | | 3 months | | | | | |
| No. of cases | 27 | 22 | 25 | 28 | 31 | 28 | 28 | 26 |
| Response rate | 37.0 | 45.4 | 32.0 | 60.7 | 45.2 | 53.6 | 14.3 | 19.2 |
| Dissolution rate | 14.8 | 13.6 | 8.0 | 10.7 | 12.9 | 17.9 | 0 | 0 |
| | | | 6 months | | | | | |
| No. of cases | 27 | 22 | 24 | 28 | 31 | 28 | 28 | 26 |
| Response rate | 70.3 | 63.6 | 45.8 | 75.0 | 55.9 | 71.5 | 28.6 | 38.4 |
| Dissolution rate | 37.0 | 31.8 | 20.8 | 25.0 | 19.4 | 28.6 | 3.6 | 3.8 |
| | | | 12 months | | | | | |
| No. of cases | 27 | 22 | 24 | 28 | 31 | 28 | 28 | 26 |
| Response rate | 74.0 | 81.9 | 70.8 | 82.2 | 70.9 | 75.0 | 46.5 | 73.1 |
| Dissolution rate | 48.1 | 45.5 | 25.0 | 53.6 | 29.0 | 35.7 | 17.9 | 26.9 |

Source: Barbara et al. [2]  * 7-8 mg/kg/day
** 14-15 mg/kg/day

Assessment and Management of Hepatobiliary Disease
Eds.: L. Okolicsányi, G. Csomós, and G. Crepaldi

**Table 2.** Sex, age, body weight, height, dosage, stones, and treatment time in 28 CDCA-treated patients

| | Sex | Age (years) | Body weight (kg) | Height (cm) | Dosage (mg/kg/day) | Stones | | Treatment time (months) |
|---|---|---|---|---|---|---|---|---|
| | | | | | | No. | Area ($cm^2$) | |
| Success | M 3<br>F 14<br>(60.7%) | 49.2<br>(21-65) | 66.2<br>(55-95) | 165.6<br>(154-175) | 15.0±1.2<br>(10.5-18.6) | 11.4<br>(1-61) | 4.8<br>(1.1-11.5) | 19<br>(7-46) |
| Failure | M 4<br>F 7<br>(39.3%) | 46.9<br>(32-67) | 64.5<br>(52-76) | 167.7<br>(157-184) | 14.3±1.3<br>(11.0-19.9) | 6.1<br>(1-46) | 5.0<br>(1.4-14.2) | - |

**Table 3.** Sex, age, body weight, height, dosage, stones, and treatment time in 135 UDCA-treated patients

| | Sex | Age | Body weight (kg) | Height (cm) | Dosage (mg/kg/day) | Stones | | Treatment time (months) |
|---|---|---|---|---|---|---|---|---|
| | | | | | | No. | Area ($cm^2$) | |
| Complete dissolution | M 19<br>F 65<br>(62.2%) | 45.9<br>(20-75) | 65.8<br>(49-89) | 167.0<br>(148-182) | 11.2±1.6<br>(8.8-14.7) | 14.2<br>(1-58) | 3.2<br>(0.3-10.0) | 16<br>(6-31) |
| Failure (total) | M 28<br>F 23<br>(37.8%) | 46.9<br>(19-72) | 61.9<br>(58-95) | 168.3<br>(158-189) | 11.4±1.1<br>(10.1-13.5) | 10.8<br>(1-35) | 4.9<br>(1.0-15.1) | - |
| Failure (with calcification) | M 5<br>F 5<br>(7.4%) | 30.1<br>(20-36) | 75.0<br>(63-95) | 170.8<br>(162-189) | 11.6<br>(10.5-13.5) | 10.1<br>(5-23) | 3.1<br>(1.0-4.5) | - |
| Failure (without calcification) | M 23<br>F 18 | 58.9<br>(42-71) | 70.3<br>(60-82) | 167.0<br>(158-172) | 11.2<br>(10.1-12.5) | 12.2<br>(1-35) | 4.2<br>(2.0-15.1) | - |

High doses of UDCA are believed to induce secondary stone calcification. The ten cases of such calcification among the 51 failures (7.4% of all patients treated) in our UDCA group all occurred in young, overweight subjects with small stones which initially dissolved rapidly. However, there was no correlation between UDCA dose and calcification; six of the ten patients received 10.0-11.9 mg/kg body weight/day. One received 13.5 mg/kg/day, but in this particular case five of six stones dissolved and only one calcified. One patient receiving the low dose of 11.0 mg/kg/day had all 12 stones calcified after initial diminution. Therapeutic failures without calcification were regularly less overweight, elderly, and had large stones (Table 3).

The side effects of CDCA and UDCA treatment are given in Table 4. A follow-up of 4 years showed recurrence rates of 35% in the CDCA group and 22% in the UDCA group.

The effect of CDCA is dose-dependent. For UDCA, Erlinger et al. [6] showed in 1984 that an increase of dosage from 2.5 to 8.4 mg/kg/day improved the stone dissolution rate. When the dosage was doubled to 16.2 mg/kg/day the results deteriorated.

**Table 4.** Side effects of CDCA and UDCA treatment

| | Elevation of transaminases | Stool | | | | Complaints improved |
|---|---|---|---|---|---|---|
| | | Normal | Soft | Diarrhea | Constipated | |
| CDCA ($n=28$) | 9 (32.1%) | 15 (53.6%) | – | 13 (46.4%) | – | 15 (53.6%) |
| UDCA ($n=135$) | 6 (4.4%) | 82 (60.7%) | 26 (19.3%) | 8 (5.9%) | 19 (14.1%) | 68 (50.4%) |

**Table 5.** Sex, age, body weight, height, and therapeutic dosage of patients treated successfully with CDCA or UDCA

| No. | CDCA group | | | | | UDCA group | | | | |
|---|---|---|---|---|---|---|---|---|---|---|
| | Sex | Age | Weight (kg) | Height (cm) | Dosage (mg/kg/day) | Sex | Age | Weight (kg) | Height (cm) | Dosage (mg/kg/day) |
| 1. | F | 64 | 62 | 160 | 16.1 | F | 31 | 68 | 166 | 11.0 |
| 2. | F | 50 | 55 | 161 | 18.6 | F | 52 | 85 | 173 | 11.8 |
| 3. | F | 33 | 62 | 169 | 16.1 | F | 31 | 68 | 165 | 14.7 |
| 4. | F | 40 | 60 | 175 | 16.7 | F | 35 | 61 | 172 | 12.3 |
| 5. | F | 65 | 66 | 156 | 15.2 | M | 75 | 60 | 171 | 12.5 |
| 6. | F | 35 | 55 | 168 | 13.6 | F | 21 | 63 | 165 | 11.9 |
| 7. | F | 21 | 55 | 172 | 18.2 | F | 40 | 73 | 160 | 10.3 |
| 8. | F | 45 | 72 | 168 | 13.9 | F | 29 | 49 | 166 | 10.2 |
| 9. | F | 46 | 61 | 166 | 16.4 | F | 35 | 63 | 164 | 11.9 |
| 10. | M | 54 | 57 | 166 | 17.5 | F | 33 | 53 | 172 | 9.5 |
| 11. | F | 62 | 65 | 160 | 11.5 | F | 30 | 74 | 166 | 13.5 |
| 12. | | | | | | F | 55 | 87 | 169 | 11.5 |
| 13. | | | | | | F | 24 | 49 | 164 | 10.2 |
| 14. | | | | | | F | 55 | 67 | 165 | 11.2 |
| 15. | | | | | | F | 56 | 56 | 162 | 13.3 |
| 16. | | | | | | F | 59 | 55 | 169 | 9.0 |
| 17. | | | | | | F | 54 | 65 | 164 | 11.5 |
| Mean | | 46.8 | 60.9 | 165.5 | 15.8 | | 42.1 | 64.5 | 166.6 | 11.5 |

Therefore the optimal dosage of UDCA is around 10–12 mg/kg/day. Northfield et al. [15] reported that UDCA in the dosage of 12.5 mg/kg/day is superior to CDCA in the same dosage concerning stone reduction within the first 6 months of treatment. In 1983 this finding was confirmed by Barbara et al. [2] at a dosage of 14 mg/kg/day for both bile acids.

However, comparing the dissolution rate of the recommended dosages of CDCA (15 mg/kg/day) and UDCA (10 mg/kg/day) for a whole treatment period ending with stone dissolution or failure, we could find no differences in stone dissolution capacity. In 11 (61%) of 18 CDCA-treated patients and 17 (85%) of 20 UDCA-treated patients the stones dissolved completely. CDCA was administered in a mean dosage of 15.8 mg/kg/day, UDCA in a mean dosage of 11.5 mg/kg/day. The two groups of successfully treated patients were closely matched in sex, age, body weight, and height (Table 5).

Although success rate (CDCA 61%; UDCA 85%) and dissolution velocity (CDCA $0.096 \pm 0.07$ cm²/month; UDCA $0.026 \pm 0.03$ cm²/month) differed for CDCA and UDCA, there was a highly significant correlation for both bile acids when dissolution velocity was correlated to mean stone area ($r_{CDCA} = 0.85$, $r_{UDCA} = 0.83$; both $p < 0.001$), showing that CDCA and UDCA are equally effective in the treatment of cholesterol gallstones.

But since a treatment time of 18-24 months, in our studies of 16-19 months, is rather long; since the therapeutic success in CDCA- or UDCA-treated patients amounted to only 60%; and since in about 10% of UDCA-treated patients stone calcification occurred, three major attempts were made to improve the results:

1. Variation of the administration time with and without a special diet.
2. Combination of the two bile acids.
3. Addition of taurin.

Lanzini and Northfield [9] tried to improve the results by bedtime administration of CDCA and UDCA. Bedtime administration of CDCA had a better effect on gallstone reduction than mealtime administration, but there was no such effect in UDCA. However, biliary saturation index (SI) could be reduced by UDCA too when given at bedtime [15]. When bedtime CDCA therapy is combined with a low-cholesterol diet, SI can be further reduced; with UDCA, such a diet induces a rise of SI. In 1982 Kupfer et al. [8] showed in gallstone patients that bedtime CDCA combined with a low-cholesterol diet would improve the dissolution rate of gallstones.

In consequence, the optimal treatment seems to be 12.5 mg UDCA/kg/day up to the 6th month, and from then on at least 12.5 mg/kg/day CDCA at bedtime in combination with a low-cholesterol diet. However, all these data have to be confirmed by further studies.

Since CDCA induces gallstone dissolution more by inhibition of HMG-CoA-reductase and by micellar cholesterol solution, and UDCA more by inhibition of cholesterol resorption in the gut and by formation of liquid crystals, it was studied whether combination of the two substances might enhance the effect. In a combination preparation, the individual bile acids and thus the side effects, such as stone calcification by ursodeoxycholic acid, could be reduced.

In 1980, Stiehl et al. [18] demonstrated that a combination of CDCA and UDCA reduces the saturation index significantly ($p < 0.05$) compared to controls on monotherapy, and the amount of the less water-soluble glycourso decreased from 58.8% (monotherapy) to 34.2% of total bile acids. There was no elevation of transaminases as seen in CDCA therapy. In 1985 and 1986 respectively, Czygan et al. [3] and Roehrkasse et al. [16] presented the first clinical data. Czygan et al. treated 24 patients with UDCA and 25 patients with a combination. With UDCA there was stone dissolution in 40.5%, with the combination in 58.3%. However, the difference was statistically not significant. Three of the 24 patients on UDCA showed stone calcification (Table 6). Roehrkasse et al. treated 16 patients for 19 months with a combination preparation. Since the stones dissolved within 24 months in only 4 out of 16 patients, the results are not convincing. No assessment of stone calcification is possible from these studies.

Another step to prevent stone calcification was administration of UDCA and taurin (TUDCA), which is better water-soluble than glyco-ursodeoxycholic acid (GUDCA). In 1985, Thistle and La Russo [19] compared a regimen of 10 mg UDCA/kg/day plus 2 g taurin to a combination therapy of UDCA 5 mg/CDCA 10 mg/kg/day. They

**Table 6.** Dissolution of cholesterol stones with UDCA alone vs UDCA+CDCA

| Patients | UDCA (12.4 mg/kg/day) 22 F 2 M | UDCA+CDCA (6.8/8.0 mg/kg/day) 22 F 3 M |
|---|---|---|
| Age (years) | 58.9 ± 10.4 | 59.9 ± 10.2 |
| Complete dissolution | 40.5% | 58.3% ($p > 0.1$) |
| Calcification | 3 (9, 11, 15 months) | - |

Source: Czygan et al. [3]

found that use of taurin would reduce the ratio glyco-ursodeoxycholate (GUDC)/tauro-ursodeoxycholate (TUDC) but no treatment regimen would increase the absolute TUDCA concentration. Combination treatment showed the best stone dissolution results and the most marked desaturation of bile. This study revealed no information with respect to prevention of stone calcification by taurin. In 1985, however, Frabboni et al. [7], describing investigations covering a total of 262 patients, reported calcification rates of 13.2% (14/106) with UDCA, 8.8% (11/125) with CDCA, and 12.9% (4/31) with TUDCA. The differences were statistically not significant.

So far, we are not convinced that combination therapy of UDCA plus CDCA will dissolve cholesterol stones better than monotherapy or really prevent calcification. Even the admixture of taurin is of no avail.

Which options do we have for treatment of cholesterol common bile duct stones? The most successful method is endoscopic stone extraction after sphincterotomy. In a total of 7316 EPTs, complete stone removal was achieved in 91% [11]. Stones that cannot be dealt with in this way can be treated with bile acid solutions or mono-octanoin. The solvents can be administered either via T-tube or by nasobiliary tube. This method will eliminate stones in 50%-60% of cases [12].

What perspectives are there for the future? In 1985, Allen et al. [1] reported the dissolution of cholesterol stones with methyl-tert-butyl-ether (MTBE). In May 1986, [20] they reported on 19 patients and up to the time of writing they had already treated 26 patients (personal communication). Treatment was administered via percutaneous transhepatic 1.7 mm pigtail catheter which was placed via the gallbladder bed. MTBE was alternately instilled and aspirated in doses of 2-5 ml. Complete or more than 90% dissolution of stones was achieved in more than 90% of cases within 1-2 days. About 70% of the patients had residual debris. All patients resumed normal activity 2 days later.

In April 1986, van Sonnenberg et al. [22] reported on one patient with a large gallstone that was impacted in the cystic duct. Treatment with MTBE was successful. Tritapepe et al. [21] used MTBE to treat three patients with common bile duct stones. In all patients the treatment had to be continued with mono-octanoin because MTBE had no effect. In May 1985 [13] we reported the MTBE treatment of one patient with several huge common bile duct stones; it was unsuccessful. After surgical removal the stones would not dissolve in MTBE, but did dissolve in a buffered 1% EDTA solution (Table 7). We believe that treatment with MTBE is an excellent method for selected patients with cholesterol gallbladder stones. The frequently remaining residue, obviously calcium bilirubinate, can be dissolved by renewed irrigation with an EDTA solu-

**Table 7.** Treatment of gallstones with methyl-tert-butyl-ether (MTBE)

| Author(s) | Patients | Site | MTBE therapy | Result | Side effects |
|---|---|---|---|---|---|
| Thistle et al. [20] | 19 | GB | 5-10 ml<br>4- 6 ×/min | Complete or >90% dissolution 18/19 | Nausea (50%), raised serum aminotransferase (4/19), duodenitis (1/19), hemolysis (1/19), anesthesia (1/19) |
| Thistle (personal communication) | 7 | GB | 5-10 ml<br>4- 6 ×/min | Complete or >90% dissolution 6/7 | Nausea, burning |
| van Sonnenberg et al. [22] | 1 | GB | 2-5 ml/ 30 min | Dissolution | Burning, tolerable pain |
| Tritapepe et al. [21] | 3 | CBD | 11 ml/6 h<br>8 ml/3 h<br>22 ml/8 h | No dissolution | Nausea, somnolence, duodenitis (1/3) |
| Leuschner et al. [13] | 1 | CBD | 2-5 ml/h | No dissolution | Nausea, anesthesia, death |

GB, gallbladder, CBD, common bile duct

**Table 8.** Composition of solvent for calcium bilirubinate sludge

| pH | Component | mmol/l | % |
|---|---|---|---|
| 9.5 | EDTA-2Na | 26.9 | 1.0 |
| | Cholic acid | 12.3 | 0.5 |
| | Ursodeoxycholic acid | 12.7 | 0.5 |
| | Carnosine | 18.0 | 0.5 |
| | Arginine | 109.0 | 1.9 |
| | Water, NaOH | | |

tion (Table 8). This solution will not only dissolve calcium bilirubinate debris, but will also disaggregate admixtures of black pigment, as we have demonstrated in vitro with brown and black pigment stones [14].

In 1986, Sauerbruch et al. [17] reported the shock-wave treatment of cholesterol gallstones in nine patients. In only one patient was fragmentation and expulsion complete, and in three of the nine cases there were residual concretions. Also in 1986, Ell et al. [5] reported on lithotripsy using a pulsating Neodym-Yag laser. Energy is transferred via a 0.3-mm-thick universally flexible glass fiber that touches the stones. This glassfiber can be introduced via any endoscope into the intrahepatic bile ducts, perhaps even into the gallbladder. In vitro experiments with approximately 200 stones have been completed. Up to now only two patients have been treated, but in about a year the instrument could be available for other groups too.

We believe that the future medical treatment of cholesterol gallstones has a sound basis. For more efficient use of the bile acids available at present, we need further epidemiologic data in order to improve patient selection. The investigations into improvement of dissolution capacity must continue. New investigations with NOR bile acids and with methylated bile acids, more resistant to bacterial 7-dehydroxylation, are on the way. Direct irrigation with potent cholesterol solvents and development of pigment solvents, per se and in combination with extracorporeal lithotripsy, will enable us to find a suitable method for every stone patient.

Prevention of gallstone recurrence after complete dissolution is still at the stage of animal experiments, but there are hints that administration of low-dosage salicylate or indomethacin might prevent stone recurrence.

## References


1. Allen MJ, Borody TJ, Bugliosi TF, May GR, LaRussow NF, Thistle JF (1985) Rapid dissolution of gallstones by methyl-tert-butyl-ether. N Engl J Med 312: 217-220
2. Barbara L, Bazzoli F, Festi D, Morselli AML, Roda E (1983) A comparative study of chenodeoxycholic acid and ursodeoxycholic acid as cholesterol gallstone dissolving agents. In: Paumgartner G, Stiehl A, Gerok W (eds) Bile acids and cholesterol in health and disease. MTP Press, Lancaster, pp367-370
3. Czygan P, Stiehl A, Raedsch R, Seitz H, Kommerell B (1985) Dissolution of cholesterol gallstones by combination therapy of urso/cheno versus urso. In: Paumgartner G, Stiehl A, Gerok W (eds) Enterohepatic circulation of bile acids and sterol metabolism. MTP Press, Lancaster, pp351-353
4. Dowling RH, Ruppin DC, Meredith T, Myszor M, Forgacs I, Murphy GM (1983) Efficacy of bile acid treatment in dissolving gallstones: collateral benefits of CDCA and UDCA therapy; gallstone recurrence and postdissolution management. In: Paumgartner G, Stiehl A, Gerok W (eds) Bile acids and cholesterol in health and disease. MTP Press, Lancaster, pp345-362
5. Ell C, Hochberger J, Müller D, Lux G, Demling L (1986) Laserlithotripsie von Gallensteinen. Fortschr Med 104: 203-204
6. Erlinger S, Go AL, Hussen JM, Fevery J (1984) Franco-Belgian cooperative study of ursodeoxycholic acid in the medical dissolution of gallstones: a double-blind randomised, dose-response study, and comparison with chenodeoxycholic acid. Hepatology 4: 308-314
7. Frabboni R, Bazzoli F, Mazzella G, Festi D, Villanova N, Roda E, Barbara L (1985) Acquired gallstone calcification during cholelitholytic treatment with chenodeoxycholic, ursodeoxycholic and tauroursodeoxycholic acids (Abstr). Hepatology 5: 1004
8. Kupfer RM, Maudgal DP, Northfield TC (1982) Gallstone dissolution rate during chenic acid therapy: effect of bedtime administration plus low cholesterol diet. Dig Dis Sci 27: 1025-1029
9. Lanzini A, Northfield TC (1984) Effect of ursodeoxycholic acid on secretory coupling of bile acid with cholesterol and phospholipid in gallstone patients. Poster at VIIIth International Bile Acid Meeting, August 31-September 2, Berne
10. Leuschner U (1984) Medikamentöse Auflösung von Gallensteinen. Arzneimitteltherapie 2: 143-152
11. Leuschner U (1986) Endoscopic therapy of biliary calculi. Clin Gastroenterol 333-358
12. Leuschner U, Baumgärtel H, Klempa J (1984) Chemical treatment of choledocholithiasis. In: Classen M, Geenen J, Kawai K (eds) Nonsurgical biliary drainage, Springer, Berlin Heidelberg New York Tokyo, pp81-85
13. Leuschner U, Baumgärtel H, Fischer H, David R, Leuschner M, Hübner K (1985) The dissolution of CBD cholesterol and pigment stones with methyl-tertiary-butyl-ether (MTBE) in vitro and in vivo (Abstr). Gastroenterology 88: 1674
14. Leuschner U, Baumgärtel H, Wosiewitz U (1985) Dissolution of black pigment stones (BPS) of the gallbladder (Abstr). Galstroenterology 88: 1674
15. Northfield TC, Lanzini A, Jazrawi R, Maudgal DP, Kupfer R (1985) Methods of improving the efficacy of litholytic therapy. In: Paumgartner G, Stiehl A, Gerok W (eds) Enterohepatic circulation of bile acids and sterol metabolism. MTP Press, Lancaster, pp335-350
16. Roehrkasse, R, Fromm H, Malavolti M, Tunuguntla AK, Ceryak S (1985) Cholelitholytic

treatment with a combination of ursodeoxycholic (UDC) and chenodeoxycholic (CDC) acids: effects on lithogenic index, bile acid pool, liver tests and gallstones (Abstr). Hepatology 5: 985
17. Sauerbruch T, Delius M, Paumgartner G, Holl J, Wess O, Weber W, Hepp W, Brendel W (1986) Fragmentation of gallstones by extracorporeal shock waves. N Engl J Med 314: 818-822
18. Stiehl A, Raedsch R, Czygan P, Götz R, Männer C, Walker S, Kommerell B (1980) Effects of biliary cholesterol saturation in gallstone patients treated with chenodeoxycholic acid and/or ursodeoxycholic acid. Gastroenterology 79: 1192-1198
19. Thistle JL, La Russo NF (1985) Combination of taurine or chenodeoxycholic acid with ursodeoxycholic acid therapy: effects on biliary lipids, bile acids and gallstones. In: Paumgartner G, Stiehl A, Gerok W (eds) Enterohepatic circulation of bile acids and sterol metabolism. MTP Press, Lancaster, pp 355-359
20. Thistle JL, Nelson PE, May GR (1986) Dissolution of cholesterol gallbladder stones (CGS) using methyl-tert-butyl-ether. Meeting of AGA, AASLD, May 18-21, San Francisco
21. Tritapepe R, di Padova C, di Padova F (1985) Methyl tertiary butyl ether fails to dissolve cholesterol retained biliary tract stones (Abstr). Hepatology 5: 981
22. Van Sonnenberg E, Hofmann AF, Neoptolemus J, Wittich GR, Princenthal RA, Willson SW (1986) AJR 146: 865-867

# Bile Acid Treatment of Cholesterol Gallstones: A Reappraisal

Flavio Lirussi, Rosa Maria Iemmolo, Rocco Orlando, Gino Nassuato, Maurizio Muraca, Mario Strazzabosco, and Lajos Okolicsányi
Institute of Internal Medicine, University of Padua, Padua, Italy

## Introduction

The options currently available for the medical treatment of symptomatic cholesterol cholelithiasis, as an alternative to cholecystectomy, include oral administration of chenodeoxycholic acid (CDCA) or ursodeoxycholic acid (UDCA), instillation of methyl-*tert*-butylether (MTBE) directly into the gallbladder via a percutaneous transhepatic catheter or retrograde endoscopic cannulation (Allen et al. 1985; Thistle et al. 1985), and fragmentation of gallstones by extracorporeal shock waves (Sauerbruch et al. 1986).

Despite being a highly effective litholytic agent, MTBE is a potentially explosive cholesterol solvent capable of producing anesthesia, hemolysis, and acute duodenitis if excessive amounts escape from the biliary tree and are absorbed systemically (Allen et al. 1985; Thistle et al. 1985). On the other hand, shock wave fragmentation requires hospitalization and general anesthesia and may be complicated by acute pancreatitis and hematuria (Sauerbruch et al. 1986). Moreover, experience with these new techniques is limited, whereas the potential benefits and side effects of medical treatment of cholesterol gallstones with bile acids are at least partly known.

This chapter reviews briefly: (a) the "revisited" criteria of eligibility for bile acid treatment; (b) the factors affecting efficacy; (c) the experience with new bile acid preparations, new litholytic bile acids, and combination therapy; (d) the problems related to gallstone recurrence and post-dissolution management.

## Patient Selection

Originally, the criteria for inclusion in a trial of therapy with litholytic bile acids were: (1) radiolucent gallstones; (2) a radiologically functioning gallbladder; (3) absence of surgical complications such as severe and/or recurrent biliary colic, and gallstone-induced pancreatitis, jaundice, cholangitis; (4) no liver and/or gastrointestinal disease; (5) no severe cardiac, pulmonary, or renal disease; (6) no concurrent treatment with potentially hepatotoxic drugs. Finally, (7) women in the reproductive age group had to have adequate mechanical contraceptive devices to be eligible for cholelitholytic therapy.

However, based on experience gained over the last 15 years, some of the above-mentioned criteria – namely 1, 2, 4, and 6 – have become progressively less strict and may be regarded, at least in some instances, as relative and not absolute.

Assessment and Management of Hepatobiliary Disease
Eds.: L. Okolicsányi, G. Csomós, and G. Crepaldi

In the American National Cooperative Gallstone Study (NCGS; Schoenfield et al. 1981), where more than 900 gallstone patients entered a 2-year trial with CDCA, complete gallstone dissolution was observed in patients who had stones containing small radiopaque nuclei at enrollment. Similarly, acquired calcification does not invariably halt gallstone dissolution (Gleeson et al. 1983).

Nonvisualization of the gallbladder does not prevent subsequent partial or complete gallstone dissolution: in the NCGS revisualization occurred in 60% of such cases by the end of the 2-year study (Schoenfield et al. 1981).

Hypertransaminasemia represents a dose-related, self-limiting complication of CDCA treatment, whereas it is virtually absent during UDCA treatment (Roda et al. 1982; Fromm et al. 1983; Erlinger et al. 1984). On these grounds, Leuschner et al. (1985) used UDCA to treat patients with cholelithiasis and histologically confirmed chronic active hepatitis. Apart from a high rate of complete gallstone dissolution, they noted that transaminase decreased significantly throughout the first year of UDCA and rose again after completion of the treatment. This is in keeping with observations by our group on the safety of short-term high-dose UDCA treatment for intrahepatic bile duct stones (Lirussi et al. 1981) and long-term CDCA administration in patients with intra- and/or extrahepatic cholesterol cholelithiasis (Okolicsanyi et al. 1982). In four of these cases bile acid therapy was started notwithstanding signs of cholestasis and/or liver cell necrosis and was associated with a progressive return to normal of liver function tests. Furthermore, reports from Maton et al. (1977) indicated that UDCA could lead to a decrease in gamma-GT and alkaline phosphatase in patients with cholesterol gallstones.

Despite the lack of controlled clinical trials, these findings would suggest that liver function test abnormalities do not contraindicate, per se, UDCA therapy and would hint that UDCA possesses a hepatoprotective effect.

Another area of continuing concern was whether bile acid therapy could be associated with lithogenic drugs such as the estrogens contained in the commonly used combination contraceptives (Heikel and Lathe 1970, Okolicsanyi et al. 1986). Theoretically, several effects of oral contraceptive administration seem to be opposite to those of litholytic bile acids (Bennion et al. 1976). However, in a recent cooperative study on gallstone dissolution with CDCA and UDCA, ten women were on oral contraceptives and stones dissolved in three of them (Erlinger et al. 1984). The possibility of pregnancy, on the other hand, still contraindicates the use of bile acids, as these drugs cross the placenta and the effects on a developing fetus are not known, at least in humans.

## Efficacy

"Drug efficacy," i.e., the potential of bile acids to dissolve gallstones under favorable circumstances, is unlikely to be over 80%, as 15%-20% of radiolucent stones are pigment stones which are not suitable for dissolution with bile acids. "Treatment efficacy," i.e., the chances of a patient on bile acid therapy achieving confirmed complete dissolution is 25%-30% after 1-2 years' treatment with either CDCA or UDCA in patients unselected for gallstone size (Fromm et al. 1983; Gleeson et al. 1983; Erlinger et al. 1984; Lirussi et al. 1986a).

Previous studies claimed that dissolution rates were twice as high as those currently reported. However, in most of these trials, subjects dropping out or withdrawing from the study were not included in the final calculation (Tokyo Cooperative Study Group 1980; Ponz de Leon et al. 1980). Expressing the results in terms of partial plus complete dissolution may also be misleading, as although the rate of partial gallstone dissolution may be high, the conversion rate from partial to complete dissolution may be low, thus defeating the aim of freeing the patient from his/her stone(s) (Gleeson et al. 1983).

Dropouts and withdrawals due to side effects (diarrhea with CDCA, acquired gallstone opacification especially with UDCA but also with CDCA) or for other reasons (lack of compliance, no change of stone diameter after 6-12 months' treatment, pregnancy, onset of surgical complications, etc.) are to be regarded as treatment failures and therefore must be taken into account when assessing treatment efficacy.

As a result of these considerations and with the goal of improving efficacy, research in the bile acid field has been recently directed at (a) definition of the characteristics of the patients (and their stones) most likely to benefit from bile acid treatment, (b) optimization of the dose and timing of bile acid administration, and (c) testing of new potentially litholytic bile acids.

## Attempts to Improve Efficacy

### Assessment of Favorable Prognostic Factors

In a retrospective analysis of 135 patients with radiolucent gallstones, given adequate doses of CDCA or UDCA for up to 2 years, we were able to identify a number of prognostic factors favoring gallstone dissolution. The "classical" logrank test (univariate analysis) showed that age less than 40 years, female sex, and, above all, gallstones less than 10 mm in diameter signficiantly improved the complete dissolution rate. When data were analyzed with the "more powerful" Cox's model (multivariate analysis), which can assess the potential combined effect of a set of variables, once again small stones, female sex, and, this time, normal gallbladder opacification were significantly linked with complete gallstone dissolution. Nondyspeptic patients treated with UDCA would also seem to do better than symptomatic patients in terms of partial plus complete dissolution rates (Lirussi et al. 1986a).

Gallstone size has been recognized by many other groups as one of the most important factors governing the efficacy of CDCA and UDCA in dissolving gallstones. Maton et al. (1982) found a nearly twofold increase in the rate of dissolution when patients with stones larger than 15 mm were excluded from the analysis. Similarly, the Tokyo Cooperative Study Group (1980) and, more recently, the Franco-Belgian Cooperative Study (Erlinger et al. 1984) showed that response to UDCA treatment was significantly greater for stones less than 5 mm in diameter than for those exceeding this size.

As a corollary to these findings, it is generally accepted that single stones are less frequently dissolved than multiple stones (Erlinger et al. 1984; Dowling 1984), whereas floating stones seem to be most suitable for bile acid treatment (Schoenfield et al. 1981; Fromm et al. 1983).

The NCGS, using a logistic regression model, also reported that the variable "female sex" contributed significantly to improving complete gallstone dissolution. This result is important, as cholelithiasis predominates in women (Friedman et al. 1966; Barbara 1984) and a potentially greater number of patients, possibly including women "on the pill" (see above) could be selected for bile acid therapy with a better chance than men of having their stones dissolved.

Further controlled clinical trials of bile acid treatment are needed to confirm the results of these analyses.

## Optimum Dosage and Timing of Bile Acid Administration

The recommended daily doses of CDCA and UDCA are approximately 15 mg/kg and 10 mg/kg respectively. The optimum dose of CDCA is about 50% more than the higher dose used in the NCGS (Schoenfield et al. 1981). This may explain, at least in part, the disappointing results obtained in that trial, with a rate of complete gallstone dissolution of 14% at 2 years. An even lower rate of dissolution (10.9%) was observed in Canada after 2 years' treatment with suboptimal doses of CDCA (Fisher et al. 1985).

The results of most, but not all (Salen et al. 1980) dose-response studies suggest that increasing the dose of UDCA to 15-16 mg/kg/day does not increase success rate (Maton et al. 1977; Roda et al. 1982; Erlinger et al. 1984).

Whether the time of drug administration – namely bedtime mealtime – may affect the gallstone dissolution rate is still controversial. Kupfer et al. (1982) first observed that bedtime administration of CDCA together with a low cholesterol diet significantly increased gallstone dissolution rate, at least in the first 6 months of therapy, when compared to the conventional regimen of divided doses at mealtime plus an unrestricted diet.

Further studies from the same group showed that bedtime administration of CDCA significantly reduced gallstone volume at 6 months by comparison with mealtime administration, but this was not true for UDCA (Northfield et al. 1985). Mazzella et al. (1983), however, have shown that UDCA given at bedtime is more effective than a mealtime schedule in decreasing the biliary cholesterol saturation index.

## New "Old" Bile Acid Preparation and New Litholytic Bile Acids

When litholytic bile acids are given at mealtimes in divided doses, two problems still remain: to maintain a desaturated bile during the overnight fast, and to improve patient compliance, which is known to affect the efficacy of a treatment, especially if long-term. In order to obviate these difficulties, a new repeated-release (immediate, and at 4 and 7 h after ingestion) preparation of UDCA has been developed (Table 2). It has been shown to possess good bioavailability (Sama et al. 1983) and to be more effective in desaturating bile than other UDCA preparations, despite a lower content of UDCA (Bazzoli et al. 1983; Mazzella et al. 1983; Zuin et al. 1984).

In a multicenter trial carried out in Switzerland and Italy on the efficacy of this new UDCA preparation, complete dissolution occurred in 31% of the patients unselected for gallstone size and in 40% of those with gallstones less than 5 mm in diameter after 6 months of treatment (Amoruso et al. 1983). The drug was well tolerated and induced partial gallstone dissolution in another 33% of the patients. However, it remains to be seen whether this new repeated-release preparation will offer significant advantages over the "conventional" immediate-release form of UDCA.

**Table 1.** Bile acids proposed for the medical treatment of cholesterol gallstones

| |
|---|
| 1. UDCA repeated-release |
| 2. Tauroursodeoxycholic acid (TUDCA) |
| 3. UDCA + taurine |
| 4. UDCA + CDCA |
| 5. Ursocholic acid (UCA) |

Table 1 shows some of the other bile acids recently proposed for the medical treatment of cholesterol gallstones.

Tauroursodexycholic acid (TUDCA) has been shown to be more soluble than glycoursodeoxycholate and therefore may be more bioavailable, more effective in forming liquid crystals and less likely to precipitate than its glyco conjugate (Igimi and Carey 1980). However, although clinical experience with this bile acid is limited, preliminary results show that TUDCA possesses no advantages over CDCA or UDCA, especially in terms of acquired stone calcification: Frabboni et al. (1986) recently reported that the frequency of gallstone calcification was 13.2%, 8.8%, and 12.9% respectively in a total of 262 UDCA-, CDCA-, and TUDCA-treated patients. A possible explanation for these disappointing results is that TUDCA seems to be deconjugated to UDCA in the intestine and then reconjugated mainly with glycine in the liver, thus failing to enrich bile with TUDCA.

Conversely, the regimen of UDCA plus taurine decreases the cholesterol saturation index significantly, induces a higher percent of litholytic bile acids than UDCA alone, and prevents an increase in the ratio of glycine to taurine (Thistle and LaRusso 1985). Taurine supplementation should therefore reduce the risk of formation of precipitates of glycine conjugates of UDCA, thereby preventing gallstone calcification. Attili et al. (1985) randomly allocated 31 patients with radiolucent gallstones to two treatment groups: UDCA plus a dietary supplementation of taurine and UDCA alone. No acquired calcification was observed in the group treated with the first regimen, whereas three UDCA-treated patients developed radiopaque shells around the stones. However, there was no significant difference between the two treatment groups in terms of gallstone dissolution rate.

The rationale for combination therapy with CDCA and UDCA is based both on the physicochemical properties of the two bile acids and on their clinical use. Micelles containing predominantly CDCA have a greater uptake rate and capacity for cholesterol than those composed mainly of its 7-beta epimer (Igimi and Carey 1980). UDCA, on the other hand, can dissolve cholesterol by liquid crystal formation as well as micellar solubilization (Park et al. 1981) and causes cholesterol gallstone dissolution at a dose which is about half as great as that of its alpha epimer (Fromm et al. 1983; Erlinger et al. 1984). Moreover, in contrast to CDCA, UDCA does not cause diarrhea or hypertransminasemia.

The combination of CDCA and UDCA at approximately half-dose each should therefore be less expensive than UDCA, cause fewer side effects than CDCA, and may be more effective than either bile acid alone.

Podda et al. (1986) reported a true efficacy of 51% with combination therapy as compared to 40% with UDCA alone at 2 years in patients with gallstones less than

15 mm in diameter. Czygan (1986) suggested that the efficacy of the combined CDCA-UDCA therapy could be further enhanced by a single daily administration at bedtime: in a prospective trial, complete dissolution occurred in 64% of the patients who received both bile acids at bedtime as compared to 50% of the patients given CDCA+UDCA in three divided doses. Thistle and LaRusso (1985) reported that 8 of 10 patients receiving a combination therapy showed continuing or complete stone dissolution and no calcification after 12–24 months of treatment. In these studies, none of the patients developed liver function test abnormalities or experienced diarrhea which required dose reduction.

UCA, the 7-beta epimer of cholic acid, is a newly synthesized bile acid which has been shown to solubilize less cholesterol than UDCA (Carulli et al. 1983). Enrichment of the bile acid pool with UCA may therefore result in decreased cholesterol solubilization and secretion and hence favor cholesterol gallstone dissolution. However, after short-term oral UCA administration: (1) the cholesterol saturation index decreases only slightly, (2) UCA constitutes 20%–30% of the biliary bile acids, and (3) deoxycholic acid becomes the predominant bile acid in bile (Howard et al. 1984; Loria et al. 1986). Preliminary results of a clinical trial in Italy show that UCA is able to dissolve gallstones in only a small percentage of patients (Lanzini et al. 1986).

Another characteristic of UCA is its marked choleretic effect, which has been demonstrated both in animals and in man (Kitany et al. 1983; Tamberi et al. 1985). This may have contributed (by means of a washout effect) to the successful outcome of short-term UCA treatment in patients with retained stones of the biliary tree (Lirussi et al. 1986b).

## Gallstone Recurrence and Post-Dissolution Management

When cholesterol gallstones have been dissolved completely and bile acid treatment is stopped, bile returns to its pretreatment state (i.e., supersaturated with cholesterol). Under these conditions, and independently of the type of treatment used to dissolve the gallstones, gallstones tend to form again, although not inevitably. The 5-year recurrence rate, calculated by actuarial analysis, is about 50% (Ruppin and Dowling 1982; Toulet et al. 1983; Thistle 1985). Dowling and coworkers, however, have recently (1986) suggested that there may be a "protected" subgroup of patients who will never develop recurrent stones: subjects who had been free of stones for more than 9 months had significantly lower recurrence rates than those who had been stone-free for less than 9 months at 1, 2, and 3 years of follow-up.

The results of post-dissolution trials, designed to identify the best type of treatment for prevention of gallstone recurrence, are controversial. Low-dose (250 mg/day) and medium-dose (375 mg/day) CDCA were ineffective in preventing gallstone recurrence (Perez-Aguilar et al. 1985; Marks et al. 1984), whereas medium-dose UDCA (300 mg/day) completely prevented gallstone recurrence in 9 patients followed up for 18 months (Perez-Aguilar et al. 1985). However, preliminary results from the British/Belgian Gallstone Study Group's post-dissolution trial (Dowling et al. 1986) suggest that neither low-dose UDCA (3 mg/kg/day) nor a diet containing a low refined carbohydrate intake plus added bran can effectively prevent recurrence.

## Summary

The gallstone patients most likely to benefit from bile acid therapy are those with small, floating radiolucent stones within an opacifying gallbladder. Women appear to respond better than men. Concurrent oral contraceptive intake or liver dysfunction does not seem to contraindicate bile acid treatment, especially with UDCA.

CDCA and UDCA are equally effective in dissolving cholesterol gallstones when given at adequate doses. Unlike CDCA, UDCA is virtually free from adverse effects such as transient diarrhea and hypertransaminasemia, but is associated with acquired gallstone calcification. Combination treatment with CDCA and UDCA at half dose each is encouraging and may offer several advantages which relate to efficacy, safety and costs of gallstone dissolution therapy. Bedtime administration of either CDCA or UDCA (immediate/repeated-release) or both seems to further enhance successful gallstone dissolution rate.

Prevention of gallstone recurrence after confirmed dissolution and post-dissolution management are under investigation.

## References

Allen MJ, Borody TJ, Bugliosi TF, May GR, LaRusso NF, Thistle JL (1985) Rapid dissolution of gallstones by methyl tert-butyl ether. N Engl J Med 312: 217-220

Amoruso A, Arnold J, Bettini L, Borel GA, Bretholds A, Capitaine A, Di Simone A, Facchinetti D, Francavilla A, Gonvers JJ, Hofstetter JR, Lanzini A, Muiesan G, Plaitano G, Realini S, Ruggeri G, Sansonno D, Viviani G (1983) A multicenter study on a new repeated-release preparation of ursodeoxycholic acid for gallstones dissolution. Curr Ther Res 33: 565-570

Attili AF, Angelico M, Alvaro D, Capocaccia L (1985) Taurine supplementation during treatment of gallstones with ursodeoxycholic acid. In: Barbara L et al. (eds) Recent advances in bile acid research. Raven Press, New York, pp 313-316

Barbara L for the Progetto Sirmione (1984) Epidemiology of gallstone disease: The Sirmione study. In: Capocaccia L et al. (eds) Epidemiology and prevention of gallstone disease. MTP Press, Lancaster, pp 23-25

Bazzoli F, Morselli Labate AM, Malvolti M, Roda A, Monti F, Rucci P, Roda E (1983) The effect of ursodeoxycholic administration on bile lipid composition in man: comparison of three different ursodeoxycholic preparations. Curr Ther Res 33: 543-550

Bennion LJ, Ginsberg RL, Garnick MB, Bennet PH (1976) Effects of oral contraceptives on the gallbladder bile of normal women. N Engl J Med 294: 189-192

Carulli N, Loria P, Medici G, Iori R, Salvioli G (1983) Ursocholic acid (UCA) cholesterol dissolving capacity and effect on bile lipid composition. Gastroenterology 84: 1367

Czygan P (1986) Efficacy of combined ursodeoxycholic and chenodeoxycholic acid treatment. Proceedings of the 9th International Bile Acid Meeting, 19-21 October 1986, Basel

Dowling RH (1984) Epidemiology and medical treatment of cholesterol gallstones: recurrence, post-dissolution management and the future. In: Capocaccia L et al. (eds) Epidemiology and prevention of gallstone disease. MTP Press, Lancaster, pp 116-128

Dowling RH, Gleeson D, Hood K, Ruppin DC and the British/Belgian Gallstone Study Group (1986) Gallstone recurrence and post-dissolution management. Proceedings of the 9th International Bile Acid Meeting, 19-21 October 1986, Basel

Erlinger S, Le Go A, Husson JM, Fevery J (1984) Franco-Belgian cooperative study of ursodeoxycholic acid in the medical dissolution of gallstones: a double-blind, randomized, dose-response study, and comparison with chenodeoxycholic acid. Hepatology 4: 308-314

Fisher NM, Roberts EA, Rosen IE, Shapero TF, Sutherland LR, Davies RS, Bacchus R, Lee SV (1985) The Sunnybrook gallstone study: a double-blind controlled trial of chenodeoxycholic acid for gallstone dissolution. Hepatology 5: 102-107

Friedman GD, Kannel WB, Dawber TL (1966) The epidemiology of gallbladder disease: observations in the Framingham study. J Chron Dis 19: 273-292

Fromm H, Roat JW, Gonzalez V, Sarva RP, Farivar S (1983) Comparative efficacy and side effects of ursodeoxycholic and chenodeoxycholic acids in dissolving gallstones. Gastroenterology 85: 1257-1264

Gleeson DC, Ruppin DC, Dowling RH (1983) Second look at ursodeoxycholic acid (UDCA): high efficacy for partial but low efficacy for complete gallstone dissolution, and a high rate of acquired stone opacification. Gut 24: A999

Heikel TAJ, Lathe GH (1970) The effects of oral contraceptive sterols on bile secretion and bilirubin Tm in rats. Br J Pharmacol 38: 593-601

Howard P, Gleeson D, Murphy GM, Dowling RH (1984) Ursocholic acid (UCA): bile acid and bile lipid dose-response studies in gallstone (GS) patients. Proceedings of the 8th International Bile Acid Meeting, 1-2 September 1984, Berne

Igimi H, Carey MC (1980) Cholesterol monohydrate (ChM) gallstones dissolve faster in chenodeoxycholate (CDC)-rich bile than in ursodeoxycholate (UDC)-rich bile. Gastroenterology 78: 1186

Kitani K, Kanai S, Sato Y, Uchida K (1983) The bile flow and biliary excretion of ursocholate in the rat. Life Sci 33: 2377-2386

Kupfer RM, Maudgal DP, Northfield TC (1982) Gallstone dissolution rate during chenic acid therapy: effect of bedtime administration plus low cholesterol diet. Dig Dis Sci 27: 1025-1029

Lanzini A, Pigozzi G, Facchinetti D, Castellano M, Bettini L, Beschi M, Muiesan G (1986) Ursocholic acid administration to gallstone patients: effect on biliary lipid composition, bile acid pattern and gallstone dissolution. Curr Ther Res 39: 8-18

Leuschner U, Leuschner M, Sieratzki J, Kurtz W, Hubner K (1985) Gallstone dissolution with ursodeoxycholic acid in patients with chronic active hepatitis and two years follow-up. Dig Dis Sci 30: 642-649

Lirussi F, Pedrazzoli S, Gerunda G, Orlando R, Venuti M, Nassuato G, Jemmolo RM, Okolicsanyi L (1981) Retained cholesterol intrahepatic bile duct stones: efficacy of high-dose short-term ursodeoxycholic acid administration. Curr Ther Res 30: 775-785

Lirussi F, Iemmolo RM, Piccoli A, Orlando R, Muraca M, Nassuato G, Strazzabosco M, Okolicsanyi L (1986a) Prognostic factors affecting cholesterol gallstone dissolution rate: who will benefit more from medical therapy? Eur J Clin Invest 16: A11

Lirussi F, Jemmolo RM, Nitti D, Lise M, Sorato R, Corsini A, Okolicsanyi L (1986b) Medical treatment of cholesterol bile duct stones with ursocholic acid. J Hepatol 3 [Suppl 1]: S141

Loria P, Carulli N, Medici G, Menozzi D, Salvioli G, Bertolotti M, Montanari M (1986) Effect of ursocholic acid on bile lipid secretion and composition. Gastroenterology 90: 865-874

Marks JW, Lan S and the Steering Committee for the National Cooperative Gallstone Study Group (1984) Low-dose chenodiol to prevent gallstone recurrence after dissolution therapy. Ann Intern Med 100: 376-381

Maton PN, Murphy GM, Dowling RH (1977) Ursodeoxycholic acid treatment of gallstones. Dose-response study and possible mechanisms of action. Lancet 2: 1297-1301

Maton PN, Iser JH, Reuben A, Saxton HM, Murphy GM, Dowling RH (1982) Outcome of chenodeoxycholic acid (CDCA) treatment in 125 patients with radiolucent gallstones. Medicine 61: 86-97

Mazzella G, Morselli Labata AM, Malavolti M, Petronelli A, Roda A, Barbara L (1983) The effects of usodeoxycholic administration on bile lipid composition in man: comparison of bed time versus meal time administration. Curr Ther Res 33: 551-557

Northfield TC, Lanzini A, Jazrawi R, Kupfer R, Maudgal DP (1985) Gallstone dissolution rate and recurrence rate during and after bile acid therapy. In: Barbara L et al. (eds) Recent advances in bile acid research. Raven, New York, pp 289-302

Okolicsanyi L, Lirussi F, Pedrazzoli S, Orlando R, Zacchi C, Naccarato R, Nassuato G, Dal Brun G (1982) Intra- and extrahepatic cholesterol cholelithiasis: efficacy of prolonged CDCA administration. Hepatogastroenterology 29: 14

Okolicsanyi L, Lirussi F, Strazzabosco M, Iemmolo RM, Orlando R, Nassuato G, Muraca M, Crepaldi G (1986) The effect of drugs on bile flow and composition. An overview. Drugs 31: 430-448

Park YH, Igimi H, Carey MC (1981) Human cholesterol (ChM) gallstones dissolve as fast in simulated urso-rich bile as in cheno-rich bile. Gastroenterology 81: 1248

Perez-Aguilar F, Breto M, Alfonso V, Martinez-Silvestre M, Berenguer J (1985) Gallstone recurrence following cessation of dissolving treatment and during prophylactic administration of either low-dose chenodeoxycholic acid (CDCA) or medium-dose ursodeoxycholic acid (UDCA). J Hepatol 1: S305

Podda M, Zuin M, de Fazio C, Dioguardi ML, Battezzati PM, Grandinetti G (1986) Efficacy of combined ursodeoxycholic and chenodeoxycholic acid treatment. Proceedings of the 9th International Bile Acid Meeting, 19-21 October 1986, Basel

Ponz de Leon M, Carulli N, Iori R, Loria P, Smeritri A, Zironi F (1980) Medical treatment of radiolucent gallstones with chenodeoxycholic acid (CDCA): follow-up report at four years. Ital J Gastroenterol 12: 17-22

Roda E, Bazzoli F, Morselli Labate AM, Mazzella G, Roda A, Sama C, Festi D, Aldini R, Taroni F, Barbara L (1982) Ursodeoxycholic acid vs. chenodeoxycholic acid as cholesterol gallstone-dissolving agents: a comparative randomized study. Hepatology 2: 804-810

Ruppin DC, Dowling RH (1982) Is recurrence inevitable after gallstone dissolution by bile acid treatment? Lancet 1: 181-185

Salen G, Colalillo A, Verga D, Bagon E, Stephen Tint G, Shefer S (1980) Effect of high and low doses of ursodeoxycholic acid on gallstone dissolution in humans. Gastroenterology 78: 1412-1418

Sama C, Morselli Labate AM, Chiodarelli C, Roda A, Briganti M, Roda E (1983) Bioavailability of a delayed-release preparation of ursodeoxycholic acid in man. Curr Ther Res 33: 558-564

Sauerbruch T, Delius M, Paumgartner G, Holl J, Wess O, Weber W, Hepp W, Brendel W (1986) Fragmentation of gallstones by extracorporeal shock waves. N Engl J Med 314: 818-822

Schoenfield LJ, Lachin JM and The Steering Committee of the National Cooperative Gallstone Study Group (1981) Chenodiol (chenodeoxycholic acid) for dissolution of gallstones: the National Cooperative Gallstone Study. Ann Intern Med 95: 257-282

Tamberi P, Alessandrini G, Saccomanno G, Mammoliti F, Cappuccio A, Maccheroni M, Servadio L (1985) Choleretic effect of ursocholic acid in man: its comparison with placebo and ursodeoxycholic acid. Curr Ther Res 38: 50-60

Thistle JL, LaRusso NF (1985) Combination of taurine or chenodeoxycholic acid with ursodeoxycholic acid therapy: effects on biliary lipids, bile acids, and gallstones. In: Barbara L et al. (eds) Recent advances in bile acid research. Raven, New York, pp 307-309

Thistle JL, May GL, Allen MJ (1985) Dissolution of gallstones by methyl tert-butyl ether. N Engl J Med 313: 386

Tokyo Cooperative Study Group (1980) Efficacy and indications of ursodeoxycholic acid treatment for dissolving gallstones. A multicenter double-blind trial. Gastroenterology 78: 542-548

Toulet J, Rousselet J, Viteau JM, Duchon Y, Pagniez R, Samain B, Vienn JL (1983) Relapses and preventive treatment of relapses after dissolution of gallstones in 22 patients. Gastroenterol Clin Biol 7: 605-609

Zuin M, Frigerio G, Ghezzi C, Andreini C, Camissasca M, De Fazio C, Podda M (1984) Effect on biliary lipids of three different preparations containing ursodeoxycholic acid (UDCA): a balanced cross-over study. Curr Ther Res 35: 93-99

# Biliary Lipid Composition after Endoscopic Sphincterotomy in Postcholecystectomy Patients: Effect of Short-Term Ursodeoxycholic Acid Administration

R. M. Iemmolo[1], F. Lirussi[1], D. Oselladore[2], R. Rossoni[2], M. Muraca[1], R. Orlando[1], G. Nassuato[1], M. Strazzabosco[1], and L. Okolicsányi[1]

[1] Istituto di Medicina Interna, Università di Padova, Italy
[2] Clinica Chirurgica I, Università di Padova, Italy

## Introduction

Endoscopic sphincterotomy (ES) of the sphincter of Oddi (SO) has been proposed as the treatment of choice in patients with stenosis of the papilla or papillary motor dysfunction, which are considered to be the major causes of the so-called postcholecystectomy syndrome (Schein and Beneventano 1968; Geenen et al. 1981; Bar Meir et al. 1984).

The SO plays an important role in the regulation of the dynamics of the enterohepatic circulation of bile acids, both in normal subjects and in cholecystectomized patients (Ashkin et al. 1978; Kurtz and Classen 1983; Greenfield et al. 1985). When the contractions of the SO are abolished by means of sphincterectomy, the storage function of the gallbladder and the bile acid pool size are reduced, the delivery of bile into the duodenum is altered and the proportion of secondary bile acids in bile is increased (Hutton et al. 1981). Furthermore, the diurnal rhythm of biliary cholesterol saturation is changed by the ablation of both the gallbladder (Roda et al. 1978) and the SO (Kurtz and Classen 1983). Sauerbruch et al. (1983) reported that the changes in the composition of the bile acid pool in cholecystectomized patients after sphincterotomy had no significant effects on the cholesterol saturation of bile, i.e., it remained abnormal. Conversely, oral administration of ursodeoxycholic acid (UDCA) in patients with gallstones has been reported to desaturate bile and to be effective in reducing the frequency and severity of specific biliary symptoms (Bachrach and Hofmann 1982; Ward 1984; Hofmann 1985; Frigerio 1979; Polli et al. 1979).

The aim of our study was threefold: (1) to study bile acid and biliary lipid composition before and after ES, in previously (1–24 years) cholecystectomized patients; (2) to investigate the effect of short-term UDCA and UDCA-RR (a new repeated-release preparation of UDCA), on bile composition after ES; and (3) to verify whether UDCA or UDCA-RR treatment could relieve specific biliary symptoms in postcholecystectomy patients undergoing ES.

## Patients

Table 1 summarizes the characteristics of the patients included in the study. Twenty-one cholecystectomized patients, 10 females (age range 54–79 years) and 11 males (age range 48–78 years), were studied. Criteria for admission to the study were:

1. Stenosis of SO documented by i.v. cholangiography and endoscopic retrograde cholangiopancreatography (ERCP);

Assessment and Management of Hepatobiliary Disease
Eds.: L. Okolicsányi, G. Csomós, and G. Crepaldi

**Table 1.** Cholecystectomized patients undergoing endoscopic sphincterotomy

| Patient no. | Age | Sex | Years after cholecystectomy | Medical treatment (mg/kg · day) |
|---|---|---|---|---|
| Group I: Placebo | | | | |
| 1 | 76 | M | 3 | – |
| 2 | 62 | M | 24 | – |
| 3 | 70 | F | 4 | – |
| 4 | 65 | M | 1 | – |
| 5 | 52 | M | 1 | – |
| 6 | 58 | F | 1 | – |
| 7 | 66 | F | 12 | – |
| Group II: UDCA | | | | |
| 8 | 54 | F | 6 | 4.6 |
| 9 | 58 | F | 3 | 5.2 |
| 10 | 68 | M | 10 | 6.6 |
| 11 | 72 | F | 10 | 7.2 |
| 12 | 65 | F | 2 | 6.9 |
| 13 | 63 | F | 3 | 6.9 |
| 14 | 79 | F | 2 | 7.7 |
| Group III: UDCA-RR | | | | |
| 15 | 54 | F | 3 | 7.4 |
| 16 | 75 | F | 6 | 7.1 |
| 17 | 48 | M | 10 | 6.0 |
| 18 | 62 | M | 20 | 5.3 |
| 19 | 78 | M | 9 | 7.1 |
| 20 | 75 | M | 2 | 5.2 |
| 21 | 69 | M | 4 | 5.4 |

2. Absence of lesions of the upper gastrointestinal tract, as determined by endoscopy;
3. Presence of one or more of the following biliary symptoms: postprandial fullness or headache, abnormal frequent belching, pyrosis and acid regurgitations, epigastric pain, right upper quadrant abdominal pain, meteorism or flatulence, or intolerance to dietary fat.

## Study Design

Immediately before ES, performed according to Classen and Demling (1974) and Kaway et al. (1974), hepatic bile samples were obtained by selective cannulation of the common bile duct and stored at −20 °C for analyses. Following ES, all patients were assigned three treatment groups according to a latin square design: group I ($n=7$) received placebo (lactose) at bedtime for 30 days; group II ($n=7$) received UDCA (450 mg/day; Deursil, Gipharmex SpA, Milan Italy) in a single bedtime administration for 30 days; group III ($n=7$) received UDCA-RR (450 mg/day; Deursil RR, Gipharmex SpA Italy) in a single bedtime administration for 30 days. At the end of the treatment period, hepatic bile samples were taken again for estimation of biliary lipids.

## Methods

Biliary total bile acids, phospholipids, and cholesterol were determined using an enzymatic spectrophotometric method (3-$\alpha$-dehydrogenase, Nieegard, Norway), an enzymatic colorimetric test (Enzycholor PL, Poli, Italy), and a colorimetric test (CHOD-PAP, Boehringer Mannheim, FRG), respectively. The cholesterol saturation index (SI) was calculated according to the equation of Thomas and Hofmann (1973) using the limits of cholesterol saturation of Hegardt and Dam (1971). In groups I and III glyco- and tauroconjugates of individual bile acids in bile were assayed using a high-pressure liquid chromatographic method (Muraca and Ghoos 1985). The concentration of each bile acid was expressed as a percentage of total bile acids.

The effect of drug administration on biliary symptoms was evaluated by means of a linear analog scale with a score ranging between 0 (absence) and 10 (severe). As a corollary to the study, routine liver function tests (alanine aminotransferase, alkaline phosphatase, and y-GT = $\gamma$ glutamyl-transpeptidase) were performed before and after treatment. Statistical significance was determined by Student's *t* test for paired data; $P<0.05$ was considered statistically significant.

## Results

Three patients (one from group I and two from group III) did not complete the study, patient 1 because of a histologically documented adenocarcinoma of the papilla of Vater requiring surgery, and patients 20 and 21 because of unsuccessful cannulation of the common bile duct at the end of the treatment period. Radiological evaluation of the biliary tree performed by ERCP one month after ES, demonstrated no dilation of the biliary tract, absence of common bile duct stones and a free passage of contrast media into the duodenum in all other patients.

As shown in Fig. 1, hepatic bile collected before ES showed a high cholesterol SI in all patients. At the end of the treatment period (Fig. 1) the cholesterol SI significantly increased in the placebo group (mean ± SD, 1.70 ± 0.7 vs 1.35 ± 0.5, $P<0.05$), while it decreased significantly in UDCA-treated patients (1.15 ± 0.4 vs 1.59 ± 0.4, $P<0.05$) and in the group receiving UDCA-RR (1.15 ± 0.3 vs 1.87 ± 0.3, $P<0.05$). The molar percentages of tauro- and glycoconjugates of biliary bile acids were not significantly modified by ES and placebo (Fig. 2); in UDCA-RR-treated patients (Fig. 3) the percentage of biliary UDCA significantly increased (6.25 ± 1.4 vs 1.37 ± 0.5, $P<0.02$), whereas the molar percentages of the other bile acids did not vary significantly.

Figure 4 shows the influence of treatment on the dyspepsia score. Biliary symptoms significantly decreased in the placebo (6.0 ± 2.5 vs 16.4 ± 8.1, $P<0.01$) as well as in the UDCA (4.8 ± 1.8 vs 12.4 ± 3.1, $P<0.001$) and UDCA-RR (4.4 ± 0.2 vs 12.4 ± 3, $P<0.05$) groups. Biochemical signs of cholestasis, which were present in all patients before ES, had improved, although not significantly, in all groups by the end of the treatment period, possibly as a result of restoration of a normal delivery of bile from the biliary tree into the duodenum.

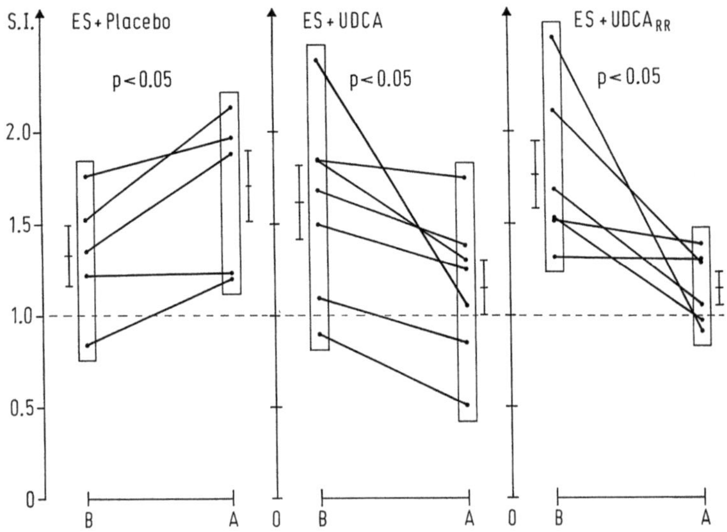


**Fig. 1.** Cholesterol saturation index (SI) in cholecystectomized patients 1 month after endoscopic sphincterotomy (ES), ES + UDCA (450 mg/day) and ES + UDCA-RR (450 mg/day) respectively (mean ± SD)

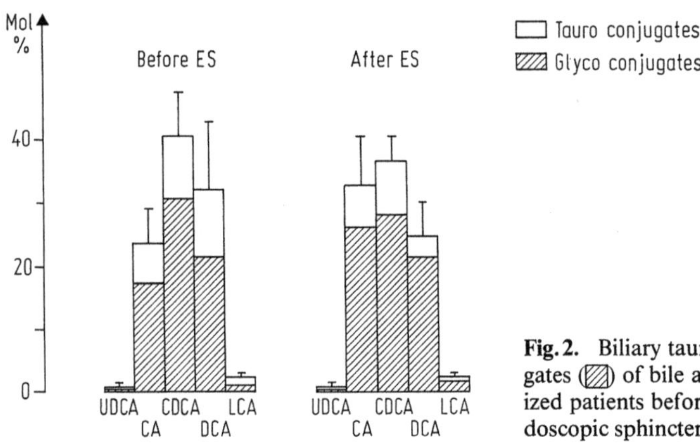


**Fig. 2.** Biliary tauro- (□) and glycoconjugates (▨) of bile acids in cholecystectomized patients before and 1 month after endoscopic sphincterotomy (ES) (mean ± SD)

## Discussion

The results of short-term UDCA administration in postcholecystectomy patients with ES indicate that UDCA is able to significantly reduce both biliary cholesterol concentration and the cholesterol SI, with only modest changes in the pattern of biliary bile acid concentration. In all patients included in the study, the initial bile samples had a high cholesterol SI. Thus, cholecystectomy alone had not succeeded in restoring a normal biliary lipid composition. This is in keeping with many reports showing biliary lithogenesis to be unaltered after cholecystectomy (Simmons et al. 1972; Boyer et al. 1974; McDougall et al. 1975; Roda et al. 1978; Kurtz and Classen 1983).

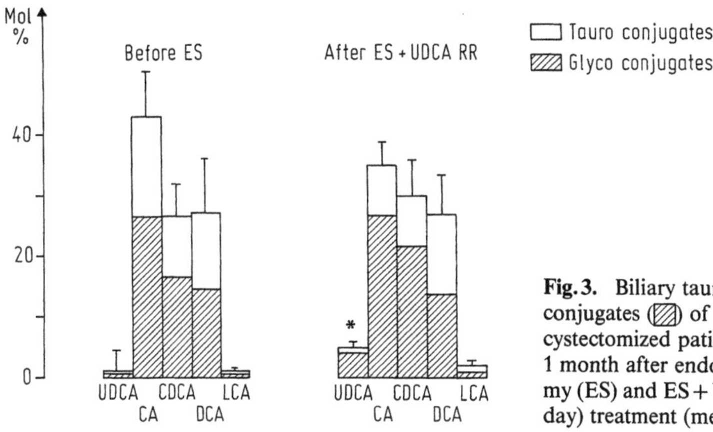


**Fig. 3.** Biliary tauro- (☐) and glyco-conjugates (▨) of bile acids in cholecystectomized patients before and 1 month after endoscopic sphincterotomy (ES) and ES + UDCA-RR (450 mg/day) treatment (mean ± SD)

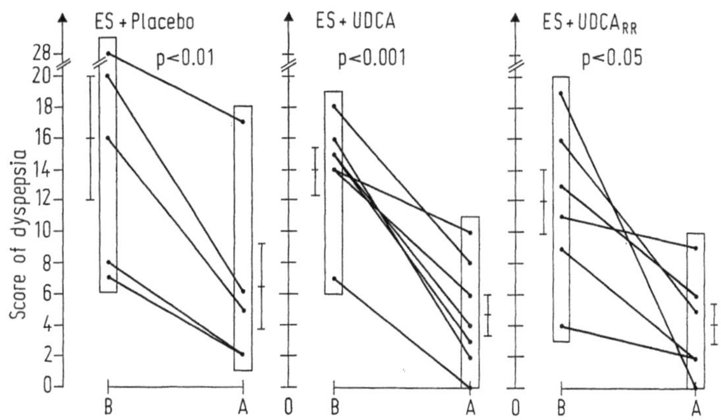


**Fig. 4.** Dyspepsia score in cholecystectomized patients before and 1 month after endoscopic sphincterotomy (ES), ES + UDCA (450 mg/day) and ES + UDCA-RR (450 mg/day) treatment (mean ± SD)

Sauerbruch et al. (1983) have recently demonstrated that ES does not modify biliary lipid composition or the biliary bile acid pool, both in patients with an intact gallbladder and cholecystectomized patients. In our hands, ES alone produced a slight but significant increase in the cholesterol SI, whereas UDCA treatment, both in the immediate-release preparation and the repeated-release preparation, significantly diminished the bile cholesterol SI. Sama et al. (1983) showed that bedtime administration of a single repeated-release capsule of UDCA in patients with gallstones induced a constant input of UDCA from the intestine into the liver, causing a decrease in biliary cholesterol secretion and, thus, a decrease in the saturation index.

Moreover, the differences in bile acid pool size between patients with an intact gallbladder and patients after cholecystectomy are essentially abolished by sphincterotomy (Sauerbruch et al. 1983). The molar percentages of tauro- and glycoconjugates of cholic, chenic, deoxycholic, and lithocholic acid were not modified after ES. Our findings are in agreement with previous observations by Sauerbruch et al. (1983), who showed that ES does not influence the pattern of biliary bile acids in cholecystectomized patients. The molar percentage of UDCA in bile increased less than expected after short-term administration of UDCA-RR. This is likely to depend on the relatively low dose given daily (450 mg) which, in our patients, corresponds to 4.6-7.7 mg/kg·day, and on the greater recycling of the bile acid pool observed after cholecystectomy (Hepner et al. 1974; Kimball et al. 1976; Roda et al. 1978; Kurtz and Classen 1983), with a resulting increased fecal loss of bile acids.

UDCA treatment was as effective at reducing biliary symptoms as the placebo, suggesting that ES per se may be beneficial in these patients. A possible explanation is that sphincterectomy decreases the enhanced pressure gradient that exists between the common bile duct and duodenum in case of stenosis of the SO (Geenen et al. 1981; Hamilton et al. 1982; Greenfield et al. 1985). A strong "placebo effect" of UDCA administration is less likely, although it has been reported in short-term clinical trials in patients with gallstones (Frigerio 1979; Polli et al. 1979). In conclusion, our short-term study shows that ES does not modify biliary lipid composition and the bile acid pattern in cholecystectomized patients. Bedtime UDCA administration seems effective in reducing biliary cholesterol saturation. Further clinical studies are needed to verify whether long-term UDCA administration may be useful in preventing common bile duct stone formation if stenosis of the distal part of biliary tree develops again.

## References

Ashkin JR, Lyon DT, Shull SD, Wagner CI, Soloway RD (1978) Factors affecting delivery of bile to the duodenum in man. Gastroenterology 74: 560-565

Bachrach WH, Hofmann AF (1982) Ursodeoxycholic acid in the treatment of cholesterol cholelithiasis. Part 1. Dig Dis Sci 27: 737-761

Bar-Meir JL, Helpner Z, Bardan E, Gilat T (1984) Frequency of papillary disfunction among cholecystectomized patients. Hepatology 4: 328-330

Boyer JL, Bloomer JR, Maddry WC (1974) Variation in hepatic bile composition following cholecystectomy in patients with previous gallstones. Yale J Biol Med 47: 211-222

Classen M, Demling L (1974) Endoskopische Sphincterotomie der papilla vateri und Steinextraktion aus ductus choledochus. Dtsch Med Wochenschr 99: 496-497

Frigerio G (1979) Ursodeoxycholic acid (UDCA) in the treatment of dyspepsia: report of a multicenter controlled trial. Curr Ther Res 26: 214-224

Geenen JE, Vennes JA, Silvis SE (1981) Resumè of a seminar on endoscopic retrograde sphincterotomy (ERS). Gastrointest Endosc 27: 31-38

Greenfield C, Cleland P, Dick R, Masters S, Summerfield JA, Sherlock S (1985) Biliary sequelae of endoscopic sphincterotomy. Postgrad Med J 61: 213-215

Hamilton I, Ruddel WS, Mitchell CJ, Lintott J, Axon AT (1982) Endoscopic retrograde cholangiograms of the normal and postcholecystectomy biliary tree. Br J Surg 69: 343-345

Hegardt FG, Dam H (1971) The solubility of cholesterol in aqueous solutions of bile salts and lecithin. Z Ernähr Wiss 10: 223-233

Hepner GW, Hofmann AF, Malagelada JR, Szczepanik PA, Klein PD (1974) Increased bacterial degradation of bile acids in cholecystectomized patients. Gastroenterology 66: 556-564

Hofmann AF (1984) Medical treatment of cholesterol gallstones by bile desaturating agents. Hepatology 4: 1995-2085

Hutton SW, Sievart CE, Vennes JA, Duane WC (1981) The effect of sphincterotomy on gallstone formation in the prairie dog. Gastroenterology 81: 663-667

Kaway K, Akasaka Y, Murakami K, Tada M, Nakajiama M (1974) Endoscopic sphincterotomy of the ampulla of Vater. Gastrointest Endosc 20: 148-151
Kimball A, Pertsemlidis D, Panvelivalla D (1976) Composition of biliary lipids and kinetics of bile acids after cholecystectomy in man. Am J Dig Dis 21: 776-732
Kurtz W, Classen M (1983) The role of the gallbladder and the sphincter of Oddi in the regulation of enterohepatic circulation and biliary lipid secretion. In: Csomós G, Thaler E (eds) Clinical hepatology. Springer, Berlin Heidelberg New York Tokyo, pp 101-111
McDougall RM, Walker K, Thurston OG (1975) Prolonged secretion of lithogenic bile after cholecystectomy. Ann Surg 182: 150-153
Muraca M, Ghoos Y (1985) Glyco-7 $\alpha$,12 $\alpha$-dihydroxy-5 $\beta$-cholanic acid as internal standard for high-pressure liquid chromatographic analysis of conjugated bile acids. J Lip Res 26: 1009-1011
Polli E, Inter-Hospital Clinical Research Group (GRRC) (1979) The effect of ursodeoxycholic acid (UDCA) on "dyspepsia" in patients with gallstones or other biliary tract anomalies. Curr Ther Res 26: 230-233
Roda E, Aldini R, Mazzella G, Roda A, Sama C, Festi D, Barbara L (1978) Enterohepatic circulation of bile acids after cholecystectomy. Gut 19: 640-648
Sama C, Morselli Labate AM, Chiodarelli C, et al. (1983) Bioavailability of a delayed-release preparation of ursodeoxycholic acid in man. Curr Ther Res 33: 558-564
Sauerbruch T, Stellaard F, Brunholzl N, Paumgartner G (1983) Bile acid pattern and cholesterol saturation of bile after cholecystectomy and endoscopic sphincterotomy. In Paumgartner G, Stiehl A, Gerok W (eds) Bile acid and cholesterol in health and disease. MTP Press, pp 279-282
Schein CJ, Beneventano TC (1968) Choledochoduodenal junction stenosis in the postcholecystectomy syndrome. Surgery 64: 1039-1046
Simmons F, Ross APJ, Bouchier AD (1972) Alterations of hepatic bile composition after cholecystectomy. Gastroenterology 63: 466-471
Thomas PJ, Hofmann AF (1973) A simple calculation of the lithogenic index of bile: expressing biliary lipid composition on rectangular coordinates. Gastroenterology 65: 698-700
Ward A (1984) UDCA. A review of its pharmacological properties and therapeutic efficacy. Drugs 27: 95-131

# Concluding Remarks

Hans Popper

A large amount of material is given in this section, which is dominated by an evaluation of bile formation and of the two major disturbances of this formation which cause groups of clinical manifestations, cholestasis and cholesterol gallstone formation. The process of bile formation is still not fully understood, particularly the site and nature of its initiation and its molecular aspects. These chapters contribute to our understanding by focusing on the results of new techniques. The study of vesicles derived from specific domains of hepatocytes and their uptake of protons, inorganic ions, and organic anions, as well as the measurement of alterations of phospholipid membranes in the specific domains are important tools. Synthesis, metabolism, and conjugation of bile acids enter into our understanding of bile formation. Progress in the field, to which effective physicochemical methods have only recently been applied, should clarify the physiology of bile formation.

In explaining the mechanism of cholestasis, it becomes clear that disturbances of many different processes in specific sites are involved. Today the emphasis is on ion pumps and the composition of the phospholipid membranes determining both transport and membrane enzyme activities. The paracellular flow and the cytoskeleton are in the foreground of our concepts of the guidance of intracellular transport and canalicular contractability. Today we assume that disturbance at any one of these at least four sites not only initiates cholestasis but also causes secondary changes at other sites, in the sense of a network disturbance.

Discrepancy in biliary secretion of bile acid and cholesterol, induced genetically or by such environmental factors as obesity, is stressed at present in cholesterol gallstone precipitation because it is therapeutically possible to dissolve gallstones by means other than direct installation of potent solvents into the biliary tract, and, more importantly, because oral administration of chenodeoxycholic acid or ursodeoxycholic acid has become a widely evaluated therapeutic modality; at this time urso seems to enjoy a slight preference, with some recommending a combination of both bile acids. It is interesting that bear (urso) bile has been a popular traditional medicine for many disease in Japan for some centuries, and this may be the reason that the Japanese were the first to recommend urso for dissolution of gallstones.

The epidemiologic studies presented here reveal important facts, and the revived interest in pigment stones is welcome because these stones occur not only in the Far East but seem to be also moderately frequent in western countries.

I would like to add two final remarks. In the last decade physiological and hydromechanical disturbances have been incriminated in both cholestasis and gallstone disease, which, interestingly, develop in combination during total parenteral nutrition, particularly in infants. Today, physical-mechanical processes re-emerge in both groups

Assessment and Management of Hepatobiliary Disease
Eds.: L. Okolicsányi, G. Csomós, and G. Crepaldi

of disease. In intrahepatic cholestasis, obstruction of bile flow in portal and periportal zones is being considered again; it is presumably not only caused by fibrosis but also by edema, probably induced by leukotrienes, the biliary secretion of which is impaired. Similarly, in the gallbladder nucleating factors are stressed. Secondly, in both cholestasis and gallstone disease we probably do not deal with defects in one specific step, which may be corrected by one specific drug, but rather we are confronted by a disturbed balance in a cascade or even better in a network which is more effectively restored by multiple procedures, including dietary as well as pharmaceutical factors.

Thus, the interesting if somewhat heavy diet presented in these chapters offers new vistas and provides a better understanding.

# Assessment of Liver Function

# Drug-Induced Liver Injury

Hans Popper

Stratton Laboratory for the Study of Liver Diseases, Mount Sinai School of Medicine of the City University of New York, New York, NY 11010, U.S.A.

The manifold aspects of adverse hepatic drug reactions which have been frequently reviewed (Kaplowitz et al. 1986; Ludwig and Axelsen 1983; Popper et al. 1972; Stricker and Spoelstra 1985; Zimmerman 1978) include (a) pharmacology, based also on the chemical constitution of the drug, (b) mechanistics, dealing with the pathogenesis of the reaction, (c) clinical manifestations, and (d) pathology, mainly as to histological features. In the following discussion the classification of the reactions will be based primarily on the morphological changes, where available in biopsy specimens, and less on the other aspects (Popper and Geller 1981). This classification serves as a guide in the solution of three main problems, namely (1) in determining the hepatotoxicity in initial animal toxicologic studies and subsequent clinical observations, (2) in weighing the risk of giving a drug to an individual patients, and (3) in establishing whether an acute or chronic disease, with or without jaundice, results from drug therapy or other factors.

## Predictability of Drug Reactions

In this approach, predictable and nonpredictable drug reactions have to be distinguished (Davidson et al. 1979; Popper et al. 1965). *Predictable (type I) reactions* are characteristically produced in experimental animals and are dose-dependent, though the effect of the dose may be influenced by stress such as lactation or pregnancy. Age has no effect. Other organs, particularly kidney and bone marrow, are frequently involved and the latent period between the last drug administration and the appearance of symptoms is usually short. In effect, these reactions can be considered as intoxications in which a risk is deliberately taken in view of other beneficial effects. Oncotherapeutic drugs represent a typical example, e.g., acute liver injury from methotrexate, with septal fibrosis rapidly developing. Chronic methotrexate injury, which can progress to cirrhosis, has been observed particularly in the treatment of psoriasis. This is complicated by the hepatic alterations in psoriasis, independent of treatment, as well as the frequent absence of laboratory abnormalities despite progression of the hepatic lesion to cirrhosis. This makes monitoring by liver biopsy important. Proper spacing of the methotrexate intake has recently been shown to reduce the incidence of these reactions. Steatosis, (small- or large-droplet) is a predictable reaction to many drugs, such as glucocorticoids, some antibiotics, valproic acid, and, of course, ethanol. In some cases, e.g., after valproic acid, the clinical significance depends greatly on associated lesions such as hepatocellular necrosis (Zimmerman and Ishak 1982). Large intravenous doses of tetracycline have produced an extensive microvesicular steatosis with

Assessment and Management of Hepatobiliary Disease
Eds.: L. Okolicsányi, G. Csomós, and G. Crepaldi

limited necrosis, particularly in pregnant women treated for pyelitis; histologically it resembles acute fatty liver of pregnancy. Otherwise, centroacinar (zone 3) necroses are typical histologic features, for instance after overdoses of acetaminophen, which requires biotransformation for activity. Since lipid peroxidation is one, (though not the most important) effect of acetaminophen, excess lipofuscin is a characteristic feature.

Unusual but predictable drug reactions include the increased tendency of cholestatic drugs, which otherwise produce nonpredictable reactions, to induce cholestasis in primary biliary cirrhosis, apparently because of increased sensitivity. However, this lack of predictability of cholestatic reactions in other circumstance concerns light-microscopic reactions, because with sensitive methods, functional alterations (and with electron microscopy, cholestatic changes) may be demonstrated regularly, for instance following androgenic/anabolic steroids.

*Nonpredictable (type II) reactions* (Popper et al. 1965) are characterized by lack of the ability to produce the typical lesion in experimental animals, and by involvement of only some of the persons exposed, with the incidence varying from as high as 60% to as low as 0.001%. Children are rarely involved, and dose dependency is absent or vague. Usually, a long latent period separates the last drug exposure from the onset of symptoms. Thus, in general, lesions may not be detected in toxicologic studies in experimental animals and are frequently recognized only after considerable clinical use following release of the drug by regulatory agencies. Various factors may account for the lack of predictability.

One is *genetic variations,* reflected in a polymorphism of the enzymes involved in drug metabolism (Küpfer 1983; Vesell 1984). Examples of the cytosolic enzymes are variations in acetylation rate, for instance of isoniazid (Yamomoto et al. 1986). Recently, emphasis has been placed on genetic variation of microsomal enzymes, particularly of one of the cytochrome $P_{450}$ species, such as a defect of 4-hydroxylation (Clark 1985), which is found in about 10% of the population of Western countries. It accounts for susceptibility to various drug reactions, including some involving the liver. The drug reaction following the antiarrhythmic perhexiline is an example (Pessayre et al. 1979); the lesion is histologically characterized by Mallory bodies, as well as excess deposition of phospholipids, which latter distinguishes it from alcoholic liver injury, to which it is otherwise similar. The 4-hydroxylation defect can be recognized by urinary metabolites after test doses of similarly metabolized drugs, such as debrisoquine, sparteine, or bufarol (Morgan et al. 1984). Another antiarrhythmic drug, amiodarone (Poucell et al. 1984; Simon et al. 1984), which is retained in the body for an unusually long time, produces similar histologic lesions, possibly as the result of a similar genetic defect. Probably, other such genetic forms of polymorphism exist.

Nonpredictable drug reactions may, furthermore, be caused by *hypersensitivity,* either on an immunologic or on a metabolic basis. Hypersensitivity is recognized by successful challenge, i.e., readministration of a reduced dose of the implicated drug after subsidence of the original reaction causes a reactivation; false-negative results have been explained by a desensitization as a result of the previous exposure. The immunologic alterations may have a humoral basis, as in the severe halothane reaction. Cellular immune reactions to drugs may be induced by HLA-dependent killer lymphocytes, HLA-independent natural killer cells, antibody dependent lymphocytes toxicity or even by macrophages; moreover, lymphokines have been incriminated, for instance cholestatic ones. Autoantibodies of various types permit classification of drug reactions

(Homberg et al 1985). In addition, secondary, non-drug-specific autoimmune reactions may complicate chronic drug-induced liver diseases. Most immunologic drug reactions show histologic features resembling viral hepatitis, particularly type B, in that lymphocytes are in close contact with, and sometimes within, hepatocytes.

Metabolic hypersensitivity, or idiosyncracy, is less well understood. In some persons or in some conditions, sometimes related to a previous administration of the same or a similar drug, the adverse reaction is unusually severe. A different type of metabolic pathway may be the reason, as in the idiosyncratic adverse reactions from benoxaprofen, predominantly in elderly females (Taggart and Alderdice 1982). This nonsteroidal anti-inflammatory drug is greatly converted to a glucuronide which, as the result of a reduced metabolic rate, precipitates in the bile canaliculi and thus produces cholestatic jaundice. Furthermore, *interactions* between different drugs may aggravate otherwise mild drug reactions. Examples are the accentuation of the acetaminophen injury in alcoholics (O'Dell et al. 1986; Seef et al. 1986) or combination with drugs inducing the cytochrome $P_{450}$ system, such as dilantin.

Finally, *carcinogenic effects* have to be mentioned, with neither mechanism, nor incidence fully established; azathioprine and cyclosporin are incriminated. A specific example is provided by sex steroids; contraceptives may produce a low incidence of hepatic adenomas, which may bleed, and possibly hepatocellular carcinoma though the evidence for this is not convincing. By contrast, androgenic/anabolic steroids, if given in high dose, produce a relatively high incidence of hepatocellular carcinoma and also angiosarcoma. Sex-steroid-induced tumors differ from others by virtue of their regression on discontinuation of the exposure and their dose dependence. Contraceptive-induced adenomas develop only after use for more than 5 years. Smaller doses of androgenic steroids, in wide use as anabolic agents, have never induced tumors, whereas large doses given in aregeneratory anemia have been followed by a high incidence of hepatocellular carcinoma.

## Drug Metabolism

An important component in almost all unpredictable reactions is the inducing or blocking influence of mainly *environmental factors* on the drug metabolizing system (Sato and Omura 1978; Singer and Grunberger 1983). The bulk of drugs administered are fat-soluble and are as a rule not bioactive in this form; they are transformed, often in several steps, to a bioactive metabolite with both beneficial (therapeutic) and toxic potencies and subsequently to water-soluble metabolites, usually inert, which are excreted by the cell and the body. Class I reactions, mostly oxidative or reductive and carried out by the mostly microsomal cytochrome $P_{450}$ system, produce bioactive intermediates, often electrophilic, on which the class II reactions act. Substrates of some class II reactions do not require preceding class I reactions. The class II reactions are mainly glucosyl-, glutathione-, and sulfoconjugases and epoxide hydrases. Only few of their products are noxious; some epoxides are carcinogenic and some glucuronides cholestatic, possibly by being precipitated. Glutathione not only participates in enzymatic reactions, but also binds (or traps) some electrophilic metabolites nonenzymatically. Glutathione-*S*-transferase represents 5%-10% of cytosolic proteins. With some metabolites, two glutathione molecules react to result in a disulfide. Glutathione, which also moves through the hepatocytic cell membrane, is now ascribed increasing importance in the metabolism of drugs and chemicals (Kaplowitz 1980; Kaplowitz et al. 1985). The intermediate metabolites of class I are toxic, because they may represent electrophilic free radicals [formed in addition to toxic oxygen species (Freeman and Crapo 1982)] which may bind covalently to macromolecules. Such binding to proteins may result in hepatocytic injury, in part immunological, by hapten formation, while binding to DNA may represent an initiation in a carcinogenic chain. Both class I and class II reactions can be influenced by environmental factors, which may either increase enzyme activity by so-called induction, particularly of the cytochrome $P_{450}$ system, or block the enzyme system. Both actions, especially induction, may result from exposure to various drugs and other factors, including ethanol, environmental agents, hepatotoxins, smoking, nutritional, and climactic factors.

Different metabolites of the some drug may be associated with different functional and morphologic lesions, sometimes simultaneously, as has been demonstrated, for instance, for halothane (Editorial 1986) and chlorpromazine (Samuels and Carey 1978). Indeed, histologically recognizable involvement of several structures in the liver raises the suspicion of a drug reaction.

## Morphologic Classification of Adverse Drug Reactions

*Nonspecific drug hepatitis,* characterized by mild parenchymal and/or portal lesions corresponding to a nonspecific reactive hepatitis, is usually accompanied by a slight elevation of serum aminotransferase activities. This is the most frequent drug reaction without jaundice. It is of limited functional significance. The many drugs incriminated include cimetidine and ranitidine. A variant with allergic manifestations follows, for instance, para-aminosalicylic acid use, and is characterized by accumulation of eosinophils in the portal tracts.

*Granulomatous drug hepatitis* shows, on biopsy, granulomas which may consist almost entirely of giant cells and are often short-lived; they may be absent on subsequent biopsy as little as 4 weeks later. This assists in the histologic differential diagnosis. The lesion is produced by long-acting sulfonamides, phenylbutazone, allopurinol, and other drugs.

*Drug-induced simple cholestasis,* i.e., without inflammatory reaction but with clinical jaundice, is mainly caused by anabolic/androgenic and less frequently by contraceptive steroids. The steroids may produce sinusoidal dilatation, also seen in pregnancy. Particularly following anabolic steroids, the dilatation may progress to severe peliosis, which has been fatal in rare instances. Discontinuation of exposure is usually followed by rapid subsidence.

*Drug-induced cholestatic hepatitis,* reflected in both cholestasis and parenchymal necroinflammation as well as in portal inflammatory infiltration, is the most frequent drug reaction with jaundice and sometimes raises a problem of differentiation from large bile duct obstruction. It followed chlorpromazine intake in about 1% of patients exposed, and also occurs, but less frequently, after other phenothiazines, sulfonyl urea derivatives, some antibiotics, and organic arsenicals. Drugs which sometimes induce nonspecific drug hepatitis occasionally cause the somewhat more severe cholestatic hepatitis. Particularly in chlorpromazine jaundice, cholestasis may outlast the inflammatory reaction by many months.

*Drug cholangitis,* also with conspicuous jaundice and usually with the features of drug-induced cholestatic hepatitis, involves small portal bile ducts after the use of the antiarrhythmic ajmalin (Börsch et al. 1984), and large bile ducts after the antidiabetic chlorpropamide.

*Drug reactions resembling viral hepatitis* in clinical, laboratory, and histologic manifestations can be divided into those with a grave prognosis and those with low acute mortality, the latter usually disappearing on discontinuation of the exposure. However, in both instances, challenge is hazardous and, in contrast to cholestatic hepatitis, should be carried out with caution if at all. Those reactions with grave prognosis are characterized by extremely high serum aminotransferase activities and bilirubin levels. There is no evidence that preceding liver disease creates a predisposition. In general, in contrast to cholestatic hepatitis, the reaction develops in extremely low incidence but is accompanied by high mortality. A series of drugs have been implicated, such as cincophen, iproniazid, some antidiabetics, and muscle relaxants, but the very low incidence has made it difficult to establish a causal relation. Once such a relation has been established, the drug is withdrawn from clinical use. An exception is halothane – it is an excellent noninflammable and safe anesthetic, and the incidence of severe, often fatal hepatitis is extremely low, apparently less frequent than nonhepatic fatal reactions to other anesthetics. The typical lesion shows, in biopsy specimens, circumscribed areas resembling viral hepatitis with abundance of lymphocytes and acidophilic bodies, and other areas in which the hepatocytes reveal rather toxic changes with macrophagic reaction and a tendency to collapse, as well recognized in silver stains. The combination of both lesions in the same liver is suggestive of a drug-induced liver injury, and specifically of halothane. Only exceptionally does chronic hepatitis result, while in autopsy specimens the massive necrosis is devoid of etiologic characteristics.

At least two metabolic pathways exist, with different outcomes. One is oxidative, leading to fluoroacetate, which is innocuous. The other is reductive, regularly producing in rodents a transient perivenous (zone 3) necrosis which is accentuated by phenobarbital and by hypoxia. It corresponds to the transient mild aminotransferase elevations which occur in 25% of humans after halothane anesthesia but have no functional or prognostic significance (Neuberger and Williams 1984). Only very rarely, in less than one out of every 1000 patients exposed, are metabolites formed in sufficient amounts to produce a severe hepatitic lesion, with a mortality rate of about 25%. These metabolites may cause direct toxicity or an immunologic hypersensitivity in which specific antibodies which also bind to hepatocytes of halothane-exposed rabbits cause an antibody-dependent cytotoxicity (Vergani et al. 1980). Moreover, specific susceptibility of the lymphocytes has been claimed (Farrell et al. 1985). Usually, both immunologic and metabolic factors are at play, and electron-microscopically, mitochondrial injury is in the foreground. The hypersensitivity character of the reaction is also indicated by the fact that the reaction is far more frequent after repetition of the halothane anesthesia. Today, therefore, first exposures to halothane are widely used, while repetition within such a short period as a year should be avoided, particularly if abnormalities develop after the first halothane anesthesia. Following halothane-related anesthetics such as enflurane and isoflurane, hepatitic reactions barely occur.

Drug hepatitis resembling viral hepatitis with *low acute mortality* is either predominantly immunologic, as after indomethacin or isoniazid, or predominantly toxic with cytoplasmic alterations and macrophages, as noted after sulfonamides or methyldopa.

However, mixed reactions are frequent. Severe cholestasis may enter into the mixture, for instance after azathioprine (DePinho et al. 1984). The reaction may develop several months after initiation of the therapy, and its continuation after hepatic lesions have appeared may induce chronic active hepatitis, progressing to cirrhosis or sometimes to fatal massive necrosis. Since the reaction is relatively rare in hypertensive treatment with methyldopa and serial hepatic tests, such as aminotransferase determinations, are usually not done, vigilance for clinical symptoms pointing to liver injury, such as fatigability, is indicated. Chronic active hepatitis, usually with low-grade aggressivity but sometimes with conspicuous autoimmune reaction, has been observed after the laxative oxyphenisatin or after methyldopa, isoniazid or nitrofurantoin, and cirrhosis has developed. Prolonged use of aspirin in collagen diseases has also led to chronic active hepatitis (Seaman et al. 1974).

## Outlook and Summary

Some reactions do not fit into the the histologic classification of adverse drug reactions, for instance, the veno-occlusive disease, mainly of small vessels, reported after azathioprine and some oncotherapeutic drugs. Moreover, the presented classification lists only the most frequent types of reactions. For instance, halothane may produce a predominantly cholestatic hepatitis, and chlorpromazine features of viral hepatitis. Thus, a scheme (Fig. 1) covering both drug- and chemical-induced liver injury emphasizes once more that the different metabolites induced by biotransformation of the same drug may produce several lesions in one patient. It also indicates that cholestasis

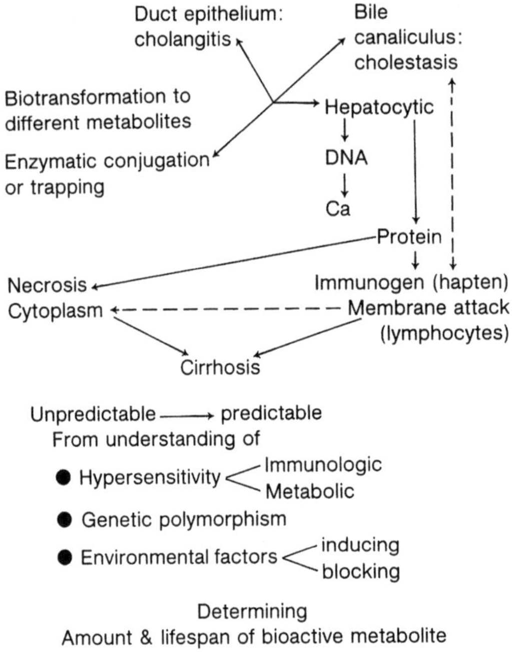


**Fig. 1.** Proposed mechanisms of drug- and chemical-induced hepatic adverse reactions

may be initiated in different sites, that cirrhosis may develop from both immunologic and metabolic hypersensitivity reactions, and that the lack of predictability results from immunologic or metabolic, but also genetic and environmental, inducing or blocking factors which are being unraveled.

In conclusion, the response of the liver to a drug, and with it the adverse reactions, depend on (1) biotransformation, influenced by genetic factors, previous drug exposure, hormones, environmental agents, and nutrition; (2) drug interactions; (3) binding to serum protein; and (4) drug clearance, influenced by blood flow and the uptake of drugs, presumably by receptors. Clarification of factors producing hypersensitivity (immunologic or metabolic), of the genetic polymorphism, and of the blockade or induction by environmental agents may eventually make nonpredictable drug reactions predictable and thus reduce the risk of adverse reactions of the majority of drugs.

## References


Börsch G, Schmidt G, Hopmann G, Surmann TH, Sabin G, Ricken D (1984) Prajmaliumbitartrate-associated liver damage. Report on seven further cases with follow-up for two to five years. Klin Wochenschr 62: 998-1000

Clark DWJ (1985) Genetically determined variability in acetylation and oxidation. Therapeutic implications. Drugs 29: 342-375

Davidson CS, Leevy CM, Chamberlayne EC (eds) (1979) Guidelines for detection of hepatotoxicity due to drugs and chemicals. US Department of Health, Education, and Welfare, Washington (NIH publication no 79-313)

DePinho RA, Goldberg CS, Lefkowitch JH (1984) Azathioprine and the liver. Evidence favoring idiosyncratic, mixed cholestatic-hepatocellular injury in humans. Gastroenterology 86: 162-165

Editorial (1986) Halothane-associated liver damage. Lancet I: 1251-1253

Farrell G, Prendergast DT, Murray M (1985) Halothane hepatitis. Detection of a constitutional susceptibility factor. N Engl J Med 313: 1310-1314

Freeman BA, Crapo JD (1982) Free radicals and tissue injury. Lab Invest 47: 412-426

Homberg J-C, Abuaf N, Helmy-Khalil S, Biour M, Poupon R, Islam S, Darnis F, Levy VG, Opolon P, Beaugrand M, Toulet J, Danan G, Beuhamou J-P (1985) Drug-induced hepatitis associated with anticytoplasmic organelle autoantibodies. Hepatology 5: 722-727

Kaplowitz N (1980) The physiologic significance of the glutathione S-transferase. Am J Physiol 239: G439-444

Kaplowitz N, Aw TY, Ookhtens M (1985) The regulation of hepatic glutathione. Annu Rev Pharmacol Toxicol 25: 715-744

Kaplowitz N, Aw TY, Simon FR, Stolz A (1986) Drug-induced hepatotoxicity. Ann Intern Med 104: 826-839

Küpfer A (1983) Inherited defects of hepatic drug metabolism. Semin Liver Dis 3: 341-354

Ludwig J, Axelsen R (1983) Drug effects on the liver. An updated tabular compilation of drugs and drug-related hepatic diseases. Dig Dis Sci 28: 651-666

Morgan MY, Reshef R, Shah RR, et al. (1984) Impaired oxidation of debrisoquine in patients with perhexiline liver injury. Gut 25: 1057-1064

Neuberger J, Williams R (1984) Halothane anaesthesia and liver damage. Br Med J 289: 1136-1139

O'Dell JR, Zetterman RK, Burnett DA (1986) Centrilobular hepatic fibrosis following acetaminophen-induced hepatic necrosis in an alcoholic. JAMA 255: 2636-2637

Pessayre D, Bichara M, Degott C, Potet F, Benhamou JP, Feldmann G (1979) Perhexiline maleate-induced cirrhosis. Gastroenterology 76: 170-177

Popper H, Geller SA (1981) Pathogenetic considerations in the histologic diagnosis of drug-induced liver injury. In: Fenoglio C, Wolff M (eds) Progress in surgical pathology, vol 3. Masson USA, New York, pp 233-246

Popper H, Rubin E, Gardiol D, Schaffner F, Paronetto F (1965) Drug-induced liver disease. A penalty for progress. Arch Intern Med 115: 128-136
Popper H, Perez V, Schaffner F (1972) Hepatic drug reactions. Prog. Liver Dis 4: 597-625
Poucell S, Ireton J, Valencia-Mayoral P, Downar E, Larratt L, Patterson J, Blendis L, Phillips MJ (1984) Amiodarone-associated phospholipidosis and fibrosis of the liver. Light, immunohistochemical, and electron microscopic studies. Gastroenterology 86: 926-936
Samuels Am, Carey MC (1978) Effects of chlorpromazine hydrochloride and its metabolites on $Mg^{2+}$ and $Na^{+}$, $K^{+}$-ATPase activities of canalicular-enriched rat liver plasma membranes. Gastroenterology 74: 1183-1190
Sato R, Omura T (eds) (1978) Cytochrome $P_{450}$. Academic, New York
Seaman WE, Ishak KG, Plotz PH (1974) Aspirin induced hepatotoxicity in patients with systemic lupus erythematosus. Ann Intern Med 80: 1-8
Seef LB, Cuccrevini BA, Zimmerman HJ, Benjamin SB (1986) Acetaminophen hepatotoxicity in alcoholics: a therapeutic misadventure. Ann Intern Med 104: 399-404
Simon JB, Manley PN, Brien JF, Armstrong PW (1984) Amiodarone hepatotoxicity simulating alcoholic liver disease. N Engl J Med 311: 167-172
Singer B, Grunberger D (1983) Molecular biology of mutagens and carcinogens. Plenum, New York
Stricker BHC, Spoelstra P (1985) Drug-induced hepatic injury. A comprehensive survey of the literature on adverse drug reactions up to January 1985. Elsevier, Amsterdam (Drug-induced disorders, vol 1)
Taggart HMcA, Alderdice JM (1982) Fatal cholestatic jaundice in elderly patients taking benoxaprofen. Br Med J 284: 1372
Vergani D, Mieli-Vergani G, Alberti A, et al. (1980) Antibodies to the surface of halothane-altered rabbit hepatocytes in patients with severe halothane-associated hepatitis. N Engl J Med 303: 66-71
Vesell ES (1984) Pharmacogenetic perspectives: genes, drugs and disease. Hepatology 4: 959-965
Yamomoto T, Takeaki S, Hirayama C (1986) Elevated serum aminotransferase induced by isoniazid in relation to isoniazid acetylator phenotype. Hepatology 6: 295-298
Zimmerman HJ (1978) Hepatotoxicity. The adverse effects of drugs and other chemicals on the liver. Appleton-Century-Crofts, New York
Zimmerman HJ, Ishak KG (1982) Valproate-induced hepatic injury: analysis of 23 fatal cases. Hepatology 2: 591-597

# Biochemical Liver Tests: Recent Developments and Challenges

Norbert Blanckaert

Department of Laboratory Medicine and Liver Center, School of Medicine, University of California, San Francisco, CA 94143, U.S.A.

Concurrent with the explosive growth of clinical laboratory testing during the last 30 years, an enormous number of biochemical tests have been proposed for diagnosis and monitoring of hepatobiliary disorders. The wealth of candidate tests obviously reflect the myriad of functions performed by the liver. Their development has also been spurred by the intense interest of clinicians who are confronted daily with the question of whether a patient has a hepatobiliary disorder. Notwithstanding this enormous and continuing activity at the drawing boards in hepatological reseach and clinical biochemistry laboratories, almost no change has occurred in the armamentarium of biochemical liver tests routinely employed in clinical practice. Assays of total bilirubin and conjugated bilirubins in serum and bilirubins in urine have been used widely for clinical purposes since the second decade of this century. Measurement of alkaline phosphatase and transaminase activities in serum became widespread in the early 1950s. Together with the one-stage prothrombin time and some form of assessment of serum albumin and gamma-globulins, these analyses continue to be the only biochemical tests to enjoy general acclaim and are considered indispensable clinical tools in the follow-up of patients with suspected or established liver disease.

A detailed discussion of the currently available biochemical liver tests, even if restricted to the aforementioned well-established assays, is clearly beyond the scope of this chapter. After a concise overview of the various biochemical approaches that are routinely used or have recently been proposed for assessment of disease activity in patients with liver disease, two themes will be discussed in somewhat more detail. Because measurements of transaminases, alkaline phosphatases, and several other serum enzymes employed for liver testing are performed by determining catalytic activity, special attention should be paid to the often overlooked standardization problems that typically arise in enzyme assays. The second topic is the clinical significance of recent developments in the field of serum bilirubins.

## Clinical Problems to Which Biochemical Tests Are Applied

An essential component of a discussion of the clinical utility of a laboratory test is identification of the problems faced by the clinician when the analysis is requested. The usefulness of a test depends on the benefit that may be derived from resolving the problem, the damage that would result if the clinician were to reach the wrong conclusion, and the actual contribution of the test result to the physician's correct or erroneous decision. It is therefore of importance first to define the questions asked by the hepatologist once the diagnosis of chronic liver disease has been made. Two types of

Assessment and Management of Hepatobiliary Disease
Eds.: L. Okolicsányi, G. Csomós, and G. Crepaldi

problems arise. The first type relates to identification of the underlying cause or causes of the chronic liver disease:

- Toxin- or drug-induced: e.g., alcohol or laxative abuse
- Viral etiology: HBV, NANB
- Metabolic disorder: hemochromatosis, Wilson's disease, $alpha_1$-antitrypsin deficiency

Elucidation of a specific disorder may lead to institution of specific treatment, and various biochemical tests can be valuable in reaching such decisions. A second series of questions pertains to assessment of the extent and progression of liver damage:

- Extent of ongoing hepatocellular injury
- Progression to decompensated state, hepatic failure
- Fibrogenesis, progression to cirrhosis
- Progression to malignancy
- Development of complications

The major determinants of the symptoms and prognosis of a patient with chronic liver disease are the degree to which hepatic failure develops and the possible progression of the disease to cirrhosis and hepatocellular carcinoma. Biochemical tests that assess these developments may therefore be helpful in clinical management of patients with liver disease.

## Assessment of Disease Activity

The following aspects of hepatic disease are monitored in patients with chronic liver disease by means of the biochemical tests indicated:

*Assessment of disease activity*

- Hepatocellular injury: transaminases
- Immunological markers: serum protein electrophoresis, serum immunoglobulins, anti-mitochondrial antibody (AMA)
- Viral infection markers: serology, DNA probes
- Fibrogenesis markers: e.g., amino-terminal propeptide of procollagen Type III, various enzymes
- Malignancy markers: e.g., alpha-fetoprotein

*Assessment of repercussions on hepatic functions*

- Excretory functions: bilirubins, alkaline phosphatase, gamma-glutamyltransferase, bile acids
- Metabolic decompensation: albumin, prothrombin time, cholinesterase, ammonia or CSF glutamine
- Portal systemic shunting: bile acids, ammonia

### Hepatocellular Injury

Because some form of liver cell damage is at the origin of almost any form of hepatic disease, and the intensity of cellular injury is a major determinant of the progression of chronic liver disease, biochemical tests to detect and assess hepatocellular injury are of key importance in patient follow-up. These tests are based primarily on an assessment of the release of intracellular substances from the injured tissue into the bloodstream. The majority of laboratory methods of hepatocellular injury are based on assaying catalytic concentrations of enzymes in serum. Because certain hepatic enzymes have a selective zonal distribution in the liver acinus, it may be possible to obtain some informations on the type of liver injury from analyzing the serum enzyme pattern. Tests of hepatocellular injury comprise cytosolic enzymes as well as mitochondrial enzymes, and the extent of enzyme release from these two intracellular locations may depend on the type and severity of liver disease. Thus both microanatomical and intracellular distribution of the enzymes may need to be considered in the selection and interpretation of clinical enzyme assays. A proposal to use glutamate dehydrogenase as a marker of liver cell damage because of its predominant activity in the centrolobular portion of the liver (where alcohol produces its major effects) and its exclusively mitochondrial location illustrates these principles (Van Waes and Lieber 1977). However, the clinical utility of the serum glutamate dehydrogenase level as an index of hepatocytic damage in patients with chronic alcoholism has been questioned (Mills et al. 1981; Jenkins et al. 1982), and the reliability of the test may be limited to patients in whom the measurement is carried out within 48 h of the last drinking episode (Worner and Lieber 1980).

Serum transaminases are unanimously accepted as the most reliable biochemical measures of hepatocellular injury and therefore constitute a cornerstone of the clinical follow-up of the patient with chronic liver disease and of every study on management and prognosis of hepatobiliary disorders. Discussion of recent developments in measurement and clinical utilization of these enzymes can be found in several recent reviews (MacNamara and Goldberg 1985; Vanderlinde 1986).

Because serum lactate dehydrogenase has poor organ specificity and is generally less sensitive than transaminases for detecting liver cell injury, measurement of this enzyme has little to offer as a liver test. Gamma-glutamyltransferase (GGT) is considered to be one of the most sensitive liver tests. In particular, this enzyme has been advocated as a highly sensitive marker for chronic alcoholism. However, the enthusiasm for GGT has waned, because there is now evidence that its sensitivity and reliability for detecting alcoholism and liver disease are not clearly superior to more conventional biochemical liver tests (Gluud et al. 1981; Rybäck et al. 1982; Eriksen et al. 1984; Nalpas et al. 1984) or questionnaires designed to reveal chronic alcoholism (Kristenson and Trell 1982; Skinner et al. 1984). Interpretation of GGT results is frequently hampered by the fact that the enzyme can be elevated by drug therapy (Lesgourgues et al. 1984). A recent report by Nalpas et al. (1984) indicates that analysis of serum aspartate aminotransferase (AST or SGOT) isoenzymes may be a more reliable biochemical marker of alcohol abuse if a precise immunoinhibition method is used for measurement of the mitochondrial isoenzyme.

## Biochemical Markers of Liver Fibrogenesis, Fibrosis, and Cirrhosis

Assessment of hepatic fibrosis and cirrhosis still depends almost completely on histological examination of liver tissue. Noninvasive biochemical tests aimed at gauging fibrogenic activity in the liver include measurements of proline and hydroxyproline in serum and urine, assay of enzymes involved in post-translational processing of collagen, and immunoassay of the amino-terminal propeptide of type III procollagen (PIIIP; for recent reviews, see Hahn 1984; Rojkind 1984; Millward-Sadler et al. 1985). The latter test has undergone further technical improvements (Rohde et al. 1983) and appears to be promising (Galambos et al. 1985), although enthusiasm for it is not universal (Roberts et al. 1986).

**Biochemical Markers of Hepatocellular Carcinoma**

Because of the increased incidence of development of hepatocellular carcinoma (HCC) in patients with liver cirrhosis and HBV infection, alcoholic liver disease, or hemochromatosis, there is continued interest in identifying a biochemical marker for early detection of malignancy in these patient groups. Screening with a combination of serum alpha-fetoprotein (AFP) and a high-resolution imaging method (usually real-time abdominal ultrasonography) may permit early detection of HCC (Kobayashi et al. 1985; Liaw et al. 1986). How sensitive such screening methods are for detection of HCC in asymptomatic patients is impossible to determine at this time. Serum AFP alone seems to be often negative in cases of early HCC (Giannoulis et al. 1984). Various other biochemical markers, including serum ferritin (Giannoulis et al. 1984; Nakano et al. 1984), serum copper (Miatto et al. 1985), fucosylated AFP (Aoyagi et al. 1985; Buamah et al. 1986), and des-gamma-carboxy prothrombin (Liebman et al. 1984) are presently under investigation.

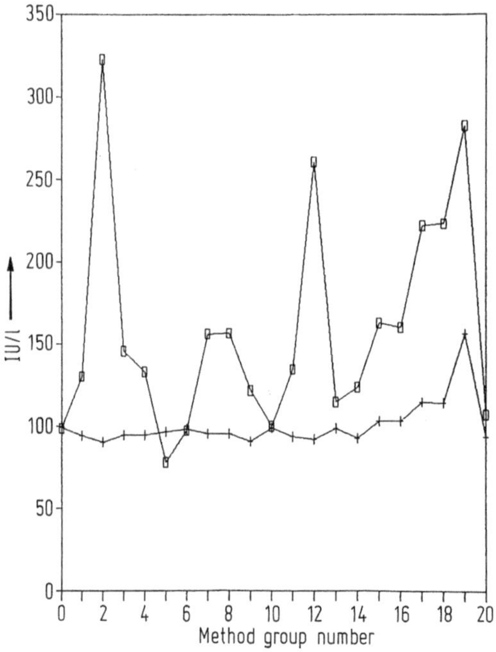


**Fig. 1.** Alkaline phosphatase activity concentration values for sample V-11 (set V-D) of 1985 CAP proficiency survey. Mean alkaline phosphatase values reported for each of 20 different method groups (shown on *abscissa*) are plotted as square symbols along the *ordinate*. Each group comprises results from 11 to 132 laboratories using the same methodology. Because authentic ICES enzyme activity values are not available for CAP samples, reported raw numeric values were converted to normalized values by the following normalization procedure, which in principle resembles the one employed in the ICES system. A correction factor was computed for each method group. The mean of the two method groups performing the enzyme assay at 30 °C was selected as primary reference value (shown as method group number 0). A correction factor was then computed for each method group by dividing the raw reported mean values by the primary reference value. Finally, raw reported values of each method group in the survey using sample V-11 were multiplied with the corresponding correction factor to obtain the normalized values plotted as + symbols

## Standardization Problems in Biochemical Liver Tests

Almost all routine biochemical liver tests involve measurement of serum enzymes. Fortunately, arbitrary units for expressing catalytic activity concentration have been almost universally replaced by international units per liter (IU/L; one IU = conversion of one micromole of substrate per minute). Physicians should realize that this does not eliminate the possibility of marked variability in the enzyme concentration values reported from different clinical laboratories and possibly even from different instruments used within the same laboratory for a single specimen. That such a situation presently exists is documented by interlaboratory proficiency surveys such as the one by the College of American Pathologists (CAP). For example, results taken from 1985 CAP surveys on serum enzymes reveal that values for alkaline phosphatase may vary by as much as 400%-450% for the same specimen (Fig. 1). Similar variability was found for GGT (211%; Fig. 2), AST (168%; Fig. 3), alanine aminotransferase (148%; Fig. 4), and amylase (260%; Fig. 5). This lack of uniformity of numerical values reflects the critical dependence of enzymatic activity on assay conditions (temperature, assay mixture composition) and the differences thereof in the methods employed on different instruments for measuring the same enzyme. Worldwide use of a single assay procedure obviously cannot be achieved. However, it would be possible to alleviate the problem, considerably and achieve reasonable numerical compatibility of enzyme results among laboratories, by introducing a unifying reference system for expression of catalytic activity concentration results based on use of human reference materials to which concentration values are assigned by state-of-the-art International Federation for Clinical Chemistry (IFCC) reference methods. Such a reference system, in which enzyme activity re-

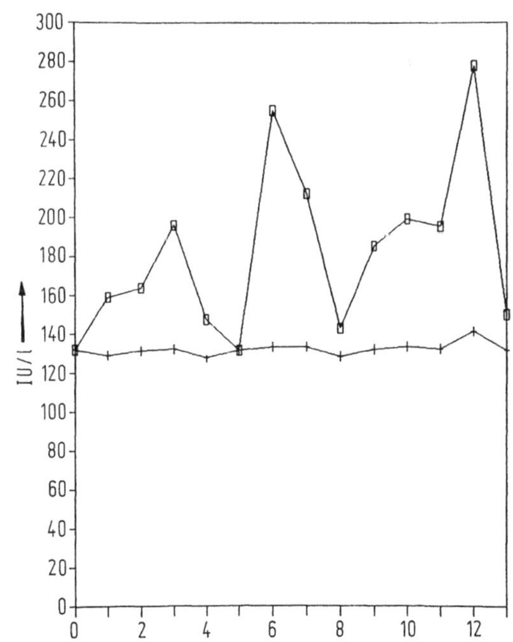


**Fig. 2.** Gamma-glutamyltransferase activity concentration values for sample V-11 (set V-D) of 1985 CAP proficiency survey. For details see Fig. 1

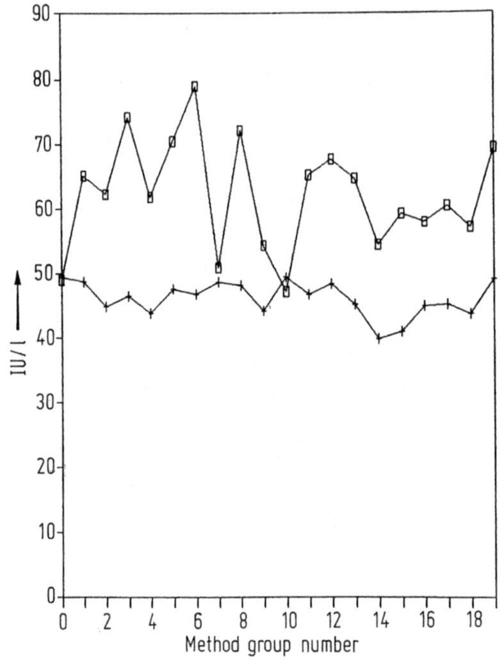


**Fig. 3.** AST activity concentration values for sample V-11 (set V-D) of 1985 CAP proficiency survey. For details see Fig. 1

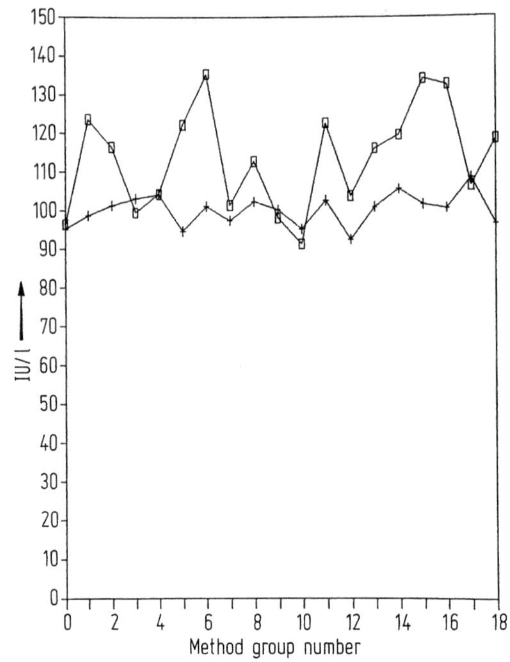


**Fig. 4.** Alanine aminotransferase activity concentration values for sample V-11 (set V-D) of 1985 CAP proficiency survey. For details see Fig. 1

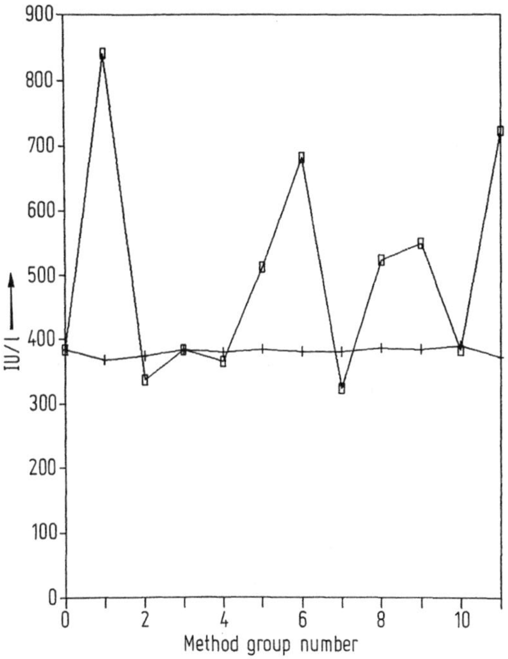


**Fig. 5.** Amylase activity concentration values for sample V-11 (set V-D) of 1985 CAP proficiency survey. For details see Fig. 1

sults would be expressed with reference to a so-called International Clinical Enzyme Scale (ICES) in IU/L (ICES) has been proposed (Bowers and McComb 1984; McComb and Bowers 1985). Specifically, implementation of the ICES system would involve production of limited amounts of human reference enzyme materials to be assayed in designated ICES references laboratories using IFCC reference methods at 29.77 °C (gallium temperature standard), to assign certified ICES enzyme activity concentration values. These *primary* reference materials would then have to be used as calibrators in secondary (e.g., reagent manufacturers') laboratories for assigning ICES enzyme activity values to *secondary* calibration standards for distribution to individual clinical laboratories. Clinical laboratories would use these secondary calibration materials in assaying patient specimens and express enzyme activity results in ICES units. That such a system might lead to markedly improved uniformity has been demonstrated by recomputation of CAP survey results (Bowers and McComb 1984; McComb and Bowers 1985). Results of similar recalculations of 1985 CAP enzyme results are shown in Figs. 1-5. Adoption of the ICES system or a similar proposal would be of importance to hepatologists, especially to those involved in developing or wishing to use clinical indices that incorporate biochemical liver test results for evaluation of severity and prognosis, and thereby provide guidance for treatment of patients with chronic liver disease. For example, recently proposed scoring systems cannot be directly used by other hepatologists, because the enzyme assay methodology and therefore the transferability of the numerical enzyme concentration values used in computation of the prognostic indices are unknown.

## Serum Bilirubins: Recent Developments

Recent evidence indicates that the complexity of the bilirubins in sera of patients with conjugated hyperbilirubinemia is far greater than previously suspected. Normal serum contains predominantly unconjugated bilirubin, small amounts of bilirubin monoglucuronide and bilirubin diglucuronide, and trace levels of bilirubin-IX-beta (Muraca and Blanckaert 1983). It has recently become evident that when hepatobiliary excretory function is impaired, the bilirubin glucuronides accumulated in serum undergo two types of secondary, most likely nonenzymatic changes (Fig. 6): hydrolysis to unconjugated bilirubin (Acocella et al. 1968; Blanckaert et al. 1980; McDonagh et al. 1984), with shifting of the bilirubin acyl group on the glucuronide moiety to form positional isomers (Compernolle et al. 1978; Blanckaert et al. 1978b), and an unidentified type of reaction with serum proteins, predominantly albumin, resulting in presumably covalent bonding of the bilirubin pigment to protein, i.e., bilirubin-protein conjugates (Lauff et al. 1982; Blanckaert and d'Argenio 1982; Weiss et al. 1983; McDonagh et al. 1984). Various confusing terms to denote this protein-linked pigment fraction have been used in recent literature: delta-bilirubin, biliprotein, bil-alb, albumin-bound bilirubin. We propose the term "bilirubin-protein conjugate" (Blanckaert et al. 1986). Two types of natural bilirubin-protein conjugates exist. An esterified bilirubin-protein conjugates corresponds with pigment that is covalently bonded to protein (probably at a propionic acid side chain) and that is also esterified, at the other propionic acid side chain, with a sugar moiety. An unesterified bilirubin-protein conjugate consists of bilirubin with one free propionic acid side chain and another propionic acid side chain linked to protein. The term "esterified bilirubins" is used to denote bilirubins in which one of both propionic acid side chains are esterified and covalent linkage of the pigment to protein is absent. "Conjugated bilirubins" comprise mono- and diesterified bilirubins, as well as the two types of bilirubin-protein conjugates.

Bilirubin-protein conjugates are not detectable in normal serum or in sera of patients with unconjugated hyperbilirubinemia, such as in physiological jaundice of the

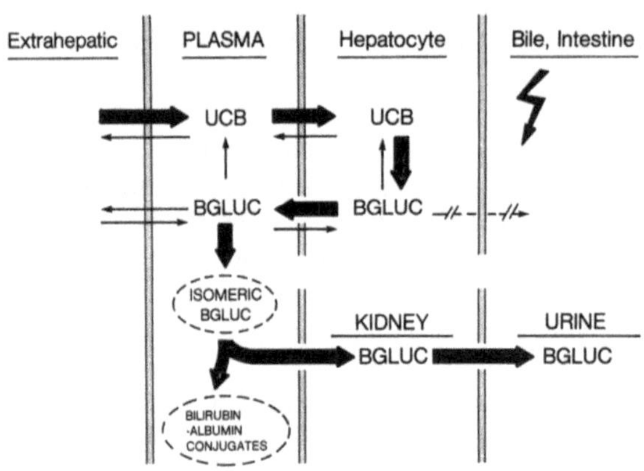


**Fig. 6.** Composition of serum bilirubins in patients with conjugated hyperbilirubinemia. Impairment of hepatobiliary excretion of bilirubin glucuronides *(BGLUC)* is indicated by the interrupted arrow for transfer of BGLUC from hepatocyte to bile. BGLUC accumulating in serum is converted to unconjugated bilirubin *(UCB)*, positional isomers of BGLUC *(isomeric BGLUC)*, and bilirubin-protein conjugates. The scheme also indicates that only BGLUC can be eliminated in urine

newborn, Gilbert's syndrome, or uncomplicated hemolytic hyperbilirubinemia. There is evidence that a precursor-product relationship exists between bilirubin glucuronides and bilirubin-protein conjugates, and that conversion of esterified bilirubins to bilirubin-protein conjugates is a nonenzymatic process that can occur in vivo as well as in vitro (Blanckaert and Servaes 1983; McDonagh et al. 1984). Thus, presence of bilirubin-protein conjugates in serum is merely an epiphenomenon of accumulation of bilirubin glucuronides in serum, independent of the cause of the conjugated hyperbilirubinemia. The clinical significance of specific measurement of bilirubin-protein conjugates in serum presently remains poorly defined, and there seems to be no need to specifically measure this pigment fraction in standard clinical practice. It is important to realize that based on the postulated nonenzymatic and nonspecific mechanism of formation of bilirubin-protein conjugates, one cannot expect that the pigment-protein conjugate fraction in serum reflects the actual status of hepatobiliary function. Only the accumulation of the esterified bilirubin precursors of the pigment-protein conjugates is a direct and immediate reflection of impaired hepatobiliary excretion. Also, removal of bilirubin-protein conjugates from blood is probably not dependent on the hepatobiliary excretory function, because the pharmacokinetic properties of this serum pigment fraction are most likely determined primarily by the plasma clearance of the albumin moiety (half-life ca 20 days). For example, it is conceivable that following complete recovery from hepatobiliary dysfunction, the total bilirubin level in serum remains temporarily elevated because of the persistence of long-lived bilirubin-protein conjugates in serum after the unconjugated and esterified bilirubin concentrations have normalized. Consequently, measurements of bilirubin-protein conjugates can provide information on the status of hepatobiliary function only in an indirect manner and with a considerable lag period.

In summary, these recent findings and considerations suggest that assay of bilirubin-protein conjugates in serum should not be used routinely for evaluation of hepatobiliary function in patients. A specific and well-validated method for determination of bilirubin-protein conjugates which can be performed in any clinical laboratory has recently become available (Blanckaert et al. 1986). Such an assay may be clinically useful under some particular circumstances, for example in patients with elevated serum total bilirubin values in whom a prior acute episode of impairment of hepatobiliary function is suspected.

## References


Acocella G, Tenconi LT, Armas-Merino R, Raia S, Billing BH (1968) Does deconjugation of bilirubin glucuronide occur in obstructive jaundice? Lancet 1: 68-69

Aoyagi Y, Isemura M, Suzuki Y, Sekine C, Soga K, Ozaki T, Ichida F (1985) Fucosylated alfafetoprotein as marker of early hepatocellular carcinoma. Lancet 1353-1354

Blanckaert N, d'Argenio G (1982) Presence of bilirubins covalently linked to albumin in serum of patients with cholestasis. Gastroenterology 82: 1222

Blanckaert N, Servaes R (1983) Formation and excretability in bile of the bilirubin covalently linked to albumin present in serum of rats with conjugated hyperbilirubinemia. Gastroenterology 84: 1364

Blanckaert N, Compernolle F, Leroy P, van Houtte R, Fevery J, Heirwegh KPM (1978) The fate of bilirubin-IXalpha glucuronide in cholestasis and during storage in vitro. Intramolecular rearrangement to positional isomers of glucuronic acid. Biochem J 171: 203-214

Blanckaert N, Gollan JL, Schmid R (1980a) Mechanism of bilirubin diglucuronide formation in intact rats. J Clin Invest 65: 1332-1342
Blanckaert N, Kabra PM, Farina FA, Stafford BE, Marton LJ, Schmid R (1980b) Measurement of bilirubin and its monoconjugates and diconjugates in human serum by alkaline methanolysis and high-performance liquid chromatography. J Lab Clin Med 96: 198-212
Blanckaert N, Servaes R, Leroy P (1986) Measurement of bilirubin-protein conjugates in serum and application to human and rat sera. J Lab Clin Med 100: 77-87
Bowers GN Jr, McComb RB (1984) A unifying system for clinical enzymology. Aspartate aminotransferase and the international clinical enzyme scale (ASAT/ICES). Clin Chem 30: 1128-1136
Buamah PK, Cornell C, Casselis-Smith AJ, Harris AL (1986) Fucosylation of alfa-fetoprotein in hepatocellular carcinomas. Lancet 922-923
Christensen E, Schlichting P, Fauerholdt L, Juhl E, Poulsen H, Tygstrup N: Copenhagen Study Group for Liver Diseases (1985) Changes of laboratory variables with time in cirrhosis: prognostic and therapeutic significance. Hepatology 5: 843-853
Compernolle F, van Hees GP, Blanckaert N, Heirwegh KPM (1978) Glucuronic acid conjugates of bilirubin-IXalpha glucuronide in cholestasis and during storage in vitro. Intramolecular rearrangement to positional isomers of glucuronic acid. Biochem J 171: 203-214
Eriksen J, Staun Olsen P, Thomsen AaC (1984) Gamma-glutamyltranspeptidase, aspartate aminotransferase, and erythrocyte mean corpuscular volume as indicators of alcohol consumption in liver disease. Scand J Gastroenterol 19: 813-819
Galambos MR, Collins DC, Galambos JT (1985) A radioimmunoassay procedure for type III procollagen: its use in the detection of hepatic fibrosis. Hepatology 5: 38-42
Giannoulis E, Arvanitakis C, Nikopoulos A, Doutsos I, Tourkantonis A (1984) Diagnostic value of serum ferritin in primary hepatocellular carcinoma. Digestion 30: 236-241
Gluud C, Andersen I, Dietrichson O, Gluud B, Jacobsen A, Juhl E (1981) Gamma-glutamyl-transferase, aspartate aminotransferase and alkaline phosphatase as markers of alcohol consumption in out-patient alcoholics. Eur J Clin Invest 11: 171-176
Hahn EG (1984) Blood analysis for liver fibrosis. J Hepatol 1: 67-73
Jenkins WJ, Rosalki SB, Foo Y, et al. (1982) Serum glutamate dehydrogenase is not a good measure of liver cell necrosis in alcoholics. J Clin Pathol 35: 207-210
Kobayashi K, Sugimoto T, Makino H, Kumagai M, Unoura M, Tanaka N, Kato Y, Hattori N (1985) Screening methods for early detection of hepatocellular carcinoma. Hepatology 5: 1100-1105
Kristenson H, Trell E (1982) Indicators of alcohol consumption. Br J Addict 77: 297-304
Lauff JJ, Kaspar MB, Wu T-W, Ambrose RT (1982) Isolation and characterization of a fraction of bilirubin in serum that is firmly bound to protein. Clin Chem 28: 629-637
Lauff JJ, Kasper ME, Ambrose RT (1983) Quantitative liquid-chromatographic estimation of bilirubin species in pathological serum. Clin Chem 29: 800-805
Lesgourgues B, Nalpas B, Berthelot P (1984) Gamma-glutamyltransferase – a simple assay but frequent misinterpretations. Gastroenterol Clin Biol 8: 99-102
Liaw Y-F, Tai D-I, Chu C-M, Lin D-Y, Sheen I-S, Chen T-J, Pao CC (1986) Early detection of hepatocellular carcinoma in patients with chronic type B hepatitis. Gastroenterology 90: 263-267
Liebman HA, Furie BC, Tong MJ, Blanchard RA, Lo K-J, Lee S-D, Coleman MS, Furie B (1984) Des-gamma-carboxy (abnormal) prothrombin as a serum marker of primary hepatocellular carcinoma. N Engl J Med 310: 1427-1731
MacNamara E, Goldberg DM (1985) Serum enzymes and enzyme profiles in the diagnosis of liver and biliary tract disease. Surv Dig Dis 3: 165-186
McComb RB, Bowers GN Jr (1985) Alkaline phosphatase and the international clinical enzyme scale. Am J Clin Pathol 84: 67-73
McDonagh AF, Palma LA, Lauff JJ, Wu T-W (1984) Origin of mammalian biliprotein and rearrangement of bilirubin glucuronides in vivo in the rat. J Clin Invest 74: 763-770
Miatto O, Casaril M, Gabrielli GB, Nicolo N, Bellisola G, Corrocher R (1985) Diagnostic and prognostic value of serum copper and plasma fibrinogen in hepatic carcinoma. Cancer 55: 774-778
Mills PR, Spooner RJ, Russell RI, et al. (1981) Serum glutamate dehydrogenase as a marker of hepatocyte necrosis in alcoholic liver disease. Br Med J 283: 754-755

Millward-Sadler GH, Hahn EG, Wright R (1985) Cirrhosis: an appraisal. In: Wright R, Millward-Sadler GH, Alberti KGMM, Karran S (eds) Liver and biliary disease, 2nd edn. Bailliere Tindall, Saunders, Eastbourne, pp 821-860
Muraca M, Blanckaert N (1983) Liquid chromatographic assay and identification of mono- and diester conjugates of bilirubin in normal serum. Clin Chem 29: 1767-1771
Nakano S, Kumada T, Sugiyama K, Watahiki H, Takeda I (1984) Clinical significance of serum ferritin determination for hepatocellular carcinoma. Am J Gastroenterol 79: 623-627
Nalpas B, Vassault A, Le Guillou A, Lesgourgues B, Ferry N, Lacour B, Berthelot P (1984) Serum activity of mitochondrial aspartate aminotransferase: a sensitive marker of alcoholism with or without alcoholic hepatitis. Hepatology 4: 893-896
Orrego H, Kalant H, Israel Y, Blake J, Medline A, Rankin JG, Armstrong A, Kapur B (1979) Effects of short-term therapy with propylthiouracyl in patients with alcoholic liver disease. Gastroenterology 76: 105-115
Roberts FD, Sanford NL, Bradbear RA, Cooksley WGE, Powell LW, Halliday JW (1986) Serum procollagen-III-peptide: failure to reflect the extent of hepatic fibrosis. J Gastroenterol Hepatol 1: 27-32
Rohde H, Langer I, Krieg T, Timpl R (1983) Serum and urine analysis of the aminoterminal procollagen peptide type III by radioimmunoassay with antibody Fab fragments. Coll Relat Res 3: 371-379
Rojkind M (1984) The value of serum amino-terminal propeptide of type III procollagen as a marker of liver fibrosis. Hepatology 4: 977-978
Ryback RS, Eckardt MJ, Felsher B, Rawlings RR (1982) Biochemical and hematologic correlates of alcoholism and liver disease. JAMA 248: 2261-2265
Seligson D, Seligson H, Wu T-W (1985) An anion-exchange chromatographic method for measuring bilirubin covalently bound to albumin. Clin Chem 31: 1317-1321
Skinner HA, Holt S, Schuller R, Roy J, Israel Y (1984) Identifikation of alcohol abuse using laboratory tests and a history of trauma. Ann Intern Med 101: 847-851
Vanderlinde RE (1986) Review of pyridoxal phosphate and the transaminase in liver disease. Ann Clin Lab Sci 16: 79-93
Van Waes L, Lieber CS (1977) Glutamate dehydrogenase: a reliable marker of liver cell necrosis in the alcoholic. Br Med J 2: 1508-1510
Weiss JS, Gautam A, Lauff JJ, Sundberg MW, Jatlow P, Boyer JL, Seligson D (1983) The clinical importance of a protein-bound fraction of serum bilirubin in patients with hyperbilirubinemia. N Engl J Med 309: 147-150
Worner TM, Lieber CS (1980) Plasma glutamate dehydrogenase, a marker of alcoholic liver injury. Pharmacol Biochem Behav 13: 107-110

# Should Serum Bile Acid Determinations Be Performed Routinely in Patients with Liver Disease?

Barbara H. Billing

Department of Medicine, Royal Free Hospital, London NW3 2QG, United Kingdom

None of the blood tests routinely used to assess liver function are ideal. Serum albumin and prothrombin time provide an index of protein synthesis by the hepatocyte, but are somewhat insensitive. Serum transaminase levels, though sensitive, reflect hepatocyte damage rather than function. Serum bilirubin and alkaline phosphatase are good indicators of cholestasis but poor indicators of hepatic function. Serum gamma glutamyl transpeptidase is a sensitive test of both cholestasis and hepatic damage but as a microsomal enzyme is susceptible to induction by certain drugs, including alcohol, so that interpretation of the results may present difficulties. There is, therefore, a need for a more specific and sensitive test of liver function.

Bile acids are both synthesised and excreted by the liver, and with the development of relatively simple techniques for their estimation their potential as a liver function test has been explored by many investigators, particularly in Italy, Scandinavia and the United States. Before examining in greater detail the value of serum bile acids as a test of liver function, it is important to consider some of the factors which control the level of bile acids in the blood; this is achieved by maintaining a balance between intestinal absorption and hepatic uptake. In hepatic disorders there may be impairment in hepatic blood flow and intrinsic clearance, which includes hepatic uptake, intracellular transport and biliary excretion. Studies in patients with cirrhosis by Islam et al. (1985) have shown that there is a significant log-log relationship between the fasting serum bile acid and the intrinsic clearance of ICG, which parallels that of bile acid as well as hepatic plasma flow. By the measurement of intrahepatic shunts, using macroaggregated albumin, it has been possible to show that in patients with moderately advanced cirrhosis, the serum bile acid level is related to the degree of intrahepatic shunting (Ohkubo et al. 1984). It is also important to mention that there is now good evidence that the fractional hepatic extraction of bile acids in an individual is relatively constant and is, therefore, independent of the load of bile acids presented. This information, in addition to the known individual variation in the time taken to achieve maximum levels of the different bile acids after a meal, provides an explanation for the current thinking that post-prandial serum bile acid determinations are not necessarily a more sensitive index of liver function than the fasting level (Van Blankenstein et al. 1983; Cravetto et al. 1985; Festi et al. 1983).

In order to determine the role of serum bile acid estimations in the assessment of liver function it is obviously necessary to know whether it matters which analytical method is employed. Few investigators have addressed themselves to this problem, and I would therefore like to mention a limited study performed at the Royal Free Hospital which was designed to determine whether serum bile acids were more sensitive for the detection of minimal liver disease than routine liver function tests (Chitranukroh et al.

Assessment and Management of Hepatobiliary Disease
Eds.: L. Okolicsányi, G. Csomós, and G. Crepaldi

1984). Bile acid determinations were performed by radioimmunoassay for conjugated primary bile acids, glycocholate and conjugated chenodeoxycholate, as well as enzymatically for 3 $\alpha$ total bile acids. The incidence of abnormal serum bile acid levels was essentially independent of the analytical method employed. It therefore appears justifiable to compare the results obtained from several studies even if different techniques have been employed.

During the last 5 years there have been several reports in which large numbers of patients with biopsy-proven liver disease have been examined with respect to the value of serum bile acid determinations in diagnosis (Linnet and Rye Andersen 1983; Rickers et al. 1982; Van Blankenstein et al. 1983; Festi et al. 1983; Ferraris et al. 1983; Cravetto et al. 1985; Van Hootegem et al. 1985). In addition to a discussion of the findings of these authors with respect to diagnosis and detection of minimal liver disease, the value of serum bile acids in prognosis, monitoring of treatment, prediction of severity of histological damage and screening will be assessed.

## Diagnosis and Detection of Minimal Liver Disease

The large scatter in serum bile acid levels seen in various types of liver disease makes it not surprising that an individual bile acid determination rarely has diagnostic value. Attempts have been made to use bile acid concentrations to discriminate between major diagnostic categories, but these have not proved successful (Rickers et al. 1982; Berry and Reichen 1983; Linnet and Rye Andersen 1983; Ferraris et al. 1983; Cravetto et al. 1985). The discrimination achieved with standard liver function tests can, however, be improved by the addition of a bile acid determination (Festi et al. 1983; Ferraris et al. 1983; Chitranukroh et al. 1984). For the detection of mild liver disease bile acids have not proved to be superior to transaminases (Festi et al. 1983; Van Blankenstein et al. 1983). Indeed, their value in anicteric patients does not appear to be as great as originally anticipated (Douglas et al. 1981; Van Hootegem et al. 1985). Although the sensitivity of bile acids may vary in the different hepatobiliary diseases (Berry and Reichen 1983; Ferraris et al. 1983), overall the sensitivity and specificity of bile acid determinations are similar to those of transaminases (Table 1).

**Table 1.** Sensitivities of serum bile acids and transaminase determinations in the detection of biopsy-proven liver disease

| Authors | No. of patients studied | Mean sensitivity (%) | |
|---|---|---|---|
| | | Bile acids | Transaminases |
| Cravetto et al. (1985) | 234 | 70 | 88 |
| Ferraris et al. (1983) | 344 | 78 | 74 |
| Festi et al. (1983) | 322 | 70 | 75 |
| Rickers et al. (1982) | 42 | 50 | 79 |
| Van Hootegem et al. (1985) | 108 | 66 | 71 |

## Screening

The studies mentioned above did not conclude that serum bile acid determinations provided a better screening test for liver disease than transaminases. There have, however, been favourable reports of their use in the detection of drug hepatotoxicity, including vinyl chloride. In this connection, Liss et al. (1985) found that serum bile acids exhibited a higher specificity for chemical liver disease than non-chemical liver disease. They did not, however, appear to be of any value in the detection of carriers of non-A non-B hepatitis (Mishier et al. 1981).

## Prognosis

The use of serum bile acid determinations as a predictor of prognosis in cirrhosis has recently been proposed (Mannes et al. 1986). Seventy-six patients with post-hepatitic and alcoholic cirrhosis were followed prospectively for 1 year. Sixteen died within the follow-up period, of whom 3 of 43 patients 7% had an initial serum bile acid concentration $<20\ \mu M$ while 6 of 9 patients 67% had values $>50\ \mu M$. Prediction of mortality based on serum bile acids was comparable with that of the Child's classification and was superior to clinical and laboratory parameters such as ascites, albumin, pseudocholinesterase, bilirubin, prothrombin time and nutritional state.

## Monitoring of Treatment

Levels of serum bile acids are often raised in the initial stages of liver disease, before the patient becomes icteric, and they tend to return to normal more quickly than other liver function tests (Berry and Reichen 1983). They may, therefore, be of value in monitoring treatment, and in chronic active hepatitis is has been shown that when steroids are withdrawn and there is a relapse, bile acid levels tend to rise before transaminases (Hofmann 1982). In tuberculous patients receiving rifampicin and isoniazid, the increases in bile acids observed in some patients were significantly greater than those of other liver function tests, which in many instance remained within the normal range (Berg et al. 1984).

## Prediction of Severity of Histological Damage

Comparisons of serum bile acids levels with pathological lesions in liver biopsies have not supported the view that these determinations constitute a sensitive test of liver function, since in the presence of a fatty liver a high proportion have normal values (Alm et al. 1982; Einarsson et al. 1985). When compared with 11 different histological characteristics, it was found that serum levels of bile acids correlated best with cholestasis, piecemeal necrosis, Kupffer cell activity and inflammation, although the association was not entirely convincing (Alm et al. 1982). Nevertheless, it has been observed in another study that the degree of elevation of serum bile acids provides a better indication as to whether the patient has moderate or minimal liver disease than the standard liver function tests (Chitranukroh et al. 1984).

## Other Uses of Bile Acid Determinations

Increased levels of bile acids may be of value in establishing a diagnosis of jaundice of pregnancy or benign recurrent intrahepatic cholestasis during the anicteric phase of the illness (Berry and Reichen 1983). On the other hand, a normal bile acid level can have diagnostic significance in differentiating Gilbert's syndrome from structural liver disease (Briheim et al. 1982; Roda et al. 1982).

## Summary and Conclusions

A review of the literature of the last 5 years has revealed that although serum bile acids and transaminases have similar sensitivity, specificity and predictive values in hepatobiliary disease, transaminases are probably more suitable as a screening test for liver disease, as the techniques are well established in all hospital laboratories. Bile acid determinations do, however, give a better indication of the severity of the histological lesion and may be of value as a prognostic indicator in cirrhosis and in the detection of chemical hepatoxicity. In agreement with Hofmann (1982), the addition of serum bile acids determination to the battery of standard liver function tests does not appear to be justified, although the assays should be available for special investigations.

## References


Alm R, Carlso J, Eriksson S (1982) Fasting serum bile acids in liver disease. A comparison with histological featues. Scand J Gastroenterol 17: 213-218

Berg JD, Pandov HI, Sammons HG (1984) Serum total bile acid levels in patients receiving rifampicin and isoniazid. Ann Clin Biochem 21: 218-222

Berry W, Reichen J (1983) Bile acid metabolism: its relation to clinical disease. Semin Liver Dis 3: 330-340

Briheim G, Fryden A, Tobiasson P (1982) Serum bile acids in Gilbert's syndrome before and after reduced caloric intake. Scand J Gastroenterol 17: 877-886

Chitranukroh A, Heady JR, Rosalki S, Summerfield JA, Billing BH (1984) The value of bile acid determinations in the detection of mild liver disease. In: Proceedings of first international symposium on bile acids in hepatobiliary and gastrointestinal diseases. IRL Press, Oxford, pp 91-94

Cravetto C, Molino G, Biondi AM, Cavanna A, Avagnina P, Frediani S (1985) Evaluation of the diagnostic value of serum bile acid in detection and functional assessment of liver diseases. Ann Clin Biochem 22: 596-605

Douglas JG, Beckett GJ, Nimmo IA, Finlayson NDC, Percy-Robb IW (1981) Clinical value of bile salts in anicteric liver disease. Gut 22: 141-148

Einarsson K, Angelin B, Bjorkhem I, Glauman H (1985) The diagnostic value of fasting individual serum bile acids in anicteric alcoholic liver disease: relation to liver morphology. Hepatology 5: 108-111

Ferraris R, Colombatti G, Fiorentini MT, Carosso R, Arossa W, de la Pierre M (1983) Diagnostic value of serum bile acids and routine liver function tests in hepatobiliary diseases. Dig Dis Sci 28: 129-136

Festi D, Labate AMM, Roda A, Bazzoli F, Frabboni R, Rucci P, Taroni F, Aldini R, Roda E, Barbara L (1983) Diagnostic effectiveness of serum bile acids in liver diseases as evaluated by multivariate statistical methods. Hepatology 3: 707-713

Hofmann AF (1982) The aminopyrine demethylation breath test and the serum bile acid level: nominated but not yet elected to join the common liver tests. Hepatology 2: 512-517

Islam S, Poupon RE, Barbare JC, Chretien Y, Darnis F, Poupon R (1985) Fasting serum bile acid level in cirrhosis. A semi-quantitative index of hepatic function. J Hepatol 1: 609-617
Linnet K, Rye Andersen J (1983) Differential diagnostic value in hepatobiliary disease of serum conjugated bile acid concentrations and some routine liver tests assessed by discriminant analysis. Clin Chim Acta 127: 217-228
Liss GM, Greenberg RA, Tamburro CH (1985) Use of serum bile acids in the identification of vinyl chloride hepatotoxicity. Am J Med 78: 68-76
Mannes GA, Thieme C, Stellard F, Wang T, Sauerbruch T, Paumgarter G (1986) Prognostic significance of serum bile acids in cirrhosis. Hepatology 6: 50-53
Mishier JM, Barbosa I, Milhalko J, McCartner H (1981) Serum bile acids and alanine aminotransferase concentrations. Comparison of efficacy as indirect means of identifying carriers of non-A, non-B hepatitis agents and of onset, severity, and duration of posttransfusion non-A, non-B hepatitis in recipients. JAMA 246: 2340-2344
Ohkubo H, Okudo K, Iida I, Ohnishi K, Ikawa S, Makino I (1984) The role of portal and splenic vein shunts and impaired hepatic extraction in the elevated serum bile acid levels in liver cirrhosis. Gastroenterology 86: 514-520
Rickers H, Christensen M, Arnfred T, Dige U, Hess Thaysen E (1982) The diagnostic value of fasting serum bile acid concentration in patients with suspected liver disease. A prospective, consecutive study. Scand J Gastroenterol 17: 565-570
Roda A, Roda E, Sama C, Festi D, Aldini R, Murselli AM, Mazzella G, Barbara L (1982) Serum primary bile acids in Gilbert's syndrome. Gastroenterology 82: 77-83
Van Blankenstein M, Frenkel M, van den Berg JWO, Ten Kate FJW, Bosman-Jacobs EP, Touw-Blommesteyn AC (1983) Endogenous bile acid tolerance test for liver function. Dig Dis Sci 28: 137-144
Van Hootegem P, Fevery J, Blanckaert N (1985) Serum bilirubins in hepatobiliary disease: comparison with other liver function tests in the postobstructive period. Hepatology 5: 112-117

# Clinical Significance of Serum Bilirubins: Recent Advances

Maurizio Muraca, Rocco Orlando, Mario Strazzabosco, Gino Nassuato, Flavio Lirussi, Rosa Maria Iemmolo, and Lajos Okolicsanyi
Institute of Internal Medicine, University of Padua, Padua, Italy

The potential clinical value of serum bilirubin cannot be fully exploited because of analytical problems affecting in particular the determination of the conjugated pigment fraction. In this review, some recent methodological advances are described which now allow direct quantitation of unconjugated bilirubin, bilirubin monoconjugate, and bilirubin diconjugate in human serum. This novel methodology has greatly improved our understanding of the mechanisms determining the levels of conjugated bilirubin in serum, and of changes occurring in pathological conditions.

## Analytical Problems

Current methods for the determination of serum bilirubins are still based on the diazo coupling of the pigments as described initially by Ehrlich (1883). The reaction is based on a nucleophilic attack of a first diazonium molecule on the carbon atom 9 or 11 of the tetrapyrrole, with formation of an azodipyrrole and of an intermediate, unstable dipyrrole which further reacts with a second diazonium molecule yielding a second azodipyrrole. Thus, in this two-stage reaction, two molecules of azodipyrrole are formed per molecule of bilirubin. The amount of azoderivatives formed in the reaction is determined spectrophotometrically. Van den Berg and Muller (1916) observed that bilirubin in bile reacts "directly", i.e., without requiring the presence of an accelerator, such as alcohol, and concluded that at least two species of bilirubin were present in biological fluids. The direct reaction was associated with bile and with the bilirubin in urine and in plasma in obstructive jaundice, while the bilirubin in plasma of patients with hemolytic disease required the presence of alcohol to give a positive diazo reaction ("indirect-reacting" bilirubin). The direct-reacting pigment was later identified as bilirubin glucuronide, and the indirect-reacting bilirubin was found to correspond to unconjugated bilirubin (Talafant 1956; Billing et al. 1957; Schmid 1957). This distinction was found to be very useful in clinical practice. However, it soon became clear that the two pigment fractions did not reflect the actual concentrations of unconjugated and conjugated bilirubin, but were influenced by the reaction conditions (such as pH or exposure to light) and by the composition of the sample (Nosslin 1960). In general, there is always a variable fraction of unconjugated pigment in plasma that behaves as direct-reacting, while the exact behavior of conjugated bilirubin has not been completely clarified, due to lack of reference standards. The determination of conjugated bilirubin is complicated by peculiar analytical problems in relation to the chemical characteristics of the compound. The ester bond between glucuronic acid and the propionic acid side chain of the pigment is very labile and can easily be hydrolyzed. During stasis in vivo

Assessment and Management of Hepatobiliary Disease
Eds.: L. Okolicsányi, G. Csomós, and G. Crepaldi

or in vitro, it can also migrate to other hydroxylic groups of the sugar residue, giving rise to a number of non-C-1-positional isomers (Blanckaert et al. 1978; Compernolle et al. 1978). In addition, both mono- and diconjugated bilirubins exist, which might react differently with the diazo reagent. The lability of the compound is the main reason why purified bilirubin 1-O-acylglucuronide is not yet available as a standard for calibration.

Several modifications of the diazo reaction have been described, none of which could substantially overcome the limitations of the original method. The ethylanthranylate procedure described by Van Roy and Heirwegh (1968) yields stable azodipyrroles which are extracted into an organic solvent, increasing the sensitivity of the assay and allowing chromatographic separation, isolation, and identification of the pigments. By this procedure, fundamental information has been obtained about the composition of bilirubins in biological samples (Fevery et al. 1972). However, it is impossible to relate the azodipyrrole derivatives to the parent rubins present in complex biological samples such as serum, and the selectivity of the reaction for the conjugated pigment is not absolute (see Heirwegh and Blanckaert 1982).

The limitation of conventional diazo methods stimulated the development of several procedures for the analysis of intact tetrapyrroles. Solvent-partition techniques were developed in an attempt to separate the unconjugated from the conjugated pigment based on their different polarity, but these procedures were not reliable and usually not more selective than conventional diazo methods. Other chromatographic techniques based on separation of pigments by column or thin-layer chromatography (TLC) are usually cumbersome, not quantitative, and have never been validated as analytical tools (see Heirwegh and Blanckaert 1982).

In summary, current methods for the determination of bilirubins are affected by the following problems.
1. Interference with compounds present in serum
2. Lack of selectivity between unconjugated and conjugated bilirubin
3. Lability of the ester linkage between glucuronic acid and bilirubin, resulting in hydrolysis and/or formation of positional isomers
4. Unavailability of pure bilirubin 1-O-acylglucuronide standards for calibration

## The Alkaline Methanolysis Procedure

The alkaline methanolysis method (Blanckaert 1980) was developed in order to circumvent these limitations. Bilirubin mono- and disugar conjugates are converted to the corresponding mono- and dimethyl esters by brief treatment with alkaline methanol. Unconjugated bilirubin is not affected by the reaction, and is extracted into chloroform together with the methyl ester derivatives. The pigments can then be separated and individually quantified by TLC or high-pressure liquid chromotography (HPLC). Since conversion of the sugar conjugates to methyl esters is virtually quantitative, this method can be calibrated with available bilirubin mono- and dimethyl esters.

An initially developed HPLC procedure for quantification of individual pigments derived from alkaline methanolysis was applied to the analysis of serum samples. No conjugated bilirubin was detected in serum of healthy controls or of patients with Gilbert's syndrome (Blanckaert et al. 1980).

Variable amounts of both bilirubin mono- and diconjugates and a moderate increase of unconjugated bilirubin were observed in sera of jaundiced patients with hepatobiliary disease (Scharschmidt et al. 1982; Van Hootegem et al. 1985). The pattern of serum bilirubin was not clearly different among the various etiologic groups, including hepatocellular dysfunction and intra- or extrahepatic cholestasis. These applications of the alkaline methanolysis procedure showed that the serum bilirubin pattern is not useful in the differential diagnosis of hepatocellular disease from biliary obstruction. The most interesting aspect of the procedure, from a clinical point of view, seems to be the possibility of quantitating low levels of bilirubin ester conjugates. Their presence in serum seemed to point to hepatobiliary disease. It was possible to detect conjugates even in 87% of 40 sera of patients with hepatobiliary disease having a total serum bilirubin below 35 μmol/l, while they could not be detected in 22 healthy individuals or in patients with Gilbert's syndrome. The presence of conjugated bilirubin was a more sensitive marker for hepatobiliary disease than all other conventional liver function tests (Van Hootegem et al. 1985). In fact, conjugated bilirubin is normally readily excreted in bile, and an increased concentration in serum, relative to total bilirubin, should therefore reflect impaired biliary excretion. The latter step is easily impaired by all hepatobiliary insults.

## A New High-Pressure Liquid-Chromatographic Procedure for Accurate Identification and Measurement of Bilirubin Ester Conjugates in Serum

As outlined above, the potential clinical value of serum bilirubin is not fully appreciated, since current methods do not allow specific determination of unconjugated and conjugated bilirubin. In fact, even the normal-phase HPLC separation of pigments derived from alkaline methanolysis, proposed by Blanckaert et al. (1980), was not sensitive enough to measure conjugated bilirubin in serum of healthy adults or of patients with unconjugated hyperbilirubinemia. More recently, a reverse-phase separation system has been developed, greatly increasing the sensitivity of the assay mainly by eliminating interference from carotenoids, which are not soluble in a polar mobile phase (Muraca and Blanckaert 1983). A satisfactory separation between unconjugated bilirubin, bilirubin monomethyl and dimethyl ester, and hemin (which is present in hemolytic samples) was obtained with methanol/phosphate buffer pH 7.4 (70/30) as mobile phase and with a C-18 bonded-phase column. The selectivity of the separation system was then optimized by developing a gradient of the mobile phase, to which the counter-ion tetrabutylammonium phosphate was added to improve the chromatography of the compounds bearing carboxylic group, such as unconjugated bilirubin and its monomethylester. Accurate quantitation of the pigments was achieved by addition of xanthobilirubic acid as internal standard. The method enabled monoconjugated and diconjugated bilirubin to be estimated in human serum in concentrations as low as 10 and 20 nmol/l respectively.

The presence of bilirubin ester conjugates in serum of healthy adults was then investigated using this procedure. Bilirubin mono- and disugar conjugates were found in all of the 43 sera tested (29 men and 14 women) ranging respectively from 0.03 to 0.25 and from 0.04 to 0.26 μmol/l. The average concentration of conjugated bilirubins was about 3.5% of total bilirubin in both sexes, but the concentration of all three pigment fractions tended to be lower in women than in men (Muraca and Blanckaert 1983). The real presence of small amounts of bilirubin 1-O-acylglucuronides in normal serum was confirmed by analysis of ethylanthranylate azoderivatives. These data demonstrate unequivocally the presence of conjugated bilirubin in normal human serum. They also provide its normal concentration ranges, giving a basis for subsequent evaluation and quantitative modifications of the various bilirubin fractions in hepatobiliary or hematologic disease and in disorders of bile pigment metabolism.

## Relationships Between Serum Bilirubins and Bilirubin Production and Conjugation

The alkaline methanolysis-reverse-phase HPLC procedure was used to study how changes of pigment production and/or conjugation would affect the individual bilirubin fractions in serum. The study was thus conducted on samples of patients affected by unconjugated hyperbilirubinemia (Gilbert's syndrome and Crigler-Najjar disease) or increased pigment production (hemolytic disease). This study allowed a series of interesting observations.

### Presence of Conjugated Bilirubin in Hyperbilirubinemic Sera of Patients with Decreased Hepatic Conjugation

Bilirubin conjugates were identified in all sera tested, including those of patients with Gilbert's syndrome and Crigler-Najjar type II disease. The conjugates were also characterized by studying their ethylanthranylate azoderivatives, and were found to correspond to 1-O-acylglucuronide. The presence of esterified bilirubin in serum of Gilbert patients had previously been questioned (Blanckaert et al. 1980), but should no longer be a matter of debate.

### The Pattern of Serum Bilirubin Associated with Pigment Overload

Both unconjugated and conjugated bilirubin were increased in sera of patients affected by hemolytic disease (Fig. 1). Because of the parallel increase of both fractions, the percentage of conjugated relative to total bilirubin was not different from that in normal controls. These findings are consistent with the concept that a small fraction of the bilirubin esters formed in the liver normally refluxes into plasma, and that an equilibrium exists between the amount of conjugates present in these two compartments (Fig. 2). When the production of conjugated bilirubin in the liver increases, as is the case in conditions of pigment overload, there is a corresponding increase in the conjugates present in plasma. It should be emphasized that such an increase is best explained as the result of an equilibrium between liver and plasma concentrations. The classical belief that the increase in direct-reacting bilirubin in serum of some patients with severe hemolysis is caused by the saturation of canalicular secretion is not consistent with our finding that the ratio of conjugated to total bilirubin was normal in all hemolytic patients examined. In fact, according to the latter hypothesis, one should expect an increase of the conjugated fraction in serum only when canalicular secretion of conjugates in bile becomes saturated.

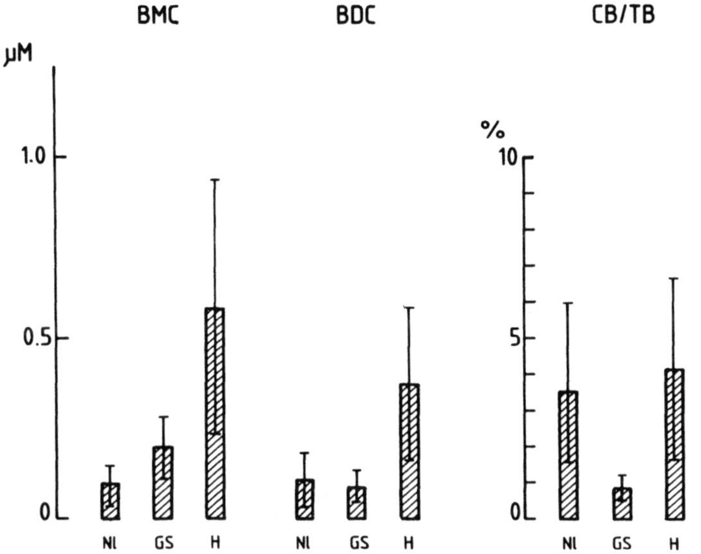


| | n | UCB (μM) | BDC/CB % |
|---|---|---|---|
| Nl | 43 | 6.2 ± 2.8 (1.8 - 12.3) | 54 ± 11 |
| GS | 22 | 31.5 ± 10.4 (18.1 - 58.3) | 33 ± 9 |
| H | 15 | 23.5 ± 7.8 (13.6 - 37.6) | 37 ± 11 |

**Fig. 1.** Bilirubin monoconjugates *(BMC)*, bilirubin diconjugates *(BDC)* and percent of conjugated to total bilirubin *(CB/TB)* in normal subjects *(Nl)* and in Gilbert's syndrome *(GS)* and hemolytic *(H)* patients. Values are means ±1 SD. The concentration of unconjugated bilirubin *(UCB)* and the percent of diconjugates to total conjugates *(BDC/CB)* in the same subjects are given in the lower part of the figure

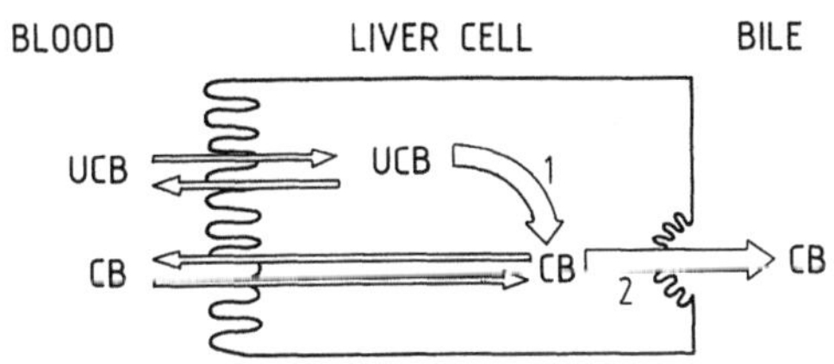


**Fig. 2.** Schematic representation of the partitioning of unconjugated *(UCB)* and conjugated *(CB)* bilirubin between blood, liver, and bile. *Thick arrows* represent the metabolic events which displace the equilibria to the right: (1) change of identity of the molecule (conjugation); (2) transfer to a different compartment (biliary excretion). In this model, the amount of conjugated bilirubin present in plasma depends on the amount formed in the liver, which in turn depends on the amount of unconjugated bilirubin reaching the liver. If one assumes that biliary excretion is not rate-limiting, the fractional exchange of conjugated bilirubin between blood and liver will be constant

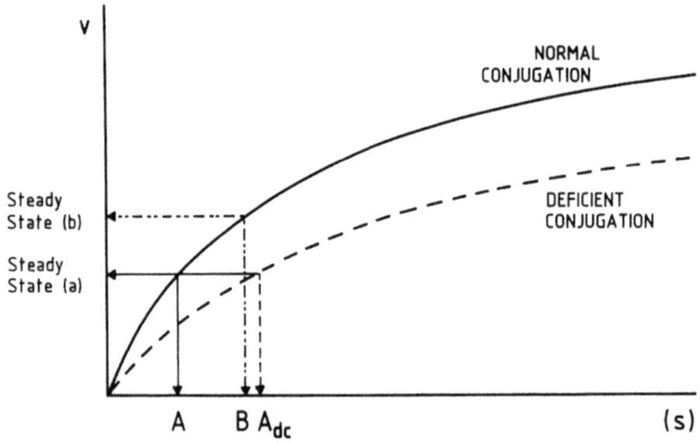


**Fig. 3.** Conjugation rate *(v)* as a function of substrate concentration *(s)*. A steady state is reached when the conjugation rate equals the rate of substrate production. In the case of normal substrate production (steady state *a*) and normal enzyme activity, such an equilibrium is reached at substrate concentration *A*. If the production of substrate is increased (steady state *b*) and conjugation is normal, a new equilibrium is reached at substrate concentration *B*. If conjugation is deficient (increased Km or decreased Vmax?), a higher concentration of substrate *(Adc)* is necessary to result in a steady state equal to normal substrate production

### The Pattern of Serum Bilirubins Associated with Decreased Hepatic Conjugation

The total concentration of esterified bilirubin in serum was normal in patients with decreased hepatic conjugation (Fig. 1). The conjugated fraction relative to total bilirubin, however, was decreased due to the elective increase of the unconjugated pigment. These findings can be explained by assuming that a steady state must be reached in the body in which the rate of bilirubin conjugation equals the rate of its production. In the presence of a lower activity of the conjugating enzyme, such an equilibrium is reached only at higher substrate concentrations. The selective increase of serum unconjugated bilirubin in Gilbert's syndrome patients might thus reflect such a mechanism (Fig. 3).

## Clinical Significance of the Present Findings

The attitude of the clinician toward serum bilirubin is to consider an isolated elevation of indirect-reacting bilirubin as related to decreased hepatic conjugation or increased pigment production, while an increased concentration of direct-reacting bilirubin is practically always regarded as an indication of cholestasis and hepatocellular damage. Our findings in patients with unconjugated hyperbilirubinemia, however, combined with the observations of Scharschmidt et al. (1982) and Van Hootegem et al. (1985) in patients with liver diseases, seem to suggest three different categories of altered bilirubin metabolism, which can be specifically identified by accurate measurement of unconjugated and conjugated bilirubin:

1. An increased concentration of unconjugated bilirubin with normal concentration of conjugates, resulting in a decreased fraction of conjugated relative to total bilirubin, is associated with decreased hepatic conjugation.

2. An increased concentration of both unconjugated and conjugated bilirubins with a normal ratio of conjugated to total pigment is associated with pigment overproduction.

3. An increased concentration of unconjugated bilirubin, but especially of the conjugates, resulting in a higher ratio of conjugated to total bilirubin, is seen in hepatobiliary diseases. This pattern has been described by Scharschmidt et al. (1982) and Van Hootegem et al. (1985) using a previous alkaline methanolysis-normal-phase HPLC method. Since our reverse-phase method is much more sensitive in detecting an increase of conjugated bilirubin, it could provide an even more powerful tool for detection of early impairment of hepatobiliary function.

## References

Billing BH, Cole PG, Lathe GH (1957) The excretion of bilirubin as a diglucuronide giving the direct Van den Bergh reaction. Biochem J 65: 774-784

Blanckaert N (1980) Analysis of bilirubin and bilirubin mono- and diconjugates. Determination of their relative amounts in biological samples. Biochem J 185: 115-128

Blanckaert N, Compernolle F, Leroy P, Van Houtte R, Fevery J, Heirwegh KPM (1978) The fate of bilirubin-IXa glucuronide in cholestasis and during storage in vitro. Intramolecular rearrangement to positional isomers of glucuronic acid. Biochem J 171: 203-214

Blanckaert N, Kabra PM, Farina FA, Stafford BE, Marton LJ, Schmid R (1980) Measurement of bilirubin and its monoconjugates and diconjugates in human serum by alkaline methanolysis and high-performance liquid chromatography. J Lab Clin Med 96: 198-212

Compernolle F, Van Hees GP, Blanckaert N, Heirwegh KPM (1978) Glucuronic acid conjugates of bilirubin-IXa in normal bile compared with postobstructive bile. Transformation of the 1-O-acylglucuronides into 2-,3-, and 4-O-acylglucuronides. Biochem J 171: 185-201

Ehrlich P (1883) Centr Klin Med 4: 721-723. Cited by With TK (1968) in: With TK (ed) Bile pigments. Chemical, biological and clinical aspects. Academic, New York, p 59

Fevery J, Van Damme B, Michiels R, De Groote J, Heirwegh KPM (1972) Bilirubin conjugates in bile of man and rat in the normal state and in liver disease. J Clin Invest 51: 2482-2492

Heirwegh KPM, Blanckaert N (1982) Analytical chemistry of rubins. In: Heirwegh KPM, Brown S (eds) Bilirubin, vol 1, chemistry. CRC Press, Boca Raton, p 125

Muraca M, Blanckaert N (1983) Liquid-chromatographic assay and identification of mono- and diester conjugates of bilirubin in normal serum. Clin Chem 29: 1767-1771

Nosslin B (1960) The direct diazo-reaction of bile pigments in serum. Experimental and clinical studies. Scand J Clin Lab Invest 12 [Suppl 49]

Scharschmidt BF, Blanckaert N, Farina FA, Kabra PM, Stafford BE, Weisiger RA (1982) Measurement of serum bilirubin and mono- and diconjugate: application to patient with hepatobiliary disease. Gut 23: 643-649

Schmid R (1957) The identification of "direct-reacting" bilirubin as bilirubin glucuronide. J Biol Chem 229: 881-888

Talafant E (1956) Properties and composition of the bile pigment giving a direct diazo-reaction. Nature 178: 312

Van den Berg AAH, Muller P (1916) Über eine direkte und eine indirekte Diazoreaktion auf Bilirubin. Biochem Z 77: 90-103

Van Hootegem P, Fevery J, Blanckaert N (1985) Serum bilirubins in hepatobiliary disease: comparison with other liver function tests and changes in the postobstructive period. Hepatology 5: 112-117

Van Roy FP, Heirwegh KPM (1968) Determination of bilirubin glucuronide and assay of glucuronyltransferase with bilirubin as acceptor. Biochem J 107: 507-518

# Enzyme Pattern Changes in Preneoplastic and Neoplastic Lesions of the Liver

K. Lapis[1], A. Jeney[1], ZS. Schaff[1], A. Zalatnai[1], I. Kovalszky[1], and A. Szécsény[2]

[1] First Institute of Pathology and Experimental Cancer Research, Semmelweiß Medical University, Budapest, Hungary
[2] First Surgical Clinic, Semmelweis Medical University, Budapest, Hungary

## Introduction

Primary hepatocellular carcinoma (PHC) is one of the ten most common cancers in the world (Editorial 1983) and one of the most fatal of all malignancies. The incidence of PHC is growing even in the so-called low-incidence countries, and thus increasing interest in PHC is justified. During recent decades experimental chemical hepatocarcinogenesis studies have shown that neoplastic transformation in the liver is a multistep process (Farber 1980; Pitot and Sirica 1980) and that well-recognizable preneoplastic alterations precede the formation of cancer. These preneoplastic alterations can be recognized most reliably by a number of functional abnormalities which are detectable by enzyme-histochemical and biochemical methods.

Studies on the pathogenesis and epidemiology of human liver cancer in accordance with the experimental observations also provide convincing evidence that precursor lesions – including most forms of chronic liver disease – also play an important role in the development of human PHC (Becker 1981). In human beings, cirrhosis, liver cell dysplasia (Anthony et al. 1973; Anthony 1976; Cohen et al. 1979; Harada et al. 1979; Ho et al. 1981; Watanabe 1983), nodular regenerative hyperplasia (Sogaard 1981), liver cell adenoma and focal nodular hyperplasia (FNH) (Christopherson and Mays 1979; Tesluk and Lawrie 1981) are regarded as possible precursor lesions. However, our knowledge concerning the nature and significance of these precursor lesions has remained rather insufficient (Schaff et al. 1986). Neither these lesions nor fully developed human liver cancer have been sufficiently studied from the point of view of enzyme-pattern changes, which, in experimental models of chemical hepatocarcinogenesis, proved to be the most reliable for the recognition and characterization of early precursor and preneoplastic lesions. Only few papers have been published on this topic (Gerber and Thung 1980; Thung and Gerber 1981; Uchida et al. 1981), and the number of the cases studied is particularly insufficient.

Our aim was to compare the enzyme-pattern changes taking place in the preneoplastic and neoplastic lesions of the human liver with those observed during experimental hepatocarcinogenesis. During the last few years this has become possible because of the improved methods of early tumour detection (Okuda et al. 1977; Takashima et al. 1982) and because more and more surgical specimens containing such lesions are becoming available to pathologists. We decided to study these specimens by applying the same enzyme-histochemical and biochemical methods which we were using in our studies on experimental hepatocarcinogenesis.

## Materials and Methods

### Experimental Hepatocarcinogenesis

Fischer 344 male rats weighing 130–150 g were obtained from LATI Breeding Centre (Gödöllő, Hungary).

The animals were maintained in plastic cages and given laboratory chow and water ad libitum. *N*-nitrosodiethylamine (DEN; Eastman-Kodak, Rochester, USA) as initiator was administered i.p. at a dose of 200 mg/kg body weight. The animals were permitted to recover for 2 weeks and then promotion was effected by administration of 5 mg/kg 2-acetyl-aminofluorene (AAF; Serva, Heidelberg, FRG) p.o. daily for 2 weeks. One week after starting promotion (i.e. 21 days after initiation) the animals were subjected to partial hepatectomy. Then the animals were killed at different time-points following this initiation-promotion procedure (Solt and Farber 1976) and their livers studied by histochemical and biochemical methods.

### Human Liver Specimens

Fourteen surgically removed human liver specimens containing preneoplastic or tumorous lesions were also studied using the same methods. The liver tissue surrounding these lesions served as control.

### Histological and Histochemical Studies

From the experimental and surgical specimens samples were taken and fixed in 8% neutral formalin and in Carnoy for the purpose of histological diagnosis. The main bulks of the rat livers and the surgical specimens – if not used immediately – were frozen and stored at −70 °C. Histological diagnosis was performed from formalin-fixed and paraffin-embedded samples that were stained with haematoxylin-eosin. The histochemical reactions were performed on cryostat sections (5–6 μm) for the following enzymes: glucose-6-phosphatase (G-6-Pase; Wachstein and Meisel 1956), $Mg^{++}$-dependent canalicular adenosine triphosphatase (ATPase; Wachstein and Meisel 1957) and gamma-glutamyl-transpeptidase (GGT; Rutenberg et al. 1968). For demonstration of the possible presence of HBsAg, orcein staining according to Shikata et al. (1974) was employed.

### Biochemical Studies

*Preparation of Tissue Samples.* One gram of liver or tumour tissue was washed and homogenized in ice-cold 50 m*M* Tris-HCl, pH 7.4, containing 1.15% KCl. Nuclei and mitochondria were removed, if whole homogenate was not used, by 600 *g* and 15000 *g* centrifugation respectively. Microsomes were pelleted by 105000 *g* centrifugation of the postmitochondrial supernatant.

*Cytochrome P-450 C=concentration.* Microsomes were resuspended in 50 m*M* Tris-HCl pH 7.6 containing 1 m*M* EDTA. Spectral measurements were performed using a Zeiss Specord UV VIS dual-beam spectrophotometer, and cytochrome P-450 concentrations were determined from reduced CO difference spectra as described by Omura and Sato (1964)

*GGT Activity.* Whole tissue homogenates were incubated with gamma-glutamyl-*p*-nitroanilide as substrate and glycyl-glycine as acceptor for 15 min at 37 °C according to the procedure reported by Szász (1969). The *p*-nitroaniline released was measured at 405 nm in an MOM spectrophotometer. Units of enzyme activity are expressed as micromoles of *p*-nitroaniline formed per minute at 37 °C.

*G-6-Pase Activity.* Whole tissue homogenates in 50 m*M* Tris-HCl pH 6.8 were incubated with glucose-6-phosphate as reported by Harper (1963). The inorganic phosphorus liberated was measured according to Fiske and Subbarow (1925).

## Results

### Studies on Experimental Hepatocarcinogenesis

Following the initiation-promotion procedure, a sequence of pathomorphological alterations – foci, nodules, PHC – developed in the liver of the rats. In the experimental model system applied in our Institute, the first foci could be detected as early as

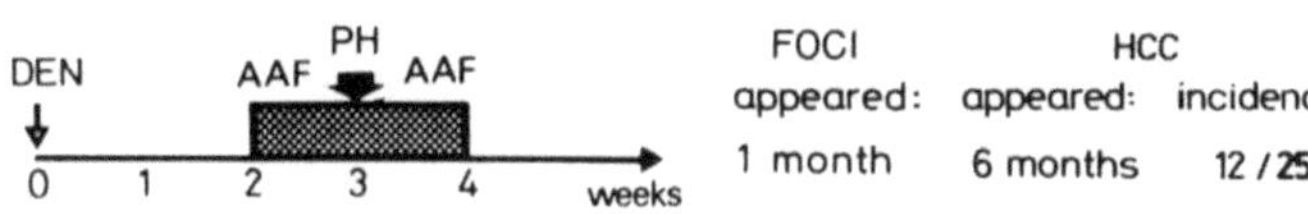


**Fig. 1.** Experimental model of hepatocarcinogenesis. *DEN*, *N*-nitrosodiethylamine; *AAF*, 2-acetyl-aminofluorence; *PH*, partial hepatectomy; *HCC*, hepatocellular carcinoma

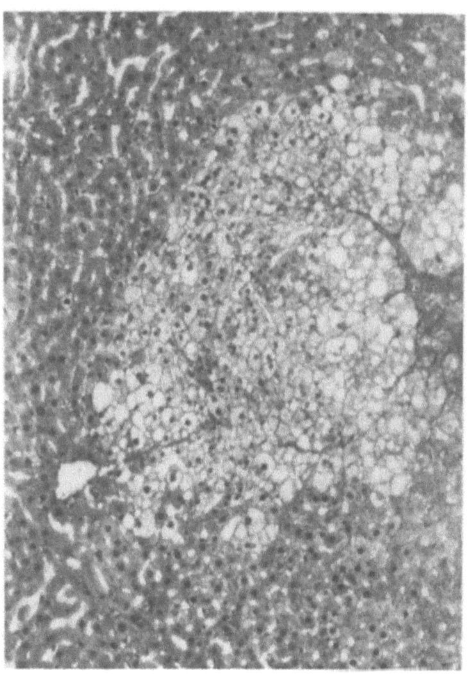

**Fig. 2.** Clear cell focus in rat liver

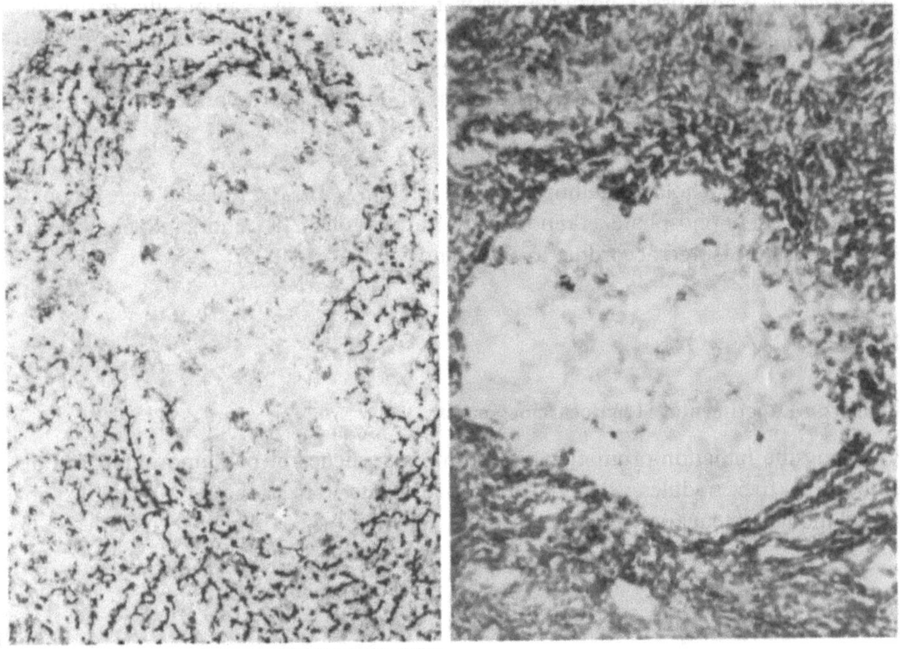

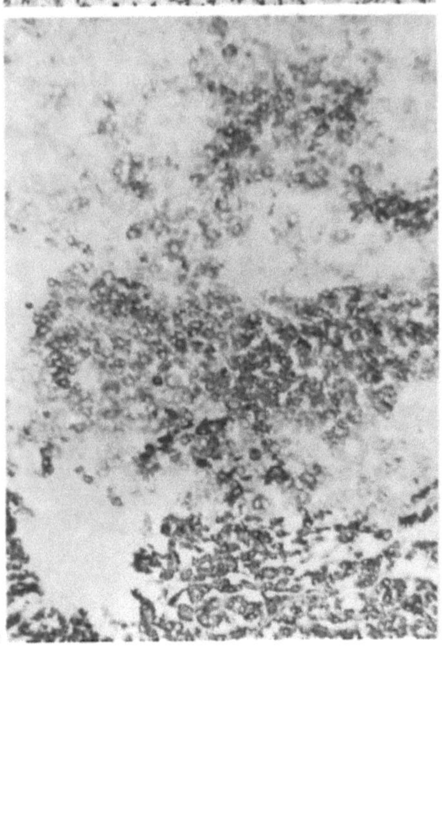

**Fig. 3a–c.** Loss of ATPase activity (**a**) and G-6-Pase activity (**b**) can be seen in rat liver in early stage of carcinogenesis. Heterogeneity of G-6-Pase activity (**c**) appears in nodules. × 150

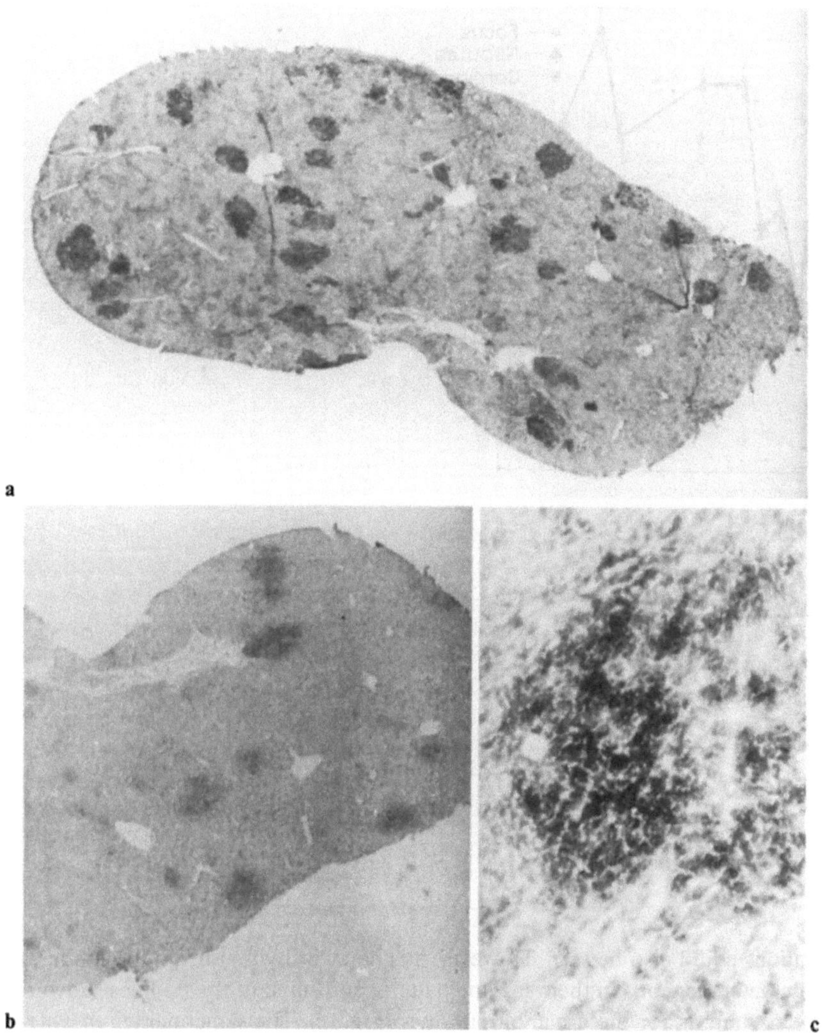

**Fig. 4a.** PAS positive foci appear in early stage of experimental hepatocarcinogenesis in rats. ×10. **b, c** GGT-positive nodules are present in rat liver 4 months after initiation with DEN. **b** ×10; **c** ×150

1 month, nodules 2 months and PHC 6 months after initiation. Histologically, clear cell, eosinophil, basophil and mixed cell foci appear at the early stage of experimental hepatocarcinogenesis (Fig. 2). Nevertheless, these lesions can be characterized much better by enzyme-histochemical techniques than by the conventional histological staining methods. The foci developed 1 month after initiation could be detected by the lack of ATPase (Fig. 3a) and G-6-Pase (Fig. 3b) activities and by the increase in GGT activity (Fig. 4b, c). PAS positivity upon fasting the animals, indicating glycogen retention, could be also a marker for early lesions (Fig. 4a). More advanced lesions in the process of experimental hepatocarcinogenesis are the neoplastic nodules, in which these enzy-

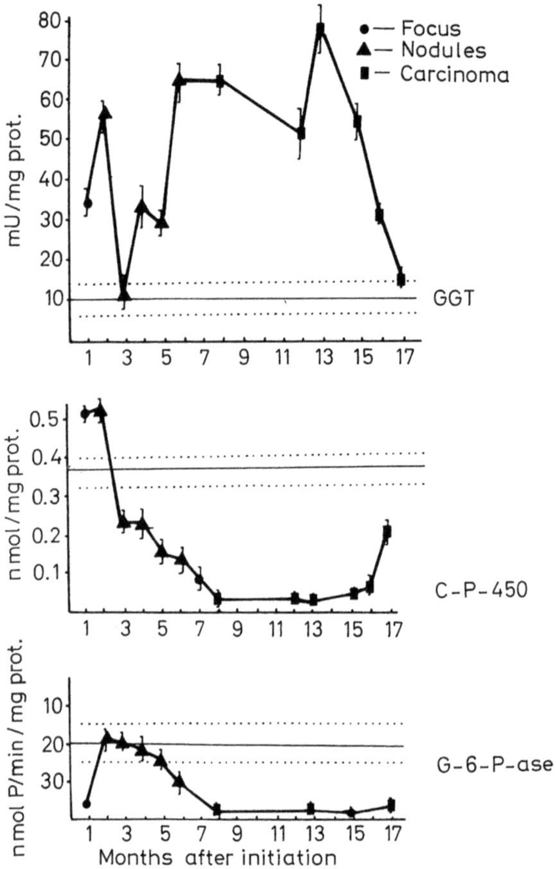


**Fig. 5.** Alterations of marker enzymes during experimental hepatocarcinogenesis

matic alterations could also be seen. However, it is noteworthy that neoplastic nodules may be more heterogeneous in their enzyme pattern, and some of the nodules show irregular patchy staining for these marker enzymes (Fig. 3c). The same marker enzymes proved also useful for the characterization of the fully developed liver cell carcinomas. The heterogeneity was particularly pronounced in the carcinomas of advanced stage. In the PHC studied 15-18 months after the initiation, increased GGT activity could be observed less frequently than in the carcinomas derived from earlier stages of hepatocarcinogenesis.

At the early stage of hepatocarcinogenesis the biochemical measurements were carried out in liver samples containing randomly distributed foci (1-4 months). At a later stage of hepatocarcinogenesis, however, when the lesions – due to their enlarged size – could be separated from the surrounding liver (5-18 months after initiation), the biochemical studies were carried out on such separated samples (nodules and carcinomas). Figure 5 shows that the activities of GGT and G-6-Pase, and also the amount of cytochrome P-450, are rather variable during the course of hepatocarcinogenesis. Although it has been well established that transformed hepatocytes are characterized by elevated GGT activity and reduced G-6-Pase activity and cytochrome P-450 levels, the

**Table 1.** Summary of enzyme alterations in human liver tumours

| Patient (case no.) | Age | Sex | Histology | HBsAg (orcein stain) | Enzyme histochemistry | | | Biochemistry | | |
|---|---|---|---|---|---|---|---|---|---|---|
| | | | | | GGT | ATPase | G-6-Pase | GGT | Cyt. P-450 | G-6-Phase |
| 155/84 | 57 | M | Adenoma | 0 | – | + | + | – | + | + |
| 1905/85 | 66 | F | Adenoma | – | ± | 0 | ++ | – | + | + |
| 914/82 | 25 | F | FNH | – | + | – | ++ | + | – | – |
| 2586/84 | 31 | F | FNH | – | ++ | + | 0 | 0 | 0 | 0 |
| 2084/83 | 37 | F | FNH | – | – | ± | ++ | + | – | – |
| 2972/85 | 40 | F | FNH | + | ++ | + | ± | + | 0 | – |
| 134/83 | 18 | F | PHC+FNH | – | ++ | 0 | – | ++ | – | – |
| 38/84 | 29 | F | PHC+FNH | – | – | – | + | – | – | + |
| 522/84 | 70 | M | PHC | – | – | ± | – | – | – | + |
| 1108/84 | 51 | F | PHC | – | – | 0 | ± | – | + | + |
| 1443/84 | 64 | M | PHC | – | – | 0 | ± | – | – | – |
| 1763/85 | 37 | F | PHC | – | + | 0 | + | + | – | + |
| 1921/85 | 47 | M | PHC | – | ++ | 0 | + | ++ | + | + |
| 444/85 | 38 | F | PHC | – | – | 0 | + | – | – | – |

– no reaction; + positive reaction; 0 not measured

results of these studies show that the level of these alterations is very much dependent on the stage of hepatocarcinogenesis. Thus quantitative measurements of GGT activity in liver samples containing foci, nodules or carcinomas showed that the highest values could be observed between 5 and 15 months after initiation. It appears especially interesting that the GGT activity returned to normal level in carcinomatous tissue taken from rats 17–18 months after they have received DEN as initiator (Fig. 5).

In our experiment the highest GGT activity was found between 5 and 15 months after initiation in the whole-liver samples containing randomly distributed foci, as well as in the nodules and carcinomas separated from the surrounding host liver tissue.

The amount of cytochrome P-450, after an early modest elevation, gradually decreased. It is again noteworthy, however, that the carcinomas at the late stages of hepatocarcinogenesis (17–18 months after initiation) contained more cytochrome P-450 than those studied at the earlier period (5–15 months) of carcinogenesis. The G-6-Pase activity was found to be the lowest at 1 month and between 8 and 17 months after initiation (Fig. 5).

## Studies on Human Liver Tumours

In the second part of our studies we addressed the question of whether the characteristic enzyme-pattern changes seen in experimental hepatocarcinogenesis also take place in preneoplastic and neoplastic lesions of the human liver, and if so, to what extent they are specific.

The studies concerning certain marker enzymes were carried out on 14 human tumorous liver specimens collected between 1982 and 1985 (Table 1). The histological examination verified two adenomas, four FNH and eight PHC. The two adenomas ap-

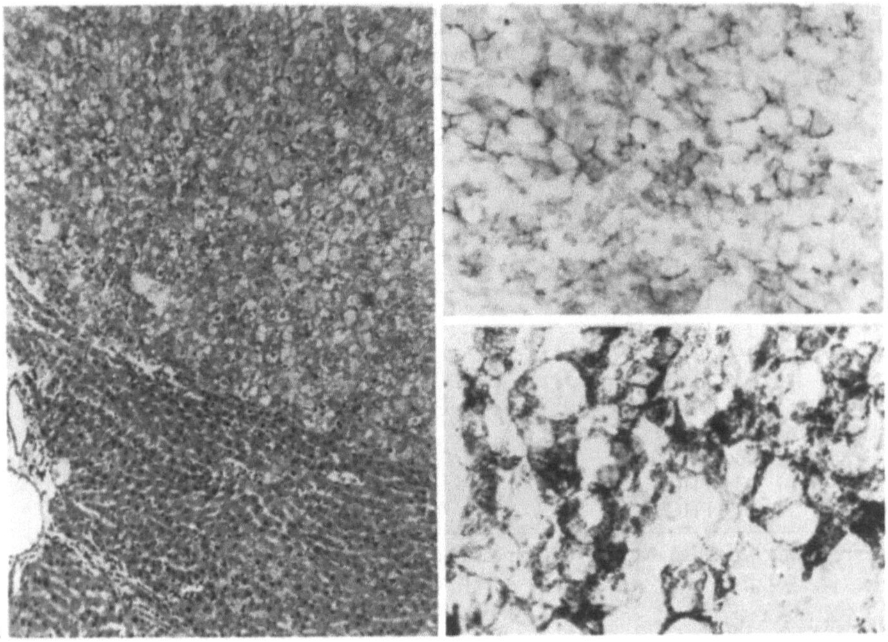
a b c

**Fig. 6 a–c.** Human liver cell adenoma. The tumour cells are larger but similar in shape and arrangement to hepatocytes (**a**). ATPase activity (**b**) and G-6-Pase activity (**c**) are well preserved. HE: **a, b** ×150; **c** ×375

peared as solitary, well-circumscribed neoplasms in the right liver lobes (Fig. 6a); one of them showed hemorrhage, whereas the other contained a large amount of fat. Interestingly, the ATPase and G-6-Pase activities were well preserved in both cases (Fig. 6b, c) as in the surrounding normal host liver. In one of the adenomas the GGT activity was only very slightly increased. The four FNH samples originated from female patients who were long-term users of contraceptive steroids. All FNH developed in noncirrhotic livers, and their most characteristic feature, a central stellate scar with connective tissue septa radiating to the periphery of the lesions, was easily recognizable (Fig. 7a). Histologically, the FNH proved to be made up of nodules of irregular size and shape in which the hepatocytes were arranged in cords of two or three cells in thickness, separated by anastomosing fibrous septa. Surprisingly, increased GGT activity was observed in all three cases studied for this enzyme, and reduced canalicular ATPase and G-6-Pase activities were found in both cases studied (Fig. 9b, c).

As for the PHC in our material, practically all histological types were represented. Histochemically, high GGT activity was observed in three of eight cases and no G-6-Pase activity was detected in four of eight cases. It is worth mentioning that in two PHC samples, increased GGT activity appeared only in the surrounding non-cancerous liver tissue, while in the tumorous tissue itself no GGT was detectable with the histochemical techniques employed (Fig. 8).

Biochemical studies were also carried out on the human liver samples, where measurements in the host liver surrounding the preneoplastic or neoplastic lesions served

a

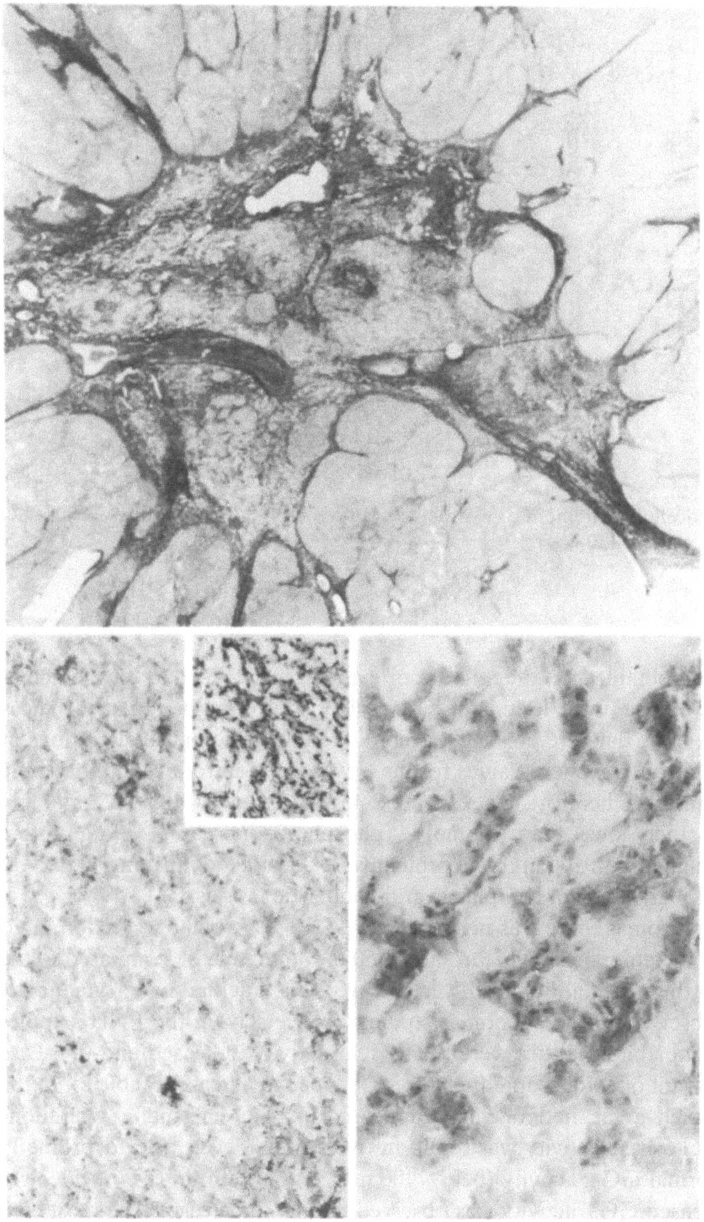

b c

**Fig. 7 a–c.** Focal nodular hyperplasia. **a** Fibrous stellate scar is located in the center of the tumour. Picrosirius staining, ×10. **b** ATPase activity is completely lost. Insert shows positive AT-Pase reaction in control liver. ×60 **c** GGT activity is partly present. ×150

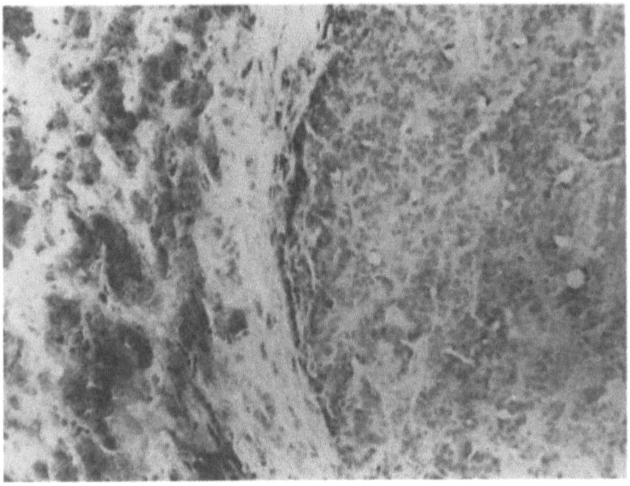

**Fig. 8.** Primary hepatocellular carcinoma. GGT activity is present in the surrounding liver tissue, but not in the tumour cells. × 150

as controls. The data obtained on the amount of cytochrome P-450 and on the activities of GGT and G-6-Pase in the lesions of human liver showed rather great variances (Table 2). However, if the data are presented according to the histological alterations of the samples and arbitrary threshold values for the enzymes are introduced, remarkable trends can be recognized. Therefore, cytochrome P-450 values lower than 0.2 nmol/mg protein, G-6-Pase activity lower than 15 μmol Pi (phosphorus inorganic)/h/mg protein and GGT activity higher than 100 mU/mg protein were considered meaningful and regarded as potential markers of preneoplastic and neoplastic lesions.

In the human adenomas there was no increase in GGT activity, no reduction in G-6-Pase activity and the amount of cytochrome P-450 did not decrease compared to the values measured in the surrounding host liver. We may conclude that no enzymatic deviation could be observed in the adenomas studied. Conversely, in the FNH samples remarkable enzymatic abnormalities were seen: GGT activity increased and G-6-Pase activity and the amount of cytochrome P-450 were reduced in all cases (Table 2). In the case of PHC, rather great heterogeneity appeared in the enzymatic alterations (Table 3). Normal G-6-Pase activity was found in five, normal levels of cytochrome P-450 in two, and normal GGT activity (below 100 mU/mg protein) in five of the eight cases studied. Increased GGT activity was observed in only three cases. The most constantly altered enzyme was the cytochrome P-450, which decreased strongly in three and slightly in two of the eight carcinoma samples studied (Table 3).

A further question was whether any consistency and uniformity could be detected in the appearance of these enzymes, i.e. whether all the marker enzyme alterations occur simultaneously in the same sample. Alterations of all three enzymes studied were seen simultaneously in only one sample, changes in two markers were observed in four samples and in two PHC only one of the three marker enzymes showed deviation from the normal values (Table 4).

**Table 2.** Enzyme studies in surgically removed liver specimens

| Patient (case No.) | Histology | Cyt. P-450 (nmol/mg protein) | | GGT (mU/mg protein) | | G-6-Pase (nmol Pi/min/mg protein) | |
|---|---|---|---|---|---|---|---|
| | | Normal | Lesion | Normal | Lesion | Normal | Lesion |
| 914/82 | FNH | 0.12 | 0.03 | 316 | 459 | 8.2 | 5.2 |
| 2084/83 | FNH | 0.22 | 0.07 | 31 | 181 | 22.5 | 0.7 |
| 2972/85 | FNH | – | – | – | 140 | – | 1.6 |
| 155/84 | Adenoma | 0.32 | 0.34 | 46 | 51 | 24.6 | 48.7 |
| 1905/85 | Adenoma | 0.58 | 0.34 | 26 | 20 | 20.1 | 15.1 |
| 522/84 | PHC | 0.18 | 0.00 | 106 | 96 | 24.8 | 25.7 |
| 1108/84 | PHC | 0.60 | 0.37 | 57 | 42 | 29.4 | 21.1 |
| 1443/84 | PHC | 0.31 | 0.16 | 115 | 35 | 32.0 | 0.8 |
| 38/84 | FNH + PHC | 0.29 | 0.04 | 30 | 30 | 29.0 | 16.0 |
| 134/83 | FNH + PHC | 0.09 | 0.00 | 109 | 688 | 11.8 | 3.0 |
| 444/85 | PHC | – | 0.12 | – | 22 | – | 8.0 |
| 1763/85 | PHC | 0.33 | 0.12 | 65 | 147 | 22.0 | 41.0 |
| 1921/85 | PHC | 0.71 | 0.35 | 67 | 534 | 26.8 | 18.1 |

**Table 3.** Evaluation of the quantitative enzymatic alterations in human liver tumours

| Enzyme | Type of changes | Histology | Number of cases studied incidence of changes |
|---|---|---|---|
| Cytochrome P-450 | Low | FNH | 2/2 |
| | | PHC | 8/6 |
| | No change | Adenoma | 2/2 |
| | | PHC | 8/2 |
| GGT | High | FNH | 3/3 |
| | | PHC | 8/3 |
| | No change | Adenoma | 2/2 |
| | | PHC | 8/3 |
| | High only in surrounding tissue | PHC | 8/2 |
| G-6-Pase | Low | FNH | 3/3 |
| | | PHC | 8/3 |
| | No change | Adenoma | 2/2 |
| | | PHC | 8/5 |

Cytochrome P-450: $\text{low} < \dfrac{0.2\ \text{nmol}}{\text{mg protein}}$

GGT: $\text{high} > \dfrac{100\ \text{mU}}{\text{mg protein}}$

G-6-Pase: $\text{low} < \dfrac{15\ \text{nmol Pi/min}}{\text{mg protein}}$

It is worth mentioning that in non-tumorous host liver tissue surrounding the preneoplastic or neoplastic lesions, in the majority of cases there was no reduction of G-6-Pase activity or of the amount of cytochrome P-450 and no increase in GGT activity. In three of the eight samples, however, GGT activity was strongly increased; furthermore, cytochrome P-450 and G-6-Pase activity proved to be reduced in one case each (Table 2).

**Table 4.** Heterogeneity of marker enzymes in human liver tumours

| Histology | Number of cases | | | | |
|---|---|---|---|---|---|
| | Total | No change | Changes in enzymes | | |
| | | | One | Two | Three |
| FNH | 2 | – | – | – | 2 |
| Adenoma | 2 | 2 | – | – | – |
| PHC | 8 | 1 | 2 | 4 | 1 |
| Total | 12 | 3 | 2 | 4 | 3 |

Cytochrome P-450 low $< \frac{0.2\ \text{nmol}}{\text{mg protein}}$

GGT high $> \frac{100\ \text{mU}}{\text{mg protein}}$

G-6-Pase low $< \frac{15\ \text{nmol Pi/min}}{\text{mg protein}}$

## Discussion

During the last couple of years we have been involved in studying chemical hepatocarcinogenesis in rats (Lapis 1983; Lapis et al. 1984) and viral hepatocarcinogenesis in chickens (Lapis 1979). In experimental hepatocarcinogenesis, studies of the changes of various enzymes proved to be rather efficient and useful in the follow-up of the steps of the neoplastic process (Fiala et al. 1972; Kalengayi and Desmet 1978; Pitot et al. 1978; Peraino et al. 1984; Scherer 1984; Hanigan and Pitot 1985). Of the broad spectrum of enzymes studied with this particular purpose, in our hands alterations of GGT activity, G-6-Pase activity and the amount of cytochrome P-450 proved to be the most relevant and reliable (Lapis 1983; Lapis et al. 1984). Our observations on the enzymatic changes taking place during chemical hepatocarcinogenesis in rats are in good agreement with the previously published data (Fiala et al. 1972; Kalengayi and Desmet 1978; Farber 1980; Peraino et al. 1984; Scherer 1984). Contrary to other authors, however, we followed up enzymatic changes until a very late stage (15–18 months after initiation) of chemical hepatocarcinogenesis. By doing so, we observed that the alterations of the studied enzymes are subject to variations during the course of hepatocarcinogenesis, and compared to the earlier stages, in this late stage a pronounced tendency toward heterogeneity did appear. The GGT activity, for example, decreased or disappeared, and the amount of cytochrome P-450 increased in these carcinomas compared to samples taken in the earlier period of hepatocarcinogenesis. This could be regarded as one aspect of tumour progression. Altogether, however, the study of the enzyme-pattern changes during chemical hepatocarcinogenesis proved to be a powerful tool in the recognition and characterization of precursor, preneoplastic and neoplastic lesions and also in clarifying the possible links between them (Farber 1980; Scherer 1984). As a result of this experience, we decided to carry out similar studies on increasing numbers of surgically removed human liver specimens arriving in our Institute for diagnostic purposes.

We think that such studies are all the more important because at present our knowledge is rather insufficient concerning the preneoplastic lesions of the primary human liver cancer; particularly scanty is our knowledge concerning the link between the supposed preneoplastic lesions and PHC. So far it is not clear whether the precancerous lesions of the human liver have enzyme activities closely similar to that of PHC, although it was concluded by Uchida et al. (1981) that they do not.

Liver cell adenoma and FNH are supposed to be preneoplastic lesions, although there is no general consensus on this point (Christopherson et al. 1977; Neuberger et al. 1980; Tesluk and Lawrie 1981). Although the progression of liver adenoma to PHC has been observed, it seems to be a very rare event, and regression of the adenoma following cessation of contraceptive steroids was reported in several cases (Foster 1982).

In the adenomas studied by us, the enzyme pattern did not differ in principle from that of the surrounding non-tumorous host liver or from the data available on the enzyme pattern of normal liver (Fujisawa et al. 1976; Selvaraj et al. 1981; Yamamoto et al. 1981). Our findings are similar to those of Gerber and Thung (1980) concerning the enzyme activities in human liver cell adenoma, seeming to support the notion that liver cell adenoma may extremely rarely transform or progress into PHC.

Concerning the nature of FNH there are rather differing views in the literature. It is not regarded as a preneoplastic lesion by Ishak (1981) or Foster (1982). On the other hand, in some cases PHC was thought to have originated from FNH (Christopherson and Mays 1979).

In all four FNH cases studied by us, enzymatic changes – increase of GGT, decrease or loss of G-6-Pase, loss of canalicular ATPase activity, decrease of amount of cytochrome P-450 – did take place which, at least in experimental hepatocarcinogenesis, are regarded as markers of the progressing neoplastic process. Similar enzyme-pattern changes were observed and published by Thung and Gerber (1981) in a case of nodular regenerative hyperplasia. The enzyme-pattern changes observed in FNH seems to indicate a closer link between this alteration and PHC. These observations support the view (Christopherson and Mays 1979) that FNH is a preneoplastic lesion. Further studies are needed to provide more evidence on the suggested link between FNH and PHC. The number of PHC studied by us (eight cases) is high enough to justify certain conclusions. Of the described observations, for us the most important seems to be the pronounced heterogeneity of enzyme-pattern changes. It is particularly surprising that simultaneous changes in all three so-called marker enzymes studied were observed in only one of the eight cases. This observation casts doubt on the marker role of the enzymes studied. Presumably these liver cancers were already in an advanced stage when they were recognized; this might explain the observed heterogeneity in enzyme pattern, which seemingly increases with progression.

## Summary

We studied the changes of certain "marker" enzymes – gamma-glutamyl-transpeptidase (GGT), glucose-6-phosphatase (G-6-Pase), canalicular adenosine triphosphatase (ATPase) and cytochrome P-450 – during chemically induced hepatocarcinogenesis in rats and in surgically removed tumorous human liver samples. Our findings concerning the changes of marker enzymes in experimental hepatocarcinogenesis are consistent with the previously published observations, except that there was no longer any increase in GGT activity in the carcinoma samples taken in the late stage (15-18 months) of hepatocarcinogenesis.

The same enzymes were studied in 14 surgically removed human liver samples: two adenomas, four focal nodular hyperplasias (FNH) and eight primary hepatocellular carcinomas (PHC). In the case of the adenomas, no changes in enzyme pattern were observed compared to the surrounding non-tumorous host liver using either biochemical or histochemical techniques. In contrast, all enzyme markers showed pronounced changes in the four FNH samples. Such changes are regarded as markers of the neoplastic process in experimental hepatocarcinogenesis. The observed enzymatic changes may be regarded as indicators of a closer link between FNH and PHC.

In the PHC great heterogeneity was found in the enzymatic changes. Surprisingly, GGT activity was increased in only three, and G-6-Pase activity was not reduced in five of the eight carcinoma samples. The most consistent changes were seen in the amount of cytochrome P-450, which was decreased in six of the eight cases.

The heterogeneous pattern of enzymatic alterations in PHC appears to support the concept of sequential genetic changes and clonal evolution underlying tumour progression.

## References

Anthony PP (1976) Precursor lesions for liver cancer in humans. Cancer Res 36: 2579-2583

Anthony PP, Vogel CL, Barker LF (1973) Liver cell dysplasia: a premalignant condition. Am J Clin Pathol 26: 217-223

Becker FF (1981) Recent concepts of initiation and promotion in carcinogenesis. Am J Clin Pathol 105: 3-9

Christopherson WM, Mays ET (1979) Relation of steroids to liver oncogenesis. In: Lapis K, Johannessen JV (eds) Liver carcinogenesis. Hemisphere, Washington, pp 37-60

Christopherson WM, Mays ET, Barrows G (1977) A clinicopathologic study of steroid related liver tumors. Am J Clin Pathol 1: 31-41

Cohen C, Berson SD, Geddes EW (1979) Liver cell dysplasia: association with hepatocellular carcinoma, cirrhosis and hepatitis B antigen carrier status. Cancer 44: 1671-1676

Editorial (1983) Prevention of primary liver cancer. Report of a meeting of a WHO Scientific Group. Lancet 1: 463-465

Farber E (1980) The sequential analysis of liver cancer induction. Biochim Biophys Acta 605: 149-166

Fiala S, Fiala AE, Dixon B (1972) $\gamma$-Glutamyltranspeptidase in transplantable, chemically induced rat hepatomas and "spontaneous" mouse hepatomas. INCI 48: 1393-1401

Fiske CH, Subbarow Y (1925) The colorimetric determination of phosphorus. J Biol Chem 66: 375-400

Foster JH (1982) Benign liver tumors. World J Surg 6: 25-31

Fujisawa K, Kurihara N, Nishikawa H, Kimura A, Kojima M, Kameda H, Taneka M (1976) Carcinoembryonic character of $\gamma$-glutamyl transpeptidase in primary hepatocellular carcinoma. Gastroenterol Jpn 11: 380-386

Gerber MA, Thung SN (1980) Enzyme pattern in human hepatocellular carcinoma. Am J Clin Pathol 98: 395-400

Hanigan MH, Pitot HC (1985) Gamma glutamyl transpeptidase – its role in hepatocarcinogenesis. Carcinogenesis 6: 165-172

Harada T, Fukumoto Y, Kodama T, Nishimura H, Nishioka M, Takemoto T (1979) Clinical significance of liver cell dysplasia in chronic liver disease. Bull Yamaguchi Med School 26: 115-121

Harper AE (1963) Glucose 6-phosphatase. In: Bergemeyer HU (ed) Methods of enzymatic analysis. Academic, New York, pp 788-792

Ho JCI, Wu PC, Mark TK (1981) Liver cell dysplasia in association with hepatocellular carcinoma, cirrhosis, and hepatitis B surface antigen in Hong Kong. Int J Cancer 28: 571-574
Ishak KG (1981) Hepatic lesions caused by anabolic and contraceptive steroids. Semin. Liver Dis. 1: 116-128
Kalengayi MMR, Desmet VJ (1978) $\gamma$-glutamyl transferase as oncofetal marker of experimental hepatocarcinogenesis in the rat. Scand J Immunol [Suppl] 8: 547-556
Lapis K (1979) Histology and ultrastructural aspects of virus-induced primary liver cancer and transplantable hepatomas of viral origin in chickens. In: Lapis K, Johannessen JV (eds) Liver carcinogenesis. Hemisphere, Washington, pp 299-332
Lapis K (1983) Morphologic expression of neoplasia in human and experimental liver tumours. In: Mirand EA, Hutchinson WB, Mihich E (eds) Thirteenth international cancer congress, part D. Research and treatment, Liss, New York, pp 67-76
Lapis K, Ujhelyi E, Gyenes M, Jeney A (1984) Alterations of markers during hepatocarcinogenesis in rats. In: Börzsönyi M, Lapis K, Day NE, Yamasaki H (eds) Models, mechanism and etiology of tumour promotion. IARC, Lyon, pp 25-36
Neuberger J, Nunnerley HB, Davis M, Portmann B, Laeuws JW, Williams R (1980) Oral-contraceptive-associated liver tumours: occurrence of malignancy and difficulties in diagnosis. Lancet 1: 273-276
Okuda K, Nakashima T, Obata H, Kubo Y (1977) Clinicopathological studies of minute hepatocellular carcinoma. Gastroenterology 73: 109-115
Omura T, Sato R (1964) The carbon monoxide binding pigment of liver microsomes. I. Evidence for its hemoprotein nature. J Biol Chem 177: 751-766
Peraino C, Staffeldt EF, Carnes BA, Ludemann VA, Blomquist J, Vesselinovitch SD (1984) Characterization of histochemically detectable altered hepatocyte foci and their relationship to hepatic tumorigenesis in rats treated once with diethylmitrosamine or benzo(a)pyrene within one day after birth. Cancer Res 44: 3340-3347
Pitot HC, Sirica AE (1980) The stages of initiation and promotion in hepatocarcinogenesis. Biochim Biophys Acta 605: 191-215
Pitot HC, Barsness L, Goldsworthy T (1978) Biochemical characterization of stages of hepatocarcinogenesis after a single dose of diethylnitrosamine. Nature 271: 456-457
Rutenberg AM, Kim H, Fischbein IW, Hanker J, Wasserburg HL, Seligman AM (1968) Histochemical and ultrastructural demonstration of $\gamma$-glutamyl-transpeptidase activity. J Histochem Cytochem 17: 517-526
Schaff Z, Lapis K, Henson DE (1986) Liver. In: Henson DE, Albores WB (eds) Incipient neoplasia. Co Saunders, Philadelphia
Scherer E (1984) Neoplastic progression in experimental hepatocarcinogenesis. Biochim Biophys Acta 738: 219-236
Selvaraj P, Balasubramanian KA, Hill PG (1981) Isolation of $\gamma$-GT from human primary hepatoma and comparison its kinetic and catalytic properties with the enzyme from normal adult and fetal liver. Enzyme 26: 57-63
Shikata T, Uzawa T, Yoshiwara N, Akatruka T, Yamazaki S (1974) Staining methods of Australia antigen in paraffin section. Detection of cytoplasm inclusion bodies. Jpn J Exp Med 44: 25-36
Sogaard PE (1981) Nodular transformation of the liver, alpha-fetoprotein, and hepatocellular carcinoma. Hum Pathol 12: 1052
Solt D, Farber E (1976) New principle for analysis of chemical carcinogenesis. Nature 263: 701-703
Szasz G (1969) A kinetic photometric method for serum $\gamma$-glutamyl transpeptidase. Clin Chem 15: 124-136
Takashima T, Matsui O, Suzuki M, Ida M (1982) Diagnosis and screening of small hepatocellular carcinomas. Comparison of radionuclide imaging, ultrasound, computed tomography, hepatic angiography, and alpha-1-fetoprotein assay. Radiology 145: 635-638
Tesluk H, Lawrie J (1981) Hepatocellular adenoma. Its transformation to carcinoma in a user of oral contraceptives. Arch Pathol Lab Med 105: 296-299
Thung SN, Gerber MA (1981) Enzyme pattern and marker antigens in nodular "regenerative" hyperplasia of the liver. Cancer 47: 1796-1799
Uchida T, Miyata H, Shikata T (1981) Human hepatocellular carcinoma and putative precancerous disorders. Their enzyme histochemical study. Arch Pathol Lab Med 105: 180-186

Wachstein M, Meisel E (1956) On the histochemical demonstration of glucose-6-phosphatase. Histochem Cytochem 4: 592
Wachstein M, Meisel E (1957) Histochemistry of hepatic phosphatase at a physiological pH with special reference to the demonstration of bile canaliculi. Am J Clin Pathol 27: 12–23
Watanabe S (1983) Morphologic studies of the liver cell dysplasia. Cancer 51: 2197–2205
Yamamoto H, Sumikawa K, Hada T, Higashino K, Yamamura Y (1981) $\gamma$-Glutamyltransferase from human hepatoma tissue in comparison with normal liver enzyme. Clin Chim Acta 111: 229–237

# The Value of Quantitation of Liver Function

H. Lösgen, J. Bircher
Division of Clinical Pharmacology, University of Göttingen, Robert-Koch-Str. 40, D-3400 Göttingen, Federal Republic of Germany

The presence and type or absence of liver disease can be assessed with high accuracy by modern biochemical, serological, and morphological tests. In contrast, assessment of severity and prognosis have remained difficult. These two aspects, however, are being accorded increasing importance with regard to therapeutic strategies, particularly regarding liver transplantation and the appreciation of the effects of pharmacological treatments.

As a guide to the problem of severity of liver diseases, e.g., for evaluation of its prognosis, clinicians have empirically established scores based on various combinations of clinical and biochemical features (Pugh et al. 1973). However, accurate measurement of a number of these features, e.g., ascites, encephalopathy, and nutritional status, is still unsatisfactory. Alternatively, they represent relatively nonspecific and insensitive parameters of liver function, e.g., serum bilirubin and serum albumin.

To overcome these problems, quantitative measurements of some specific functions of the liver have been established with the suggestion that such tests are better reflections than the clinical signs and scores of the physiological derangements of the diseased liver.

Quantitative liver function tests (QLFT) are direct or modified applications of the clearance principles in regard to hepatic handling or metabolism of some defined exogenous compounds. The tests used most frequently are:

1. Indocyanine green plasma elimination, e.g., the fractional clearance (ICG-k; 0.5 mg ICG/kg b.w., i.v.), considered to be a reflection of hepatic blood flow
2. Galactose elimination capacity (GEC; 0.5 g galactose/kg b.w., i.v.), measuring cytosolic metabolic capacity of the liver
3. Aminopyrine breath test (ABT; 1.5 μCi dimethyl $^{14}C$-aminopyrine i.v.), measuring functional capacity of the microsomal cytochrome P-450 system
4. Antipyrine plasma clearance (ACl; 10 mg antipyrine/kg b.w., p.o.), measuring functional capacity of the cytochrome P-450 system
5. Caffeine plasma clearance (CCl; 3–5 mg caffeine/kg b.w., p.o.), measuring functional capacity of the microsomal P-448 system

The clinical implications of these tests have been reviewed by Bircher (1983) and Preisig (1986). Using the results of the ABT, the value of quantitating liver function may be demonstrated with the following examples:

1. *Evaluation of severity of liver disease.*
   In alcoholic liver disease (Schneider et al. 1980), chronic active hepatitis (Monroe et al. 1982), and cirrhosis of different etiology (Carlisle et al. 1979) the ABT showed a close correlation with the histological severity. In paracetamol intoxication (Saun-

Assessment and Management of Hepatobiliary Disease
Eds.: L. Okolicsányi, G. Csomós, and G. Crepaldi

ders et al. 1980) the ABT was a good indicator of the extent of liver damage compared to biochemical parameters.

2. *Evaluation of prognosis of liver disease.*
   a) Short-term survival: In alcoholic hepatitis (Schneider et al. 1980), cirrhosis of different etiology (Henry et al. 1985), and paracetamol intoxication (Saunders et al. 1980) the ABT served as an efficient predictor of outcome.
   b) Clinical improvement: In alcoholic liver disease ABT predicted clinical improvement more reliably than conventional liver parameters (Schneider et al. 1980).
   c) Surgical risk: In patients with different liver diseases ABT was shown to predict operative risk clearly (Gill et al. 1983).

These examples illustrate that quantitation of liver function yields information about severity and short-term survival in patients with advanced liver diseases. The long-term prognostic value has not yet been determined, and no critical comparison with clinical and laboratory indices of severity has yet been carried out.

## References

1. Bircher J (1983) Quantitative assessment of deranged hepatic function: a missed opportunity? Semin Liver Dis 3: 275-284
2. Carlisle RA, Galambos JT, Warren WD (1979) The relationship between conventional liver tests, quantitative function tests, and histopathology in cirrhosis. Dig Dis Sci 24: 358-362
3. Gill RA, Goodman MW, Golfus GR et al. (1983) Aminopyrine breath test predicts surgical risk for patients with liver disease. Ann Surg 198: 701-704
4. Henry DA, Kitchingman G, Langman MJS (1985) $^{14}$C-Aminopyrine breath analysis and conventional biochemical tests as predictors of survival in cirrhosis. Dig Dis Sci 30: 813-818
5. Monroe PS, Baker AL, Schneider JF et al. (1982) The aminopyrine breath test and serum bile acids reflect histologic severity in chronic hepatitis. Hepatology 2: 317-322
6. Preisig R (1986) Clinical evaluation of liver function. In: Thomas HC, Joneks EA (eds), Recent advances in hepatology 2. Churchill Livingstone, London
7. Pugh RNH, Murray-Lyon IM, Dawson JL et al. (1973) Transection of the oesophagus for bleeding oesophageal varices. Br J Surg 60: 646-649
8. Saunders JB, Wright N, Lewis KO (1980) Predicting outcome of paracetamol poisoning by using $^{14}$C-aminopyrine breath test. Br Med J 280: 279-280
9. Schneider JF, Baker AL, Haines NW et al. (1980) Aminopyrine N-demethylation: a prognostic test of liver function in patients with alcoholic liver disease. Gastroenterology 79: 1145-1150

# Quantitation of Liver Function: Antipyrine Metabolism, an Update

Henrik E. Poulsen[1,2] and Steffen Loft[1]

[1] Department of Pharmacology, University of Copenhagen, 20, Juliane Maries Vej, 2100 Copenhagen, Denmark
[2] Department of Medicine A2152, Rigshospitalet, 9, Blegdamsvej, 2100 Copenhagen, Denmark

## Introduction

For the majority of drugs, hepatic metabolism is a necessary pathway of elimination. Due to large inter- and intraindividual variations in hepatic metabolism of drugs, it is difficult to predict the actual elimination rate of a therapeutic agent. For many years it was believed that the rate of metabolism of any individual could be estimated from the elimination of a test drug; however, the failure of the antipyrine test to predict the rates of other drugs has demonstrated the inadequacy of such a simple approach. In the case of antipyrine this is probably due to its metabolism by a multiplicity of hepatic cytochrome P-450 enzymes.

Antipyrine was synthesized at the end of the last century, became one of the first important synthetic drugs, and remained popular until the 1930s. In the late 1940s Brodie (Brodie et al. 1949) Axelrod (Brodie and Axelrod 1950), and Soberman et al. (1949) performed the original studies on antipyrine metabolism in man. They determined the elimination half-life of antipyrine, showed that it is rapidly and completely absorbed following oral administration, determined its volume of distribution to be total body water, and established that it is eliminated almost exclusively by biotransformation. A large number of studies emerged concerning the influence of inheritance, and up to and during the 1970s antipyrine was extensively used in studies on the influence of inheritance, environmental factors, diseases, other drugs, etc. One of the driving forces was Elliot Vesell, who contributed many original papers and comprehensive reviews (Vesell 1979, 1982).

Huffmann et al. (1973) hypothesized that each of the antipyrine metabolites was formed in the liver by a single selective form of the mixed-function oxidase isozyme, cytochrome P-450. This hypothesis is now generally accepted and the underlying experiments have recently been reviewed (Danhof and Teunissen 1984).

In the last 10 years antipyrine has become more widely used and a large variety of factors influencing its elimination have emerged due to improved designs and measurements of individual metabolic pathways.

In the present review we shall give details of the present state of knowledge regarding (1) the pharmacokinetics of antipyrine, (2) determination of antipyrine using a single time-concentration point, and (3) quantitative assessment of liver function by antipyrine clearance.

Assessment and Management of Hepatobiliary Disease
Eds.: L. Okolicsányi, G. Csomós, and G. Crepaldi

## Pharmacokinetics of Antipyrine

After intravenous administration, the decay of antipyrine in plasma can be described by the sum of two exponentials, suggesting two-compartment kinetics (Greisen and Andreasen 1976). The oral systemic bioavailability of antipyrine is almost complete (Andreasen and Vesell 1974; Danhof et al. 1982a). After oral administration the absorption and distribution of antipyrine occur very rapidly compared with the elimination, and the clearance determined from postabsorption/distribution data according to a one-compartment model is not different from that determined from the area under the complete plasma concentration-time curve (Greisen and Andreasen 1976; Danhof et al. 1982a). The volume of distribution equals total body water and the protein binding is negligible (Brodie and Axelrod 1950; Soberman et al. 1949). Independently of the rate of secretion and pH, saliva holds concentrations of antipyrine close to plasma and can act as a substitute in kinetic studies (Welch et al. 1975; Vesell et al. 1975). The clearance of antipyrine is independent of liver blood flow and of the dose, at least within the common range, from 250 to 1000 mg (Ohnhaus et al. 1976; Danhof and

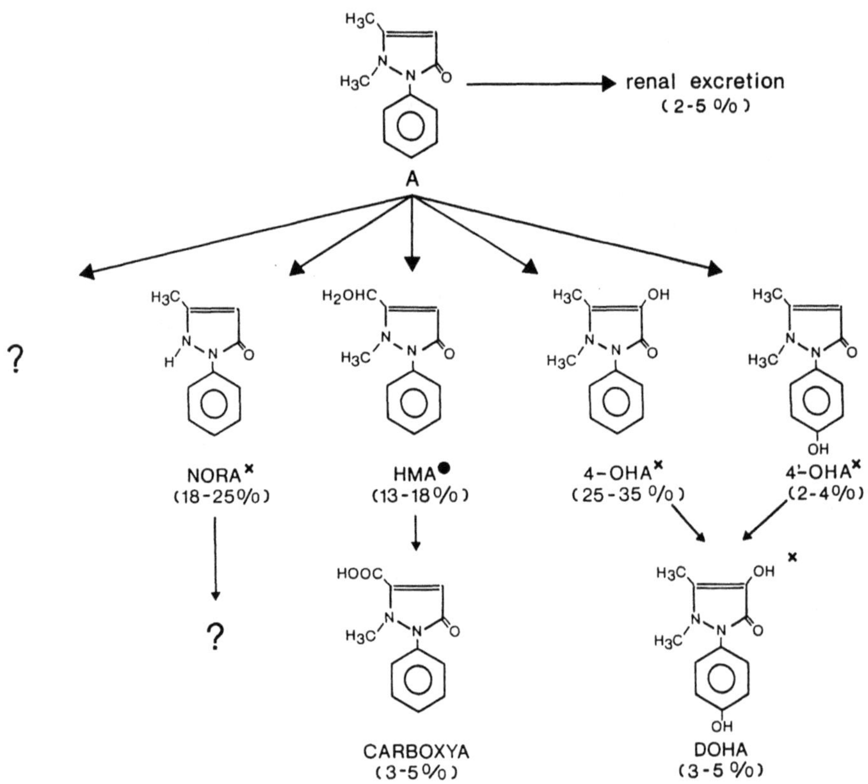


× excreted as glucuronide or sulfate.

● partly excreted as conjugates.

**Fig. 1.** Fate of antipyrine in man

Breimer 1979). In the isolated perfused pig liver, saturation kinetics has been demonstrated at very high antipyrine concentrations (Andreasen et al. 1977).

Antipyrine is almost completely metabolized by hepatic cytochrome P-450 enzymes, leaving only a few percent to be excreted unchanged into urine (Brodie and Axelrod 1950). About 99% of radiolabeled doses of antipyrine has been recovered in urine (Böttcher et al. 1981; Uchino et al. 1983). The excretion into urine of unchanged antipyrine and the three major metabolites (Fig. 1) – the *N*-demethylated (NORA), the 4-hydroxylated (OHA), and the 3-methylhydroxylated (HMA) – account for 65%-70% of the dose (Danhof et al. 1979a, 1982a, c). Minor metabolites are 3-carboxy antipyrine formed from HMA, 4'-hydroxy-antipyrine, and 4,4'-dihydroxyantipyrine (DOHA), each accounting for 5% of the dose or less in man (Danhof et al. 1979a, b, 1982a, b; Inaba et al. 1981; Böttcher et al. 1981). In the rat, the excretion of DOHA accounts for about 15% of the dose administered (Danhof et al. 1979a, b; Böttcher et al. 1981). Other possible metabolic pathways include 1-phenyl-4,5-dioxypyrazoline, formed from NORA, and epoxidation may also take place (Zietz et al. 1978; Eichelbaum et al. 1981). All the 4-hydroxylated metabolites and NORA are almost completely conjugated to glucuronic acid in man, leaving a few percent to be excreted as sulphates or free metabolites (Danhof et al. 1979 a, b; Böttcher et al. 1982). In the rat, sulphate conjugates predominate (Böttcher et al. 1982). About half of the excreted amount of HMA is conjugated to glucuronic acid, whereas the other half and carboxy-antipyrine are excreted as free metabolites (Danhof et al. 1982a-c). HMA may to some extent be subject to enterohepatic recirculation (Aarbakke 1978). The excretion into urine of the three major metabolites of antipyrine has been shown to reflect their rate of formation (Boobis et al. 1981; Teunissen et al. 1985). There is increasing evidence that the formation of each of the three main antipyrine metabolites is dependent on one or more selective form(s) of cytochrome P-450. The evidence is based mainly on the differential changes in the rates of metabolite formation observed in man and rat after administration of some enzyme-inducing or -inhibiting agents (Danhof et al. 1979b, 1982b; Toverud et al. 1981; Teunissen et al. 1985). Accordingly, the saliva or plasma clearance of antipyrine reflects the aggregate activity of at least three different hepatic cytochrome P-450 drug-metabolizing isozymes. By measuring the excretion of metabolites into urine, the activity of each isozyme can be assessed.

## Determination of Antipyrine Using a Single Time-Concentration Point

Since antipyrine elimination follows first-order kinetics and can be described by a one-compartment model, the minimum requirement for information to estimate antipyrine clearance (APC) is the elimination constant $(k)$ and the volume of distribution $(Vd)$. In order to estimate $k$, two time-plasma concentration points are needed. Suppose that $Vd$ is given from body weight, height, age, and sex, and that the dose of antipyrine is $D$, then the theoretical plasma concentration at time $t=0$ is $D/Vd$ and can be used as one point. If the plasma antipyrine concentration $C_T$ is determined at a time $t=T$, then the elimination constant is given by $[\ln(D/VD) - \ln C_T]/T$ and APC can be calculated

$$\mathrm{APC} = Vd \cdot [\ln (D/Vd) - \ln C_T]/T$$

Intuitively, the longer the time interval $T$ between dosing and sampling, the smaller the variation of the determination. From mathematical-statistical considerations

(Døssing et al. 1983) it can be shown that the optimal time for taking the one sample is

$$t = (1 + \sigma^2/\omega^2)/k$$

where $\sigma^2/\omega^2$ is the ratio between the variation of the concentration determination and the variation of *Vd*. Calculated this way, the optimal time is about 24 h (Døssing et al. 1983b), which is in agreement with our empirical estimate from a study of 142 persons (Døssing et al. 1982). It should be noted that a dramatic increase in the variance of the estimate occurs when one sample is taken too early, whereas only a slight increase occurs when the sample is taken late (Døssing et al. 1983), and that bias on the *Vd* has a relatively small influence (Pilsgaard and Poulsen 1984).

The one-sample method can be used as a noninvasive test if saliva is collected instead of plasma, since the concentrations are almost identical (Welch et al. 1975; Vesell et al. 1975).

In our experience, patients and volunteers can perform the test at home, write the necessary information on a data sheet, and mail the saliva sample for analysis if they have performed the test once under supervision. The concentration of antipyrine in saliva is constant for 14 days at room temperature. The saliva sample is easily obtained if a piece of Para-Film is chewed; in our laboratory, conventional chewing gum gives interfering peaks when the saliva is analyzed by HPLC.

The one-sample method only gives information as to clearance. If another parameter is to be estimated, e.g., *Vd*, or if large changes in *Vd* are expected, conventional multiple sampling of plasma or saliva is preferred.

We have also determined the optimal method for multiple sampling in order to minimize the variation of the clearance determination (Døssing et al. 1983): the average sampling time should equal $1/k$. If the half-life of antipyrine is about 12 h, the corresponding optimum sampling time is about 17 h. Preferentially, the sampling times should be spaced equally around the optimum time.

Until recently, many investigators collected the samples for determination of antipyrine kinetics within 12 h after administration (Ballinger et al. 1972; Døssing and Andreasen 1981; Elin et al. 1975; Vessel and Page 1968; Uppal et al. 1980). In such cases the variation coefficient of antipyrine clearance will be at least 8%. If the half-life is 24 h and the samples are taken within 12 h the coefficient of variation will be at least 20%. If the samples are collected optimally, i.e., spaced around 1/k, which is 17.3 h in the first example and 34.6 h in the second, then the coefficient of variation of antipyrine clearance is reduced, at best, to 2.5%.

Assuming that *Vd* changes very little in repeated measurements in a subject under stable environmental conditions, then one can calculate the number of samples needed to estimate antipyrine clearance by the conventional method for comparison with the one-sample method (Døssing et al. 1983). Quite surprisingly, 26 blood or saliva samples are required. One might doubt the one-sample method, but in our experience it is useful when studying adults (Døssing et al. 1983; Loft et al. 1986), children (Loft et al. 1985), and animals (Pilsgaard and Poulsen 1984; Poulsen and Pilsgaard 1985; Poulsen 1985; Hansen and Poulsen 1986a, b).

## Quantitative Assessment of Liver Function by Antipyrine Clearance

Liver disease causes a sequential loss of hepatic function. It has been put forward that the "functional hepatic mass" is reduced as the disease progresses (Tygstrup and Vilstrup 1983) until a minimal residual function is reached incompatible with survival.

Eliminated almost exclusively by hepatic metabolism, antipyrine is an ideal model drug to investigate hepatic function. As intrinsic clearance is a measure of drug-metabolizing enzyme activity, this parameter is the most attractive for estimating hepatic function (Rowland 1972; Andreasen et al. 1974).

Quantitative assessment of liver function by antipyrine clearance is not of much diagnostic value, especially in the initial stage of the disease. According to the concept of functional hepatic mass, quantitative assessment can estimate (1) severity of disease, (2) prognosis, (3) risk, e.g., exposure to hepatotoxins, (4) time course, (5) need for treatment, and (6) results of therapy.

The prognostic value of antipyrine clearance is well established in the case of acute viral or toxic hepatitis (Andreasen and Ranek 1975; Ramsøe et al. 1980; Bremmelgård et al. 1983). The minimal residual function is about 10%-20% of control value, which is consistent with animal experiments, where 90% reduction in antipyrine clearance from subtotal hepatectomy is associated with mortality of about 10% (Poulsen 1985).

In patients with alcoholic liver cirrhosis, antipyrine clearance is reduced (Andreasen et al. 1974) compared with other measures of functional liver mass (Vilstrup 1980). As such, antipyrine is considered to be predictive for survival of patients with liver cirrhosis; however, completed long-term studies are still lacking, though some are in progress.

It remains to be established whether an estimate of the individual metabolic pathways in patients with liver diseases is more informative than antipyrine clearance per se.

## References


Aarbakke J (1978) Disposition and oxidative metabolism of antipyrine in the rat. Acta Pharmacol Toxicol (Copenh) 42: 63-68

Andreasen PB, Vesell ES (1974) Comparison of plasma level of antipyrine, tolbutamide and warfarin after oral and intravenous administration. Clin Pharmacol Ther 16: 1059-1065

Andreasen PB, Ranek L (1975) Liver failure and drug metabolism. Scand J Gastroenterol 10: 293-297

Andreasen PB, Ranek L, Statland BE, Tygstrup N (1974) Clearance of antipyrine dependence of quantitative liver function. Eur J Clin Invest 4: 129-134

Andreasen PH, Tønnesen K, Rabøl A, Keiding S (1977) Michaëlis-Menten kinetics of phenazone elimination in the perfused pig liver. Acta Pharmacol Toxicol (Copenh) 40: 1-13

Ballinger B, Browning M, O'Malley K, Stevensen IM (1972) Drug-metabolizing capacity in states of drug dependence and withdrawal. Br J Pharmacol 45: 638-643

Böttcher J, Bässmann M, Schüppel R (1981) Direct quantitation of urinary conjugates of 3-14-C-antipyrine metabolism in man. Naunyn Schmiedebergs Arch Pharmacol [Suppl R5] 316

Boobis AR, Brodie MJ, Kahn GC, Toverud EL, Blair IA, Murray S, Davies DS (1981) Comparison of the in vivo and in vitro rates of formation of the three main oxidative metabolites of antipyrine in man. Br J Clin Pharmacol 12: 771-777

Bremmelgård A, Rank L, Bahnsen M, Andreasen PB, Christensen E (1983) Cholic acid conjugation test and quantitative liver function in acute liver failure. Scand J Gastroenterol 18: 797-802

Brodie BB, Axelrod J (1950) The fate of antipyrine in man. J Pharmacol Exp Ther 98: 97-104
Brodie BB, Axelrod J, Soberman R, Levy BB (1949) The estimation of antipyrine in biological materials. J Biol Chem 179: 25-29
Danhof M, Breimer DD (1979) Studies on the differential metabolic pathways of antipyrine in man. I. Oral administration of 250, 500 and 1000 mg to healthy volunteers. Br J Clin Pharmacol 8: 529-537
Danhof M, Teunissen MWE (1984) Antipyrine as a model drug to assess oxidative drug metabolizing activity in man. Pharm Int 5: 11-15
Danhof M, de Groot-van der Vis E, Breimer DD (1979) Assay of antipyrine and its primary metabolites in plasma, saliva and urine by HPLC, and some preliminary results in man. Pharmacology 18: 210-223
Danhof M, van Zeilen A, Boeijinga JK, Breimer DD (1982a) Studies on the metabolic pathways of antipyrine in man: oral versus i.v. administration and the influence of urinary collection time. Eur J Clin Pharmacol 21: 433-441
Danhof M, Verbeck RMA, van Boxtel CJ, Boijinga JK, Breimer DD (1982b) Differential effects of enzyme induction on antipyrine metabolite formation. Br J Clin Pharmacol 13: 379-386
Danhof M, Teunissen MWE, Breimer DD (1982c) 3-hydroxymethyl-antipyrine excretion in urine. A reconsideration of previously published data and synthesis of a pure reference substance. Pharmacology 24: 181-184
Døssing M, Andreasen PB (1981) Ethanol and antipyrine clearance. Clin Pharmacol Ther 30: 101-104
Døssing M, Poulsen HE, Andreasen PB, Tygstrup N (1982) A simple method for determination of antipyrine clearance. Clin Pharmacol Ther 32: 392-396
Døssing M, Vølund A, Poulsen HE (1983) Optimal sampling times for minimum variance of clearance determination. Br J Clin Pharmacol 15: 231-235
Eichelbaum M, Sontag B, Dengler HJ (1981) HPLC determination of antipyrine metabolites. Pharmacology 23: 192-202
Elin RJ, Vesell ES, Wolff SM (1975) Effects of etiocholanolone-induced fever on plasma antipyrine half-lives and metabolic clearance. Clin Pharmacol Ther 17: 447
Greisen G, Andreasen PB (1976) Two-compartment analysis of plasma elimination of phenazone in normals and in patients with cirrhosis of the liver. Acta Pharmacol Toxicol (Copenh) 38: 49-58
Hansen BA, Poulsen HE (1986a) Changes in the hepatic capacity of urea-N synthesis, galactose elimination and antipyrine clearance following 70% hepatectomy in the rat. Scand J Clin Lab Invest 46: 233-237
Hansen BA, Poulsen HE (1986b) The capacity of urea-N synthesis as a quantitative measure of the liver mass in rats. J Hepatol 2: 460-474
Huffman DH, Shoeman DW, Pentikäinen P, Azarnoff DL (1973) The effect of spironolactone on antipyrine metabolism in man. Pharmacology 10: 338-344
Inaba T, Uchino H, Kalow W (1981) Identidication of *p*(4')-hydroxyantipyrine as a metabolite of antipyrine in man. Res Commun Chem Pathol Pharmacol 33: 3-8
Loft S, Haxholdt O, Døssing M (1985) Antipyrine clearance in children from single saliva sample. Br J Clin Pharmacol 19: 698-700
Loft S, Sonne J, Pilsgaard H, Døssing M, Poulsen HE (1986) Inhibition of antipyrine elimination by disulfiram and cimetidine: the effect of concomitant administration. Br J Clin Pharmacol 21: 75-77
Ohnhaus EE, Cominx S, Ramos M, Noel PPU (1976) Liver blood flow and enzyme induction in man. Eur J Clin Invest 6: 325
Pilsgaard H, Poulsen HE (1984) A one-sample method for antipyrine clearance determinations in rats. Pharmacology 29: 110-116
Poulsen HE (1985) One sample antipyrine clearance after 90% partial hepatectomy in the rat. Liver 5: 200-204
Poulsen HE, Pilsgaard H (1985) Antipyrine metabolism during hepatic regeneration in the rat. Liver 5: 196-199
Ramsøe K, Andreasen PB, Ranek L (1980) Functioning liver mass in uncomplicated and fulminant acute hepatitis. Scand J Gastroenterol 15: 65-72
Rowland M (1972) Application of clearance concepts to some literature data on drug metabolism in the isolated perfused liver preparation and in vivo. Eur J Pharmacol 17: 352-356

Soberman R, Brodie BB, Levy BB, Axelrod J, Hollander V, Steele JM (1949) The use of antipyrine in the measurement of total body water in man. J Biol Chem 179: 31-42
Teunissen MWE, Kampf D, Roots I, Vermeulen NPE, Breimer DD (1985). Antipyrine formation in patients with chronic renal failure. Eur J Clin Pharmacol 28: 589-595
Toverud EL, Boobis AR, Brodie MJ, Murray S, Bennett PN, Whitmarsh V, Davies DS (1981) Differential induction of antipyrine metabolism by rifampicine. Eur J Clin Pharmacol 21: 155-160
Tygstrup N, Vilstrup H (1983) Functional evaluation of the hepatocyte. In: Simon Beker G (ed) Diagnostic procedures in the evaluation of hepatic disease. Liss, New York
Uchino H, Inaba T, Kalow W (1983) Human metabolism of antipyrine labelled with 14-C in the pyrazolone ring or in the *N*-methyl group. Xenobiotica 13: 155-162
Uppal R, Sharma PR, Nair CR, Chaudhury RR (1980) Enhanced antipyrine metabolism in cigarette smokers in Indian population. Int J Clin Pharmacol Ther Toxicol 18: 269-271
Vesell ES (1979) The antipyrine test in clinical pharmacology: conceptions and misconceptions. Clin Pharmacol Ther 26: 275-286
Vesell ES (1982) On the significance of host factors that affect drug disposition. Clin Pharmacol Ther 31: 1-7
Vesell ES, Page JG (1968) Genetic control of drug levels in man: antipyrine. Science 161: 72-73
Vesell ES, Passananti I, Glenwright PA, Dvorchik BH (1975) Studies on the disposition of antipyrine, aminopyrine and phenacetine using plasma saliva and urine. Clin Pharmacol Ther 18: 259-272
Vilstrup H (1980) Synthesis of urea after stimulation with amino acids: relations to liver function. Gut 21: 990-995
Welch RM, DeAngelis RL, Wingfield M, Farmer TW (1975) Elimination of antipyrine from saliva as a measure of metabolism in man. Clin Pharmacol Ther 18: 249-258
Zietz E, Eichelbaum E, Dengler HJ, Spiteller G (1978) Zum Metabolismus von Antipyrin beim Menschen. Arzneimittelforsch 28: 315-318

# Antipyrine Clearance: Evaluation of Simplified Methods in Chronic Liver Diseases

M. Strazzabosco[1], M. Muraca[1], M. Venuti[1], A. Varotto[1], G. Nassuato[1], R. M. Iemmolo[1], R. Orlando[1], F. Lirussi[1], C. Manzati[2], T. Crimella[2], E. Iaccheri[2], R. Bernardi[2], and L. Okolicsányi[1]

[1] Istituto di Medicina Interna, Policlinico Universitario, Università di Padova, Via Giustiniani 2, 35122 Padova, Italy
[2] Laboratori Boehringer Biochemia Robin, Viale Libertà Km 0.750, 20052 Monza, Italy

## Introduction

Antipyrine exhibits unique kinetic properties: given orally it is rapidly and completely absorbed, its binding to plasma proteins is negligible and its distribution volume equals total body water (Soberman et al. 1949; Stevenson 1977; Vessell 1979). Moreover, the drug is extensively metabolized by hepatic microsomal enzymes, its disposal can be described by a one-compartment model, and it is not influenced by hepatic blood flow (Stevenson 1977; Vessell 1979; Danhof and Tennissen 1984). Therefore, the determination of antipyrine clearance is being increasingly used to assess hepatic drug metabolism and as a quantitative test of liver function (Branch et al. 1973; Andreasen et al. 1974; Vessell 1979; Bircher 1983; Tygstrup and Vilstrup 1983). Due to a number of factors, antipyrine clearance shows a large interindividual variation, therefore the test is not useful for the diagnosis of liver disease. However, its use in clinical hepatology seems to be promising for prognostic purposes, for the assessment of surgical risk, and for the follow-up of liver patients (e.g., to assess the need and timing of transplantation; Andreasen and Ranek 1975; Ramsoe et al. 1980; Poulsen 1985; Poulsen and Loft 1986).

The procedure usually performed is cumbersome and requires repeated blood sampling for at least 27 h. Much effort has recently been spent to devise simpler procedures. The possibility of determining antipyrine kinetics from saliva samples (Van Boxtel et al. 1975; Frazer et al. 1976; Brooks et al. 1976; Danhof et al. 1979; Loft et al. 1985) is of great interest in this respect as it is the proposed method to assess antipyrine clearance from a single plasma or saliva sample (Dossing et al. 1982).

The aim of our work was to evaluate, in a series of patients, the applicability of antipyrine clearance calculated from one or two serum or saliva samples by using a newly available kit that includes a spectrophotometric assay suitable for clinical laboratories.

## Patients and Methods

### *Patients*

Sixty-eight hospitalized patients (54 males, 14 females, mean age $49 \pm 8$ years) were studied. Thirty of them presented no signs or symptoms of liver disease and had not received drugs for at least 2 weeks before the study. The other 38 were affected by chronic liver disease of varying clinical severity. They were classified as decompensated ($n = 24$) if they presented at least two of the following features: bilirubin > 1.2 mg/dl,

Assessment and Management of Hepatobiliary Disease
Eds.: L. Okolicsányi, G. Csomós, and G. Crepaldi

albumin $<3.2$ g/dl, ascites, and portal hypertension. A careful drug history was recorded. Most of the patients were treated with various drugs during the study. However, no patient taking hypnotic drugs or known enzyme inducers was admitted to the study. The only drug known to influence antipyrine clearance that was administered to a limited number of patients was spironolactone. In 15 patients with liver disease the procedure was repeated at 6-month intervals, so that a total 90 tests was performed. Informed consent was obtained from each patient.

*Methods*

Antipyrine, 18 mg/kg body weight (Welch et al. 1975) as an aqueous solution, was given orally after overnight fasting. After the administration of the drug, blood samples were taken at 3-h intervals up to the 27th hour. Samples were kept at $-20\,°C$ until the time of the assay.

Antipyrine concentrations in biological fluids were determined both by spectrophotometric and high-pressure liquid chromatographic (HPLC) methods. The spectrophotometric assay was derived from Brodie et al. (1949; Davidson and MacIntyre 1956; Greenblatt and Locnisar 1979). The method is based on the estimation of the absorbance at 350 nm of a nitro-derivative of antipyrine, after precipitation of plasma proteins by zinc sulfate in diluted sulfuric acid, and subsequent addition of sodium hydroxide.

For the HPLC assay, a Hewlett-Packard chromatograph model 1084 was used. The column was an Sph ODS of 5 μm (Violet, Rome, Italy); the elution was isocratic during the antipyrine analysis and then a solvent program was carried out to clean the column of serum impurities. The two components of the eluting mixture were acetonitrile and sodium acetate buffer (2 g/l, pH 3 with acetic acid). The antipyrine peak was detected at 252 nm. Samples of both serum and saliva were prepared by mixing 1 ml acetonitrile with 500 μl biological fluid and then centrifuging for 10 min at 6000 rpm. The method showed a good recovery (more than 98%) and a good reproducibility (CV less than 2.5%).

*Calculations*

In all patients antipyrine clearance (ApCl) and apparent volume of distribution ($V_d$) were calculated by the three following procedures:

1. The standard procedure: this takes into account the whole series of concentrations determined and clearance (Cl) is calculated as:

$$\mathrm{Cl} = K \times V_d = (\mathrm{d}C/\mathrm{d}T) \times (D/C_0) \tag{1}$$

where $C$ is the concentration, $T$ is time, $D$ is the dose given, $C_0$ is the extrapolated concentration at time 0, and $K$ is the elimination constant estimated from the linear regression of the logarithm of $C$ on $T$.

2. The one-sample procedure: this is based on the same principle, but $C_0$ is estimated from a postulated $V_d$ and $K$ is assessed from $C_0$ and $C_t$.

$$\mathrm{Cl} = \frac{\ln (D/V_d) - \ln C_t}{t} \times V_d \tag{2}$$

In each patient, for each of the seven samples determined, ApCl was calculated both assuming a $V_d$ of 40 l and by approximating it from age, sex, body weight, and height, using the formula of Bruce et al. (1980). The latter estimation was possible since the volume of distribution of antipyrine can be considered equal to total body water.

3. The two-sample procedure: in this case antipyrine clearance was calculated from Eq. 1, utilizing only two time-concentration points. $V_d$ was estimated from the administered dose and the extrapolated $C_0$.

At any calculated point, the values of one-sample and two-sample clearances were tested for correlation with the values obtained from the whole set of data by least-squares analysis.

## Results

### *Spectrophotometric vs HPLC Methods*

The reaction was linear from 2 to 50 μg/ml. Hemolyzed or hyperlipidemic sera did not interfere with the reaction, nor did bilirubin, up to a concentration of 50 mg/dl (data not shown).

An excellent correlation was found in serum between antipyrine concentration determined by HPLC and by colorimetric assay ($r=0.97$, $n=250$, $P<0.001$, $y=1.03+0.96x$). Employing the HPLC method, serum values correlated well with those obtained from saliva ($r=0.89$, $n=143$, residual variance$=15.81$). However, a systematic error was present, leading to underestimation of saliva concentrations (mean values 19.77±9.35 vs 15.85±7.80 ml/min, $y=1.54+0.72x$). Moreover, when using the spectrophotometric assay in saliva, the accuracy of the method was lower and possible interference from unidentified substances was found. Therefore, only re-

**Table 1.** Linear regression analysis of antipyrine clearance (ApCl) calculated using the one- and two-sample methods and clearance calculated from multiple samples

| Sampling time (h) | No. of samples | $r$ | Slope of regression | Intercept of regression | Residual variance | ApCl (ml/min) (mean ± SD) |
|---|---|---|---|---|---|---|
| One-sample method | | | | | | |
| 3 | 52 | 0.24 | 0.62 | 30.06 | 887.5 | 47.69 ± 30.44 |
| 6 | 60 | 0.44 | 0.68 | 16.70 | 262.4 | 35.42 ± 17.88 |
| 9 | 57 | 0.69 | 0.88 | 8.31 | 110.0 | 33.81 ± 14.37 |
| 12 | 54 | 0.82 | 0.88 | 6.93 | 50.8 | 31.65 ± 12.56 |
| 24 | 61 | 0.92 | 0.98 | 0.45 | 23.6 | 27.90 ± 12.40 |
| 27 | 53 | 0.93 | 1.06 | −0.10 | 21.4 | 27.76 ± 13.03 |
| Two-sample method | | | | | | |
| 3- 6 | 58 | 0.34 | 0.41 | 20.63 | 188.2 | 31.64 ± 14.48 |
| 24-27 | 39 | 0.26 | 0.31 | 11.72 | 176.0 | 20.18 ± 13.59 |
| 6-12 | 52 | 0.88 | 1.00 | 1.12 | 41.6 | 28.75 ± 13.60 |
| 3-12 | 54 | 0.87 | 0.85 | 6.26 | 33.9 | 29.16 ± 11.94 |
| 12-24 | 48 | 0.96 | 0.98 | −1.15 | 11.0 | 27.31 ± 12.29 |
| 6-24 | 53 | 0.97 | 0.98 | −0.76 | 8.1 | 27.35 ± 11.90 |
| 3-24 | 57 | 0.96 | 0.98 | −0.31 | 11.8 | 26.77 ± 12.41 |
| 6-27 | 50 | 0.97 | 1.05 | −1.04 | 6.3 | 27.24 ± 12.41 |
| 3-27 | 49 | 0.97 | 1.03 | −0.05 | 7.5 | 26.49 ± 12.62 |

Whole-series clearance = 27.79 ± 11.56 ml/min

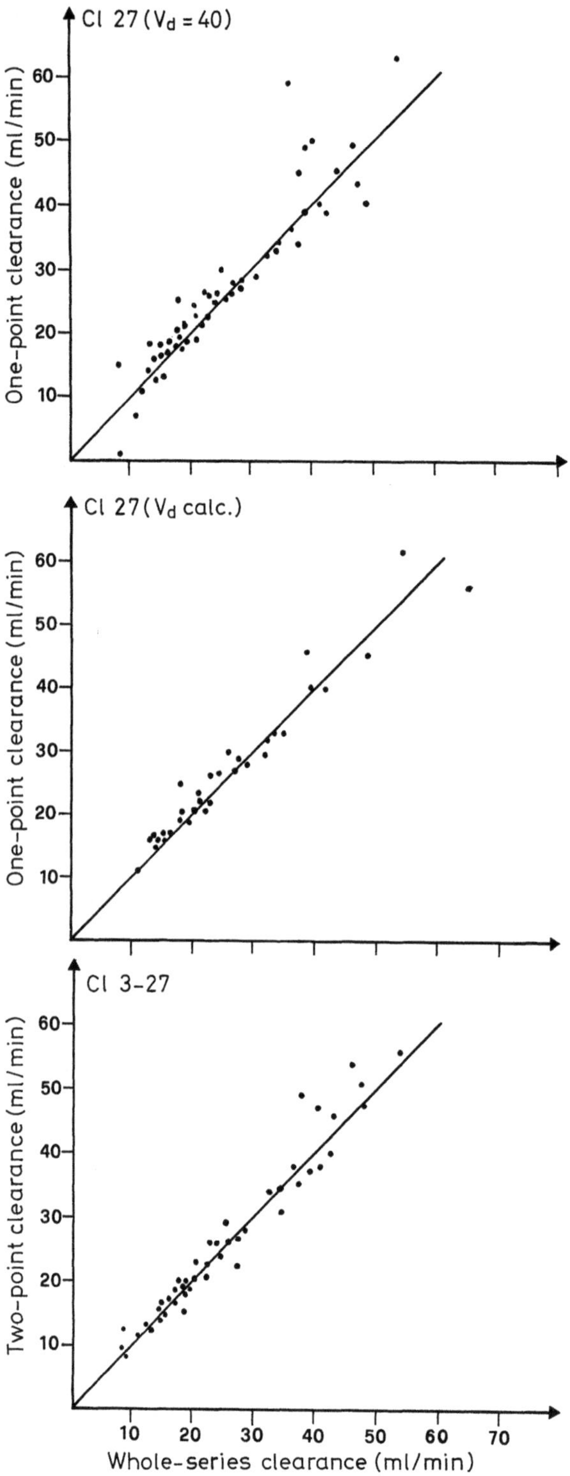


**Fig. 1.** Correlation between simplified methods and clearance calculated employing the whole series of plasma samples. For the one-sample method, results were obtained using the 27th hour as sampling point both assuming a $V_d$ of 40 l and by calculating it from Bruce formula ($V_d$ *calc*). For the two-sample method the results obtained with the 3rd and 27th hours as sampling points are shown

sults obtained from serum samples with the spectrophotometric assay will be considered for further discussion.

*One-Point Method*

The results of regression analysis (Table 1) indicate that the longer the time interval between administration and sampling, the better the correlation with the clearance calculated on the whole series of plasma samples. As shown in Fig. 1, the 27th hour time point gave the best correlation coefficient, using both a fixed $V_d$ of 40 l and the one calculated from Bruce's formula ($r=0.93$ and 0.92 respectively). When separating our patients according to the presence or absence of liver disease, the one-sample method was also found to be reliable in patients with liver disease. Assuming that the 27th hour is the best sampling point, mean antipyrine clearance values were $34.5 \pm 12.8$ vs $37.4 \pm 13.7$ ml/min (standard calculation vs one-point, $r=0.91$) in the control group and $22.8 \pm 9.7$ vs $24.7 \pm 9.8$ ml/min ($r=0.97$) in patients with liver disease. Data obtained employing Bruce's formula were comparable.

*Two-Point Method*

The regression analysis of the two-sample method is also shown in Table 1. The longer the interval between the two samples, the better the correlation was with the clearance calculated from the whole series of plasma samples. The 3rd–27th hour pair of time points appeared to be the best combination ($r=0.97$; see Table 1).

The simplified method also gave reliable results when dividing our patients according to the presence or absence of liver disease ($34.5 \pm 12.8$ vs $33.5 \pm 14.9$ ml/min, $r=0.98$ in controls, and $22.8 \pm 9.7$ vs $24.2 \pm 11$ ml/min in patients with liver disease).

Moreover, as shown in Fig. 2, the two-sample method allowed an accurate estimation of the apparent volume of distribution of antipyrine ($r=0.95$, $P<0.001$). In our

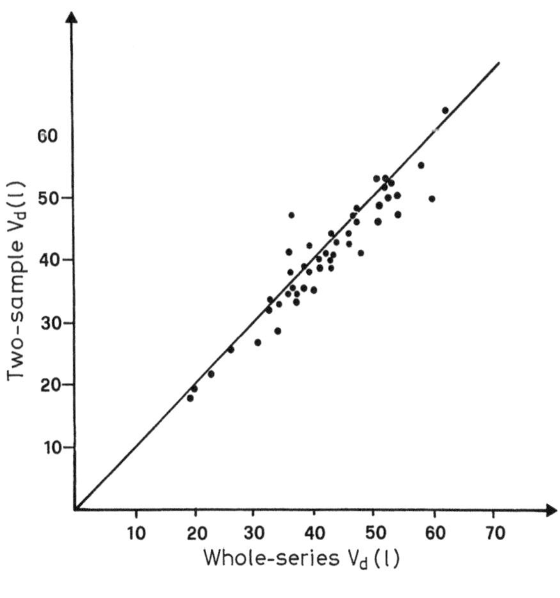


**Fig. 2.** Correlation between antipyrine $V_d$ calculated with the two-sample method and $V_d$ calculated from the whole series of samples

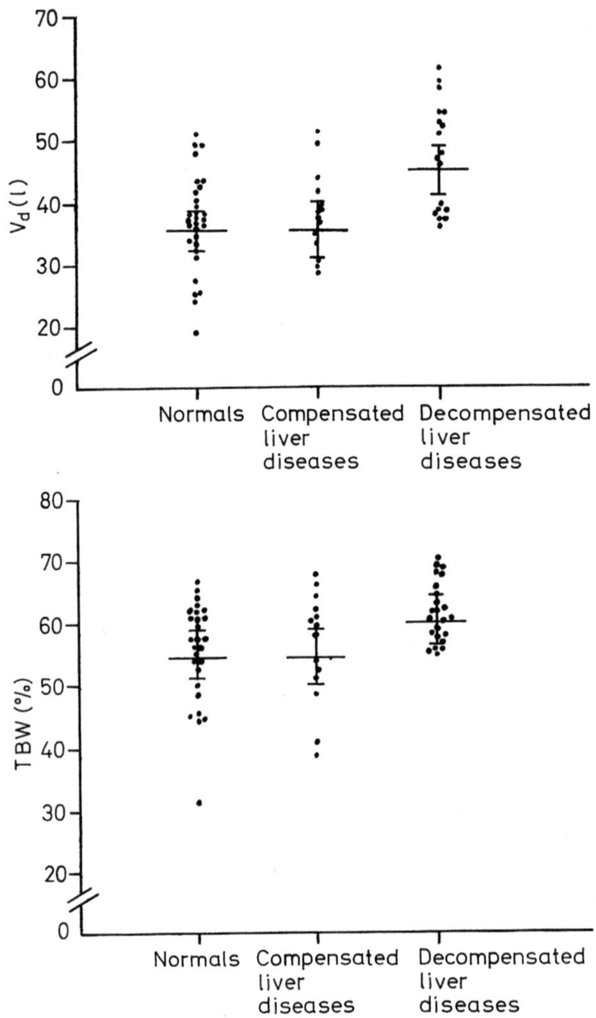


**Fig. 3.** $V_d$ and total body water *(TBW)* values in normal subjects and in patients with liver disease of differing clinical severity. Normal subjects and patients with decompensated liver disease differed significantly in both cases ($P < 0.025$)

series, the mean apparent volume of distribution of the group of patients with liver disease was significantly different from that of the control group (43.6 ± 9.3 vs 36.9 ± 9.0 l, $P < 0.025$); total body water was significantly higher in decompensated patients than in compensated or normal subjects (60.5 ± 4.2 vs 54.75 ± 8.9 and 54.5 ± 8.4% respectively, $P < 0.025$) (Fig. 3).

## Discussion

In the present work we tested two simplified methods for the determination of antipyrine clearance in a series of normal subjects and patients with liver disease. Moreover, we evaluated the applicability of the classical spectrophotometric method of Brodie et al. (1949) with respect to an HPLC assay of blood and saliva.

The results of the one-sample method confirmed the results obtained by Dossing et al. (1982) in a series of patients with chronic liver disease of varying clinical severity. The correlation between one-point ApCl and ApCl calculated from the whole series of plasma samples was highly significant and the mean variance of the clearance is minimal if the sampling time is correctly placed at $1/K$ (on average about 24 h after medication; Dossing et al. 1983). As already mentioned, with this method, $V_d$ can be assumed to be equal to 40 l or it can be approximated from the age, sex, body weight, and height of the patient (Bruce et al. 1980). The bias in clearance values due to the approximation of $V_d$ is negligible (Pilsgaard and Poulsen 1984). However, the one-point method can only be applied to patients in a stable condition, and frequently this is not the case in patients with liver disease. Moreover, since water retention commonly occurs in liver disease, the determination of total body water (i.e., antipyrine $V_d$) could be important in such conditions.

With the two-sample method, we obtained a highly significant correlation with ApCl calculated on the whole series of samples, the 3rd and 27th hours being the best pair of time-concentration points. The possibility of performing the antipyrine test with only two plasma samples was first suggested by McPherson et al. (1982), who applied it to the calculation of antipyrine halflives. We propose the two-sample method for the assessment of clearance since this is the most appropriate parameter to describe drug disposition (Gibaldi and Koup 1981).

Moreover, we obtained an accurate estimation of distribution volume. This is of particular interest since clearance and $V_d$ are two independent pharmacokinetic variables (Gibaldi and Koup 1981). In our series, the mean $V_d$ of antipyrine was higher in the group of patients with decompensated liver disease, than in compensated patients or normal subjects. Nevertheless, the potential value of estimating antipyrine $V_d$ in the follow-up of patients with liver disease remains to be established.

When determining antipyrine concentration in blood, the spectrophotometric assay of Brodie et al. (1949) is accurate enough to be employed with the simplified method which requires high analytical accuracy and reproducibility. Its sensitivity limits are satisfactory for most clinical pharmacokinetic studies. On the other hand, for saliva the accuracy of the method was lower, interference from unidentified substances being present. Therefore, if antipyrine concentrations have to be determined in saliva, we recommend HPLC or gas-liquid chromatographic methods (Velch et al. 1975; Van Boxtel et al. 1976; Frazer et al. 1976).

In conclusion, the simplified methods considered in the present work can correctly assess antipyrine clearance in patients with liver disease, even when using a spectrophotometric assay. We propose that the two-sample method should be preferred when using ApCl in the follow-up of patients with liver diseases since it also allows an accurate determination of volume of distribution.

## References

Andreasen PB, Ranek L (1975) Liver failure and drug metabolism. Scand J Gastroenterol 10: 293-297

Andreasen PB, Ranek L, Statland BE, Tygstrup N (1974) Clearance of antipyrine dependence of quantitative liver function. Eur J Clin Invest 4: 129-134

Bircher J (1983) Quantitative assessment of deranged hepatic function: a missed opportunity? Semin Liver Dis 3: 275-284

Branch RA, Herbert CH, Read AE (1973) Determinants of serum antipyrine half-lives in patients with liver disease. Gut 14: 569-573

Brodie BB, Axelrod J, Soberman R, Levy BB (1949) The estimation of antipyrine in biological materials. J Biol Chem 179: 25-29

Brooks PM, Bell MA, Burns H (1976) Salivary antipyrine half-life: a useful measure of hepatic drug metabolism. Br J Clin Pharmacol 3: 945-946

Bruce A, Anderson M, Arvidson B, Isaksson B (1980) Body composition prediction of normal body potassium, body water and body fat in adults on the basis of body height, body weight and age. Scand J Clin Lab Invest 40: 461-463

Danhof M, De Groot E, Van der Vis E, Breimer DD (1979) Assay of antipyrine and its primary metabolites in plasma, saliva and urine by HPLC, and some preliminary results in man. Pharmacology 18: 210-223

Danhof M, Tennissen MWE (1984) Antipyrine as a model drug to assess oxidative drug metabolizing activity in man. Pharmacol Int 5: 11-15

Davidson D, MacIntyre I (1956) Estimation of antipyrine in plasma. Biochem J 62: 37p

Dossing M, Poulsen HE, Andreasen PB, Tygstrup N (1982) A simple method for determination of antipyrine clearance. Clin Pharmacol Ther 32: 392-396

Dossing M, Volund A, Poulsen HE (1983) Optimal sampling times for minimum variance of clearance determination. Br J Clin Pharmacol 15: 231-235

Frazer HS, Mucklow JC, Murray S, Davies DS (1976) Assessment of antipyrine kinetics by measurement in saliva. Br J Clin Pharmacol 3: 321-325

Gibaldi M, Koup JR (1981) Pharmacokinetic concepts – Drug binding, apparent volume of distribution and clearance. Eur J Clin Pharmacol 20: 299-305

Greenblatt DJ, Locnisar A (1979) Spectrophotometric assay of antipyrine in plasma: a reevaluation. Int J Clin Pharmacol Biopharmacy 17: 401-404

Loft S, Haxholdt O, Dossing M (1985) Antipyrine clearance in children from single saliva samples. Br J Clin Pharmacol 19: 698-700

McPherson GAD, Benjamin IS, Boobis AR, Brodie MG, Hampden C, Blumgart LH (1982) Antipyrine elimination as a dynamic test of hepatic functional integrity in obstructive jaundice. Gut 23: 734-738

Pilsgaard H, Poulsen HE (1984) A one-sample method for antipyrine clearance determination in rats. Pharmacology 29: 110-116

Poulsen HE (1985) One sample antipyrine clearance after 90% partial hepatectomy in the rat. Liver 5: 200-204

Poulsen EP, Loft S (1986) Antipyrine metabolism, an update. Abstract in International symposium on assessment and management of hepatobiliary disease, 28-31 May 1986, Padova, Italy

Ramsoe K, Andreasen PB, Ranek L (1980) Functioning liver mass in uncomplicated and fulminant acute hepatitis. Scand J Gastroenterol 15: 65-72

Stevenson IH (1977) Factors influencing antipyrine elimination. Br J Clin Pharmacol 4: 261-265

Soberman R, Brodie BB, Levy BB, Axelrod J, Hollander V, Steele JM (1949) The use of antipyrine in the measurement of total body water in man. J Biol Chem 179: 31-42

Stevenson IH (1977) Factors influencing antipyrine elimination. Br J Clin Pharmacol 4: 261-265

Tygstrup N, Vilstrup H (1983) Functional evaluation of the hepatocyte. In: Simon Beker G (ed) Diagnostic procedures in the evaluation of hepatic disease. Liss, New York

Van Boxtel CJ, Wilson JT, Lindgren S, Sjoqvist F (1975) Comparison of the half-life of antipyrine in plasma, whole blood and saliva of man. Eur J Clin Pharmacol 9: 327-332

Vessell ES (1979) The antipyrine test in clinical pharmacology: conceptions and misconceptions. Clin Pharmacol Ther 26: 275-286

Welch RM, De Angelis RM, Wingfield M, Farmert TW (1975) Elimination of antipyrine from saliva as a measure of metabolism in man. Clin Pharmacol Ther 18: 249-258

# Preoperative Care of Adult Patients Chosen for Liver Transplantation

G. Brunner, W. Lauchart, B. Ringe, H. Freyberger, and R. Pichlmayr

Department of Gastroenterology and Hepatology, Department of Abdominal and Transplant Surgery, Department of Psychosomatic Medicine, Medizinische Hochschule, 3000 Hannover, Federal Republic of Germany

## Introduction

Liver transplantation has found its place as an accepted therapy in end-stage liver disease. It is no longer considered an experimental procedure [6, 9, 10–12]. However, the chance of immediate and long-term survival is still far from ideal. Low-risk and high-risk (elective and non-elective) patients are offered to the transplant surgeon, and it is well known that the best results are achieved in the elective or low-risk patients [9, 11, 12] (Fig. 1). Therefore surgeons urge the internist to send patients earlier. The internist, however, tends to keep the patient on conservative regimes as long as possible before he makes such a far-reaching decision. This often results in a situation where the patient becomes an extremely high operative risk.

Since from the nature of his education even the progressive internist will "always" be (relatively) late in sending the patient for liver transplantation, it is his task to prepare the patient in the best possible way once the decision has been made to offer this mode of therapy.

## Preoperative Care of Urgent Patients

One must distinguish between elective, urgent, and emergency patients (Table 1). *Elective* patients are usually those in good or excellent clinical condition who happen to have a malignant or benign primary tumor in the liver which cannot be completely re-

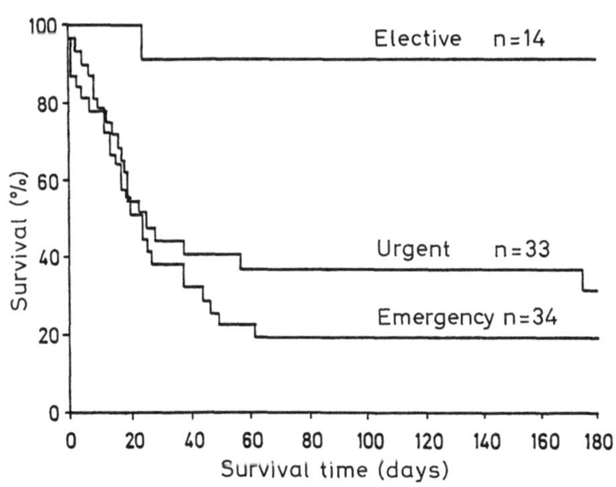


**Fig. 1.** Survival of 81 adult patients with benign liver disease grafted between 1972 and 1985

Assessment and Management of Hepatobiliary Disease
Eds.: L. Okolicsányi, G. Csomós, and G. Crepaldi

**Table 1.** Categories of indication for liver transplantation

| Category | Status | Type of preoperative care |
|---|---|---|
| Elective | Liver tumors, compensated cirrhosis. No extrahepatic disease-related organ complications | Outpatient |
| Urgent | Decompensated deteriorating cirrhosis | Inpatient |
| Emergency | Acute liver failure<br>Acute on chronic failure<br>Severe decompensation in cirrhosis<br>Acute form of Wilson's disease | Intensive care |

sected. These patients usually need no special preoperative training and care except for vaccination and occasional psychosomatic aid. The same applies to some patients with well-compensated cirrhosis.

*Urgent* patients are persons who are progressively deteriorating clinically as well as in liver function but may well live, or rather "vegetate," for some more months. Ascites and edema may have developed but are kept under control with spironolactone and/or diuretics without significant impairment of kidney function. An episode of encephalopathy may have appeared but can be reversed or kept under control by restriction of protein intake or the use of lactulose and/or neomycin. Blood clotting may be impaired but can be kept in balance on a lower scale.

*Muscle Wasting.* This is the gravest sign and problem. The immediate postoperative period after liver transplantation demands good respiratory muscle function and for remobilization good skeletal muscle strength is also essential. Very often, patients with advanced liver cirrhosis are not able to do knee bends or walk upstairs normally. Therefore, physical training of increasing intensity is organized for these patients, as well as respiratory training. The progress during this intensive, guided training also motivates the patient for transplantation and often stabilizes his labile mental state. During the 4–8 weeks the patient has to wait for a suitable liver, we have regularly observed a significant increase in muscle strength and volume.

*Vaccination.* Only a small number of patients coming up for liver transplantation are carriers of hepatitis B antigen or antibody. The majority have primary biliary cirrhosis, primary sclerosing cholangitis, postnecrotic non-A non-B cirrhosis, Wilson's disease, or liver tumors. These patients must be protected against transfusion hepatitis B, which may arise from the large number of transfusions necessary during transplantation. Thus active immunization is performed with double the usual dose of hepatitis B vaccine at 4-weekly intervals until a sufficient antibody titer has developed. An additional active immunization is done directly before operation if no sufficient antibody titer has developed by the date of transplantation.

*Psychosomatic Aid.* Psychoanalytic exploration of patients selected for liver transplantation has revealed that beside direct fear, there is often hidden uncertainty about the decision for transplantation and the outcome of the operation. There is sometimes also tension, misunderstanding, or controversy between the patient and his family concerning the transplantation. Therefore every patient selected for transplantation undergoes psychosomatic investigation and is offered help, which some patients gladly accept. This help is often also extended to family members. Patients have repeatedly stated that the psychosomatic guidance has been of great help concerning their attitude toward transplantation.

*Medical Care.* In most patients standard medical care is sufficient. Patients receive a protein-restricted diet, an aldosterone antagonist, lactulose and/or neomycin, and vitamin K. Rantidine is given for prophylaxis of gastric or duodenal ulcers and of acid reflux into the esophagus. If variceal bleedings occur or are imminent, sclerotherapy is performed. In severe endogenous intoxication and in unbearable pruritus in patients with primary biliary cirrhosis, plasma exchange is carried out at weekly to monthly intervals [4, 7, 8].

## Preoperative Care Before Emergency Transplantation

With increasing acceptance of liver transplantation among physicians and the general population, and with more transplantation centers being instituted, less emergency transplantation will have to be carried out in the future. But there will always be patients with sudden rapid deterioration of previous stable chronic liver disease, as well as acute liver failure or acute Wilson's disease. For these emergencies a long training program is not possible. The patients just have to be kept alive until a donor liver can be found. Beside intensive care, intermittent plasma exchange every 2nd or 3rd day and daily hemodialysis will support the three main functions of the liver: detoxification, synthesis, and regulation [3, 5]. Exchanging the patient's plasma will remove endogenous toxins, resulting in an improvement of encephalopathy. Replacing the toxic and deficient plasma with fresh frozen plasma from healthy donors will replace many missing products of liver synthesis, such as coagulation factors, proteins, and lipids.

However, this "optimal" support of liver functions has its limitations. If applied daily, it will cause serious lung and brain side effects [1, 2] resulting from protein aggregates, in analogy to polytransfused patients after severe trauma. Therefore, plasma exchange is performed approximately every 2nd or 3rd day, while hemodialysis, which has almost no severe side effects, is carried out daily. Hemodialysis will remove water-soluble toxins and especially many serum amino acids, which are grossly elevated in severe liver disease and which present as the precursors of most endogenous "liver" toxins. With this combination of intermittent plasma exchange and daily hemodialysis patients can be kept alive for periods ranging from several days up to a few weeks.

## Summary

While 2-year survival after liver transplantation is 80% for elective patients, it is below 30% after urgent and emergency transplantation. Therefore, preoperative care is of extreme importance to prepare the patient for this severe operation. High-risk patients who have advanced liver cirrhosis with jaundice, ascites, impaired coagulation, and extreme muscle wasting are admitted to a pretransplantation program including psychosomatic investigation and care, improvement of coagulation and ascites, and intensive physiotherapy and muscle training. During this 4- to 8-week preoperative training period the patient's physical and mental condition improves significantly and the postoperative period is tolerated better.

Patients with liver failure and signs of encephalopathy are treated with a combination of intermittent plasma exchange and dialysis until a suitable donor organ has been found.

## References


1. Akamatsu K, Tada K, Okada S, Ohkubo H, Mukai J, Ohta Y (1982) A new method of plasma exchange for acute hepatic failure: filtration of fresh frozen plasma. In: Oda T (ed) Therapeutic plasmapheresis II. Schattauer, Stuttgart, pp 365-367
2. Akamatsu K, Tanaka Y, Tada K, Okada S, Mukai J, Hashimoto H, Ohkubo H, Ohta Y (1983) Pulmonary microembolism due to the exchange transfusion of fresh-frozen plasma containing microaggregates. In: Oda T (ed) Therapeutic plasmapheresis III. Schattauer, Stuttgart, pp 95-100
3. Brunner G What is needed for an artificial liver? In: Progress in Artificial Organs. 1985 edited by Y. Nose, L. Kjellstrand and P. Ivanovitch. ISAO Press, Cleveland 1986
4. Brunner G, Lösgen H (1983) Plasma exchange in liver disease. In: Lysaght MJ, Gurland HJ (eds) Plasma separation and plasma fractionation. Karger, Basel, pp 115-123
5. Brunner G, Lösgen H (1985) Artificial liver support 1985. Leber Magen Darm 15 (5): 186-191
6. Calne RY (1983) Liver transplantation. Grune and Stratton, London
7. Erikson S, Lindgren S (1980) Plasma exchange in primary biliary cirrhosis. N Engl J Med 302: 809
8. Keeling PW, Bull J, Kingston P, Thompson RPH (1981) Plasma exchange in primary biliary cirrhosis. Postgrad Med J 57: 433
9. Pichlmayr R, Brölsch C, Wonigeit K, Neuhaus P, Siegismund S, Schmidt FW, Burdelski M (1984) Experiences with liver transplantation in Hannover. Hepatology 4 (1): 56S-60S
10. Pichlmayr R, Neuhaus P, Ringe B, Wonigeit K, Burdelski M, Verner L, Lauchart W, Schmidt FW (1985) Development in liver transplantation. Jpn J Surg 15 (6): 409-419
11. Starzl TE, Iwatsuki C, van Thiele D, Gartner J, Zitelli B, Malatack J, Schade R, Shaw B, Hakala T, Rosenthal J, Porter K (1982) Evolution of liver transplantation. Hepatology 2: 614
12. Starzl TE, Iwatsuki S, Shaw BW Jr, van Thiel DH, Gartner JC, Zitelli BJ, Malatack JJ, Schade RR (1984) Analysis of liver transplantation. Hepatology 4 (1): 47S-49S

# Assessment of Liver Function Before and After Liver Transplantation

Ellen R. Gordon

Liver Center, Department of Internal Medicine, Yale University School of Medicine, New Haven, CT 06510, U.S.A.

Bilirubin is the end product of heme catabolism and has no physiological function, yet it has been the subject of intense investigation, with millions of dollars being spent yearly by clinicians and scientists [1]. From its structure (Fig. 1 a), one would predict that it was very water-soluble; however, at pH 7.4 its solubility is in the nanogram range. Chemists explain this occurrence as a result of bilirubin forming a "ridge tile" through the diacid state with six intramolecular hydrogen bonds [2, 3]. This renders bilirubin insoluble (Fig. 1 b). Thus bilirubin is not secreted in urine, but is converted to conjugates within the liver. These appear in bile, mainly as bilirubin diglucuronide with minor components of bilirubin monoglucuronide and a diester containing monoglucuronide and monoglucoside [4, 5].

In vitro, the conjugation of bilirubin occurs in two sequential steps. First, bilirubin monoglucuronide is formed from bilirubin with uridine diphosphate (UDP) glucuronate as the glucuronyl donor catalyzed by a microsomal bilirubin UDP transferase.

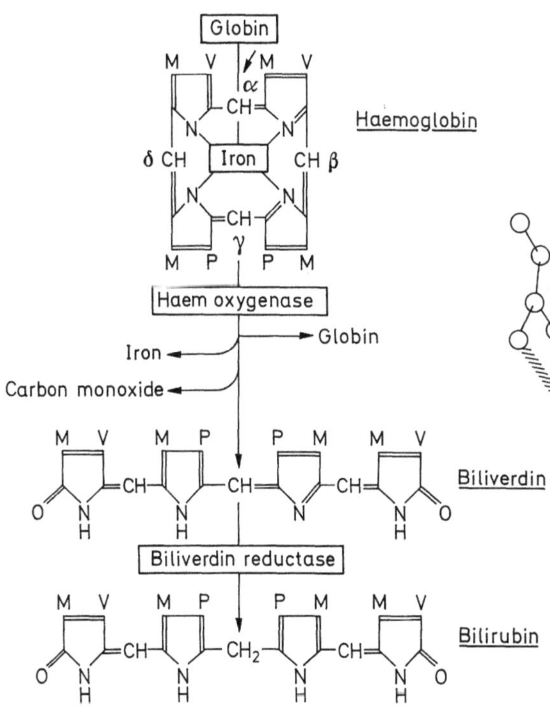


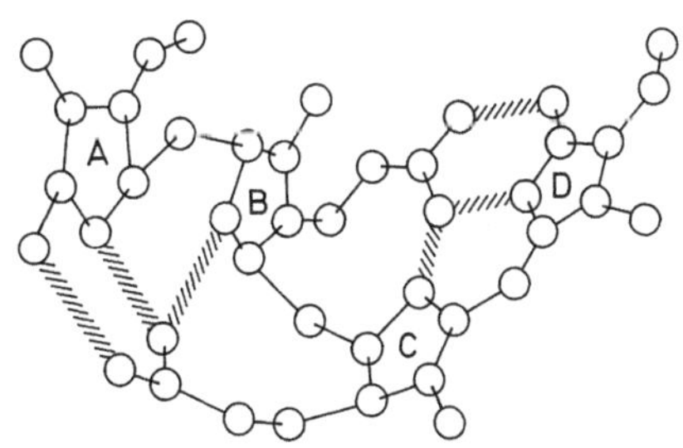


**Fig. 1.** The *upper* diagram illustrates the formation of bilirubin from hemoglobin. The *lower* diagram indicates the tile formation of bilirubin at physiological pH 7.4

Assessment and Management of Hepatobiliary Disease
Eds.: L. Okolicsányi, G. Csomós, and G. Crepaldi

Second, bilirubin monoglucuronide is converted to bilirubin diglucuronide. In the early 1980s the catalytic site for the conversion remained questionable. Initially, bilirubin monoglucuronide was detected as the only product formed from bilirubin in the hepatic microsomes [6]. Then we and Blanckaert and Schmid lowered the concentration of bilirubin from over 100 $\mu M$ to a level of 10–20 $\mu M$ and found that hepatic microsomes formed bilirubin diglucuronide quite efficiently [7, 8]. However, at the same time, Jansen et al. [9] and Roy Chowdhury et al. [10] investigated another site in the liver for the formation of bilirubin diglucuronide. An enzyme was purified from hepatic plasma membranes enriched in canaliculi and was named glucuronide glucuronyltransferase [11]. The reaction occurred in the absence of UDP glucuronic acid and took 2 mol bilirubin monoglucuronide and converted it to 1 mol bilirubin diglucuronide and 1 mol bilirubin [11].

It now appeared that within the liver there may be two hepatocelullar sites for the formation of bilirubin diglucuronide. This led us to study the other hepatocellular site, the canalicular plasma membrane preparations, for the formation of bilirubin diglucuronide. Highly purified canalicular plasma membrane was isolated from 100 g rat liver by rate zonal flotation procedures and then subjected to high-speed centrifugation in a discontinuous sucrose gradient. Vesiculated liver plasma membrane preparations of the canaliculi were located at the 31% (W/W) sucrose gradient layer and the vesiculated liver plasma membrane preparations of basolateral were located at the 38% (W/W) site of the sucrose layer. Marker enzymes were measured to ascertain the degree of contamination of the liver plasma membranes with other organelles, and included succinate and NADH cytochrome c reductase for mitochondria, NADPH cytochrome c reductase for microsomes, acid phosphatase for lysosomes, and galactosyltransferase for Golgi membrane [12].

The relative enrichment of marker enzyme activity over that of homogenate ranged from 0.1 to 0.9, except for acid phosphatase, where it was 1.1. Since lysosomes represent 2% of the total homogenate and endoplasmic reticulum represents 24%, these values indicate that the canalicular liver plasma membrane was contaminated with endoplasmic reticulum more than with lysosomes. Differences in the enzyme content of the canalicular and basolateral liver plasma membranes were also measured. The canalicular membranes did not contain activity for $Na^+K^+$ ATPase or for the glucagon-stimulated adenylate cyclase system, but had high levels of leucylnapthylamidase, $\gamma$-glutamyl transpepidase, alkaline phosphatase, $Mg^{2+}$ ATPase, and alkaline phosphodiesterase I. These enzyme localizations indicated that our purification of the canalicular liver plasma membrane preparations was good [12].

We then took the canalicular liver plasma membrane preparations and assessed their capacity to glucuronidate bilirubin monoglucuronide. First, we tested the system in untreated microsomes and with no UDP glucuronate, and there was no conversion of bilirubin [13]. If UDP glucuronate is added, bilirubin is converted to bilirubin monoglucuronide [13] (Fig. 2). However, if a perturbant with a specific amount (0.35 mg digitonin/mg protein or 0.5 m$M$ CHAP/mg protein) is added to the hepatic microsomes, bilirubin diglucuronide and bilirubin monoglucuronide are formed in the presence of UDP glucuronic acid. At the level of 12 $\mu M$ bilirubin, the microsomes perturbed by digitonin formed 50% bilirubin diglucuronide and monoglucuronide, while the microsomes perturbed with CHAPS formed 70% bilirubin diglucuronide and 30% bilirubin monoglucuronide. If the concentration of bilirubin was lowered, the percentage of bili-

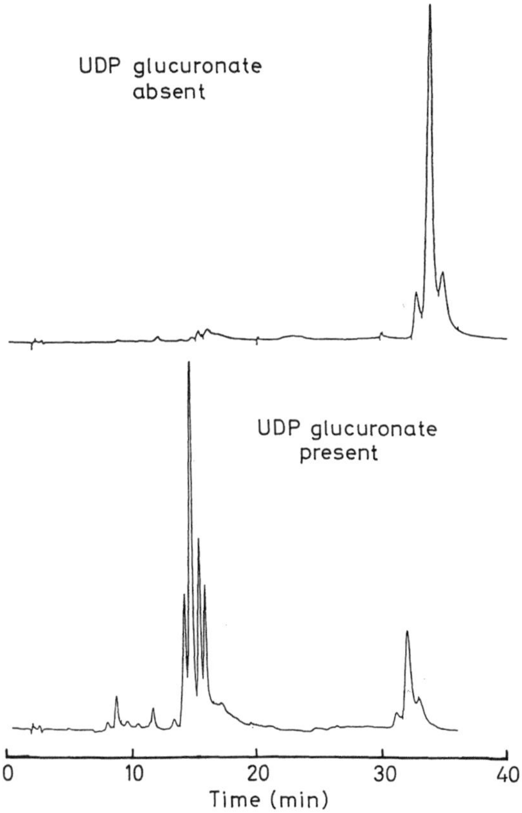


**Fig. 2.** Rat liver microsomes were incubated at 37 °C in the presence of bilirubin (12.0 μ*M*) with or without UDP glucuronate. The high-pressure liquid chromatographic tracings indicates bilirubin 1 X$\alpha$ and its two isomeric forms 111 $\alpha$ and X 111 $\alpha$ at 31-32 mins (*above,* not conjugated without UDP glucuronate; *below,* with UDP glucuronate) bilirubin. In the presence of UDP glucuronate, bilirubin monoglucuronide forms four isomeric peaks at 14-17 min *(below)*

rubin diglucuronide formed in the perturbed hepatic microsomes was greater [13] (Fig. 3). Therefore, bilirubin monoglucuronide was prepared from bile excreted by the rat [14], and in the presence of perturbed microsomes and UDP glucuronate, it was converted to bilirubin diglucuronide (Fig. 4).

However, no evidence was found that canalicular liver plasma membrane preparations had any capacity to glucuronidate bilirubin monoglucuronide. The reaction was carried out with and without treatment of the canalicular liver plasma membrane preparation with perturbants, in the presence and absence of UDP glucuronate, with varying concentrations of bilirubin monoglucuronide (9.4-17.0 μ*M*), and at different pH levels. None of these conditions resulted in the conversion of bilirubin monoglucuronide to diglucuronide either through catalytic activity of an enzyme or by dipyrrole exchange (Fig. 5) [15].

Therefore, to discover if any inactivation of the catalytic activity of the dismustase occurred, we isolated rat hepatic microsome using the same conditions that are used to prepare the canalicular liver plasma membrane preparations (1 m*M* $NaHCO_3$). When the perturbed microsomes were suspended in 1 m*M* $NaHCO_3$, bilirubin monoglucuronide was not further glucuronidated. However, if we suspended the perturbed microsomes in 0.25 *M* sucrose, rather than 1 m*M* $NaHCO_3$, bilirubin monoglucuronide was converted to bilirubin diglucuronide [15].

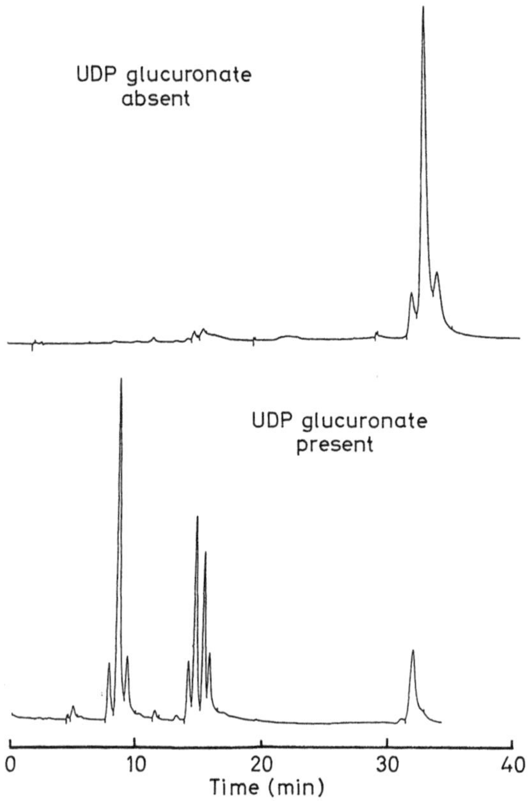


**Fig. 3.** Rat liver microsomes pretreated with digitonin (0.35 mg/mg microsomal protein) were incubated at 37 °C in the presence of bilirubin (12.5 μ*M*) with or without UDP glucuronate. The high-pressure liquid chromatographic tracings show that bilirubin 1X$\alpha$ and two isomers 111 $\alpha$ and X111$\alpha$ at 31–32 min is not conjugated without UDP glucuronate *(above)* but is conjugated with UDP glucuronate *(below)* to form bilirubin monoglucuronide (four isomeric peaks at 14–17 min) and bilirubin diglucuronide (three isomeric peaks at 9–11 min)

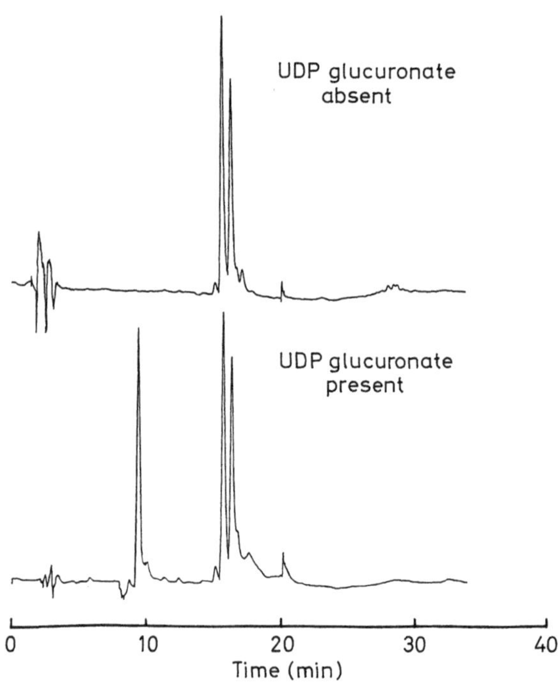


**Fig. 4.** Rat liver microsomes were pretreated with digitonin (0.35 mg/mg microsomal protein) and incubated at 37 °C in the presence of bilirubin monoglucuronide (9.4 μ*M*) with or without UDP glucuronate. Bilirubin diglucuronate was formed only in the presence of UDP glucuronate *(below)*

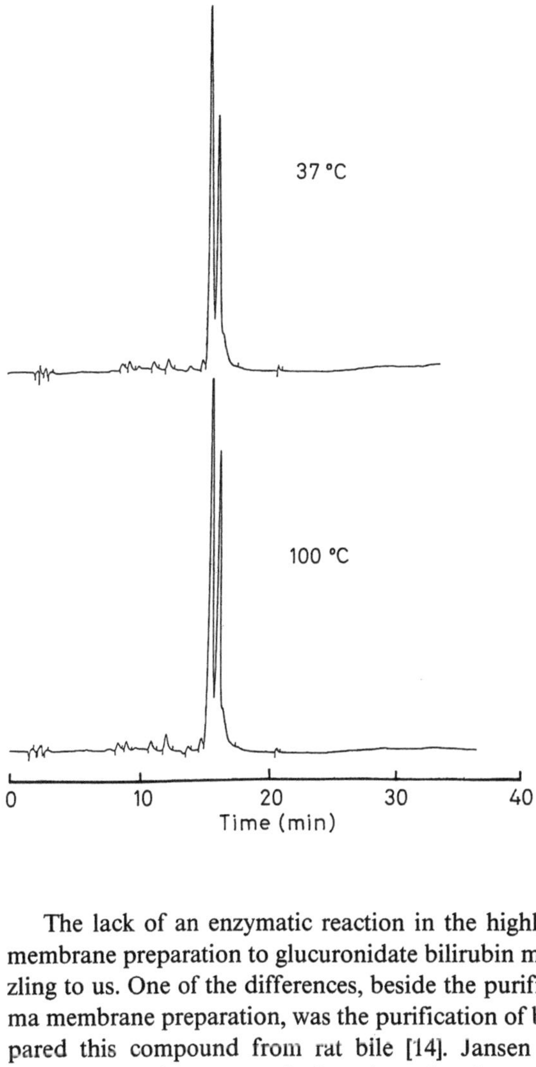


**Fig. 5.** Rat liver canalicular membranes were either denatured at 100 °C or left untreated, and were then incubated with bilirubin monoglucuronide (9.4 μ*M*) at 37 °C. No conversion to bilirubin diglucuronide occurred under either condition

The lack of an enzymatic reaction in the highly purified canalicular liver plasma membrane preparation to glucuronidate bilirubin monoglucuronide was of course puzzling to us. One of the differences, beside the purification of the canalicular liver plasma membrane preparation, was the purification of bilirubin monoglucuronide. We prepared this compound from rat bile [14]. Jansen et al. [9] prepared their bilirubin monoglucuronide enzymatic from hepatic microsomes. We therefore prepared bilirubin monoglucuronide from hepatic microsomal UDP bilirubin transferase and noted that this preparation was contaminated. It caused scrambling of the substrate, forming both bilirubin and bilirubin diglucuronide. This scrambling occurred in the presence of canalicular or basolateral liver plasma membrane preparation as well as the blank. This reaction was shown by Sieg et al. [16], Blanckaert et al. [7] and ourselves [15] to be the result of an nonenzyme scrambling of bilirubin monoglucuronide. Therefore, the conjugation of bilirubin occurs within the hepatic microsomes. If there is no defect in the secretion of the conjugates of bilirubin from the microsomes and the canalicular membranes, their formation reflects the functions of the microsomes.

These are characteristic differences between normal subjects and patients with Gilbert's syndrome in the pattern of secretion of bile pigments in bile. In normal patients, the proportion of bilirubin diglucuronide is 80%, in the Gilbert's patient only 68%. Bil-

**Table 1.** Distribution of bile pigments in biliary aspirates from normal control subjects and patients with Gilbert's syndrome (mean ± SD)

| Bilirubin tetrapyrrole | Relative content (%) | |
|---|---|---|
| | Normal subjects ($n = 13$) | Patients with Gilbert's syndrome ($n = 16$) |
| Bilirubin diglucuronide | 87.6 ± 4.3 | 67.8 ± 9.3* |
| Bilirubin monoglucuronide monoglucoside diester | 2.2 ± 3.7 | 3.6 ± 3.4 |
| Bilirubin monoglucuronide | 6.8 ± 4.7 | 23.4 ± 9.4* |
| Bilirubin | 4.4 ± 3.5 | 5.0 ± 2.7 |

* $P < 0.001$ (t-test)

irubin monoglucuronide increases from 7% in normals to 30% in the Gilbert's patients (Table 1). The differences in the proportions of the conjugates in the Gilbert's patients appears to reflect a dysfunction of the catalytic site of the bilirubin UDP transferase. Low activity of this enzyme has been demonstrated in liver biopsy preparations from these patients [17, 18]. If there is just one bilirubin UDP transferase, as shown by Burchell and Blanckaert [19], to form both conjugates of bilirubin, it would appear that the addition of the second glucuronic acid to bilirubin may be at fault in patients with Gilbert's syndrome.

Biliary fistulae were inserted at the time of operation in some subjects during liver transplantation. This permitted us to collect bile every 2–4 h after operation. Samples were collected with EDTA or ascorbic acid and extracted with chloroform containing 10 m*M* heptylammonium chloride and analyzed by high-pressure liquid chromatography [20]. Analysis of these bile pigments gave us some indications of the function of these livers.

The first patient had a hepatoma. Immediately following the operation, the alkaline phosphatase dropped rapidly and SGOT levels were within normal limits. The total serum bilirubin was not abnormal before the operation, but rose slightly and then dropped gradually to normal levels by 8 days after the operation. The HIDA scan of the liver was essentially normal, as indicated by the uptake and immediate excretion of the radioactive isotope by the liver. Analysis of the excretion of the pigments in bile revealed the following pattern: Bilirubin was barely detected. In the first bile sample collected, 2 h after operation, there was 60% bilirubin diglucuronide, 38% bilirubin monoglucuronide, and less than 11% bilirubin monoglucuronide monoglucoside. This pattern rapidly changed, returning to normal levels within 80 h after the operation (80% bilirubin diglucuronide and less than 10% of both conjugates bilirubin monoglucuronide and the diester) (Fig. 6a).

The second patient had non-A, non-B chronic active viral hepatitis. Serum bilirubin levels were above 30 mg/100 ml at the time of operation and slowly dropped over the next few weeks to normal levels. Initially, the HIDA scan was abnormal, as indicated by the poor secretion of the radioactive material. Analysis of the bile for conjugates of bilirubin demonstrated that bilirubin monoglucuronide predominated, in some cases accounting for over 60% of the total bile pigment excreted. After the first 2 weeks the pattern changed; bilirubin diglucuronide predominated and levels of the diester and bilirubin monoglucuronide dropped to below 10% each (Fig. 6b).

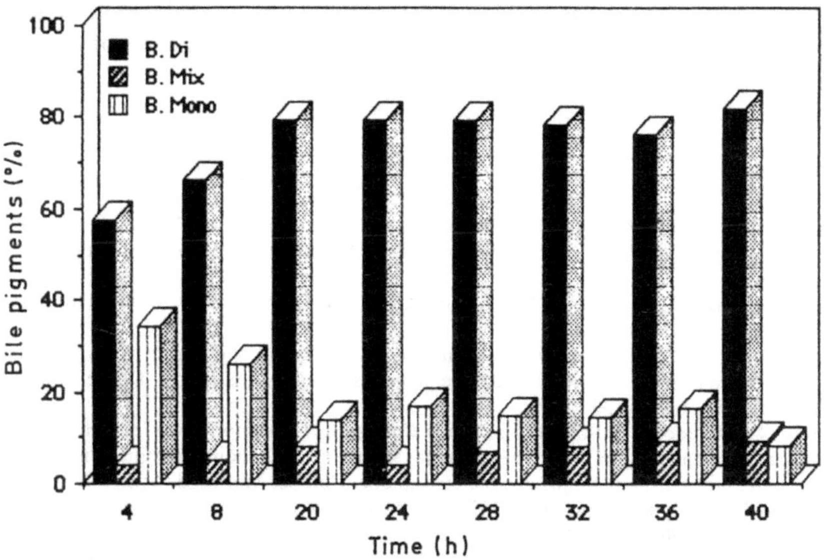


a

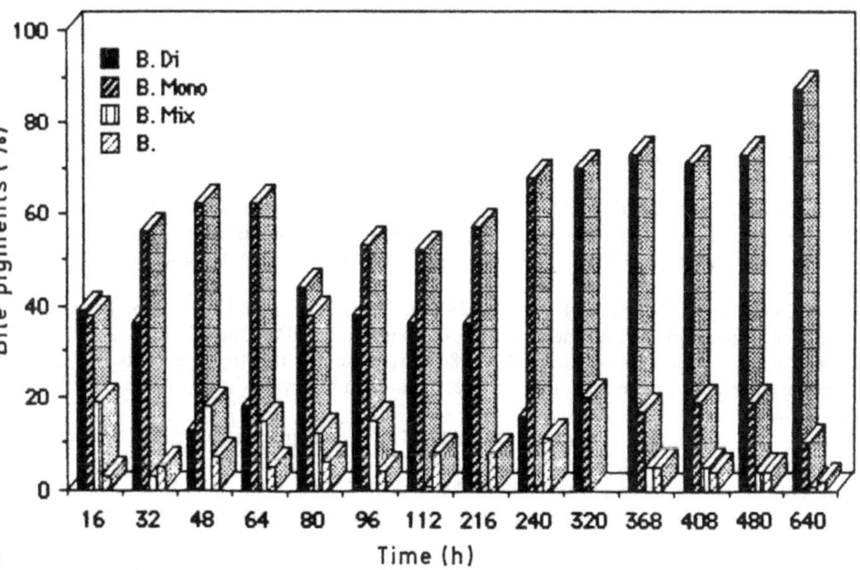


b

**Fig. 6 a and b.** The pattern of excretion of bile pigments following liver transplantation. **a** Normal pattern with 80% bilirubin diglucuronide, less than 10% each of bilirubin monoglucuronide and bilirubin monoglucuronide monoglucoside *(B. Mix)*. **b** Abnormal pattern with bilirubin monoglucuronide initially forming over 60%

The etiology of these changes in conjugates of bilirubin in bile is not known. One can postulate that if there is one enzyme in the hepatic microsomes to form both bilirubin monoglucuronide and bilirubin diglucuronide, then the microenvironment of the microsomes of the enzyme is apparently not adequate. In vitro, the formation of bilirubin monoglucuronide is not influenced markedly by changes in the microenvironment, whereas bilirubin diglucuronate is affected.

*Acknowledgements.* I thank Dr. M. W. Flye for permitting me to analyze bile pigments in the bile of liver transplant subjects and Annabel Shih for the analysis of these pigments.

## References

1. Blanckaert N, Schmid R (1982) The physiology and pathophysiology of bilirubin metabolism. In: Hepatology. A textbook of liver disease. Zakim D, Boyer T (ed) W.B. Saunders + Co. Phil. USA
2. Bonnett R, Davis JE, Hursthouse MB, Sheldrick GM (1978) The structure of bilirubin. Proc R Soc Lond [Biol] 202: 249-268
3. Carey MC, Spivak VV (1986) Physical chemistry of bile pigment and porphyrins with particular reference to bile. In: Ostrow JD (ed) Bile pigments and jaundice. Marcel Dekker, Inc. New York. NY. USA, pp 81-130
4. Goresky CA, Gordon ER, Schaffer E, Parei P, Carassavas D, Aronoff A (1978) Definition of a conjugation dysfunction in Gilbert's syndrome: studies of the handling of bilirubin loads and of the pattern of bilirubin conjugates secreted in bile. Clin Sci Mol Med 55: 63-71
5. Cornelius CE, Kelly KC, Hines JA (1975) Heterogeneity of bilirubin conjugates in several animal species. Cornell Vet 65: 90-99
6. Heirwegh KPM, van de Vijver M, Fevery F (1972) Assay and properties of digitonin-activated bilirubin uridine diphosphate glucuronyltransferase from rat liver. Biochem J 129: 605-618
7. Blanckaert N, Gollan J, Schmid R (1980) Mechanism of bilirubin diglucuronide formation in the intact rat. J Clin Invest 65: 1332-1342
8. Gordon ER, Goresky CA (1980) The formation of bilirubin diglucuronide by rat liver microsomal preparation. Can J Biochem 58: 1302-1310
9. Jansen PLM, Roy Chowdhury JR, Fischberg EB, Arias IM (1977) Enzymatic conversion of bilirubin monoglucuronide to diglucuronide by rat liver plasma membrane. J Biol Chem 252: 2710-2716
10. Roy Chowdhury J, Jansen PLM, Fischberg EB, Daniller A, Arias IM (1978) Hepatic conversion of bilirubin monoglucuronide to diglucuronide in uridine diphosphate glucuronyl transferase deficient man and rat by bilirubin glucuronide glucuronosyltransferase. J Clin Invest 62: 191-196
11. Roy Chowdhury J, Fischberg EB, Arias IM (1979) Purification and partial characterization of rat liver bilirubin glucuronoside glucuronosyltransferase. J Biol Chem 254: 8336-8339
12. Meier P, Sztul E, Reuben A, Boyer JL (1984) Structural and functional polarity of canalicular and basolateral plasma membrane vesicular isolated in high yield from rat liver. J Cell Biol 98: 991-1000
13. Gordon ER, Sommerer V, Goresky CA (1983) The hepatic microsomal formation of bilirubin diglucuronide. J Biol Chem 258: 15208-15036
14. Gordon ER, Chan TK, Sanodai K, Goresky CA (1977) The isolation and further characterization of bilirubin tetrapyrroles in bile containing human duodenal juice and dog gall bladder bile. J Biochem 155: 477-486
15. Gordon ER, Meier PJ, Goresky CA, Boyer JL (1984) Mechanism and subcellular site of bilirubin diglucuronide formation in rat liver. J Biol Chem 259: 5500-5506
16. Sieg A, van Hees GP, Heirwegh KPM (1982) Uridine diphosphate-glucuronic acid-independent conversion of bilirubin monoglucuronide to diglucuronide in presence of plasma membrane from rat liver nonenzymatic. J Clin Invest 69: 347-357
17. Black M, Billing B (1969) Hepatic bilirubin UDP glucuronyl transferase activity in liver disease and Gilbert's syndrome. N Engl J Med 280: 1266-1271
18. Black M, Sherlock S (1970) Treatment of Gilbert's syndrome with phenobarbitone. Lancet 1: 1359-1362
19. Burchell B, Blanckaert N (1984) Bilirubin mono- and diglucuronide formation by purified rat liver microsomal bilirubin UDP-glucuronyltransferase. Biochem J 223: 461-465
20. Gordon E, Goresky CA (1982) A rapid and quantitative high performance liquid chromatographic method for assaying bilirubin and its conjugates in bile. Can J Biochem 60: 1050-1057

# Hormones and Liver: Some Aspects of the Problem

M. Langer[1] and L. Chiandussi[2]

[1] Istituto di Patologia Medica, Università di Sassari, Italy
[2] Istituto di Patologia Medica B, Università di Torino, Italy

There are very tight interactions between the endocrine system and the liver. Hormones control many metabolic reactions and many processes of protein synthesis in the liver. The liver, on the other hand, is the major site for hormone metabolism. In the liver hormones may either be transformed into more active compounds (e.g., thyroxine into the four times as active triidothyronine, vitamin D3 into its 25-OH form) or be inactivated, catabolized and disposed of. Liver also influences hormone blood levels, being the site of transport protein synthesis. It is also the major source of hormone-dependent growth factors and of their inhibitors. These complex interactions between hormones and liver occur via receptors. Accordingly, specific membrane, cytoplasmic, and nuclear receptors for many hormones have been identified in liver tissue [1]. The effectiveness of hormonal actions depends on the presence of specific receptors and is modulated by their concentration. The receptor binding capacity can be modified by the specific binding hormone and by other hormones as well. For example, estrogens may increase both estrogen and prolactin (PRL) receptors while testosterone decreases estrogen and PRL binding. Receptors for sexual hormones with properties similar to those in hormone-dependent sexual target tissues are present in the liver [2-5]. Very interesting studies carried out in the rat have shown sex-linked differences in some liver functions: there are differences in male and female steroid-metabolizing enzymes in the liver; male livers have more oxidizing enzymes and female livers have more reducing enzymes [6, 7]; females have estrogen and PRL receptors; males, beside estrogen, have also androgen but not PRL receptors. Furthermore, male livers synthesize a male-specific protein – a male estrogen binder (MEBP) [3, 7] which is not a receptor – and a protein excreted with the urine, the $\alpha$-2u globulin [8]. These sex-linked differences are determined in the fetus at birth by androgen "imprinting" at the hypothalamic level, which represses a pituitary feminizing factor which has been identified as growth hormone [9]. Interestingly, growth hormone (GH) is secreted with a different pattern in male and female rats; this might be the signal which regulates the sexual dimorphism of these liver functions.

Exogenous and endogenous estrogen excess (e.g., oral contraceptives and pregnancy) may effect several liver functions. It increases the synthesis of several proteins, such as hormone-transport proteins, ceruloplasmin, renin substrate, some drug-metabolizing enzymes, aminolevulinic acid synthetase, etc. Both estrogens and androgens seem to play a role in hepatic regeneration [10-12]. There is clinical evidence for an association between liver focal nodular hyperplasia and hepatocellular adenoma on one hand and oral contraceptive or anabolic steroid intake on the other [7, 13]; elevated estrogen-binding capacity was found in liver adenoma tissue [14]. Hepatocellular carcinoma is

Assessment and Management of Hepatobiliary Disease
Eds.: L. Okolicsányi, G. Csomós, and G. Crepaldi

less frequently associated with estrogen excess, but cytosolic and nuclear estrogen receptors have been identified in these tumors as well [15].

There are data suggesting that androgenic anabolic steroids may induce or promote the growth of both hepatocellular adenoma and carcinoma [16, 17]. Androgen-binding receptors have been identified in tumor tissue [18]. However, more data are needed to assess the role of sexual steroids in hepatic regeneration and carcinogenesis.

Considering the multiple interrelationships between hormones and the liver, it is not surprising that multiple abnormalities in the endocrine balance occur in patients with liver disease. The most impressive clinical aspect of this is the well-known syndrome of hypogonadism and feminization occurring mainly in patients with alcoholic liver cirrhosis. Both alcohol toxicity and liver damage can affect several endocrine functions. Therefore it is difficult to identify clearly the sequence of events which eventually lead to the clinical picture of menstrual abnormalities and sterility in the female and in the male to infertility, testicular atrophy, decreased libido, impotence, gynecomastia, female hair and fat distribution and spider angiomata. However, a great deal of experimental work done in the last few years has shed some light on the mechanism by which alcohol and liver disease interfere with hypothalamo-pituitary-gonadal function. While in the past gonadal dysfunction was mainly attributed to estrogen excess brought about by impaired estrogen catabolism by the diseased liver, recent research has focused mainly on alcohol abuse. Alcohol exerts a direct, both acute and chronic, toxic effect at the testicular level, interfering with the activation of vitamin A, necessary for spermatogenesis, and with several enzyme activities necessary for testosterone synthesis [19–21]. There is also evidence that alcohol inhibits luteinizing hormone (LH) secretion, acting at the hypothalamic-pituitary level; plasma LH levels and their response to the releasing factor LHRH are found to be inadequately low in face of the low testosterone levels [22–24]. There is evidence that alcohol stimulates the adrenal secretion of the weak androgens androstenedione and dehydroepiandrosterone, which in peripheral tissues are then aromatized to estrogens, mainly estrone, a biologically weak estrogen [25–27]. The aromatizing enzyme is induced by alcohol [28]. Thus alcohol contributes strongly to increased estrogen production; this has been demonstrated to occur in patients with alcoholic liver cirrhosis [24]. There is, however, evidence that hypogonadism and ferminization may also occur, though less frequently, in nonalcoholic chronic liver disease [29].

Experimental data from the Pittsburgh group have given some insight into this issue, and have led to the following hypothesis [29, 30]: in portal hypertension with portosystemic shunting, weak androgens escape the enterohepatic circulation and reach peripheral tissues, where they are aromatized to estrogens. These inhibit LH secretion and therefore depress testosterone production. Gonadotropin secretion can also be deranged by the alterations in neurotransmitter metabolism which occur in patients with portosystemic shunting and hepatic encephalopathy.

Thus alcohol and liver disease can, independently or together, contribute to the clinical syndrome of hypogonadism and feminization in male patients with alcoholic cirrhosis. The same abnormalities of the hypothalamic-pituitary-gonadal axis occur in female patients, causing ovulatory failure, loss of breast and pelvic fat, menstrual abnormalities, and infertility. However, the slight increase in mainly weak estrogens caused by alcohol and liver disease can hardly account for the full-blown feminizing syndrome. Therefore the presence of an "amplifying system" has been envisaged. It has been shown, in rat liver, that alcohol administration, estrogen excess, and androgen deficiency alter the tissue estrogen-binding capacity, increasing estrogen receptors and decreasing the male-specific estrogen binder, which is supposed to act as an estrogen "scavenger" protecting the organism from excess estrogen [7, 31]. This results in an enhancement of estrogen sensitivity. Thus even small increases in weak estrogen levels can elicit marked biologic effects at peripheral levels [31]. Estrogens also markedly increase the production of sex hormone binding globulin (SHBG), which binds testosterone with greater affinity than estrogens, thus reducing free testosterone available for biological action. This increase in SHBG can occur at doses of estrogens which do not influence other proteins; it therefore seems to be a receptor-amplified response [32].

Beside gonadotropin, other pituitary functions may be deranged in patients with liver disease and in chronic alcoholics.

*Growth Hormone.* Acute and chronic alcohol consumption suppresses the sleep-related nocturnal GH secretory episodes [33] and GH responses to arginine and insulin infusion [34]. Blood concentrations of GH are significantly increased in patients with liver cirrhosis, mainly in those with decompensated liver disease. Thyrotropin-releasing hormone (TRH), which does not affect GH secretion in normal subjects, elicits and abnormal increase in GH levels in cirrhotic patients [34, 35]. Again, the response evoked by TRH was significantly higher in the decompensated patients than in the compensated ones. Hyperglycemia, which normally depresses GH levels, also elicits a paradoxical increase in GH levels in cirrhotic patients.

In order to evaluate the respective roles of alcohol abuse and liver damage in determining GH secretory abnormalities in cirrhotic patients, we measured GH levels and their response to TRH, hyperglycemia, and levodopa, a dopaminergic drug normally used as a diagnostic provocative test, in patients with compensated, decompensated, alcoholic, and nonalcoholic liver cirrhosis. Chronic alcoholics without cirrhosis were also evaluated. Severe liver damage, but not alcohol abuse, was associated with abnormal GH levels and responsiveness to TRH (Fig. 1). Alcoholism also had no effect on GH response to hyperglycemia and levodopa. Paradoxical GH increase after hyperglycemia was more frequent in severely ill patients than in those with the compensated form of the disease. GH response to levodopa was slightly blunted in decompensated cirrhotics and significantly depressed in patients with hepatic encephalopathy. Alter-

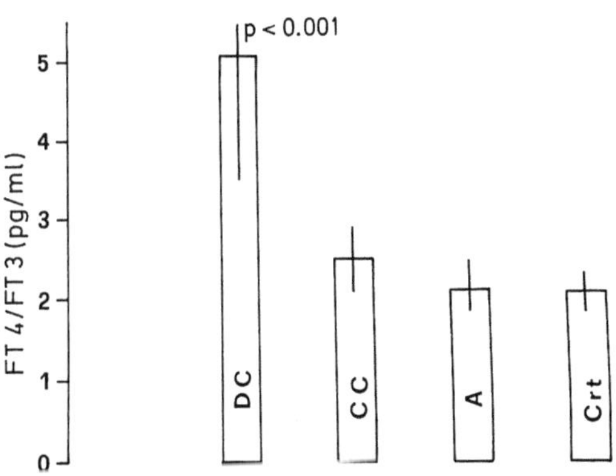


**Fig. 1.** Basal and TRH stimulated serum Growth Hormone (GH) levels in patients with alcoholic, non alcoholic, compensated (CC), and decompensated (DC) liver cirrhosis, in non cirrhotic alcoholics (A), and in normal control subjects (Crt).

**Table 1.** Mean Prolactin serum concentrations (ng/ml) in basal conditions and maximum increase after TRH (200 μg i.v.) in non cirrhotic alcoholics (CA), in patients with compensated (CLC) and decompensated (DLC) liver cirrhosis, and in normal control subjects

| | CA (12) | CLC (22) | DLC (36) | Ctrls (20) |
|---|---|---|---|---|
| Basal | 7.6 ± 2.5 | 8.8 ± 2.9 | 12.4 ± 4.3 | 6.5 ± 4.5 |
| TRH | 20.1 ± 8.0 | 48.1 ± 22.0 | 63.3 ± 37.1 | 32.3 ± 5.1 |

ations in GH secretory patterns therefore seem to be related to the severity of liver disease rather than to alcohol abuse. The mechanisms are as yet hypothetical. A derangement in central control mechanisms of GH secretion due to abnormalities in hypothalamic peptidergic hormones and neurotransmitter metabolism is supported by a range of clinical and experimental data [36–39]. Other factors such as impaired feedback regulation due to impaired somatomedin production, estrogen excess, or malnutrition may also play a role. Whether the altered GH secretory pattern plays a role in the feminization of the cirrhotic male, as might be suggested by some experimental data in the rat [9], is not known.

*Prolactin.* Increased plasma PRL concentrations have been reported in a varying percentage of patients with liver cirrhosis, together with an exaggerated response to TRH, a potent PRL releaser [35, 38–40]. A reduced suppression by levodopa has been described [38]. We found that mean basal PRL serum concentrations were moderately elevated in male patients with decompensated cirrhosis, but were normal in the compensated form of the disease and in noncirrhotic chronic alcoholics. PRL response to TRH, a potent PRL releaser, was increased in cirrhotic patients, mainly in decompensated ones, whereas it was blunted in some of the noncirrhotic alcoholic men. There was, however, great individual variability; differences were therefore not significant (Table 1). It has been suggested that the alterations in PRL secretion found in patients with liver disease are due to estrogen excess or to a derangement of the normal inhibitory dopaminergic control mechanism. In agreement with the latter hypothesis, higher PRL levels were found in patients with hepatic encephalopathy [41]. We found that Nomifensine, a dopaminergic drug which inhibits endogenous catecholamine reuptake, was unable to significantly depress PRL levels in these patients [42]. A relationship between gynecomastia and PRL hypersecretion is questionable.

*Adrenocorticothropic Hormone (ACTH)* has been shown to increase in alcoholics, who occasionally present Cushing-like features [43, 44]. In hepatic encephalopathy and in severely ill patients, cortisol levels are elevated and circadian rhythmicity is abolished [45].

Thyrotropin (TSH) serum concentrations are found to be normal or only slightly elevated in liver cirrhosis, in spite of the marked derangement in thyroid function parameters. After stimulation with its specific releaser TRH, the maximum increase in TSH may be normal, but is often greater than normal, delayed, and sustained; a similar pattern has been described in hypothalamic disorders. We found a delayed and sustained response mainly in patients with decompensated liver disease. In about 50% of the chronic alcoholics without cirrhosis the responses of TSH were at the lower limit of the normal range, although the mean value in the whole group did not significantly differ from the normal controls. In patients with hepatic encephalopathy instead, the TSH responses to TRH were significantly lower than in all the other groups of patients [46].

The liver plays a very important role in thyroid hormone metabolism and transport. Therefore, abnormalities in thyroid function parameters are very frequent in patients with impaired liver function and are correlated to the severity of the disease. Liver is the most important site for extrathyroid conversion of thyroxine (T4) into triiodothyronine (T3) and into reverse triiodothyronine (rT3), an activating and an inactivating process respectively, T3 being about four times as active as T4 and rT3 being almost devoid of metabolic activity. Furthermore, thyroid-hormone-binding proteins are synthesized in the liver and circulating thyroid hormone levels depend on binding protein concentrations. Although this concept has been challenged recently [47], only the small free fractions of thyroid hormones are believed to be biologically active. Thyroid hormone disposal also occurs mainly in the liver.

Patients with liver cirrhosis mostly present low total and free plasma T3 concentrations, due to reduced production rate from T4, and normal or high rT3 concentrations, due mainly to a decreased metabolic clearance rate [48, 49]. This pattern is the well-known "low T3 syndrome;" it occurs in other situations as well, such as systemic illnesses, starvation, surgery and fetal life, and after several drugs, e.g., propranolol, amiodarone, and desamethasone, and is due to impaired 5′-monodeiodination. Total T4 can also be decreased in severely ill patients [47, 50]. This "low T3, low T4 syndrome" is due to low binding-protein synthesis by the liver or to impaired protein binding affinity caused by the presence of an inhibitor in the serum [51]. This inhibitor also impairs the binding of thyronines to solid matrices, yielding an artificially low free T4 (FT4) level, and to the cells, reducing the T4 available for deiodination in the tissues. A low substrate availability of T4 could be the cause for the unexpected low rT3 levels that we found in some very severely ill patients (Table 2). FT4 levels are normal and often elevated [48, 50]. The low serum T3 and FT3 levels, the low T4, the high rT3 and rT3/T3 ratio correlate with the severity of the disease and have been considered to have prognostic value [50, 52, 53]. We found that the FT4/FT3 ratio (measured after separation on Sephadex LH 20) also increases with the severity of the disease (Fig. 2) and is negatively correlated with the survival rate. While the rT3/T3 ratio is also elevated in patients with compensated liver cirrhosis, the FT4/FT3 ratio is increased in severely ill patients only [54] (Table 2). Binding abnormalities occur in other severe illnesses as well (euthyroid sick syndrome) [50]. However, considering the role the liver plays in thyroid hormone metabolism it is probable that at least some of these abnormalities are due to liver function impairment and not only to an aspecific impairment of health. Patients are clinically euthyroid due to normal FT4 levels. Diagnostic problems may arise in individual patients: hyperthyroidism can be masked by the low T3 and/or T4 syndrome, and low thyroid hormone concentrations may mimic hypothyroidism. Measurement of TSH, its response to TRH, free thyroid hormones, and rT3 may contribute to a correct diagnosis. In noncirrhotic chronic alcoholics total T3 and T4 decrease moderately, but free fractions are normal. Normalization occurs with alcohol withdrawal [55, 56].

Hyperthyroxinemia due to increased serum thyroxine binding globuline (TBG) can occur during acute and chronic active hepatitis and biliary cirrhosis because of TBG leakage from the damaged liver [57]. Hashimoto thyroiditis is frequently associated

**Table 2.** Low T3, low T3 and T4, low T3, T4 and rT3 syndromes in patients with liver cirrhosis. Figures in parenthesis refer to patients who died within the first year of observation.

| | | | | | | |
|---|---|---|---|---|---|---|
| ↓*T3* | ↓FT3 | N↑rT3 | ↑rT3/T3 | N T4 | N FT4 | 20pts (2) |
| ↓T3 | ↓FT3 | N↑rT3 | ↑rT3/T3 | ↓*T4* | N↑FT4 | 24pts (12) |
| ↓T3 | ↓FT3 | ↓*rT3* | N↑rT3/T3 | ↓T4 | N↑FT4 | 4pts (3) |

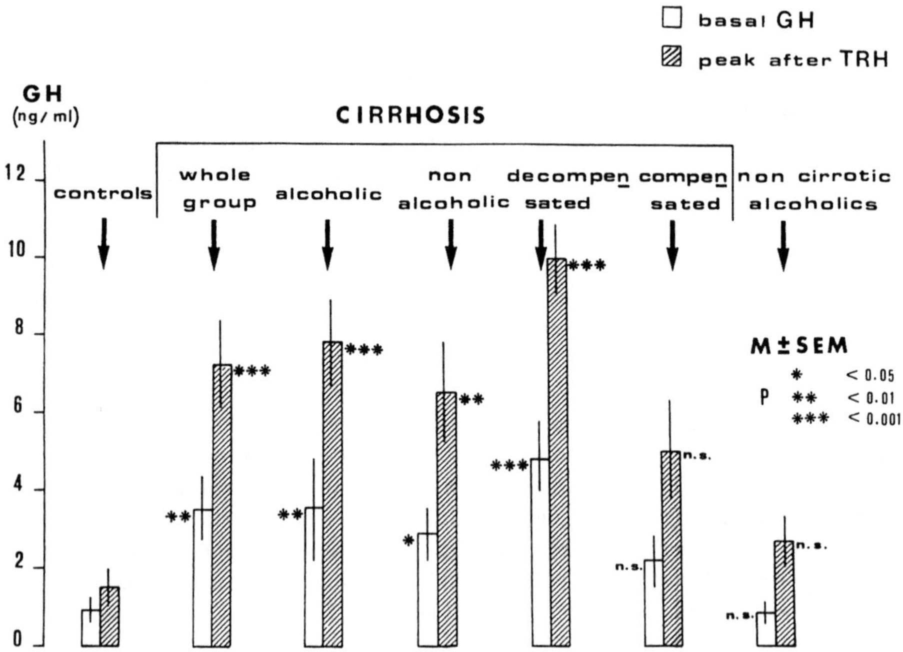


**Fig. 2.** The FT4/FT3 ratio in patients with decompensated (DC), compensated (CC) liver cirrhosis, in non cirrhotic chronic alcoholics (A) and in normal controls

with chronic active hepatitis and biliary cirrhosis [58]. Therefore real hypothyroidism can occur in these diseases.

Symptomatic hypocalcemia, although mainly due to cholestatic liver disease, may occasionally occur in non cholestatic liver disease, probably due to impaired 25-hydroxylation of Vitamin D.

## Conclusion

Complex interrelationships exist between the liver and the endocrine system, and thus multiple endocrine abnormalities occur in patients with liver disease. They are brought about either by the liver disease itself or by the damaging agent which is also the cause of liver damage. Hormone secretion, transport, and metabolism can all be affected. Clinically, only the sexual abnormalities are really relevant. Other hormone abnormalities may cause diagnostic problems. Thyroid function parameters can be of prognostic value Dynamic studies of hypothalamic-pituitary function in patients with hepatic encephalopathy may be helpful in evaluating the neurotransmitter abnormalities occurring in this situation.

## References


1. Levey GS, Pollet RJ (1985) Hormone receptors and the liver. Semin Liver Dis 5: 1-7
2. Eisenfeld AJ, Aten R, Weinberger MJ, Hasselbacher JK, Helper VK, Krakoff L (1976) Estrogen receptor in the mammalian liver. Science 191: 862-865
3. Eagon PK, Fischer SE, Imhoff AF, Poter LE, Stewart RR, van Thiel DH, Lester R (1980) Estrogen binding proteins in male liver. Arch Biochem Biophys 201: 286-499
4. Lefebvre YA, Morante SJ (1982) Binding of dihydrotestosterone to a nuclear envelope-fraction from the male rat liver. Biochem J 202: 225-230
5. Aten RY, Eisenfeld AJ (1984) Androgen and estrogen receptors in human liver (Abstr 245 A). 7th International Congress of Endocrinology, Quebec
6. Colby HD (1980) Regulation of hepatic drug and steroid metabolism by androgens and estrogens. In: Thomas JA, Singal RL (eds) Advances in sex steroid research. Urban and Schwarzenberg, Baltimore, pp 27-71
7. Eagon PK, Porter LE, Francavilla A, DiLeo A, van Thiel DH (1985) Estrogen and androgen receptors in liver: their role in liver disease and regeneration. Semin Liver Dis 5: 59-69
8. Roy AK, Chatterjee B, Demyan WF, Price GF (1983) Hormone and age dependent regulation of alpha 2u globulin gene expression. Recent Prog Horm Res 39: 425-461
9. Gustafsson JA, Enroth P, Hokfelt T, Mode A, Norstedt GV (1982) Studies on the hypothalamo-pituitary-liver axis, a novel concept in regulation of steroid and drug metabolism. In: Langer M, Chiandussi L, Chopra IJ, Martini L (eds) The endocrines and the liver. Academic, New York, pp 9-34
10. Francavilla A, DiLeo A, Eagon PK, Wu SQ, Ove P, van Thiel DH, Starzl TE (1984) Regenerating rat liver: correlation between estrogen receptor localization and deoxyribonucleic acid synthesis. Gastroenterology 86: 552-567
11. Fischer R, Qundes H, Saffer EA, Shu Z (1984) Relation of estrogen and its receptors to rat liver growth and regeneration. Cancer Res 64: 2410-2415
12. Vic P, Saint-Aubert B, Astre C, Bories C, Bonardet A, Descamps B, Hurneau C, Yoyeux H (1982) Complete liver regeneration in one stage 90% hepatectomized rats treated with testosterone. Hepatology 2: 247-248
13. Fechner RE (1977) Benign hepatic lesions and orally administered contraceptives. Hum Pathol 8: 255-268
14. Porter LE, Elm MS, van Thiel OH, Eagon PK (1984) Estrogen receptors in human liver nuclei. Hepatology 4: 1085
15. Iqbal MJ, Wilkinson ML, Johnson PJ, Williams R (1983) Sex steroid proteins in foetal, adult and malignant human liver tissue. Br J Cancer 48: 791-796
16. Westby D, Portman B, Williams R (1983) Androgen related primary hepatic tumors in non-Fanconi patients. Cancer 51: 1947-1952
17. Ziegenfuss J, Carabasi R (1973) Androgens and hepatocellular carcinoma. Lancet 1: 262
18. Nagasue N, Ito A, Yukaya H, Ogawa Y (1985) Androgen receptors in hepatocellular carcinoma and surrounding tissue parenchyma. Gastroenterology 89: 643-647
19. Van Thiel DH, Lester R (1976) Alcoholism: its effect on hypothalamic-pituitary-gonadal function. Gastroenterology 71: 318-327
20. Van Thiel DH, Cobb CFT, Herman GB, Perez HA, Estes L, Gavaler JS (1981) An examination of various mechanisms for ethanol-induced testicular injury; studies utilizing the isolated perfused rat tissues. Endocrinology 109: 2009-2015
21. Cobb CF, Gavaler JS, van Thiel DH (1981) Is ethanol a testicular toxin? Clin Toxicol 18: 149-154
22. Van Thiel DH (1983) Ethanol, its adverse effects upon the hypothalamic-pituitary-gonadal axis. J Lab Clin Med 101: 21-33
23. Gavaler JS, Gay V, Egler KM, van Thiel DH (1983) Evaluation of the differential in vivo toxic

effects of ethanol and acetaldehyde on the hypothalamic-pituitary-gonadal axis using 4-methylpyrazole. Alcoholism (NY) 7: 332-336
24. Kley HK, Peerenboom H, Wagner KK, Kruskemper HL (1982) Origin and effect of oestrogens in liver cirrhosis. In: Langer M, Chiandussi L, Chopra IJ, Martini L (eds) The endocrines and the liver. Academic, New York, pp 101-115
25. Gordon CG, Olivo L, Rafii F, Southren AL (1975) Conversion of androgens to estrogens in cirrhosis of the liver. J Clin Endocrinol Metab 40: 1018-1026
26. Cobb CT, van Thiel DH (1982) Mechanism of alcohol induced adrenal stimulation. Alcoholism (NY) 6: 202-206
27. Van Thiel DH, Loriaux DL (1979) Evidence for an adrenal origin of plasma estrogen in alcoholic men. Metabolism 28: 536-541
28. Gordon CG, Southren AL, Vittek J, Lieber CS (1979) The effect of alcohol ingestion on hepatic aromatase activity and plasma steroid hormones in the rat. Metabolism 28: 20-24
29. Stremmel W, Kley HK, Kruskemper HL, Strohmeyer G (1985) Differing abnormalities in estrogen and androgen and insulin metabolism in idiopathic hemochromatosis versus alcohol liver disease. Semin Liver Dis 5: 84-93
30. Van Thiel DH, Gavaler JS, Slone FL, Cobb CF, Smith WI, Bron KM, Lester RR (1980) Is feminization in alcoholic men due in part to portal hypertension? A rat model. Gastroenterology 78: 81-91
31. Eagon PK (1982) Alcohol induced changes in estrogen binding proteins. In: Langer M, Chiandussi L, Chopra IJ, Martini L (eds) The endocrines and the liver. Academic, New York, pp 63-76
32. Eisenfeld AJ, Aten RF (1982) Estrogen receptor in the mammalian liver. In: Langer M, Chiandussi L, Chopra IJ, Martini L (eds) The endocrines and the liver. Academic, New York, pp 49-62
33. Prinz PN, Roehrs TA, Vitaliano PT, Linnoila M, Weitzman ED (1980) Effect of alcohol on sleep and night-time plasma growth hormone and cortisol concentrations. J Clin Endocrinol Metab 51: 759-762
34. Andreani D, Tamburrano G, Javicoli M (1976) Alcohol hypoglycemia, hormonal changes. Horm Metab Res [Suppl 99] 6: 65-70
35. Panerai AE, Salerno F, Manneschi M, Cocchi D, Muller E (1977) Growth hormone and prolactin response to thyrotropin releasing hormone in patients with severe liver disease. J Clin Endocrinol Metab 45: 13
36. Salerno F, Cocchi D, Lampertico M, Monza G, Muller E (1982) Effects of hypophysiotropic stimuli and neuroactive drugs on growth hormone secretion in cirrhotic patients. In: Langer M, Chiandussi L, Chopra IJ, Martini L (eds) The endocrines and the liver. Academic, New York, pp 289-301
37. Munkgaard S, Kelbaek H, Tronier B (1981) Elevated plasma somatostatin in cirrhosis of the liver. N Engl J Med 304: 1429
38. Borzio M, Caldera R, Ferrari C, Barbieri C, Borzio F, Ramussi M (1981) Growth hormone and prolactin secretion in liver cirrhosis, evidence for dopaminergic dysfunction. ACTA Endocr Copenh 97: 441-447
39. Langer M, Masala A, Alagna S, Rassu S, Madeddu G, Solinas A, Chiandussi L (1981) Growth hormone secretion in hepatic encephalopathy. Clin Endocrinol (Oxf) 14: 189-192
40. Morgan MY (1982) Basal and dynamic prolactin secretion in liver disease. In: Langer M, Chiandussi L, Chopra IJ, Martini L (eds) The endocrines and the liver. Academic, New York, pp 303-320
41. McClain CJ, Kromhout JP, Elson MK, van Thiel DH (1981) Hyperprolactinemia in portal systemic encephalopathy. Dig Dis Sci 26: 353-357
42. Masala A, Alagna S, Rovasio PP, Deplano A, Anania V, Chiandussi L, Langer M (1985) Failure of Nomifensine to reduce serum prolactin levels in patients with hepatic encephalopathy. J Endocrinol Invest 8: 25-30
43. Smals AG, Kloppenbor PW (1977) Alcohol-induced Cushingoid syndrome. Lancet 1: 1369
44. Rees LH, Besser GM, Jeffcoate W (1977) Alcohol induced pseudo-Cushing syndrome. Lancet 1: 726-728
45. Ventura E, Zeneroli ML, Tempieri A, Pinelli G, Licari F, Gollini F, Cremonini C, Ricci P, Casalgrandi G, Baraghini G, Marrama P (1984) Chronobiological study of circadian variations

of plasma free tryptophan and of cortisol in liver cirrhosis with severe degree of encephalopathy. Ital J Gastroenterol 16: 1-5
46. Langer M, Rovasio PP, Masala A, Alagna S, Rassu S, Solinas A, Deplano A, Madeddu G, Chiandussi L (1985) Impaired thyrotrophin (TSH) response to thyrotrophin releasing hormone (TRH) in hepatic encephalopathy. Ital J Gastroenterol 17: 69-72
47. Chopra IJ, Hershman JM, Pardridge WM, Nicoloff JT (1980) Thyroid function in nonthyroidal illness. Ann Intern Med 98: 946-957
48. Chopra IJ, Solomon DH, Chopra U, Yong RT, Chua Teco GH (1974) Alterations in circulating thyroid hormones and thyrotropin in hepatic cirrhosis: evidence for euthyroidism despite subnormal serum triiodothyronine. J Clin Endocrinol Metab 39: 501-551
49. Chopra IJ (1976) An assessment of daily production and significance of thyroid secretion of reverse T3 in man. J Clin Endocrinol Metab 58: 32-40
50. Hepner GW, Chopra IJ (1979) Serum thyroid hormone levels in patients with liver disease. Arch Intern Med 139: 1117-1120
51. Oppenheimer JH, Schwartz HL, Mariash CN, Kaiser FE (1982) Evidence for a factor in the sera of patients with nonthyroid disease which inhibits iodothyronine binding by solid matrices, serum proteins and rat hepatocyte. J Clin Endocrinol Metab 54: 757-766
52. Janni A, d'Azzo GB, Pinzello G, di Stefano G, Garofalo P, Norato A (1982) The prognostic value of thyroid parameters in liver cirrhosis. In: Langer M, Chiandussi L, Chopra JI, Martini L (eds) The endocrines and the liver. Academic, New York, pp 233-237
53. Van Thiel DH, Manendra U, Shade RR, Sanghvi A, Starzl TE (1985) Prognostic value of thyroid hormone levels in patients evaluated for liver transplantation. Hepatology 5: 862-866
54. Langer M, Rovasio PP, Masala A, Alagna S, Rassu S, Solinas A, Deplano A, Madeddu G, Chiandussi L (1983) The predictive value of the thyroid hormones in patients with liver cirrhosis. IRCS Med Sci 11: 806
55. Geurts J, Demester-Mirkine D, Glinoer D, Prigogine T, Fernandez-Deville M, Corvilain J (1981) Alterations in circulating thyroid hormones and thyroxine binding globulin in chronic alcoholism. Clin Endocrinol (Oxf) 14: 113-118
56. Langer M, Rassu S, Rovasio PP, Masala A, Alagna S, Madeddu G, Solinas A, Chiandussi L (1982) Free thyroid hormone concentrations in chronic alcoholics with liver steatosis. In: [redacted] Advanced course in free hormone assays and neuropeptides. RIA 82. PROC, Venice, p 23
57. Borst GC, Eil C, Burman KD (1983) Euthyroid hyperthyroxinemia. Ann Intern Med 98: 366-378
58. Schussler GC, Schaffner F, Shapiro J, Henley F (1979) Thyroid function in primary biliary cirrhosis (Abstr) Clin Res 271: 259

# Effects of Thyroid Hormone Administration and of Thyroidectomy on the Metabolism of Bilirubin in Rats

W. van Steenbergen and J. Fevery

Department of Internal Medicine and Medical Research, U.Z. Gasthuisberg, 3000 Leuven, Belgium

## Introduction

Disturbances of thyroid function may lead to jaundice in man. Jaundice with increased conjugated bilirubin levels is known to occur in severe thyrotoxicosis complicated by congestive heart failure [1, 2], but also in hyperthyroidism in the absence of thyroid storm [3, 4]. Unconjugated hyperbilirubinemia has also been reported in hyperthyroid patients [5]. The suggestion was that the patients had an underlying defect in their bilirubin metabolism, such as Gilbert's syndrome, which was aggravated by the complicating thyrotoxicosis.

Hypothyroidism may lead to significant neonatal hyperbilirubinemia or significantly prolonged neonatal jaundice with unconjugated hyperbilirubinemia [6–8]. A single case of hypothyroidism-associated cholestasis with conjugated hyperbilirubinemia has also been described [9]. Experimental studies in rats have shown an effect of thyroid hormone status on hepatic bilirubin UDP-glucuronosyltransferase activity (UDP-GTA) [10, 11] and on so-called bile-salt-independent canalicular bile flow [12]. Hyperthyroidism is known to stimulate bile-acid-independent bile flow [12] and to decrease hepatic bilirubin UDP-GTA [10, 11]. Hypothyroidism decreases bile-acid-independent bile flow [12], whereas bilirubin glucuronide formation in vitro is either unaffected or increased [10].

In the present work, hepatic bilirubin UDP-GTA in vitro, maximal hepatic excretion of bilirubin in vivo, and the relative amounts of bilirubin and its conjugates in bile, liver, and serum have been studies in thyroidectomized and thyroid-hormone-treated normal Wistar rats.

## Material and Methods

### Experimental Design

Male Wistar R/A rats, 10 weeks old, having free access to food and water, were used. Five groups of rats were studied. Control animals received 1 ml 0.15 *M* NaCl intraperitoneally (IP) daily for 5 days before the in vivo experiments, whereas hyperthyroidism was produced in two groups of rats by IP administration of sodium levothyroxine ($T_4$) 6.26 or 12.52 nmol.day$^{-1}$.100 g$^{-1}$ body weight (b.wt.) dissolved in 1 ml 0.15 *M* NaCl for 5 consecutive days. All animals were studied 24 h after the last injection of thyroid hormone. Sham-operated controls and thyroidectomized rats were also studied. These operations were performed at 8 weeks of age under light ether anesthesia. Thyroidectomy was performed using a microsurgical technique [13].

Assessment and Management of Hepatobiliary Disease
Eds.: L. Okolicsányi, G. Csomós, and G. Crepaldi

Under sodium pentobarbital anesthesia (6 mg/100 g b.wt. IP), rats were provided with a bile cannula and a jugular vein catheter. The animals were then put in restraining cages and transferred to a premature infant incubator to keep body temperature constant at 37.5°-38 °C. During recovery, loss of water and electrolytes was compensated for by intravenous infusion of glucose 5% (w/v) in 0.15 *M* NaCl at a rate of 3.8 ml/h. Three hours after cannulation of the bile duct, when the rats had fully recovered from anesthesia, three 10-min bile samples were collected in the dark into preweighed plastic tubes kept on melting ice (basal samples). Unconjugated bilirubin (Merck, Darmstadt, FRG) 3.42 µmol/100 g b.wt. dissolved in 0.1 *M* NaOH and brought to pH 8.5 with 0.15 *M* HCl was then injected followed by a continuous infusion of the same pigment at a dosage of 256 $nmol \cdot min^{-1} \cdot 100\ g^{-1}$ b.wt., administered over a period of 1 h, to obtain maximal bilirubin output (Tm) conditions [14, 15]. Throughout this experimental period, six 10-min bile samples were collected as described above. The bilirubin output during the period from 30 to 60 min was taken as representative of the apparent maximal bilirubin transport capacity of the liver. At the end of the experiment, the rats were anesthetized with pentobarbital (1 mg/100 g b.wt.) and exsanguinated via the abdominal aorta. The serum was stored in the dark at −20 °C. The liver was flushed with ice-cold 0.15 *M* NaCl, injected via the hepatic veins, and stored at −20 °C until further assay.

### Analytical Methods

Bile volume was measured gravimetrically. The concentration of bilirubin conjugates in bile was measured by the ethyl-anthranilate method at pH 2.7 [16]. Bilirubin UDP-GTA was assayed in digitonin-activated liver homogenates [17]. Relative amounts of unconjugated bilirubin (UCB) and its monoconjugates (BMG) and diconjugates (BDG) were determined by alkaline methanolysis and reverse-phase high-performance liquid chromatography in basal and Tm bile samples, in liver homogenates, and in serum [18].

### Statistical Methods

Results are expressed as mean ± S.D. The significance of the differences among the groups was analyzed using the Mann-Whitney U-test.

## Results

### Effects of Hyperthyroidism and of Hypothyroidism on Bile Flow and Biliary Excretion of Bilirubin

Table 1 summarizes the effects of thyroid hormone administration and of thyroidectomy on bile flow, biliary bilirubin concentration, Tm, and the relative amount of diconjugates as a percentage of total conjugates present in bile. The excretion rates of UCB, BMG, and BDG in bile are shown in Table 2.

**Table 1.** Bilirubin conjugation and biliary secretion in control, thyroid-hormone-treated, and thyroidectomized Wistar rats

| | Saline-treated controls ($n=7$) | $T_4$-treated 6.26 nmol.day$^{-1}$·100 g$^{-1}$ ($n=8$) | $T_4$-treated 12.52 nmol.day$^{-1}$·100 g$^{-1}$ ($n=6$) | Sham-operated controls ($n=9$) | Thyroid ectomized ($n=9$) |
|---|---|---|---|---|---|
| UDP-glucuronyltransferase (μmol·h$^{-1}$·g$^{-1}$ of liver) | 2.3± 0.6 | 1.9± 0.2* | 1.6± 0.3* | 2.9± 0.4 | 4.2± 0.6*** |
| Bile flow (μl·min$^{-1}$·100 g$^{-1}$) | | | | | |
| Basal[a] | 9.2± 1.5 | 11.2± 0.7* | 11.0± 1.4* | 7.6± 1.1 | 4.5± 1.2*** |
| At Tm[b] | 9.3± 1.2 | 11.4± 1.6** | 12.9± 1.3*** | 9.0± 1.3 | 4.3± 1.3*** |
| Biliary bilirubin concentration | | | | | |
| Basal[a] (μmol·l$^{-1}$) | 85.1±35.2 | 65.5±11.0 | 73.4±10.9 | 85.9±25.0 | 85.3±17.3 |
| At Tm[b] (mmol·l$^{-1}$) | 11.7± 1.7 | 10.1± 1.1* | 9.0± 0.9** | 13.3± 1.3 | 14.9± 2.8 |
| Maximal bilirubin output (Tm) (nmol·min$^{-1}$·100 g$^{-1}$) | 110.5±10.9 | 113.9±13.4 | 115.2±13.4 | 121.1±17.2 | 64.9±23.9*** |
| Biliary bilirubin conjugates (% of total conjugates) | | | | | |
| Basal[a] | 51± 4 | 50± 2 | 44± 3** | 55± 4 | 58± 4 |
| At Tm[b] | 43± 2 | 39± 2** | 34± 2*** | 40± 2 | 52± 6*** |

Mean values ± SD are given. Significance with regard to control animals: * $P \leqslant 0.05$; ** $P \leqslant 0.01$; *** $P \leqslant 0.001$

[a] In each animal, the mean of three 10-min basal bile samples was taken;
[b] In each animal, the mean of three 10-min Tm bile samples (period 30-60 min after onset of bilirubin infusion) was taken

**Table 2.** Biliary excretion of UCB, BMG, and BDG during bilirubin Tm conditions in control, thyroid-hormone-treated, and thyroidectomized Wistar rats

| | Saline-treated controls ($n=7$) | $T_4$-treated 6.26 nmol·day$^{-1}$·100 g$^{-1}$ ($n=8$) | $T_4$-treated 12.52 nmol·day$^{-1}$·100 g$^{-1}$ ($n=6$) | Sham-operated controls ($n=9$) | Thyroidectomized ($n=9$) |
|---|---|---|---|---|---|
| UCB (nmol·min$^{-1}$·100 g$^{-1}$) | 9.4±3.5 | 13.9±2.8** | 18.5±3.2*** | 3.8±1.1 | 2.1± 0.4 |
| BMG (nmol·min$^{-1}$·100 g$^{-1}$) | 57.6±5.8 | 61.0±8.6* | 63.1±4.6* | 70.6±9.9 | 30.2±11.8*** |
| BDG (nmol·min$^{-1}$·100 g$^{-1}$) | 43.8±5.8 | 39.0±7.0 | 33.6±1.9** | 46.7±8.0 | 32.5±13.5* |

In each animal, the mean of three 10-min Tm bile samples (period 30-60 min after onset of bilirubin infusion) was taken. Mean values ± SD are given. Significance with regard to control animals: * $P \leqslant 0.05$; ** $P \leqslant 0.01$; *** $P \leqslant 0.001$

## Bile Pigments in Serum

The concentrations of bilirubin present in serum at the end of the experiment are shown in Table 3.

**Table 3.** Serum bilirubin concentration and composition in control, thyroid-hormone-treated, and thyroidectomized Wistar rats

| | Saline-treated controls ($n=7$) | $T_4$-treated 6.26 nmol·day$^{-1}$·100 g$^{-1}$ ($n=8$) | $T_4$-treated 12.52 nmol·day$^{-1}$·100 g$^{-1}$ ($n=6$) | Sham-operated controls ($n=9$) | Thyroidectomized ($n=9$) |
|---|---|---|---|---|---|
| Total bilirubin (mmol·$^{-1}$) | 0.56±0.13 | 0.48±0.08 | 0.56±0.04 | 0.70±0.13 | 1.09±0.21*** |
| Unconjugated (mmol·l$^{-1}$) | 0.51±0.12 | 0.45±0.08 | 0.53±0.04 | 0.63±0.12 | 0.84±0.17* |
| Conjugated (mmol·l$^{-1}$) | 0.05±0.03 | 0.02±0.01* | 0.03±0.02 | 0.07±0.03 | 0.25±0.07*** |
| BMG (mmol·l$^{-1}$) | – | – | – | 0.05±0.02 | 0.14±0.03*** |
| BDG (mmol·l$^{-1}$) | – | – | – | 0.02±0.01 | 0.11±0.04*** |

Sera were obtained after 1 h infusion of bilirubin to obtain Tm conditions. Mean values ± SD are given. Significance with regard to control animals: * $P<0.05$; ** $P<0.01$; *** $P<0.001$

**Table 4.** Liver bilirubin concentration and composition in control, thyroid-hormone-treated, and thyroidectomized Wistar rats

| | Saline-treated controls ($n=7$) | $T_4$-treated 6.26 nmol·day$^{-1}$·100 g$^{-1}$ ($n=8$) | $T_4$-treated 12.52 nmol·day$^{-1}$·100 g$^{-1}$ ($n=6$) | Sham-operated controls ($n=9$) | Thyroid ectomized ($n=9$) |
|---|---|---|---|---|---|
| Total bilirubin (μmol·g$^{-1}$liver) | 0.46±0.11 | 0.44±0.14 | 0.42±0.10 | 0.81±0.18 | 1.16±0.14** |
| Unconjugated (μmol·g$^{-1}$liver) | 0.31±0.06 | 0.29±0.08 | 0.32±0.10 | 0.51±0.11 | 0.58±0.07 |
| Conjugated (μmol.g$^{-1}$liver) | 0.15±0.05 | 0.14±0.07 | 0.09±0.02* | 0.31±0.09 | 0.59±0.14** |
| BMG (μmol·g$^{-1}$liver) | – | – | – | 0.22±0.06 | 0.29±0.06 |
| BDG (μmol·g$^{-1}$liver) | – | – | – | 0.09±0.03 | 0.30±0.09** |

Livers were obtained after 1 h infusion of bilirubin to obtain Tm conditions. Mean values ± SD are given. Significance with regard to control animals: * $P<0.05$; ** $P<0.001$

### Activity of Hepatic Bilirubin UDP-Glucuronosyltransferase and Composition of Bile Pigments in the Liver

As shown in Table 1, hepatic bilirubin UDP-GTA, as assayed in digitonin-activated liver homogenates, significantly decreased in hyperthyroid and significantly increased in thyroidectomized rats. The concentrations of bilirubin pigments present in the liver at the end of the experiment are shown in Table 4.

## Discussion

In this study, a significant increase of hepatic bilirubin UDP-GTA, as assayed in digitonin-activated liver homogenates, could be demonstrated in thyroidectomized hypothyroid Wistar rats, whereas a significant decrease in enzyme activity could be observed in thyroid-hormone-treated hyperthyroid rats. It is well known that rat liver contains at least two groups of UDP-glucuronosyltransferases which have distinct substrate specificities and different patterns of perinatal development [19]. It has been demonstrated that the formation of orthoaminophenol glucuronide in vitro is markedly decreased following thyroidectomy [10], whereas the para-nitrophenol conjugating capacity significantly increases after treatment with triiodothyronine ($T_3$) [11]. Both these enzyme activities belong to the "late fetal" group. The bilirubin UDP-GTA which belongs to the "neonatal" enzyme group, decreased after treatment with $T_3$ in the study of Chowdhury et al. [11] and with $T_4$ in the present work. An increase of bilirubin UDP-GTA could not clearly be shown in hypothyroid rats by Gartner and Arias [10], but in their study digitonin was not added to liver homogenates. However, they did find a significant increase of hepatic bilirubin UDP-GTA in hypophysectomized rats when digitonin-activated liver homogenates were studied. As such, heterogeneity of rat liver UDP-glucuronosyltransferases is further characterized by different responses to hypo- and hyperthyroidism.

In our rats, thyroidectomy resulted in a 50% decrease of bile flow, as was also found by others [10, 12]. In the study by Layden and Boyer [12], the decrease in bile flow was paralleled by a 50% decrease in liver plasma membrane $Na^+$, $K^+$-ATPase activity, whereas bile salt excretion remained unchanged from control values, suggesting that the reduced bile secretion was secondary to an inhibition of the bile-salt-independent flow. In hypothyroid animals, the concentration of bilirubin achieved in basal as well as in Tm bile was unchanged from control values. However, a 47% reduction in bilirubin Tm was observed 2 weeks after thyroidectomy. In the study by Gartner and Arias [10], a 60% reduction in the hepatic capacity to excrete bilirubin was found 5 weeks after thyroidectomy. A decreased excretion rate was found for all three bilirubin pigments in hypothyroid rats. However, the decrease was much more pronounced for BMG than for BDG. The amount of BDG excreted decreased to 69% whereas the excretion rate of BMG decreased to 43% of control values. As such, the amount of diconjugates, expressed as a percentage of total conjugates present in Tm bile, increased significantly from 40% in controls to 53% in hypothyroid rats. This relative increase of biliary BDG might be the result of the increased hepatic UDP-GTA. Furthermore, the bilirubin diglucuronide formation by microsomal preparations in vitro is increased by a prolonged incubation time [20]. This could be paralleled in vivo by a relative increased formation of BDG in hypothyroidism, which represents a cholestatic condition with prolonged retention of bilirubin in the hepatocytes. The relative increase of BDG in bile might also result from a readier reflux of BMG from the liver to the plasma [21] or from decreased $\beta$-glucuronidase activity with decreased deconjugation of bilirubin diglucuronides.

In the study by Gartner and Arias [10], no changes in the concentration of conjugated and unconjugated bilirubin were observed in liver and serum of thyroidectomized rats at the end of a continuous bilirubin infusion. However, at the end of our experiments, total bilirubin concentrations in liver and serum had significantly increased in hypothyroid rats. In serum, the increase was mainly due to a pronounced enhancement of both bilirubin mono- and diglucuronides.

The proportion of conjugates amounted to 23% of total serum bilirubin, in contrast to only 10% in sham-operated controls. The enhanced bilirubin concentration in liver was mainly due to a pronounced increase of BDG; BMG showed only a slight increase and UCB remained unchanged. These data could also fit in with a readier reflux of BMG from the hepatocytes to the plasma.

Hyperthyroid rats were characterized by a marked increase in bile flow, whereas the maximal hepatic bilirubin secretion capacity was unchanged from control values. The increase in bile flow in hyperthyroid animals was paralleled by an increase in liver plasma membrane $Na^+$, $K^+$-ATPase activity, as demonstrated by Layden and Boyer [12]. Under basal conditions, the relative amount of diconjugates significantly decreased from 51% in controls to 44% in rats treated with the highest dose of $T_4$. During maximal bilirubin secretion, this value decreased significantly from 43% in the controls to 39% in the group treated with the lower dose of $T_4$ ($P<0.001$) and even further to 34% in rats which received the higher dose of $T_4$ ($P<0.001$). This finding could be the result of the decreased conjugated capacity, as the same findings in bile have been observed in other conditions with decreased bilirubin UDP-GTA, e.g., in Gilbert's syndrome and in heterozygous Gunn rats.

## Summary

Thyroidectomized rats are characterized by increased hepatic bilirubin UDP-glucuronosyltransferase activity (UDP-GTA) and by cholestatic features such as decreases in bile flow and in maximal bilirubin output and an increase of the absolute and relative amounts of bilirubin conjugates in serum and liver. The increase of biliary bilirubin diconjugates (BDG) as a percentage of total conjugates present in bile might be the result of the increased bilirubin UDP-GTA, prolonged retention of bilirubin in the hepatocytes, predominant reflux of bilirubin monoconjugates (BMG) to the plasma, or decreased $\beta$-glucuronidase activity in bile. The increase of bilirubin conjugates in liver and serum is characterized by an increased concentration of BDG in liver and increased concentrations of BDG and BMG in serum. This could also be the result of a readier reflux of BMG from liver to plasma.

Hyperthyroid rats are characterized by decreased bilirubin UDG-GTA, increased bile flow, and unaffected total biliary bilirubin output. The observed decrease of biliary BDG as a percentage of total conjugates could represent the result of the decreased conjugating capacity.

## References

1. Schaffer JM (1940) Disease of the liver in hyperthyroidism. Arch Pathol 29: 20-30
2. Waldstein SS, Slodki SJ, Kaganiec I, Bronsky DA (1960) A clinical study of thyroid storm. Ann Intern Med 52: 626-642
3. Erven W, Flendrig JA (1973) Een geval van hyperthyreoidie verwikkeld met icterus (A case of hyperthyroidism associated with icterus). Tijdschr Geneesk 18: 895-900
4. Jansen PLM, Froeling PGAM, Schade RWB, Kloppenborg PWC, Yap SH, van Haelst UJG (1982) Intrahepatic cholestasis in hyperthyroidism and the effect of anti hyroid and betablocking drugs. Neth J Med 25: 318-324
5. Greenberger NJ, Milligan FD, de Groot LJ, Isselbacher KJ (1964) Jaundice and thyrotoxicosis in the absence of congestive heart failure. Am J Med 36: 840-846
6. Akerren Y (1954) Prolonged jaundice in newborn associated with congenital myxedema. Acta Paediatr 43: 411-425
7. Christensen JF (1956) Prolonged icterus neonatorum and congenital myxedema. Acta Paediatr 45: 367-371

8. Weldon AP, Danks DM (1972) Congenital hypothyroidism and neonatal jaundice. Arch Dis Child 47: 469-471
9. Ariza CR, Frati AC, Sierra I (1984) Hypothyroidism-associated cholestasis. JAMA 252: 2392
10. Gartner LM, Arias IM (1972) Hormonal control of hepatic bilirubin transport and conjugation. Am J Physiol 222: 1091-1099
11. Chowdhury JR, Chowdhury NR, Moscione D, Shouval R, Tukey R, Arias IM (1981) Separation, purification and radio immunoassay of UDP-glucuronyltransferase: evidence for separate regulation of subclasses (Abstr). Hepatology 1: 503
12. Layden TJ, Boyer JL (1976) The effect of thyroid hormone on bile salt-independent bile flow and $Na^+$, $K^+$-ATP-ase activity in liver plasma membranes enriched in bile canaliculi. J Clin Invest 57: 1009-1018
13. Waynforth HB (1980) Experimental and surgical technique in the rat. Academic, London, pp 207-208
14. Van Steenbergen W, Fevery J (1982) Maximal biliary secretion of bilirubin in the anaesthetized rat: dependence on UDP-glucuronosyltransferase activity. Clin Sci 62: 521-528
15. Muraca M, de Groote J, Fevery J (1983) Sex differences of hepatic conjugation of bilirubin determine its maximal biliary excretion in non-anaesthetized male and female rats. Clin Sci 64: 85-90
16. Van Roy FP, Heirwegh KPM (1968) Determination of bilirubin glucuronide and assay of glucuronyltransferase with bilirubin as acceptor. Biochem J 107: 507-518
17. Heirwegh KPM, van de Vijver M, Fevery J (1972) Assay and properties of digitonin-activated bilirubin uridine diphosphate glucuronyltransferase from rat liver. Biochem J 129: 605-618
18. Muraca M, Blanckaert N (1983) Liquid-chromatographic assay and identification of mono- and diester conjugates of bilirubin in normal serum. Clin Chem 29: 1767-1771
19. Blanckaert N, Schmid R (1982) Physiology and pathophysiology of bilirubin metabolism. In: Zakim D, Boyer TD (eds) Hepatology. A textbook of liver diseases. Saunders, Philadelphia, pp 246-296
20. Fevery J (1985) The bilirubin diglucuronide controversy. J Hepatol 1: 437-442
21. Fevery J, Blanckaert N (1986) What can we learn from analysis of serum bilirubin? J Hepatol 2: 113-121

# Comparison of Some Parameters of the Drug-Metabolizing Enzyme System and Liver Function Tests in Different Hepatic Diseases

T. Horváth

First Department of Medicine, University Medical School, Pécs, Hungary

## Introduction

The classification of various chronic liver diseases has been theoretically resolved with respect to biotransformation and elimination of drugs. Consequently there are flow-sensitive, flow-insensitive restrictive, and flow-insensitive nonrestrictive drugs, and patients with various degree of disturbance of liver blood flow, liver cell function, and level and composition of serum proteins [1, 12, 13, 15, 17]. Because of the complexity of these disturbances, quantitative adaptation of the known relations is not yet possible. The aim of the study was the quantitative investigation of the functions of some pathways of biotransformation and enzyme induction in five histologically defined groups of patients with various chronic liver diseases and in normal controls.

## Material and Methods

Investigations were carried out in five groups of patients (alcoholic fatty liver, chronic persistent hepatitis, chronic active hepatitis, alcoholic cirrhosis, Gilbert's syndrome) and in healthy controls, using exogenous test materials and measuring excretion of the endogenous metabolite, D-glucaric acid. Liver function tests were performed as usual in clinical practice. The following parameters were examined: antipyrine (AP) kinetics [4, 18], menthol loading [2, 19], sulphadimidine (SD) kinetics [3, 6, 20], and D-glucaric acid excretion [11]. The clinical studies were performed as follows.

Antipyrine kinetic studies were performed after oral administration of 20 mg/kg AP. Blood samples were taken at 3, 6, 9, and 12 h after ingestion. The results were expressed in terms of half-life ($T_{½}$), and metabolic clearance rate (MCR). Analysis and calculations were done according to Brodie and Soberman.

Menthol loading was examined after oral administration of 2 g menthol. The clinical conditions were consistent with the procedure of Szabó and Ébrey, the analytic conditions with that of Bitter and Muir. The results were expressed as the amount of menthol glucuronide measured in urine collected for 5 h.

Estimation of D-glucaric acid excretion in samples from 24 h urinary collection was performed according to Marsh with minor modifications. The results were expressed in the total value.

For the SD kinetic studies two methods were used, the second of them (b) only as control of influencing role of renal elimination:

a) After intravenous administration of 1 g SD, blood samples were taken at ½, 1, 2, 4, 6, 8, and 12 h and $T_{½}$, volume of distribution ($V_d$) and total body clearance ($Cl_b$, ac-

Assessment and Management of Hepatobiliary Disease
Eds.: L. Okolicsányi, G. Csomós, and G. Crepaldi

**Table 1.** Parameters of biotransforming ability (B), elimination (E), and enzyme induction (I)

| Parameter | Method of measurement | Function |
|---|---|---|
| Antipyrine kinetics (p.o.) | MCR ($ml \cdot h^{-1} \cdot kg^{-1}$) | B+I |
| | $T_{1/2}$ (h) | E |
| Menthol loading (p.o.) | Menthol glucuronide excreted with urine ($mg \cdot 5\ h^{-1}$) | B+I |
| Sulphadimidine kinetics | $T_{1/2}$ (h) (i.v.) | E |
| | $Cl_b$ $ml \cdot h^{-1}$ (i.v.) | E |
| | $Cl_r$ $ml \cdot h^{-1}$ (p.o.)* | E |
| | Acetylated SD in 4th h in serum (i.v.) in % of total SD | B |
| | Acetylated SD in 4th h in serum (p.o.) in % of total SD* | B |
| | Acetylated SD excreted with urine collected during 8 h (p.o.) in % of total SD* | B |
| D-glucaric acid | Excreted with urine ($mmol/l \cdot 24\ h^{-1}$) | I |

MCR, metabolic clearance rate; $T_{1/2}$, biological half-life; $Cl_b$, total body clearance; $Cl_r$, renal clearance

* Parameter used only by reclassification of patient (discriminance analysis)

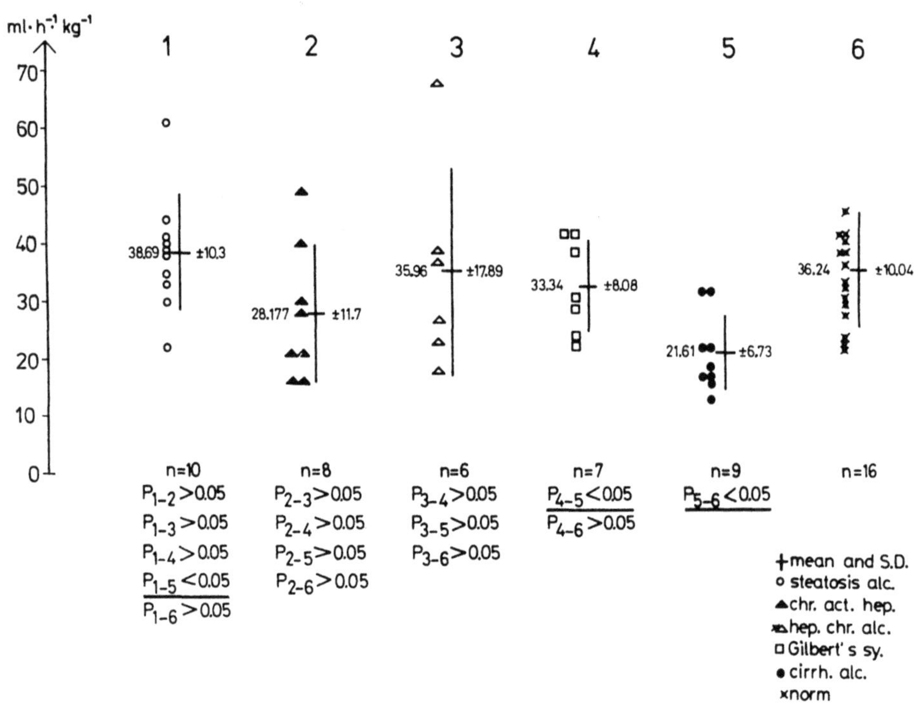


**Fig. 1.** Significant differences in $AP_{MCR}$ values (underlined) were found in three connections: the cirrhotic group shows lower values than the normal controls and the group with Gilbert's syndrome, and the steatotic group shows higher values than the cirrhotic group

cording to Talseth and Landmark) were calculated. The proportion of acetylated SD (AcSD) was calculated on the basis of measurement of total and nonacetylated SD from the 4-h blood samples.

b) SD was administered in an oral dose of 500-1500 mg, depending on body weight. Urine was collected for 8 h. Blood samples were taken at ½, 1, 2, 4, 8, 12, 18, and 24 h after ingestion. Renal clearance ($Cl_r$) of total SD was calculated by the integration of the areas under the curves of the urine and blood samples. For SD analysis the method described by Bratton and Marshall [3] was applied.

Metabolic ($AP_{MCR}$, menthol, AcSD%) and kinetic ($AP_{T_{½}}$, $SD_{T_{½}}$, $SD_{Cl_b}$) parameters measured and/or calculated from these data can be seen in Table 1. Biochemical and/or genetical interpretation of the given parameters has been published yet [7, 8]. Some of the data were used only as one of the variables of discriminance analysis [9] (Table 1).

The result of various groups were compared using variance analysis. Relevant connections between parameters of biotransformation and biochemical tests were studied with correlation analysis, and discriminance analysis was based upon biotransforming ability and the results of biochemical liver tests [14]. Patients of both sexes, between 20 and 60 years of age showed similar ratio in the studied groups.

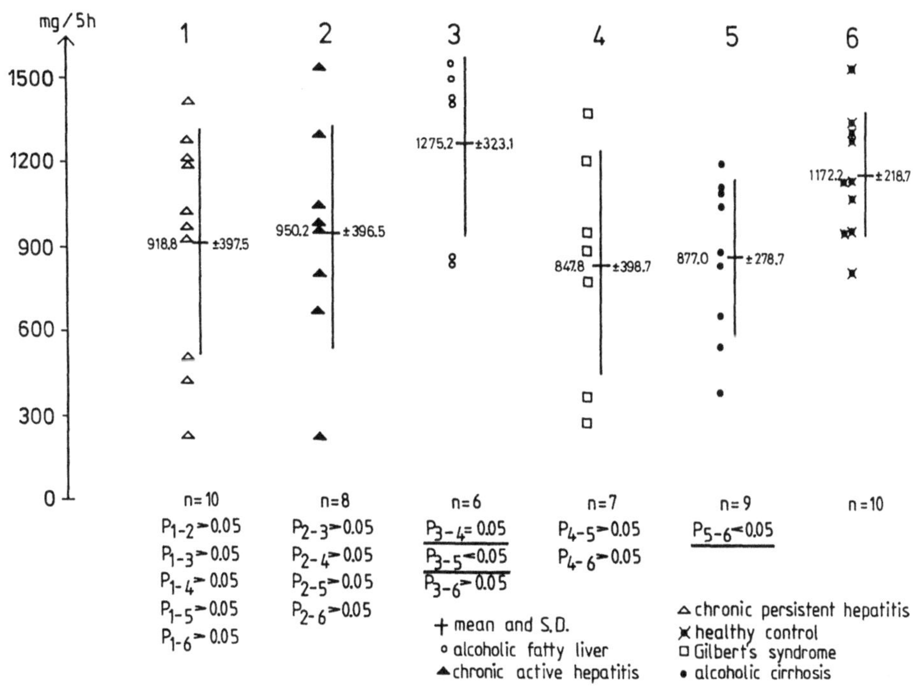


**Fig. 2.** Significant differences in menthol glucuronide excretion (underlined) were found in three connections: the cirrhotic group shows lower values than the normal controls, and the steatotic group shows higher values than the cirrhotic and Gilbert's syndrome groups

## Results

The $AP_{MCR}$ is demonstrated in Fig. 1; it shows a significant diminution compared to the normal control values only in the cirrhotic group. Glucuronidation capacity, as detected by the menthol test was diminished significantly only in the cirrhotic group (Fig. 2). D-glucaric acid excretion was higher in all groups of liver diseases than in the normal controls, but the difference was significant only in alcoholic fatty liver (Fig. 3).

Total body clearance of total SD showed no significant differences between the groups studied (Fig. 4). The ratio of total SD to AcSD was remarkably low in Gilbert's syndrome and in cirrhosis (Fig. 5).

The correlation between serum albumin level and the studied inducible pathways was significant only in the case of $AP_{MCR}$ (Fig. 6). The three parameters of inducible pathways showed no tendency toward correlation (Fig. 7).

The biological $T_{1/2}$ of SD correlated only with the serum bilirubin level, independent of disease (Fig. 8).

Discriminance analysis was carried out in two ways. In the first method both the biochemical tests and the special parameters of biotransformation and induction were used, while in the second the parameters of biotransformation and enzyme induction were used exclusively. Histologic diagnosis was given in the case of the classification matrix but not given in the case of the jack-knifed classification. The results of discriminance analysis with the use of all parameters show that the hit rate was 100% if the

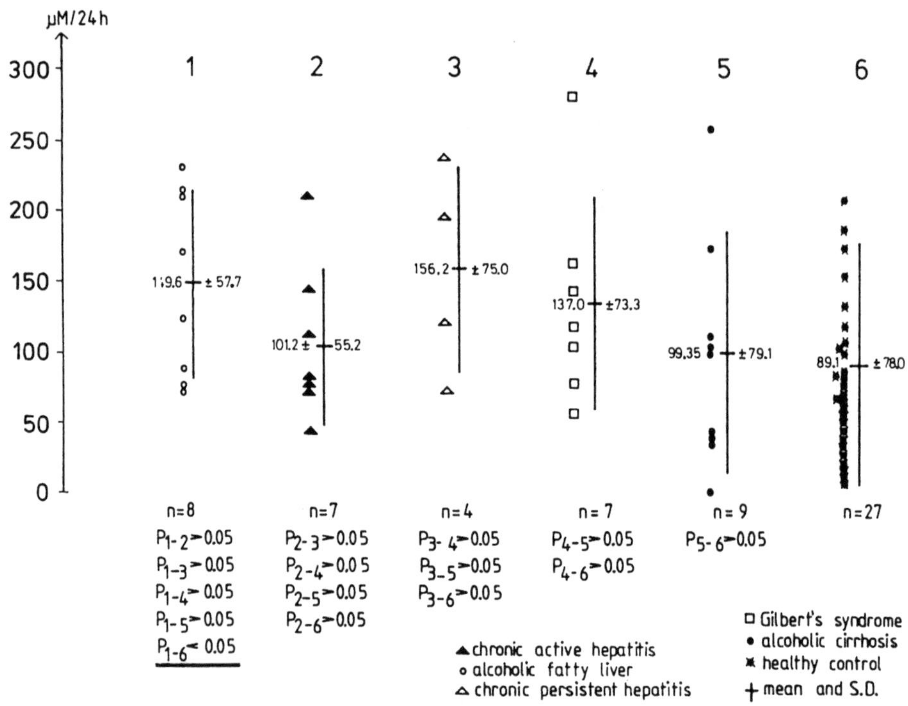


**Fig. 3.** Significantly elevated values of D-glucaric acid excretion were found only in the alcoholic fatty liver group

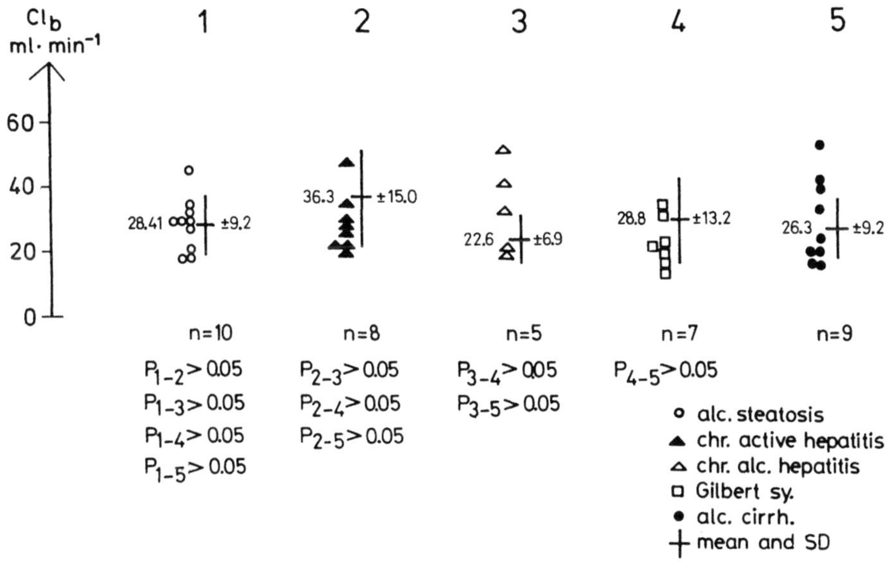


**Fig. 4.** Total body clearance, of total SD showed no significant differences between groups

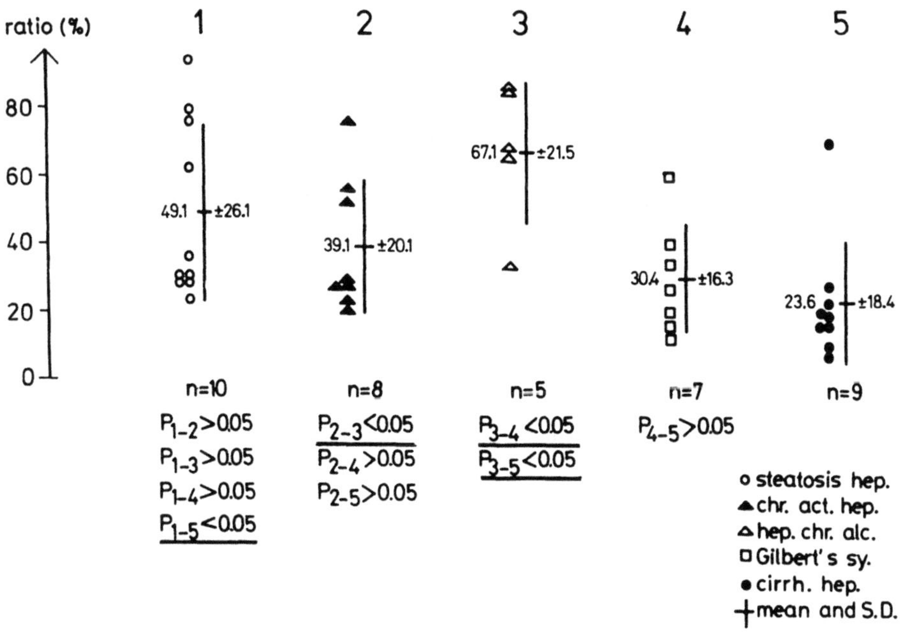


**Fig. 5.** Significant differences in the ratio of total SD to AcSD (underlined) were found in four connections. The cirrhotic group shows lower values than the alcoholic fatty liver group. The persistent hepatitis group *(3)* shows the highest values

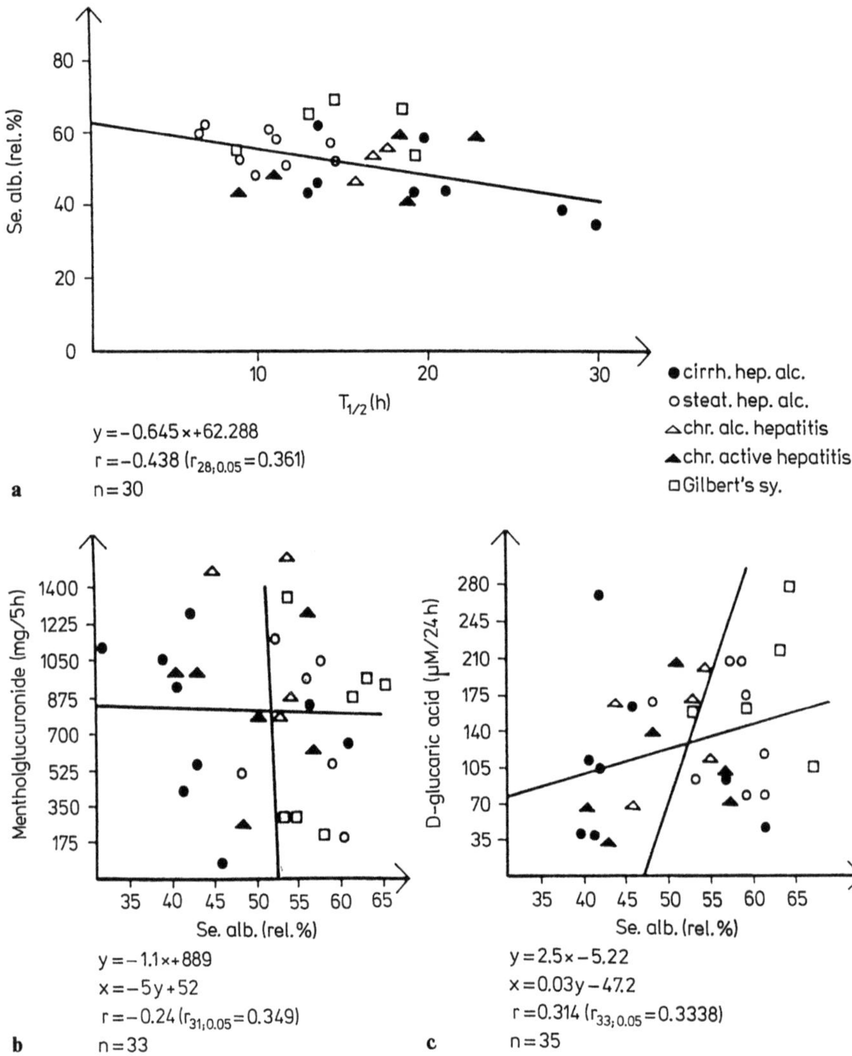


**Fig. 6 a–c.** Antipyrine kinetics (**a**) shows a correlation with serum albumin level, but two other parameters of enzyme induction, menthol loading (**b**) and D-glucaric acid excretion (**c**), do not

histologic diagnosis was given and varied between 0% and 83% if the histologic diagnosis was not given (Table 2). Diagrammatic representation of the results demonstrates the separation of groups with the help of this method (Fig. 9).

The hit rate of reclassification is much lower if only the parameters of biotransformation and enzyme induction are used, amounting to between 16% and 88% in the case of the classification matrix and between 0% and 77% in the case of jack-knifed classification. The hit rate of the cirrhotic group is the highest in all reclassifications (Table 3). Diagrammatic representation of the results shows that the middle points of the groups were closer then when all the parameters were used (Fig. 10).

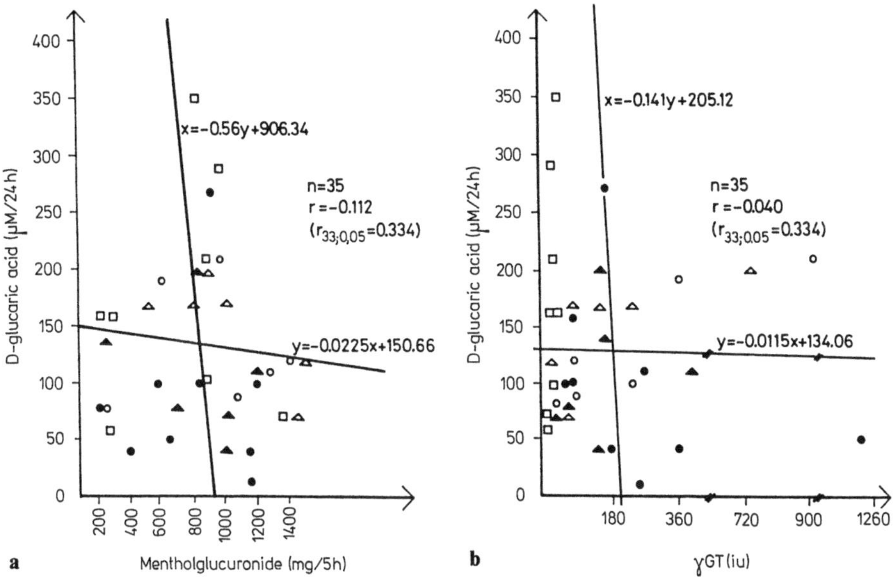


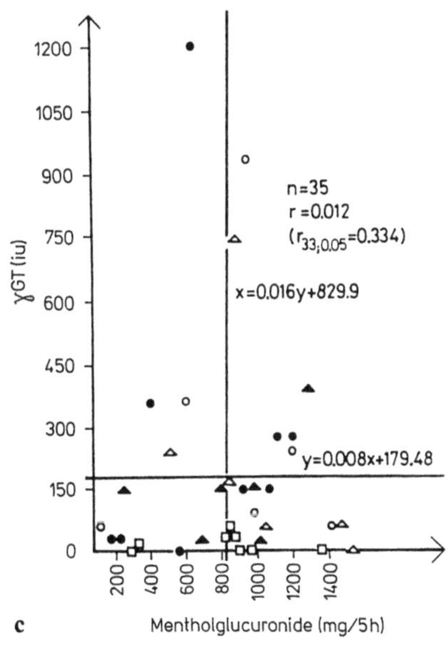


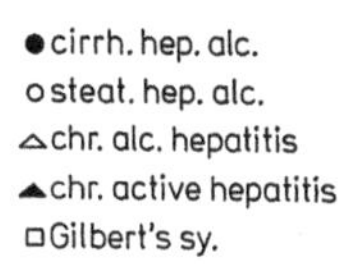


**Fig. 7.** D-glucaric acid excretion and menthol glucuronide excretion correlate neither with each other nor with $\gamma$GT activity in the serum, which is the parameter of enzyme induction used in clinical practice

## Conclusions

The most important results can be summarized as follows: Comparison of biotransforming ability using variance analysis of many parameters in various groups of chronic liver diseases shows a small number of significant differences. Most of the significant differences was found when the cirrhotic group was compared with the other groups. Correlation between parameters of biotransforming capacity and biochemical tests was significant in special connections only, and showed no general validity for

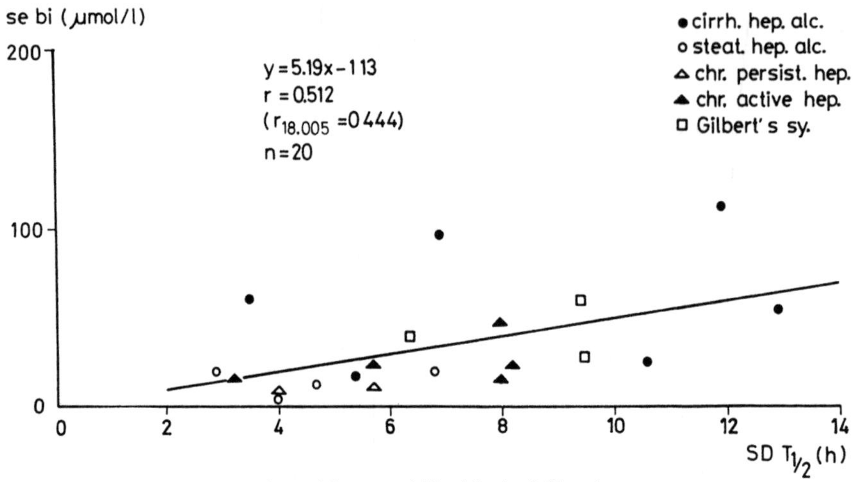


**Fig. 8.** $SD_{T½}$ shows correlation with serum bilirubin *(se bi)* level

**Table 2.** Reclassification using routine biochemical tests (12 variables) and with biotransformation and induction (10 variables)

Classification matrix

| Group | Classification (% right) | Classification of cases | | | | |
|---|---|---|---|---|---|---|
| | | ▲ | △ | □ | ● | ○ |
| ▲ | 100.0 | 6 | 0 | 0 | 0 | 0 |
| △ | 100.0 | 0 | 2 | 0 | 0 | 0 |
| □ | 100.0 | 0 | 0 | 4 | 0 | 0 |
| ● | 100.0 | 0 | 0 | 0 | 6 | 0 |
| ○ | 100.0 | 0 | 0 | 0 | 0 | 6 |
| Sum | 100.0 | 6 | 2 | 4 | 6 | 6 |

Jack-knifed classification

| Group | Classification (% right) | Classification of cases | | | | |
|---|---|---|---|---|---|---|
| | | ▲ | △ | □ | ● | ○ |
| ▲ | 50.0 | 3 | 0 | 0 | 2 | 1 |
| △ | 0.0 | 0 | 0 | 0 | 0 | 2 |
| □ | 75.0 | 0 | 0 | 3 | 0 | 1 |
| ● | 83.3 | 1 | 0 | 0 | 5 | 0 |
| ○ | 66.7 | 0 | 2 | 0 | 0 | 4 |
| Sum | 62.5 | 4 | 2 | 3 | 7 | 8 |

▲, chronic active hepatitis; △, chronic persistent hepatitis; □, Gilbert's syndrome; ●, alcoholic cirrhosis; ○, alcoholic fatty liver

Discriminance analysis with 12 parameters of routine biochemical tests and with 10 parameters of pharmacokinetical studies (calculator R22; program BMDP 7M).

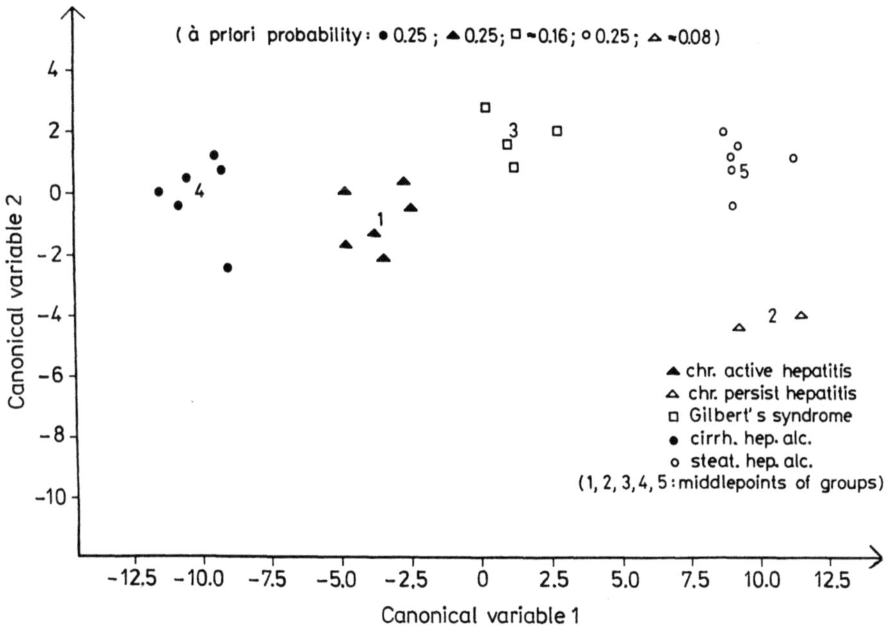


**Fig. 9.** The positions of the mid-points of the five groups of patients show an order of succession according to biochemical severity: Gilbert's syndrome occupies a position between active hepatitis and alcoholic fatty liver

**Table 3.** Reclassification using 10 parameters of biotransformation and enzyme induction

Classification matrix

| Group | Classification (% right) | Classification of cases ▲ | △ | □ | ● | ○ |
|---|---|---|---|---|---|---|
| ▲ | 16.7 | 1 | 0 | 1 | 3 | 1 |
| △ | 50.0 | 0 | 1 | 0 | 1 | 0 |
| □ | 20.0 | 2 | 0 | 1 | 1 | 1 |
| ● | 88.9 | 0 | 0 | 0 | 8 | 1 |
| ○ | 85.7 | 0 | 0 | 0 | 1 | 6 |
| Sum | 58.6 | 3 | 1 | 2 | 14 | 9 |

Jack-knifed classification

| Group | Classification (% right) | Classification of cases ▲ | △ | □ | ● | ○ |
|---|---|---|---|---|---|---|
| ▲ | 0.0 | 0 | 0 | 1 | 3 | 2 |
| △ | 0.0 | 0 | 0 | 0 | 1 | 1 |
| □ | 20.0 | 2 | 0 | 1 | 1 | 1 |
| ● | 77.8 | 0 | 0 | 1 | 7 | 1 |
| ○ | 57.1 | 1 | 0 | 1 | 1 | 4 |
| Sum | 41.4 | 3 | 0 | 4 | 13 | 9 |

Symbols ar in Table 2

Discriminance analysis with ten parameters of pharmacokinetical studies (calculator R22; program BMDP 7M).

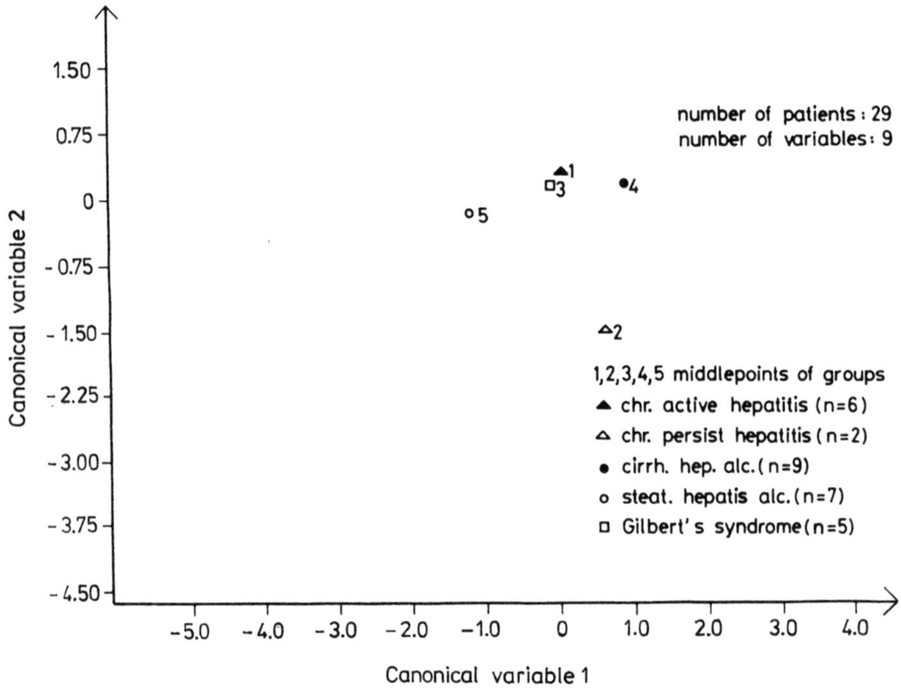


**Fig. 10.** The positions of the mid-points of the five groups of patients are nearer to each other than when the routine biochemical tests are wed as well. The order of succession of the mid-points corresponds with the severity of biochemical disturbances: Gilbert's syndrome is between active hepatitis and alcoholic fatty liver

practical use. Discriminance analysis showed that biotransforming ability and enzyme induction are less sensitive as liver function tests than the biochemical parameters. As discriminance analysis proves, the discriminative function of biochemical tests was not influenced if parameters of biotransformation and induction were included in the calculations.

Considerable dose reduction is necessary in general in the cirrhotic group; however, knowledge of relevant connections must be taken into account when considering dosage in the other groups as well. These relevant connections, for example the relation between serum bilirubin level and sulphadimidine kinetics, and the genetic characteristics of Gilbert's disease, must be borne in mind when assessing indications [5, 10, 16].

## Summary

The aim of the study was the quantitative investigation of the functions of some pathways of biotransformation and enzyme induction in five histologically defined groups of patients with chronic liver diseases. The following methods of studying biotransforming ability and enzyme induction were employed: antipyrine kinetics [4, 18], menthol loading [2, 19], sulphadimidine kinetics [3, 20], and D-glucaric acid excretion [11]. These data and the results of the usual biochemical tests were analyzed using variance analysis, correlation analysis, and discriminance analysis. The main conclusion on the basis of the findings is that considerable dose reduction is generally necessary in the cirrhotic group. Relevant connections between biochemical data and parameters of biotransforming ability must be assessed when considering indications.

## References

1. Bircher J, Blanckart R, Halpern A, Hacki W, Laissue J, Preisig R (1973) Criteria for assessment of functional impairment in patients with cirrhosis of the liver. Eur J Clin Invest 3: 72-85
2. Bitter T, Muir HM (1962) A modified uronic acid carbazole reaction. Anal Biochem 4: 330-334
3. Bratton AC, Marshall EK (1939) A new coupling component for sulphanilamide determination. J Biol Chem 128: 537-550
4. Brodie BB, Axelrod J, Soberman R, Levy BB (1949) The estimation of antipyrine in biological materials. J Biol Chem 179: 25-29
5. D'Arcy PF, Griffin JP (1972) Iatrogenic diseases. Oxford University Press, Oxford, p 208
6. Fine A, Summer DJ (1975) Determination of acetylator status in uraemia. Br J Clin Pharmacol 2: 475-476
7. Horváth T, Pár A, Past T, Tapsonyi Z, Ruzsa C, Kádas I, Jávor T (1982) Drug metabolism in alcoholic liver disease. Acta Med Sci Hung 39: 169-177
8. Horváth T, Past T, Tatai Z, Pár A, Kádas I, Tapsonyi Z, Jávor T (1984) Investigation of biotransformation capacity in patients with chronic liver diseases by pharmacokinetic methods: experimental trials. Pol J Pharmacol Pharm 36: 361-371
9. Horváth T, Tatai Z, Past T, Pár A, Kádas I, Jávor T (1984) Multivariate statistische Untersuchungen zur Diskriminierungsfähigkeit von pharmakokinetischen Parametern einiger Testsubstanzen und von Meßwerten der hepatischen Enzyminduktion. Depotarbeit Zentralbl Pharm Pharmakother Laboratoriumsdiagn AG 118/218/85: 8-9
10. Macklon AF, Savage RL, Rawlins MD (1979) Gilbert's syndrome and drug metabolism. Clin Pharmacokinet 4: 223-232
11. Marsh CA (1963) Metabolism of D-glucuronolactone in mammalian systems. Identification of D-glucaric acid as a normal constituent of urine. Biochem J 86: 77-86
12. Meier PJ (1982) Arzneimitteltherapie bei Leberkrankheiten. Schweiz Med Wochenschr 112: 258-263
13. Münst GJ, Bircher J (1978) Pharmakotherapie bei Leberpatienten – Sind Dosisanpassungen nötig? Ther Umsch 35: 756-760
14. Nilius R, Neef L, Otto L, Zipprich B, Busse HJ, Peters JE, Speck HJ (1980) Multivariate statistische Untersuchungen zur Diskriminierungsfähigkeit von klinischen-chemischen Tests in der hepatologischen Diagnostik. Hepatologie 53: 343-356
15. Baumgartner G (1980) Einfluß von Lebererkrankungen auf Bioverfügbarkeit und Clearance von Medikamenten. Internist/Berlin 21: 718-723
16. Platzer R, Küpfer A, Bircher J, Preisig R (1978) Polymorphic acetylation and aminopyrine demethylation in Gilbert's syndrome. Eur J Clin Invest 8: 219-223
17. Roberts RK, Branch RA, Desmond PV, Schenker S (1979) The influence of liver diseases on drug disposition. Clin Gastroenterol 8: 105-121

18. Soberman RBB, Brodie BB, Levy J, Axelrod V, Hollander J, Steele M (1949) The use of antipyrine in the measurement of total body water in man. J Biol Chem 179: 31-42
19. Szabó L, Ébrey P (1963) Studies on the inheritance of Crigler-Najjar's syndrome by the menthol test. Acta Pediatr Sci Hung 4: 153-158
20. Talseth T, Landmark KH (1977) Polymorphic acetylation of sulphadimidine in normal and uraemic men. Eur J Clin Pharmacol 11: 33-36

# Interaction of Ethanol with Hepatic Drug Metabolism

E. Altomare, G. Vendemiale, T. Trizio, G. Pallasciano, and O. Albano
Istituto di Clinica Medica I, Università di Bari, Italy

The microsomal ethanol-oxodizing system (MEOS), an accessory pathway of ethanol metabolism in the liver, shares many properties with other microsomal drug-metabolizing enzymes, including utilization of cytochrome P-450, NADPH, and $O_2$ [1]. This explains many of the alcohol-drug interactions which have been observed. In this respect the acute and chronic effects of ethanol are usually opposite.

## Microsomal Enzyme Induction

It is well known that repeated ethanol administration results in increased activity of a variety of microsomal drug-detoxifying enzymes [2]. Ethanol consumption also increases the content of microsomal cytochrome P-450 and the activity of NADPH cytochrome P-450 reductase. Therefore the increase in the activity of microsomal drug-detoxifying enzymes and in the content of cytochrome P-450 induced by ethanol ingestion provides a good explanation for the observation that ethanol consumption enhances the rate of drug metabolism (Fig. 1). Indeed, it has been shown that the rate of drug clearance from the blood is enhanced in alcoholics [3]. It must be pointed out, however, that the increased drug metabolism does not always result in enhanced drug detoxification, because the increased activity of hepatic microsomal enzymes may enhance the toxicity of agents that are converted to toxic metabolites in the microsomes (metabolic activation).

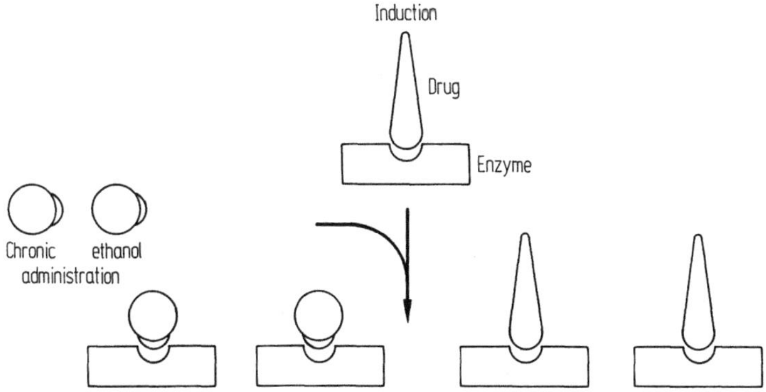


**Fig. 1.** Mechanism of microsomal enzyme induction. Repeated ethanol administration results in microsomal proliferation and increased activity of microsomal drug-detoxifying enzymes

Assessment and Management of Hepatobiliary Disease
Eds.: L. Okolicsányi, G. Csomós, and G. Crepaldi

## Inhibition of Microsomal Drug-Metabolizing Systems

### Competitive Inhibition

Unlike chronic ethanol ingestion, the principal effect of the acute presence of ethanol is inhibition of drug metabolism. The main mechanism involved appears to be competition for a partially common detoxification process, including competition for binding with cytochrome P-450 [4] (Fig. 2). The inhibitory effects of acute ethanol may explain the observation that simultaneous administration of ethanol and drugs slows the rate of drug metabolism [5].

We have studied the effects of both acute and chronic ethanol-drug interaction by means of an analgesic and antipyretic agent, acetaminophen (paracetamol, *N*-acetyl-*p*-aminophenol). This agent, generally safe when taken in recommended doses, represents a good model of "metabolic activation" (Fig. 3).

### Ethanol-Drug Interaction

Our first step was to evaluate the effects of acute and chronic ethanol administration on acetaminophen (APAP) metabolism and toxicity in subhuman primates. In our experiment 12 female baboons were pair-fed a nutritionally adequate liquid diet containing either ethanol as 50% of total calories (ethanol diet) or an isocaloric carbohydrate (control diet) for at least 18 months [6]. On the eve of each experiment, the baboons were fasted from 4 p.m. to eliminate ethanol. The experiment was started the following day preceded by slight anesthesia for insertion of a urinary catheter and two intravenous catheters, for infusion and blood sampling. During the experiment a 5% dextrose solution was infused to meet the caloric needs of the animals. After anesthesia a saline solution of APAP (40 mg/kg) was administered i.v. Blood samples were taken every 30 min for 6 h to evaluate APAP blood levels and urinary excretion.

APAP and its principal metabolites were separated in blood and urine samples by high-pressure liquid chromatography (HPLC) according to Buckpitt et al. [7] and Howie et al. [8].

In baboons fed ethanol chronically, APAP half-life was significantly shorter than in pair-fed controls ($t½$: 63.5 +/− 4 min vs 76.8 +/− 4 min, $p < 0.01$). The urinary excretion of APAP mercapturate was significantly greater in baboons fed ethanol chronically than in controls (1.2 +/− 0.2 vs 0.3 +/− 0.08% of injected dose, $p < 0.05$).

Figure 3 shows the metabolism of APAP. In addition to glucuronate and sulphate conjugation, this drug is also metabolized in the liver by the microsomal P-450-dependent drug-metabolizing system. The latter biotransformation yields an active metabolite highly toxic to the liver which is normally trapped by glutathione (GSH) and excreted with urine as APAP mercapturate, but is capable, in case of GSH depletion or APAP overdose, of causing hepatotoxicity through covalent binding to cell protein [9].

It seems clear, therefore, that in our experiment the pretreatment with inducers of microsomes (such as ethanol) enhanced the toxicity of APAP through an increased production of toxic metabolite.

In the next experiment, the same pair-fed baboons were used after an interval of 2–3 months. In this case ethanol was infused 30 min before APAP injection (40 mg/kg i.v.) at a dose of 1.5 g/kg. After the drug administration, ethanol infusion was main-

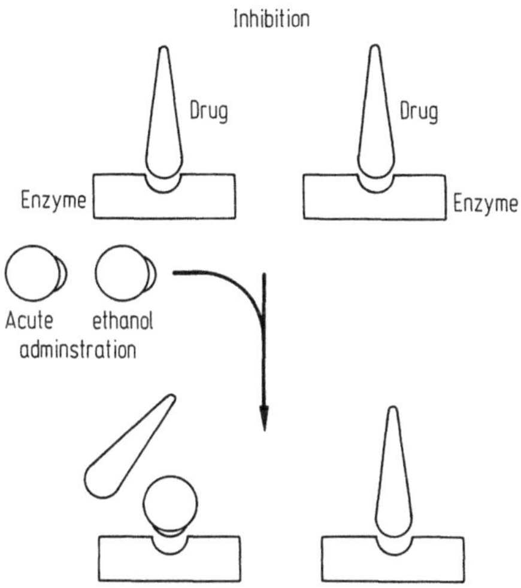


**Fig. 2.** Mechanism of microsomal enzyme inhibition. Acute ethanol administration results in inhibition of drug metabolism. The main mechanism involved appears to be competition for a partially common detoxification process

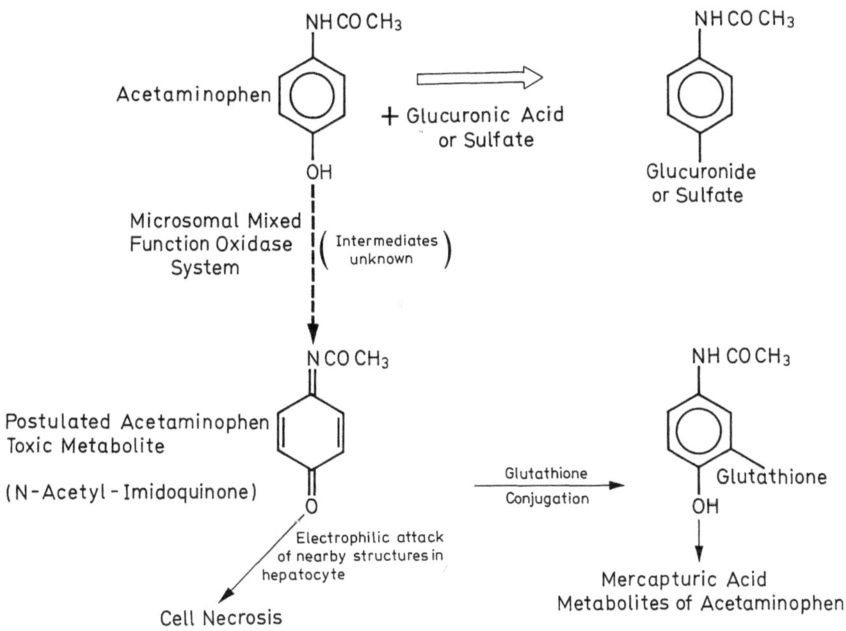


**Fig. 3.** Metabolism of acetaminophen

tained at a constant rate of 120–160 mg/kg/h. The remaining procedures were the same as in the first experimental design.

Acute ethanol infusion resulted in a slower plasma APAP disappearance (Fig. 4) and decreased APAP mercapturate urinary excretion (Fig. 5) in both baboons fed ethanol chronically and their pair-fed controls.

Our data show that chronic ethanol feeding enhances, while acute ethanol infusion reduces, APAP hepatotoxicity in subhuman primates [10]. These results are consistent

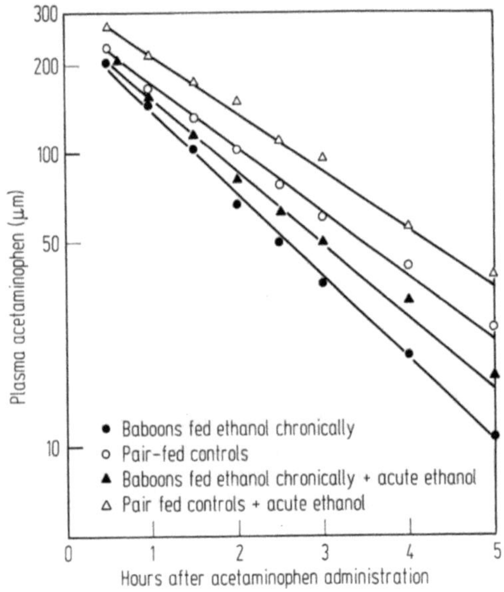


**Fig. 4.** Plasma elimination of acetaminophen after i.v. injection of 40 mg/kg of the drug in baboons fed ethanol chronically and their pair-fed controls. In another experiment, the same baboons received 1.5 g/kg ethanol i.v. 30 min before acetaminophen administration (40 mg/kg) and ethanol infusion was continued at the rate of 120–160 mg/kg/h. Blood samples were taken at 30-min intervals for 6 h. Values are means +/− SEM of six animals (From Altomare et al. 1984 [10])

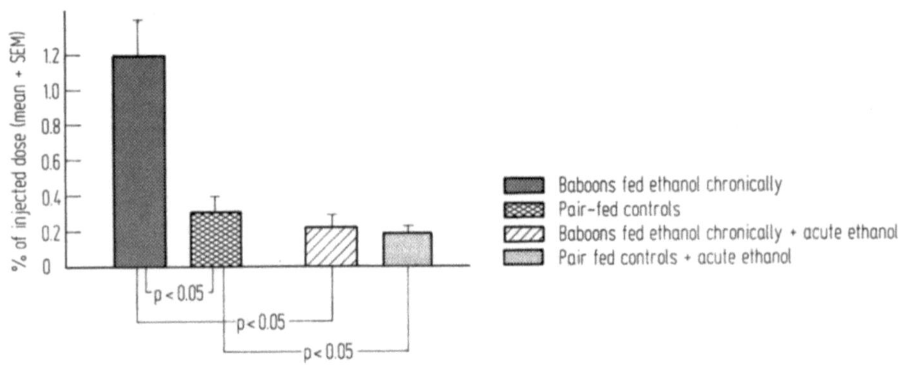


**Fig. 5.** Effect of chronic ethanol administration on the urinary excretion of acetaminophen mercapturate during the 6 h following acetaminophen injection (40 mg/kg i.v.) with and without ethanol infusion (120–160 mg/kg/h). Values are mean +/− SEM of six animals (From Altomare et al. 1984 [10])

with previous studies showing the opposite effects of acute and chronic ethanol administration on APAP hepatotoxicity [11–13].

In another study, our aim was to determine whether there is also an alteration in the biliary elimination of APAP after chronic ethanol feeding. We used male Sprague-Dawley rats pair-fed a liquid diet containing either ethanol as 36% of total energy (ethanol diet) or an isocaloric carbohydrate (control diet) for 4–6 weeks [6]. One day after bile duct cannulation, APAP (250 mg/kg) was given i.p. and drug metabolism was studied for 5 h. The biliary excretion of APAP and its metabolites was assessed every 30 min for 5 h after drug administration. The biliary excretion of both total APAP and

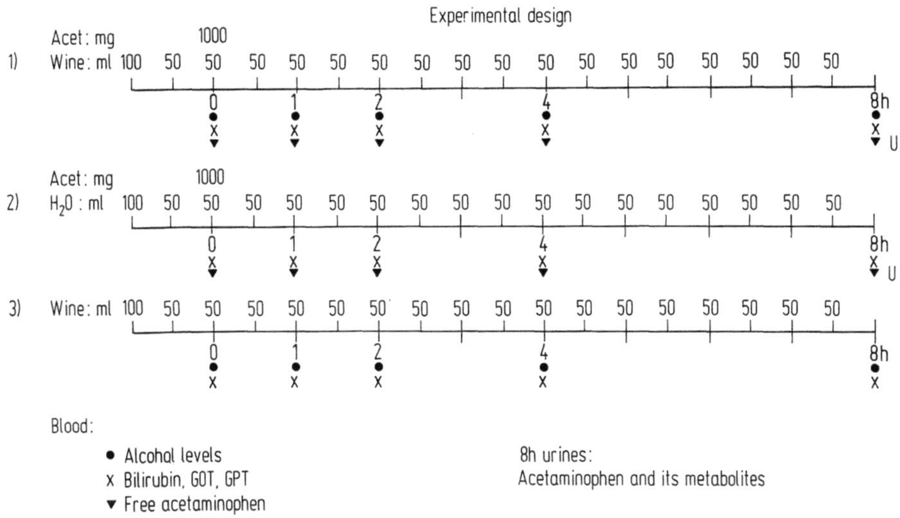


**Fig. 6.** Design of three experiments performed to study the interaction between ethanol and acetaminophen in humans. For details see text. ●, serum alcohol; ×, serum bilirubin, GOT, GPT; ▼; serum free acetaminophen

its conjugates was significantly decreased in alcohol-fed rats compared to pair-fed controls.

We also measured total biliary GSH output before and after APAP administration. The biliary GSH output before drug administration was significantly lower in alcohol-fed rats than in controls (0.03 + / − .01 vs 0.11 + / − .02 μmol/30 min/100 g, $p < 0.005$). After APAP injection the biliary output of total GSH increased in both groups and the rise was comparable. However, the cumulative excretion of GSH was lower in alcohol-fed animals than in pair-fed controls (1 + / − 0.3 vs 2.2 + / − 0.2 μmol/100 g, $p < 0.025$). The hepatic GSH concentration was also lower in rats fed ethanol chronically than in pair-fed controls (1.9 + / − 0.6 vs 3.3 + / − 0.4 μmol/g liver, $p < 0.05$). These data suport the possibility that diminished hepatic GSH and biliary excretion of the drug may contribute to the increased hepatotoxicity of APAP after chronic ethanol feeding [14].

While there have been a number of case reports showing that both laboratory animals and humans have increased susceptibility to APAP hepatotoxicity after chronic ethanol consumption [11–14], the protection afforded by acute ethanol administration in humans has been observed only in a preliminary study in which acute ethanol was given before APAP administration [15]. This prompted us to confirm the prevention of APAP toxicity afforded by acute ethanol in humans by means of three experimental designs (Fig. 6).

In the first one eight healthy male volunteers received 80 g ethanol (in the form of Italian white wine) starting 1 h (100 ml wine) prior to the ingestion of APAP (1 g) and continuing every 30 min (50 ml each time) for 9 h. In the second experiment (performed after a 15-day interval) the same subjects received APAP and water (instead of wine) according to the same regimen. In the third experiment (carried out after another 15-day interval) the volunteers consumed alcohol alone (80 g ethanol over 9 h).

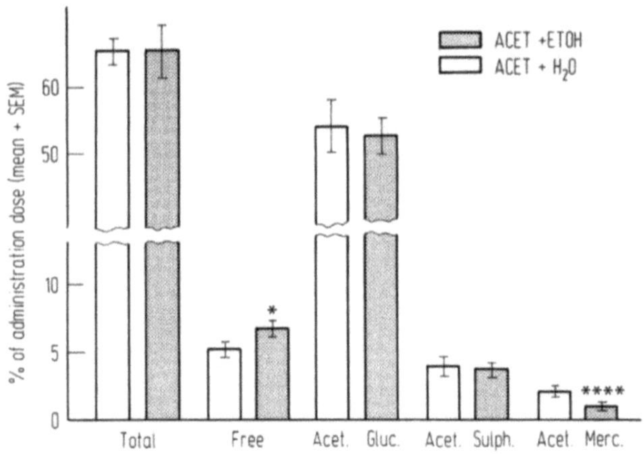


**Fig. 7.** Urinary excretion of acetaminophen and its metabolites in two groups of eight subjects receiving acetaminophen 1 g p.o. and ethanol 80 g over 8 h (▣) or acetaminophen 1 g p.o. and water according to the same regimen (□). Urines were collected over 8 h. Values are mean+/−SEM. *$p<0.05$; ****$p<0.001$ compared to the other group (From Altomare et al. 1986 [18])

In all experiments the subjects were overnight fasted and urinated before APAP ingestion.

Blood samples were taken at the time of APAP administration and after 1, 2, 4, and 8 h. Urines were collected throughout the experimental period. APAP and its metabolites were determined in blood and urine by HPLC [7-8]. Blood alcohol levels were measured by gas-liquid chromatography [16], and SGOT, SGPT, and bilirubin were assessed with a colorimetric test.

It was found that ethanol ingestion significantly increased APAP half-life (280.1 +/−11 min in the ethanol group vs 242.4+/−5 min in the control group $p<0.005$). The urinary excretion of APAP mercapturate proved to be significantly lower in the ethanol group than in the control group (water instead of alcohol) (Fig. 7). These results are in agreement with previous studies showing decreased formation of toxic APAP metabolite after acute ethanol administration. However, we also found a slight but significant increase in SGOT in the group treated with APAP and ethanol (Fig. 8). This rise was probably due to APAP-ethanol interaction, since the administration of APAP or alcohol alone produced no change in serum enzyme activities. Therefore the postulated prevention of APAP hepatotoxicity by acute ethanol in humans remains to be confirmed [17].

The interaction of ethanol and drugs is further complicated, during chronic alcohol abuse, by the degree of liver disease, which may affect the liver's capacity for detoxification. It is well known that GSH offers one of the mechanisms for the scavenging of toxic free radicals; a severe reduction in GSH favors lipid peroxidation [18] and the damage may possibly be compounded by the increased generation of active radicals by the induced microsomes following chronic ethanol consumption.

Both acute and chronic ethanol administration have been reported to cause decreased hepatic GSH content in rodents and baboons [19, 20]. However, the results of similar studies in humans have been conflicting or difficult to evaluate, mostly because

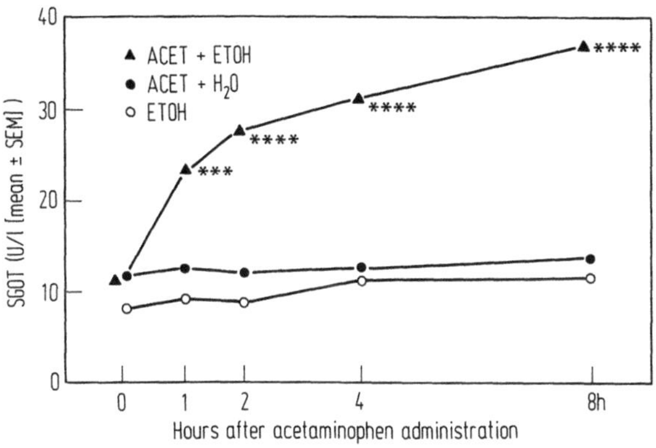


**Fig. 8.** Time course of SGOT in three groups of eight subjects receiving: ▲ = acetaminophen (1 g p.o.) + ethanol (80 g in 9 h); ● = acetaminophen (1 g p.o.) + water (some regimen); ○ = ethanol alone (80 g in 9 h). Values are mean +/− SEM. ***$p < 0.005$; ****$p < 0.001$ compared to the other two groups (From Altomare et al. [18])

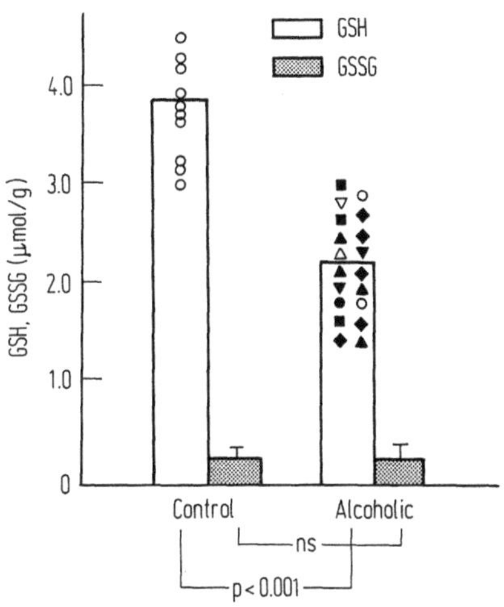


**Fig. 9.** GSH and GSSG concentration in hepatic tissues from control and alcoholic patients. Median values are indicated by the column heights, and the range is shown either by the bars (GSSG) or distributions of symbols (GSH). Each symbol represents one patient as follows: *open symbols*, subjects with normal values for all standard blood biochemical tests; *filled symbols*, patients with one or more blood changes; ●, no histologic changes; ▲, mild or moderate steatosis only; ■, severe steatosis only; ▼, hepatitis without extensive necrosis; ◆, hepatitis with extensive necrosis (From Altomare et al. 1986 [23])

of varying criteria for selection of control and alcoholic patients and, in some cases, unspecific GSH assay methods [21]. Therefore we carried out a study in order to evaluate both reduced (GSH) and oxidized (GSSG) glutathione by means of HPLC in liver biopsies from a group of selected chronic alcoholic patients ($n = 20$) and a group of appropriate controls ($n = 10$). Our results were also correlated with independent histology reports and blood chemistry values from the same subjects.

The GSH values obtained from liver biopsies of the control group (median 3.88 µmol/g liver) were found to comprise 93%-97% of the total soluble glutathione, the remainder being in the GSSG form. In all cases, the gross and microscopic appearance of the tissue was normal, as were hematologic tests of liver function. The small range of these data indicates that the control group was homogeneous in composition and appropriate as a standard for comparison with the alcoholic group. The glutathione values obtained from hepatic samples of the alcoholic group were found to be significantly lower than the controls (2.2+/−0.7 µmol/g liver vs 3.3+/−0.6, -< 0.001) (Fig. 9). This decrease was due to loss of GSH, since the GSSG concentration remained the same (median values: control = 0.18 vs 0.19 µmol/g liver for alcoholics). It must be pointed out, however, that alcoholic patients showed a high GSSG/(GSH + GSSG) ratio, which may be physiologically significant.

Since hepatic GSH plays an important role in detoxification of exogenous compounds by the liver, as well as in protection against oxidative injury induced by ethanol metabolism, the reported hepatic GSH depletion [22] may be an important contributory mechanism in the pathogenesis of alcoholic liver disease and may put alcoholic patients at higher risk of hepatotoxicity from a number of xenobiotic compounds.

## References

1. Lieber CS, de Carli LM (1970) Hepatic microsomal ethanol-oxidizing system: in vitro characteristics and adaptive properties in vivo. J Biol Chem 245: 2505-2512
2. Rubin E, Lieber CS (1968) Hepatic microsomal enzymes in man and rat: induction and inhibition by ethanol. Science 162: 690-691
3. Kater RMH, Roggin G, Tobon F (1969) Increased rate of clearance of drugs from the circulation of alcoholics. Am J Med Sci 258: 35-39
4. Rubin E, Lieber CS, Alvares AP, Levin W, Kuntzmann R (1971) Ethanol binding to hepatic microsomes: its increase by ethanol consumption. Biochem Pharmacol 20: 229-231
5. Whitehouse LW, Paul CJ, Coldwell BB, Thomas BH (1975) Effect of ethanol on diazepam distribution in rat. Res Commun Chem Pathol Pharmacol 12: 221-241
6. Liever CS, de Carli LM (1982) The feeding of alcohol in liquid diet: two decades of applications and 1982 update. Alcoholism Clin Exp Res 6: 523-531
7. Buckpitt AR, Rollins DE, Nelson SD, Franklin RB, Mitchell JR (1977) Quantitative determination of the glutathione, cysteine and N-acetyl cysteine conjugates of acetaminophen by high performance liquid chromatography. Anal Biochem 83: 168-177
8. Howie D, Adriaeussens PI, Prescott LF (1977) Paracetamol metabolism following overdosage: application of high performance liquid chromatography. J Pharm Pharmacol 29: 235-237
9. Jollow DJ, Mitchell JR, Potter WZ, Davis DC, Gillette JR, Brodie BB (1973) Acetaminophen-induced hepatic necrosis II. Role of covalent binding. J Pharmacol Exp Ther 187: 195-202
10. Altomare E, Leo MA, Sato C, Vendemiale G, Lieber CS (1984) Interaction of ethanol with acetaminophen metabolism in the baboon. Biochem Pharmacol 33: 2207-2214
11. Sato C, Matsuda Y, Lieber CS (1981) Increased hepatotoxicity of acetaminophen after chronic ethanol consumption in the rat. Gastroenterology 80: 140-148
12. Sato C, Nakano M, Lieber CS (1981) Prevention of acetaminophen induced hepatotoxicity by acute ethanol administration in the rat: comparison with carbon tetrachloride induced hepatotoxicity. J Pharmacol Exp Ther 218: 805-810
13. Altomare E, Leo MA, Lieber CS (1984) Interaction of acute ethanol administration with acetaminophen metabolism and toxicity in rats fed alcohol chronically. Alcoholism Clin Exp Res 8: 405-408
14. Vendemiale G, Altomare E, Lieber CS (1984) Altered biliary excretion of acetaminophen in rats fed ethanol chronically. Drug Metab Dispos 12: 20-24

15. Wright N, Prescott LF (1973) Potentiation by previous drug therapy of hepatotoxicity following paracetamol overdosage. Scott Med J 18: 56-58
16. Banda PW, Quart BD (1982) The effect of mild alcohol consumption on the metabolism of acetaminophen in man. Res Commun Chem Pathol Pharmacol 38: 57-70
17. Korsten MA, Matsuzaki S, Feinman L, Lieber CS (1975) High blood acetaldehyde levels after ethanol administration in alcoholics. N Engl J Med 292: 386-389
18. Altomare E, Vendemiale G, Trizio T, Albano O (1986) Does acute ethanol really protect against acetaminophen hepatotoxicity? Am J Gastroenterol 81: 91-93
19. Wendel A, Feuerstein S, Konz KH (1979) Acute paracetamol intoxication of starved mice leads to lipid peroxidation in vivo. Biochem Phys 28: 2051-2055
20. Guerri C, Grisolia S (1980) Changes in glutathione in acute and chronic intoxication. Pharmacol Biochem Behav [Suppl 1] 13: 53-61
21. Shaw S, Jayatilleke E, Ross WA, Gordon ER, Lieber CS (1981) Ethanol induced lipid peroxidation: potentiation by chronic alcohol feeding and attenuation by methionine. J Lab Clin Med 98: 417-424
22. Hissen PJ, Hilf R (1976) A fluorometric method for determination of oxidized and reduced glutathione in tissues. Anal Biochem 74: 214-226
23. Jewell SA, di Monte D, Gentile A, Guglielmi A, Altomare E, Albano O (1986) Decreased hepatic glutathione in chronic alcoholic patients. J Hepatol (in press)

# Antioxidant and Immunomodulant Effect of Hepatoprotective Drugs

János Fehér[1], Ágnes Cornides[2], and Géza Csomós[3]

[1] Second Department of Medicine, Semmelweis University, Budapest, Hungary
[2] First Department of Medicine, County Hospital, Székesfehérvár, Hungary
[3] Madäus Clinical Research, Hamburg, Federal Republic of Germany

## Introduction

The problems in the therapy of chronic liver diseases have not been solved. Owing to the variety of the causal factors in the pathogenesis of chronic liver lesions, various drugs are being used. Some of them are applied in inflammatory reactions of the liver, others are used as cytoprotective agents in toxic liver cell alterations. However, there is no specific and unequivocally effective drug for these conditions.

In general we use drugs against viral and bacterial infections, drugs for immune correction (for immune suppression or in other cases for immune stimulation), drugs for substitution (e.g., folic acid), and drugs for liver cell protection. The effectiveness of this treatment, however, can hardly be assessed either in human examinations or in animal experiments.

In this paper we demonstrate our results in various experimental models in the field of toxic liver lesions and in the therapy of chronic liver diseases.

## Materials and Methods

Ten patients (six man and four women, mean age 44 ± 10 years) suffering from chronic alcoholic liver disease were involved in the study. Peripheral blood mononuclear cells (PBMC) were separated from heparinized venous blood on a Ficoll (Pharmacia) Uromiro (Bracco) gradient (Bøyum 1968).

The naturally occurring flavonolignone silymarin (Fig. 1) (Legalon, Madäus, Cologne) was studied in the in vitro lymphocyte blast transformation test system in a concentration range of 0.1-10.0 µg/ml, corresponding to the usual therapeutic doses of the drug calculated according to the formula of Hirschaut (1969). Silibinin was present in the medium during the whole incubation period.

For the lymphocyte blast transformation test the separated PBMC were resuspended in TC-199 medium supplemented with 10% heat-inactivated fetal calf serum (Human, Budapest), antibiotics, and 25 m*M* HEPES (Serva). Then $2 \times 10^5$ cells in five replicates were placed into flat-bottomed microplates (Greiner). Con A (Calbiochem) or PHA (Pharmacia) was added to a final concentration of 25 µg/ml (Con A) or 2 µg/ml and 10 µg/ml (PHA). The cultures were kept in a humidified atmosphere at 37 °C for 72 h. Eight hours before harvesting, 0.5 µCi $^3$H-thymidine (UVVVR, Czechoslovakia) was added to each well. The cultures were sucked off into glass fiber filters (Whatman GF/c). Isotope determination was made in a Nuclear Chicago Isocap 300 counter and the results were expressed in cpm.

Assessment and Management of Hepatobiliary Disease
Eds.: L. Okolicsányi, G. Csomós, and G. Crepaldi

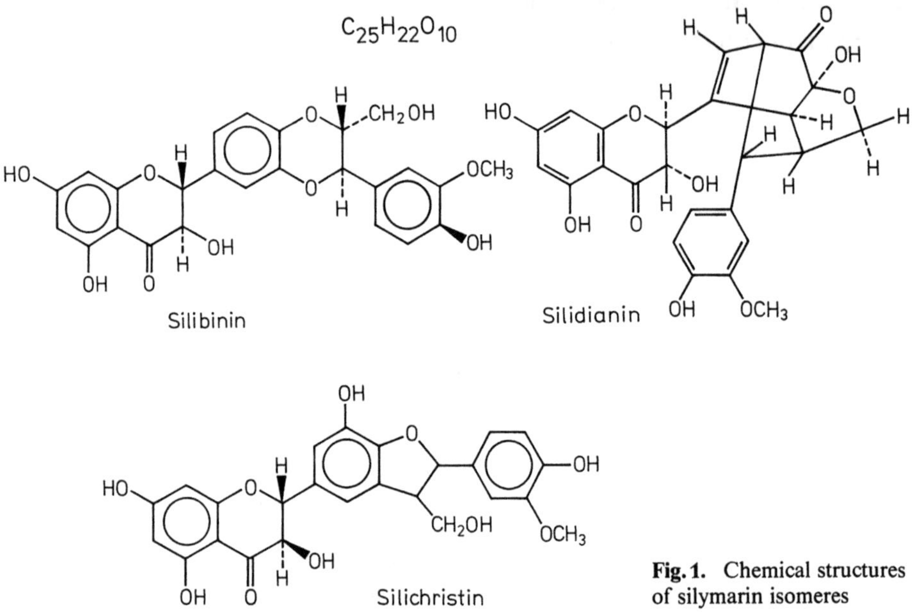


**Fig. 1.** Chemical structures of silymarin isomeres

The superoxide dismutase CSOD; E.C. 1.15.1.1) activities of erythrocytes and lymphocytes were determined by the method of Misra and Fridovich (1972). The method is based on the spontaneous auto-oxidation of epinephrine to adrenochrome in the presence of air at pH 10.2. The inhibition of this process depends on the amount of SOD. Results are given in units. One unit refers to the amount of enzyme causing a 50% inhibition of auto-oxidation during 1 min. Spectrophotometric measurements were performed with Spectromom 204 equipment at 37 °C and 480 nm.

*Erythrocyte* lysates from patients and healthy individuals were prepared by adding distilled water to packed erythrocytes previously washed with isotonic saline solution. Hemoglobin was precipitated with a chloroform-ethanol mixture. The pale-yellow supernatant obtained after centrifugation was used for estimating the specific activity of SOD (McCord and Fridovich 1969; Vanella et al. 1983).

*Lymphocytes* were separated from heparinized venous blood on a Ficoll-Uromiro gradient (Bøyum 1968). Phagocytic cells were removed by carbonyl-iron treatment. Viability as judged by the trypan blue test was greater than 98%. Monocyte contamination was less than 2%. Cells were suspended in PBS. Lymphocyte membranes were disrupted by sonication in ice-cold PBS. After centrifugation, enzyme analysis was performed from the supernatants. All data were expressed as units of total SOD per milliliter of sample.

The in vivo effect of silibinin on the Con A-induced blast transformation of rat spleen cells and on liver lysosomal fraction, as well as on enzymatically induced lipid peroxidation in rat microsomes, were studied in animals fed an atherogenic diet. Details of the methods are found in our previous publications (Fehér et al. 1982, 1985a, b; Somogyi et al. 1986).

Statistical analysis was performed using Student's *t*-test. The distribution of mean values of the total results (± SE) was determined.

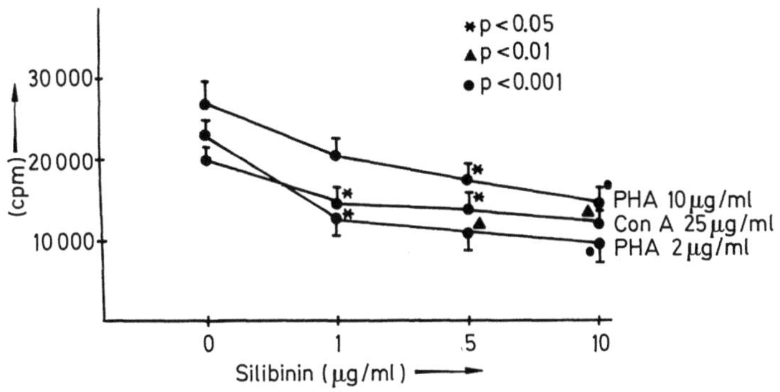


**Fig. 2.** Effect of in vitro treatment with silibinin on the lectin-induced lymphoblast transformation of healthy subjects

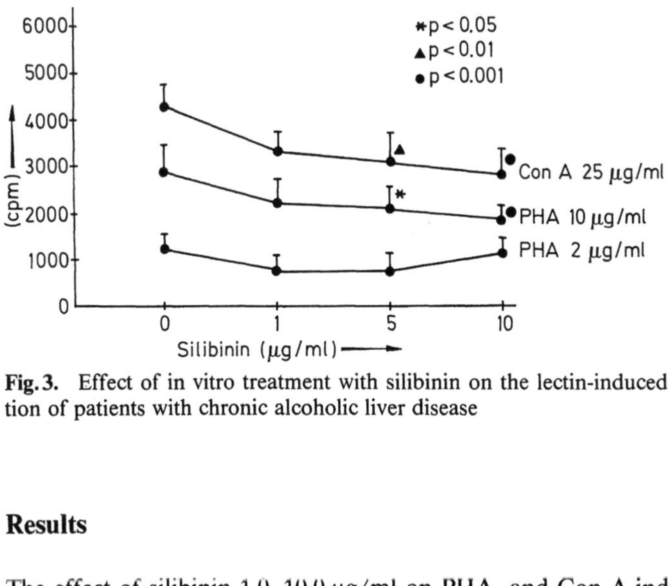


**Fig. 3.** Effect of in vitro treatment with silibinin on the lectin-induced lymphoblast transformation of patients with chronic alcoholic liver disease

## Results

The effect of silibinin 1.0–10.0 µg/ml on PHA- and Con A-induced lymphocyte blast transformation of normal individuals and of patients with chronic alcoholic liver disease is shown in Figs. 2 and 3. Using a suboptimal dose of PHA, silibinin exerted no significant effect on blastogenesis in a concentration range corresponding to the usual in vivo therapeutic concentration. However, using an optimal stimulatory dose of PHA, silibinin significantly decreased $^3$H-thymidine incorporation at a concentration of 10.0 µg/ml (1889 ± 507 vs 2979 ± 885 cpm, $p < 0.05$). In the presence of 25 µg/ml Con A, silibinin inhibited in vitro lymphocyte blast transformation of the patients in a dose-dependent fashion.

Total SOD activities of the erythrocytes and lymphocytes of patients and of healthy individuals are summarized in Fig. 4. Patients with chronic alcoholic liver disease had significantly lower mean erythrocyte and lymphocyte SOD activities than the healthy control group. After 1 month treatment with silibinin the originally decreased SOD values of the patients increased significantly both in erythrocytes and in lymphocytes.

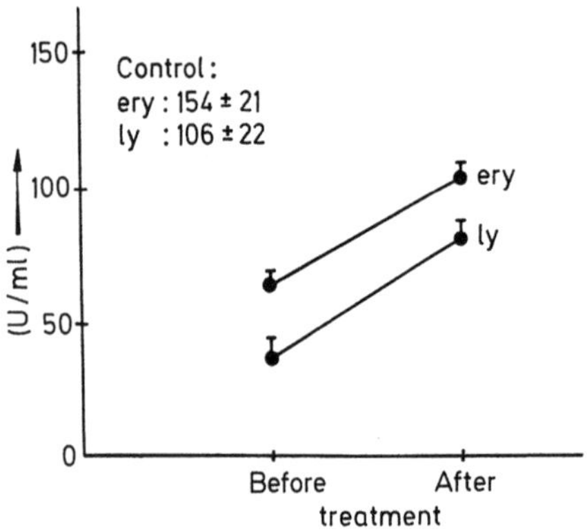


**Fig. 4.** Effect of treatment with silibinin on erythrocyte and lymphocyte SOD activity (U/ml) of patients with chronic alcoholic liver disease. *ery*, erythrocyte; *ly*, lymphocyte

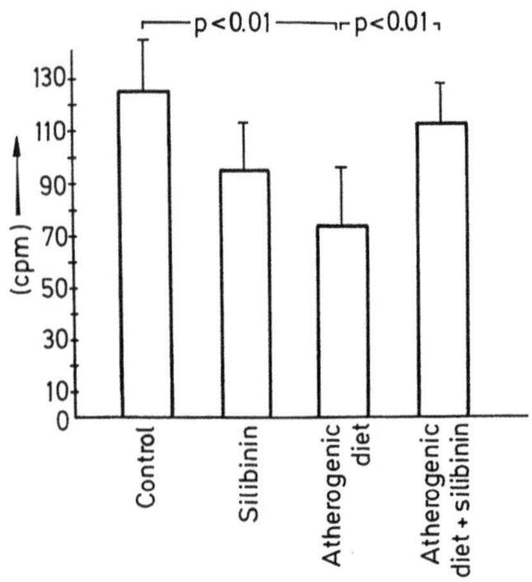


**Fig. 5.** In vivo effect of silibinin on the Con A-induced (10 μg/ml) blast transformation of rat spleen cells

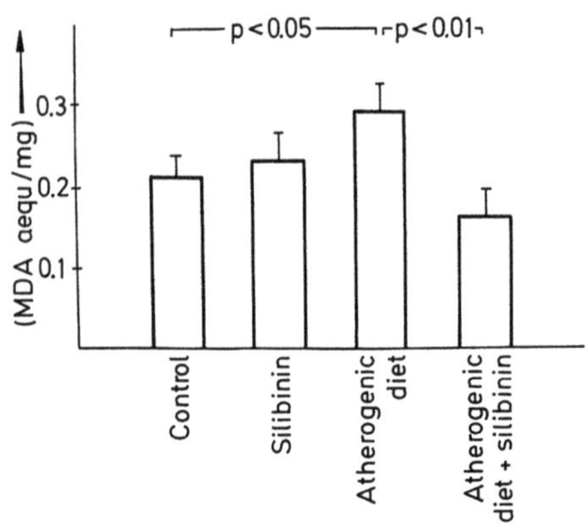


**Fig. 6.** Effect of silibinin on liver lysosomal fraction of rats on atherogenic diet

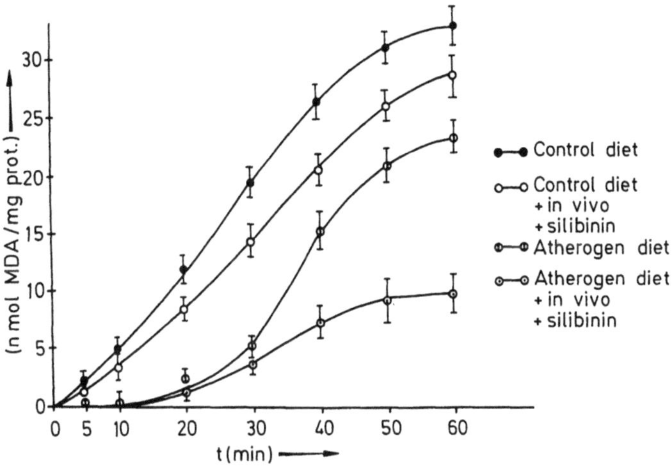


**Fig. 7.** In vivo inhibitory effect of silibinin on NADPH + Iron-induced lipid peroxidation in rat microsomes (dose: 25 mg/kg × 5 days)

The atherogenic diet highly significantly inhibited the Con A-induced blast transformation of rat spleen cells in the in vivo experiments. The silibinin was able to prevent this reaction (Fig. 5). A similar effect of silibinin was found in the lysosomal examinations of rat liver. The malondialdehyde (MDA) equivalent content of liver lysosomal membrane was increased in the animals fed an atherogenic diet. The silibinin treatment normalized the MDA equivalent content of lysosomes (Fig. 6). The enzymatically induced lipid peroxidation was inhibited with in vivo silibinin treatment both in the control animals and in rats fed an atherogenic diet (Fig. 7).

## Discussion

Prospective drugs for the treatment of chronic liver diseases should act through one or more of the following mechanisms: stabilization of the membrane of hepatocytes, protection against "oxygen stress" via the free radical scavenger effect, and support of the immunological defense of the organism. The two extensively used hepatoprotective agents, silibinin ad (+)-cyanidanol-3, are known for their membrane-protecting and antioxidant effects (Bindoli et al. 1977; Fehér et al. 1985a); furthermore, immunomodulating activity of the latter has also been demonstrated. However, sporadic occurrence of immune hemolytic anemia as a side effect of (+)-cyanidalol-3 has recently restricted its clinical use (Neftel et al. 1981). Silibinin has normalized decreased hepatic functions in experimental cases of liver damage and has also exerted beneficial effects in clinical studies (Fehér et al. 1986). We studied its effect on cellular immune reactivity in the lectin-induced lymphocyte blast transformation assay. Using optimal stimulatory doses of lectins, silibinin inhibited both PHA- and Con A-induced blastogenesis of lymphocytes from patients with chronic alcoholic liver disease in a dose-dependent fashion.

Our present results suggest that suppression of cellular immune reactivity might be one of the factors of the hepatoprotective activity of silibinin.

The mechanisms by which the advantageous antioxidant effects of silibinin in lipid peroxidation and lysosomal activity are exerted are not yet completely clear. More stable lysosomal membranes seem to protect against lysosomal breakdown, which causes tissue injury, and at the same time make lysosomal digestion of harmful materials, including cholesterol, more complete. Another antiatherosclerotic characteristic of antioxidant therapy is the raised prostacyclin level and inhibition of formation of some harmful endoperoxides (Fehér et al. 1984).

## Summary

Silibinin is one of the most frequently used hepatoprotective drugs. Its effect on the cell membrane was studied in both in vitro and in vivo models. Because the hepatoprotective drugs have their effect partly as free radical scavengers, partly as immunomodulators, we applied the following tests: blast transformation, suppressor cell activity, expression of superoxide dismutase (SOD) on lymphocytes with cytofluorimetry, measurement of SOD activity in erythrocytes and lymphocytes. The examinations were carried out on cells from healthy persons and from patients with chronic alcoholic liver disease. The in vivo effect was studied after silibinin treatment in patients with alcoholic liver disease. The silibinin produced a dose-dependent inhibition of lectin-induced blast transformation both in healthy persons and in patients with liver diseases in vitro. The in vivo treatment with silibinin restored the originally decreased SOD activity of erythrocytes and lymphocytes in chronic liver disease. In addition, the effect of silibinin on lipid peroxidation and lysosomal function was studied in rats fed an atherogenic diet. The silibinin in vivo was able to prevent the pathological effect of the atherogenic diet. On the basis of these data the antioxidant and immunomodulant effects of silibinin play a role in liver cell protection.

## References

Bindoli A, Cavallini L, Siliprandi N (1977) Inhibitory action of silymarin on lipid peroxide formation in rat liver mitochrondria and microsomes. Biochem Pharmacol 26: 2405

Bøyum A (1968) Separation of lymphocytes from blood and bone marrow. Scand J Clin Lab Invest 21 [Suppl 97]: 1-109

Fehér J, Bär-Pollák Z, Stéter L, Fehér E, Toncsev H (1982) Biochemical markers in carbontetrachloride- and galactosamine-induced acute liver injuries: the effects of dihydroquinoline-type antioxidants. Br J Exp Pathol 63: 394-400

Fehér J, Sulyok S, Pollák Z, Toncsev H, Cornides A, Blázovics A, Szondy É, Geró S (1984) The effect of a recently developed dihydroquinoline-type radical scavenger in cholesterol induced hyperlipidaemia. In: Lenzi S, Descovich GC (eds) Atherosclerosis and cardiovascular diseases. Editrice Compositori, Bologna

Fehér J, Blázovics A, Cornides A, Vereckei A (1985a) Effect of (+)-cyanidanol-3 on rat brain lipid peroxidation. Br J Exp Pathol 66: 161-164

Fehér J, Kiss Á, Blázovics A, Szondy É, Toncsev H, Mathiász D, Gerő S (1985b) Hypolipaemic effect and inhibition of lipid peroxidation by glunicate in rats on atherogenic diet. Drugs Exp Clin Res 11 (6): 413-419

Fehér J, Láng I, Nékám K, Csomós G, Müzes G, Deák G (1986) Effect of silibinin on the activity and expression of superoxide dismutase (SOD) in lymphocytes from patients with chronic alcoholic liver disease. Free Radical Res Comm

Hirschaut Y, Weiss BM, Perry S (1969) The use of long-term human leucocyte cell cultures as models for the study of antileukemic agents. Cancer Res 29: 1732

McCord JM, Fridovich I (1969) Superoxide dismutase: an enzymic function for erythrocuprein (hemocuprein). J Biol Chem 244: 6049-6055

Misra HP, Fridovich I (1972) The role of superoxide anion in the autooxidation of epinephrine and a simple assay for superoxide dismutase. J Biol Chem 247: 3170-3175

Neftel KA, Japp H, Diem P, Walti M (1981) (+) Cyanidanol-3 induced immune haemolytic anaemia. In: Conn HO (ed) International workshop on (+) cyanidanol-3 in diseases of the liver. Academic, London, p 223

Somogyi A, Rhenso Conzáles-Cabello, Szondy É, Blázovics A, Gergely P, Fehér J (1986) (to be published) Allergologia et Immunopathologia

Vanella A, Geremia E, Pinturo R, Piriolo P (1983) Superoxide dismutase activity and reduced glutathione content in erythrocytes of uremic patients on chronic dialysis. Acta Haematol 70: 312-315

# Stimulating Influence of a Flavonolignane Derivative on Proliferation, RNA Synthesis and Protein Synthesis in Liver Cells

J. Sonnenbichler and I. Zetl

Department of Membrane Biochemistry, Max-Planck-Institut für Biochemie, 8033 Martinsried, Federal Republic of Germany

Extracts of the plant *Silybum marianum* have been used for better recovery in cases of liver disease for many centuries. As active principle, Wagner et al. (1965) and also Pelter and Hänsel (1968) isolated the flavonolignane derivative silibinin.

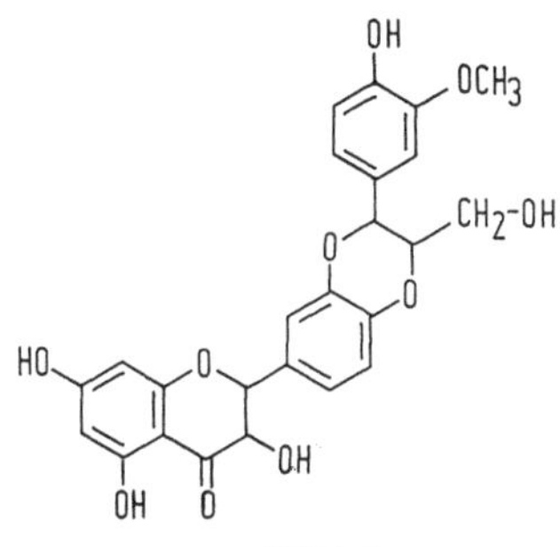


Silibinin

In 1980 Fintelmann and Albert and some other groups published clinical data which clearly demonstrate that silibinin increases the regeneration potency of damaged livers. From the biochemical point of view, regeneration potency of a tissue means stimulation of the metabolic pathway in a cell in connection with influences on the synthesis of macromolecules. To investigate this hypothesis we measured protein synthesis in rat livers in vivo following the incorporation of $^{35}$S-methionine or $^{14}$C-leucin as precursors into protein in the presence and absence of silibinin.

From Fig. 1 it can be seen that after application of silibinin protein synthesis is indeed increased by about 40%. The right columns furthermore demonstrate that even damage of the livers by D-galactosamine in amounts which reduce protein synthesis dramatically can be neutralized. We observed similar effects with hepatocytes in vitro.

In order to get more insight into the molecular biology of this stimulatory effect we asked if there might be specific effects on definite polypeptides. All liver proteins were isolated and fractionated in one-dimensional and two-dimensional electrophoretic systems with autoradiographic detection. We could find no differences in the pattern or in the labeling of distinct proteins. The conclusion had to be drawn that protein synthesis in general is increased by some mechanism but without preference of specific polypeptides.

At this point our intention was to elucidate the molecular mechanism by which the flavonolignane silibinin stimulates the macromolecular synthesis. It will be shown that silibinin primarily increases the enzyme activity of RNA polymerase I, thus stimulating rRNA synthesis either in isolated organelles or in hepatocytes and in rat livers (Son-

Assessment and Management of Hepatobiliary Disease
Eds.: L. Okolicsányi, G. Csomós, and G. Crepaldi

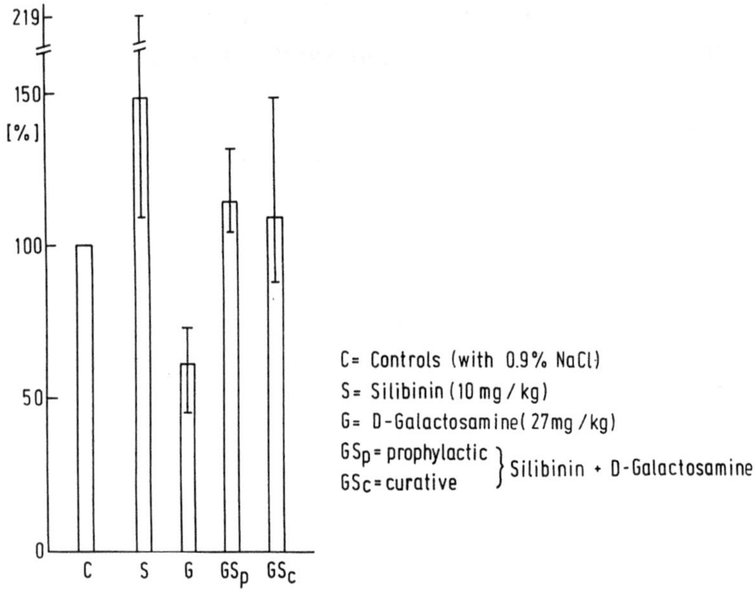


**Fig. 1.** [14]C-Leu incorporation (1.5-h pulse) into rat liver proteins after application of various drugs (3 h before killing)

nenbichler and Zetl, 1984). As a result of this stimulation the formation of ribosomes is accelerated; consequently protein synthesis, and in regenerating livers even DNA replication, is increased.

To explain the background for our biochemical experiments concerning nucleic acid and protein synthesis I would like to refer to the basic processes of gene transcription and translation (Fig. 2).

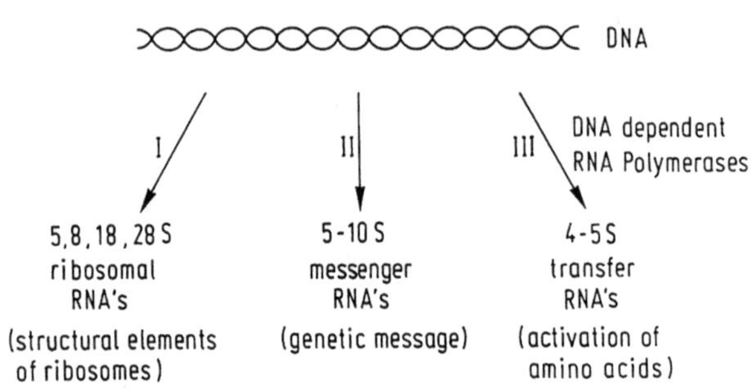


**Fig. 2.** Gene transcription

In eukaryotic cells the DNA is transcribed by the DNA-dependent RNA polymerases I, II, and III to different RNA types. Polymerase I is competent for the transcription of the rRNAs which are constituents of the ribosomes. Polymerase II synthesizes the mRNAs which bear the genetic information, and polymerase III forms the small tRNAs which are necessary to activate the amino acids during the translation process in protein synthesis. Protein synthesis then follows RNA synthesis. Specific precursors for all macromolecules can be used with a radioactive label as indicators for synthesis.

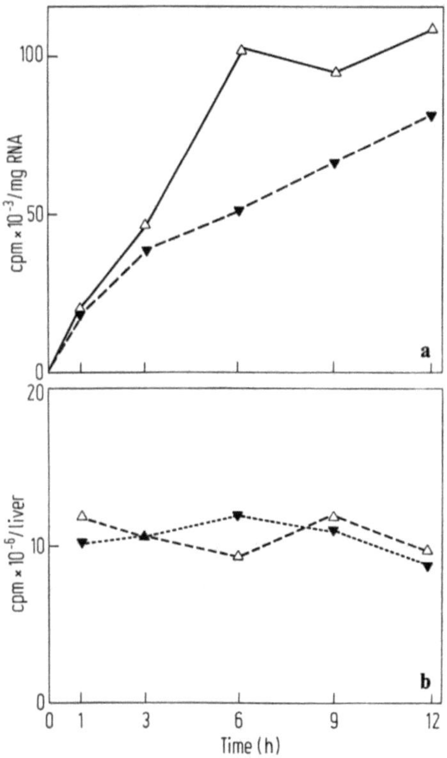


**Fig. 3a.** Specific radioactivities of liver RNA. **b** Precursor concentrations (cpm/g liver) △, after treatment with Silibinin; ▼, controls

The question was whether silibinin already influences the transcription process which precedes protein synthesis. We therefore investigated RNA synthesis in vivo in a series of experiments with rats and measured the dose and time dependence of uridine incorporation after intraperitoneal application of silibinin. As precursor, radioactive orotic acid was given. After defined times the livers were resected and the RNA was isolated. Parallel to the analysis of the specific radioactivity of the RNA, it had to be checked that the pools of radioactive precursor were the same in the livers with and without silibinin treatment, otherwise differences in the specific radioactivity of the newly synthesized RNA would have resulted (Fig. 3).

From Fig. 3 it can be seen that the precursor pools in the livers are quite similar and independent of the application of (small doses of) silibinin. In the presence of the flavonoligane, however, the rate of RNA synthesis is significantly higher than in the controls. In the experiments a maximum stimulation effect can be observed with about 25 mg silibinin/kg rat (Sonnenbichler and Zetl 1984).

The question had to be asked whether the increase in RNA synthesis is a general one concerning all RNA species or whether this stimulatory effect is specific, for instance affecting only the rRNA or mRNA or tRNA species.

After isolation the RNAs were fractionated by electrophoresis on agarose gels or by sucrose gradient centrifugations and the specific radioactivities were analyzed (Table 1).

From Table 1 it can be seen that the specific radioactivities of the RNA from sili-

**Table 1.** Specific radioactivities (cpm/mg) of RNAs from silibinin-treated rats and controls

a) rRNA

| | Total RNA | 28S RNA (43%) | 18S RNA (23%) |
|---|---|---|---|
| Treated with silibinin | 138800 | 83250 | 74000 |
| Controls | 69700 | 64750 | 42310 |

b) Small RNAs

| | Cytoplasmic RNA | tRNA (7.2%) | 5S RNA (1.4%) | 5.8S RNA (1.2%) |
|---|---|---|---|---|
| Treated with silibinin | 282000 | 105560 | 91220 | 67230 |
| Controls | 223000 | 104260 | 89050 | 50410 |

c) mRNA

| | Cytoplasmic RNA | Nuclear RNA | mRNA (cytoplasma) (1.3%) | mRNA (nuclei) (0.7-2%) |
|---|---|---|---|---|
| Treated with silibinin | 282000 | 626000 | 908900 | 68500 (2%) |
| Controls | 223000 | 402200 | 1042000 | 73900 (0.7%) |

binin-treated and untreated rats are quite similar in the case of the mRNAs, the small tRNAs, and the 5S RNA, but remarkable different for 5.8S RNA, 18S RNA, and 28S RNA. Also, great differences have been found for the 45S RNA species, which is not listed in the table but which represents the primary transcription product for the 5.8, 18S, and 28S RNAs. The data show that silibinin specifically stimulates the transcription rate of rRNA.

Hepatocytes in culture can also be used to study RNA synthesis. With tritium-labeled uridine as one of the nucleotide precursors, the time-dependent course of RNA formation can be measured, and we found that in the presence of silibinin the RNA synthesis in hepatocytes is also stimulated (Fig. 4).

Optimal stimulatory effects can be seen with 2–5 μg silibinin/ml medium. In this range an increase of RNA synthesis of about 40% is observed (Sonnenbichler et al. 1976).

To follow up the question of by what molecular mechanism the drug can accomplish the effect on RNA synthesis, a series of experiments was done in vitro with isolated nuclei and also nucleoli which still have the ability to synthesize RNA. Indeed, the time-dependent rate of RNA synthesis in isolated nuclei is affected in the presence of different silibinin concentrations (Fig. 5). With nuclei a maximum of stimulation can be seen with about 5 μg silibinin/ml.

In the following experiments the isolated RNA polymerases I and II were used with pure DNA from calf thymus as a template in buffer with tritium-labeled uridine triphosphate to perform RNA synthesis (Fig. 6).

With polymerase II (inhibited by amanitin and competent for the production of mRNA) we could find no effect of silibinin on the time course of transcription. With

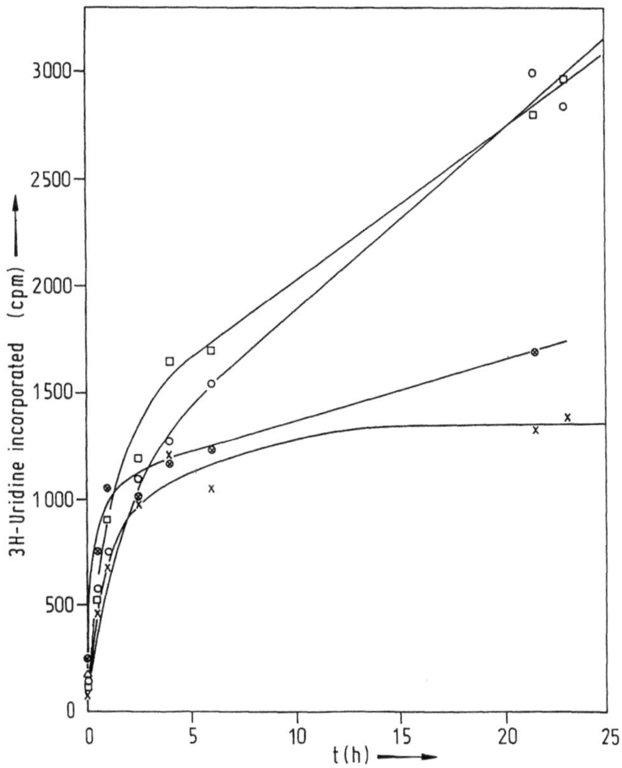


**Fig. 4.** Time-dependent course of RNA formation with $^3$H-uridine as one of the precursors ($5 \times 10^3$ hepatocytes/ml). ○, silibinin in DMSO/$H_2O$ 1:1; □, silibinin dihemisuccinate in $H_2O$; ⊗, control with DMSO/$H_2O$ 1:1; ×, control with $H_2O$

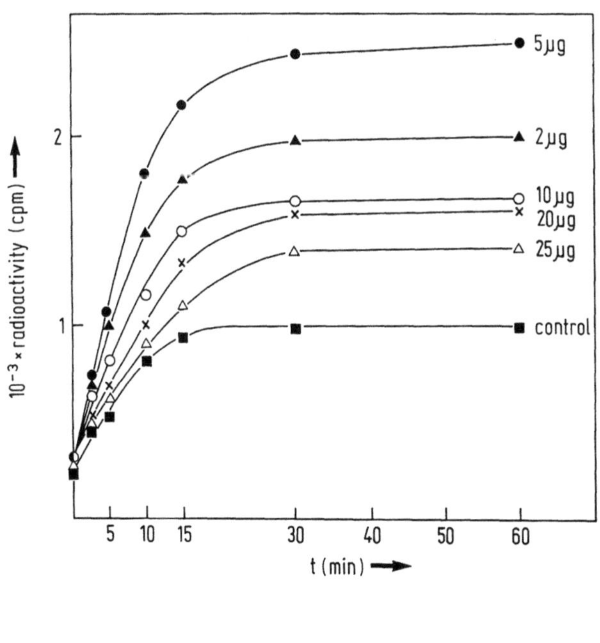


**Fig. 5.** Effect of various doses of silibinin on the time-dependent rate of RNA

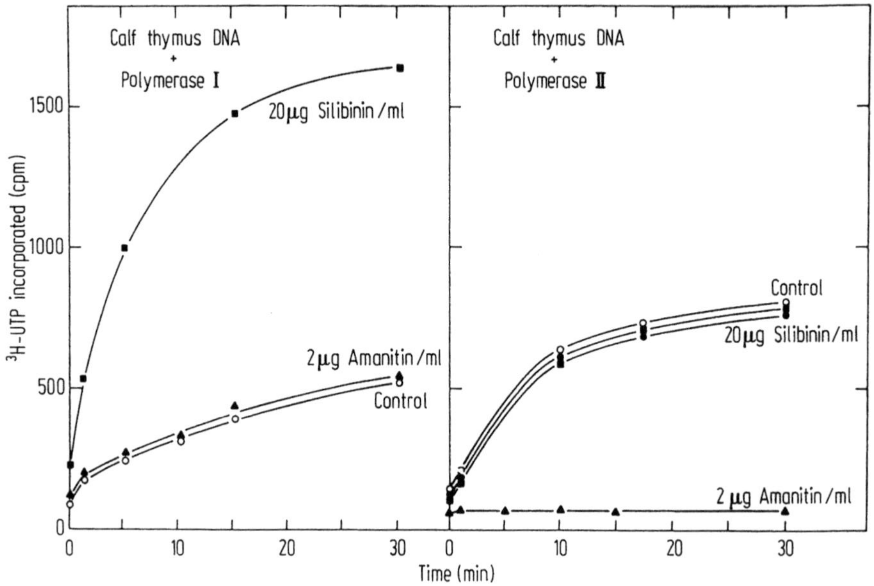


**Fig. 6.** Effect of silibinin on time course of transcription when isolated RNA polymerases I and II were used with pure calf thymus DNA as template in buffer with tritium-labeled uridine triphosphate *($^3$H-UTP)*

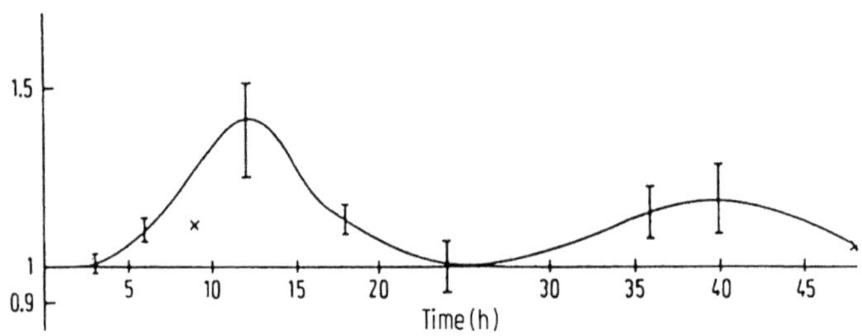


**Fig. 7.** Quotient specific radioactivity of RNA (silibinin-treated/controls)

polymerase I (not sensitive to amanitin and competent for the transcription of the ribosomal genes) a remarkable increase in the rate of synthesis was found (Machicao and Sonnenbichler 1977). From corresponding Michaelis-Menten plots with the purified polymerases it can be deduced that the enzyme is activated by the drug to an extent comparable with the action of some stimulatory enzyme effectors.

rRNA synthesis is a primary step for ribosome formation. Ribosomes are built from the rRNAs together with about 84 proteins and can be considered as the "sewing machine" within the cytoplasma for protein synthesis. Does the effect of silibinin on rRNA transcription consequently influence ribosome synthesis?

In Fig. 7 the relative increase in ribosome formation is plotted vs time of application of the drug. One can see that there are two waves of response, one (the larger) about 12 h after application of silibinin and the second after about 35 h.

**Table 2.** DNA synthesis in (a) normal livers, (b) after partial hepatectomy (68%) with and without silibinin treatment

| Silibinin 2′, 3-dihydrogensuccinate sodium salt (mg/kg body weight) | Number of Rats | $10^{-3}\times$ dpm/mg DNA | Precursor pool: radioactivity $10^{-3}\times$ dpm/g liver tissue (containing about 3 mg DNA) |
|---|---|---|---|
| a) 0 (controls) | 16 | 105 ± 12 | 1109 ± 18 |
| 17 | 3 | 127 ± 26 | 1017 ± 27 |
| 30 | 10 | 99 ± 9 | 1210 ± 9 |
| 50 | 3 | 118 ± 16 | 1314 ± 41 |
| b) 0 (controls) | 10 | 1922 ± 287 | 10285 ± 1003 |
| 0 | 10 | 1921 ± 338 | 10339 ± 1636 |
| 27 | 10 | 2367 ± 326 | 10261 ± 1846 |
| 27 | 10 | 2306 ± 290 | 9343 ± 1304 |

Results expressed as mean ± SD

When the rate of ribosome synthesis is accelerated, the potential of the "sewing machine" for translation is increased; therefore, effects on protein synthesis can be expected, as was shown at the beginning of this paper. The above-described experiments give us detailed information on the basis of the molecular action of the drug.

As stated before, it is known from clinical findings that silibinin supports the regeneration activity of liver tissue after intoxication. From the biochemical point of view, regeneration activity means an increase in protein synthesis, which has been demonstrated, but also in proliferation and DNA synthesis. Protein synthesis and RNA synthesis are prerequisites for DNA synthesis. So it seemed reasonable that DNA synthesis might also be influenced by the flavonolignane derivative.

To measure DNA synthesis, radioactive thymidine was given to rats as a precursor (Table 2). In livers of normal rats we could detect no effect of silibinin, either on the rate of proliferation or on the rate of DNA synthesis. In livers of hepatectomized rats, however, a significant effect of silibinin was observed. From Table 2 it can be seen that after hepatectomy the rate of DNA synthesis in liver cells increases dramatically. The increase after treatment with silibinin is still greater, by about 25%–30%. This means that if the trigger for DNA synthesis and proliferation is once given, the stimulation of RNA and protein synthesis by silibinin also increases the rate of DNA synthesis. This confirms the clinical finding of Fintelmann and Albert (1980).

The described effect of silbinin on such a fundamental process as transcription is fascinating, because here we find the action of a plant drug on an animal enzyme system. The question arises of what structures of the silibinin molecule might be responsible for the effect and whether there is any relationship to known enzyme effectors in animal cells.

In transcription systems with nuclei and hepatocytes the influence of about 40 flavonoids and flavonolignane compounds on RNA synthesis was investigated. Only four of these compounds showed an effect similar to that of silibinin (Sonnenbichler and Pohl 1980). We had tried to elaborate the partial structure which seems to be essential. On the basis of this work the speculation was raised that there might be a relationship to some steroid hormones which are well-known effectors in the regulation of animal

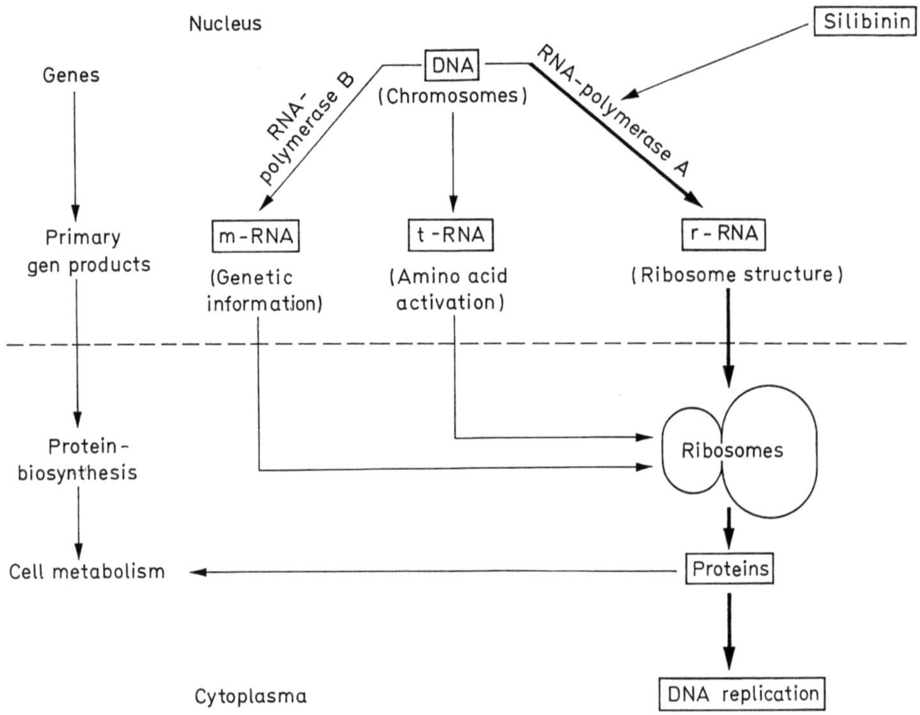


**Fig. 8.** Summary of results

cells but which also show effects on polymerase I similar to those of silibinin. This hypothesis is now proved. Silibinin fits into a specific binding site on the enzyme and in this way causes the observed stimulation of rRNA synthesis, ribosome formation, protein synthesis, and also proliferation.

The described drug does indeed seem interesting for liver therapy.

## References

Fintelmann V, Albert A (1980) Nachweis der therapeutischen Wirksamkeit von Legalon bei toxischen Lebererkrankungen im Doppelblindversuch. Therapiewoche 30: 5589-5594

Pelter A, Hänsel R (1968) The Structure of Silybin (Silibum Substance $E_6$), the first Flavonolignan. Tetrahedron Lett 2911-2916

Machicao F, Sonnenbichler J (1977) Mechanism of the Stimulation of RNA Synthesis in Rat Liver Nuclei by Silybin. Hoppe-Seylers Z Physiol Chem 358: 141-147

Sonnenbichler J, Mattersberger J, Rosen H (1976) Stimulierung der RNA-Synthese in Rattenleber und in isolierten Hepatozyten durch Silybin, einen antihepatotoxischen Wirkstoff aus Silybum marianum L. Gaertn Hoppe-Seyler's Z Physiol Chem 357: 1171-1180

Sonnenbichler J, Pohl A (1980) Untersuchungen zum Wirkungsmechanismus von Silybin IV[1] Struktur-Wirkungsbeziehungen. Hoppe Seyler's Z Physiol Chem 361: 1757-1761

Sonnenbichler J, Zetl I (1984) Untersuchungen zum Wirkungsmechanismus von Silibinin, V [1] Einfluß von Silibinin auf die Synthese ribosomaler RNA, mRNA und tRNA in Rattenlebern in vivo. Hoppe Seyler's Z Physiol Chem 365: 555-566

Wagner H, Hörhammer L, Münster R (1965) Über die Struktur eines neuen Flavonoids aus den Früchten von Carduus Marianus L. (Mariendistel). Naturwissenschaften 52: 305

# Renal Functional Impairment in Cirrhosis*

P. Gentilini, G. Laffi, G. La Villa, M. Pinzani, and F. Cominelli
Clinica Medica IV, Università degli Studi di Firenze, Firenze, Italy

The term "liver-kidney syndrome" was introduced into the medical literature to describe acute renal failure in patients undergoing surgery for cholestasis (Heyd 1931). Later, the term "hepatorenal syndrome" (HRS) was extensively used to indicate many pathological conditions affecting both liver and kidney (Lichtman and Sohval 1937). Renal functional impairment in acute and chronic liver disease was also included. However, without a clear definition, the inclusion of different types of liver and kidney disease under the same terminology is confusing. More recently, a clear classification of all diseases affecting both liver and kidney has been suggested and is listed in Table 1. The term "hepatorenal syndrome" has been proposed to define only renal functional impairment (RFI) of cirrhosis, i.e., the last situation included under part "C" of the table. In fact, HRS can be defined as an unexplained renal failure occurring in patients with cirrhosis in the absence of clinical or anatomical evidence of other known causes of renal failure (Vaamonde and Papper 1979). All the other clinical situations listed in Table 1 have also been described as pseudo-HRS (Conn 1973). One of the most important features of the pseudo-HRS syndromes is prerenal azotemia, a reduction of renal blood flow and glomerular filtration rate which follows a decrease of effective plasma volume induced by factors such as bleeding, intractable vomiting, profuse diarrhea, inappropriate diuretic administration, and paracentesis. The clinical features of prerenal azotemia are very similar to those of HRS. The two forms, however, can be distinguished easily on the basis of the response to plasma expanders, which leads to a recovery of renal function only in prerenal azotemia. The lack of response to plasma volume expansion should be recognized after both acute and chronic expansion, the latter being effective in some cases (Gentilini and Migone 1981).

Two different phases of RFI in cirrhosis (HRS) can be observed, the first being a less severe, pre-azotemic state, which can be defined as latent HRS, and the second being the clinically evident stage, as reported in Table 2.

The second stage need not necessarily follow the first, but may occur abruptly and spontaneously, especially if a sudden reduction of plasma volume takes place due to bleeding, intractable vomiting, etc. In this case, however, the latter have no etiological significance but act as precipitating factors, and plasma expansion is unable to reverse the clinical course of renal failure.

No alteration in renal morphology is observed in either phase of RFI (Gentilini et al. 1984). Moreover, kidney transplant or liver graft is followed by complete recovery of renal function.

* The work was supported by grants from the Ministero Pubblica Istruzione, Progetto Nazionale Cirrosi Epatica (1984) and from the Consiglio Nazionale delle Ricerche (no. 85.00757).

Assessment and Management of Hepatobiliary Disease
Eds.: L. Okolicsányi, G. Csomós, and G. Crepaldi

**Table 1.** Classification of pathological situations involving both the liver and the kidney

A. Disorders with simultaneous liver and kidney involvement
 1. *Congenital*
  Polycystic disease
  Caroli's syndrome
  Sickle cell anemia
 2. *Toxic agents*
  Vegetable toxins (toadstools)
  Drugs (tetracyclin, halothane, sulfamides, streptomycin, paracetamol, etc.)
  Industrial toxins (carbon tetrachloride, copper sulfate, chromium)
 3. *Systemic*
  Infections (yellow fever, sepsis, miliary tuberculosis, hepatitis B, etc.)
  Connective tissue diseases
  Circulatory alterations (heart failure, shock)
  Unknown Aetiology (amyloidosis, sarcoidosis, Reye's syndrome)

B. Disorders with primary renal and secondary hepatic involvement
  Hypernephroma
  Sarcoma
  Xanthogranulomatous pyelonephritis
  Acute renal failure

C. Disorders with primary hepatic and secondary renal involvement
  Intra- and extrahepatic cholestasis with secondary renal involvement
  Chronic liver disease with glomerulonephritis
  Renal tubular acidosis
  Prerenal azotemia
  Renal functional alterations in chronic liver disease: latent and open hepatorenal syndrome

**Table 2.** Diagnostic criteria of renal functional impairment in cirrhosis

*Stage I. Latent or preclinical stage*
a) Marked reduction of renal plasma flow and glomerular filtration rate ($\geqslant 50\%$)
b) Hypoperfusion of renal cortex with diversion of flow by opening of arteriovenous shunts
c) Opsiuria
d) Frequent reduction of sodium and water excretion (with positive balance and ascites)

*Stage II. Open or clinical stage* (hepatorenal syndrome)
a) Azotemia $>1$ g/l
b) Creatininemia $>1.5$ mg/dl (often $>4$ mg/dl)
c) Oliguria
d) Very marked reduction of sodium excretion ($<10$ mEq/l)
e) $U_{osm}/P_{osm} > 1$
f) $U_{Cr}/P_{Cr} > 30$
g) Lack of response to diuretic treatment and plasma expansion

The first stage of RFI is found much more frequently than the second. In fact, about 50% of patients with advanced cirrhosis may show some degree of renal impairment (Epstein 1983), whereas the open HRS is present in only about 4% of patients (Gentilini and Migone 1981). In contrast, sodium retention is always found in patients with cirrhosis who are developing ascites (Fig. 1).

In patients with RFI, the renal cortex is hypoperfused and blood is diverted from the outer to the inner cortex and medulla, probably because of persistent arterial vasoconstriction and the opening of arteriovenous shunts. The latter were demonstrated by

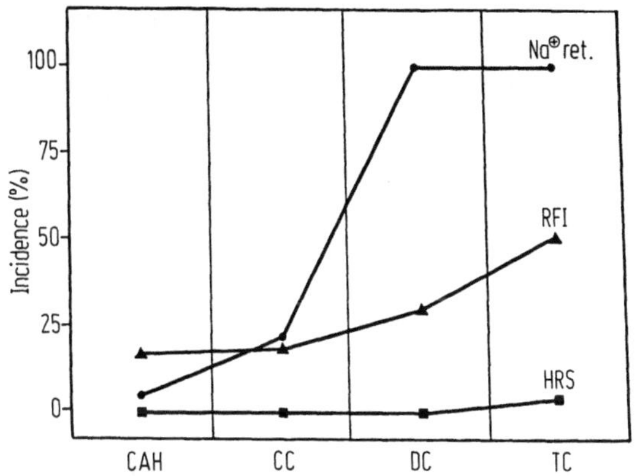


**Fig. 1.** The incidence of sodium retention *($Na^+$ ret.)*, renal functional impairment (*RFI;* stage I) and hepatorenal syndrome (*HRS;* stage II) in different stages of liver cirrhosis. *CAH*, chronic active hepatitis; *CC*, compensated cirrhosis; *DC*, decompensated cirrhosis; *TC*, terminal cirrhosis

infusing microspheres of labeled albumin directly into the renal artery (Gentilini et al. 1980).

Although overt HRS may also be present in other liver diseases (acute alcoholic hepatitis, liver cancer, acute liver failure), it generally occurs in patients with advanced cirrhosis who have already developed portal hypertension and refractory ascites. These patients usually present a characteristic alteration of systemic hemodynamics (low blood pressure, reduced systemic resistances, high cardiac output) and progressive sodium retention, the latter demonstrating the maintenance of tubular function.

## Pathogenetic Hypotheses

Several hypotheses have been proposed to explain the worsening of renal function in patients with cirrhosis. The most important are the following:

1. Active vasoconstriction in the renal cortex
2. Decrease of effective plasma volume
3. Opening of intrarenal arteriovenous shunts
4. Compression of renal blood vessels by ascites
5. False neurotransmitters
6. Endotoxemia
7. Activation of the renin-angiotensin-aldosterone system
8. Altered balance of vasoactive substances

Activation of the renin-angiotensin-aldosterone system, following a decrease in effective plasma volume, has been considered an important factor in inducing sodium retention and RFI in cirrhosis, as it can induce active vasoconstriction of renal blood vessels. However, the activation of this system might also be the result of renal cortical ischemia.

Intrarenal arachidonic acid metabolism is involved in overall regulation of renal function in healthy subjects and in many disease states. Patients with cirrhosis and ascites show an activation of the intrarenal prostaglandin (PG) system, as demonstrated by increased PGE2 levels in the renal vein (Gentilini et al. 1980) and increased urinary excretion of PGE2, PGF$2_\alpha$, 6-keto-PGF$1_\alpha$, and TxB2 (the latter two are non-enzymatic derivatives of PGI2 and TxA2 respectively) (Laffi et al. 1986b). This phenomenon has been shown to maintain renal function despite increased vasoconstrictive stimuli to the kidney. In fact, inhibition of PG synthesis with indomethacin is followed by an acute transient deterioration of renal function (Laffi et al. 1986a). An impairment of intrarenal PG synthesis may be involved in the onset of clinically overt HRS, as an evident reduction of urinary PGE2, PGF$2_\alpha$, 6-keto-PGF$1_\alpha$, and TxB2 excretion has recently been observed. In these patients, urinary PGE2 and PGF$2_\alpha$ levels are also markedly reduced when compared to healthy subjects, whereas 6-keto-PGF$1_\alpha$ and TxB2 levels are similar to controls. A relative maintenance of renal TxA2 synthesis, in a setting of increased levels of angiotensin II and other vasoconstricting factors and decreased renal synthesis of vasodilating PGs, may be of pathogenetic relevance.

Kinins synthesized in the kidney are involved in the modulation of renal blood flow and sodium handling. Reduced kinin synthesis may contribute to the abnormalities of renal function in advanced cirrhosis. According to this hypothesis, a reduced urinary excretion of kallikrein, which is thought to be a reliable index of intrarenal kinin synthesis, has been observed in patients with cirrhosis and renal impairment (Perez-Ayuso et al. 1984).

Antidiuretic hormone (ADH) is also increased, but only in patients with severe water and sodium retention, probably because of a reduction in plasma volume. However, circulating ADH levels are not significantly decreased in ascitic patients with a LeVeen shunt who excrete hypo-osmolar urine with correction of hyponatremia. The improvement of renal function observed in those cirrhotic patients with LeVeen shunt was probably due to plasma volume expansion (Reznick et al. 1983).

A severe renal impairment of both functional and anatomical type has been observed following endotoxin administration. The role of endotoxins in the pathogenesis of functional renal alterations in cirrhotics, however, is still unclear. In fact, conflicting results have been obtained in these patients with the Limulus test, a recently developed technique for endotoxin detection which does not appear to be specific (Fulenwider et al. 1980).

## Therapeutic Approach

No treatment is currently available for HRS, although some patients may respond to chronic plasma expansion (Gentilini and Migone 1981). During the first stage, the treatment for renal impairment is similar to that for sodium retention and ascites and a standard therapy has been developed as follows (Gabuzda 1970; Conn 1982; Galambos 1979; Epstein 1983):

a) Bed rest and strict regulation of dietary sodium (20 mEq/24 h),
b) The above treatment + aldosterone antagonists,
c) The above treatment + administration of loop diuretics,
d) The above treatment + plasma expansion.

We recently applied this sequential therapeutic regimen to a group of 144 patients with liver cirrhosis and ascites (Gentilini et al. 1986). All patients included in the study

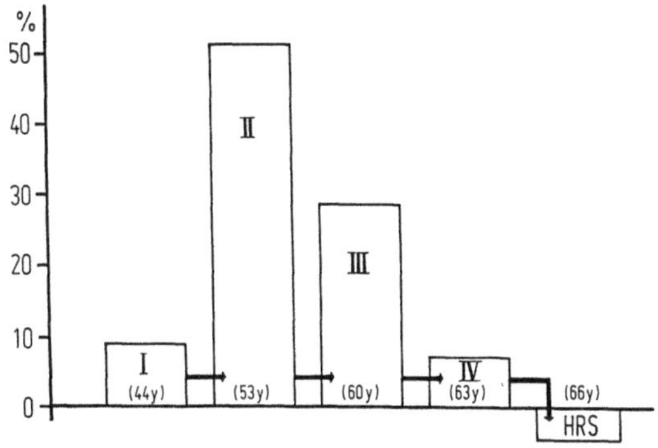


**Fig. 2.** Percentage of responders out of 144 patients to different stages of sequential treatment (mean age).
I = sodium-restricted diet and bed rest
II = sodium-restricted diet and bed rest + spironolactone
III = sodium-restricted diet and bed rest + spironolactone + furosemide
IV = sodium-restricted diet and bed rest + spironolactone + furosemide + plasma expansion
HRS = untreatable ascites hepatorenal syndrome

were submitted to the first step and those who failed to improve then went on to the following step and so on. The precentages of patients responding to each step, with their mean ages, are reported in Fig. 2; response decreased with age. Patients who did not respond to the final stage and prolonged plasma expansion were considered to have refractory ascites and all of them eventually developed open HRS.

Renal functional impairment during cirrhosis is not the only factor involved in the resistance to diuretic treatment of ascites. In fact, recently, the reduced diuretic action of furosemide has been attributed mainly to an altered pharmacokinetics of the drug, which was not related to renal clearances, and urinary sodium and PG excretion. This phenomenon was thought to be due to an alteration of tubular furosemide transport (Pinzani et al. 1986).

Increased renal synthesis of vasoconstricting TxA2 has been reported in patients with functional renal failure (Zipser et al. 1983) and in patients with cirrhosis and ascites (Gentilini et al. 1984; Laffi et al. 1986). The factors involved in determining the augmented renal synthesis of TxA2 are still unknown.

Angiotensin, catecholamines, and vasopressin do not stimulate TxA2 synthesis in experimental studies in vitro, nor are they correlated with urinary TxB2 excretion in vivo (Scharschmidt and Dunn 1983). The augmented renal vein pressure following clamping of the renal vein provokes augmented synthesis of renal TxA2 in rabbits (Zipser et al. 1980). In cirrhotics, increased renal venous pressure cannot be considered a causative factor of augmented renal TxA2 synthesis. In fact, evacuative paracentesis, a maneuver which relieves renal vein compression due to tense ascites, does not affect renal TxB2 excretion to any significant extent (Gentilini et al. 1986).

In order to evaluate the benefical effect of the suppression of renal TxA2, Zipser et al. (1984) administered dazoxiben, a thromboxane synthase inhibitor, to some patients with HRS without any significant results, despite a 50% inhibition of urinary TxB2 excretion.

**Table 3.** Effect of chronic OKY 046 administration on urinary TxB2 (UTxB2) excretion, creatinine clearance ($C_{Cr}$), sodium excretion (UNaV) and diuresis in six cirrhotic patients with ascites

| | Basal | After OKY 046 |
|---|---|---|
| UTxB2 | 32.6 ± 4.2 | 5.4 ± 1.2 ng/h* |
| $C_{Cr}$ | 71.4 ± 11.4 | 86.1 ± 21.0 ml/min |
| UNaV | 11.2 ± 6.7 | 6.3 ± 2.8 mEq/24 h |
| Diuresis | 885 ± 170 | 860 ± 165 ml/24 h |

* $p < 0.001$

We used OKY 046 (Ono Pharmaceuticals, Kyoto) 200 mg tid for 4 days, in six patients with cirrhosis and ascites. Urinary TxB2, PGE2, PGF2$_\alpha$, and 6-keto-PGF1$_\alpha$ excretion, creatinine clearance, diuresis, and daily sodium excretion were measured both before and during drug administration. Urinary TxB2 excretion, a reliable index of renal TxA2 production, was reduced by about 83% ($p < 0.001$), but no significant changes in other arachidonic acid metabolites, creatinine clearance, diuresis, or sodium excretion were observed (Table 3).

The above results suggest that TxA2 is not the most important factor in the impaired sodium excretion and renal function in cirrhotic patients. These conditions are likely to be due to an altered balance between vasodilatory and vasoconstricting factors, TxA2 being only one of the latter group.

*Acknowledgements.* The authors gratefully acknowledge Dr. K. Crowshaw (Ono Pharmaceutical Company, Osaka, Japan) for the generous gift of OKY 046 and Ms. Susan Lees for expert editorial assistance.

## References

Conn HO (1973) A rational approach to the hepatorenal syndrome. Gastroenterology 65: 321-340
Conn HO (1982) Cirrhosis. In: Schiff L, Schiff E (eds) Diseases of the liver, 5th edn. Lippincott, Philadelphia, pp 847-978
Epstein M (1983) Renal sodium handling in cirrhosis. Semin Nephrol 3: 225-240
Fulenwider JT, Sibley C, Stein SF, Evatt B, Nordlinger BM, Ivey GL (1980) Endotoxaemia in cirrhosis: an observation now substantiated. Gastroenterology 78: 1001-1004
Gabuzda GJ (1970) Cirrhosis, ascites and edema. Clinical course related to management. Gastroenterology 58: 546-553
Galambos JT (1979) Cirrhosis. Saunders, Philadelphia
Gentilini P, Migone L (1981) La sindrome epato-renale. L'insufficienza funzionale renale dell'epatopatico cronico. 82nd Congress Soc It Med Int Pozzi, Rome
Gentilini P, Laffi G, Buzzelli G, Stefani R, Scarpelli P, Paladini S, Smorlesi C, La Villa G, Forti G (1980) Functional renal alterations in chronic liver disease. Digestion 20: 73-78
Gentilini P, Laffi G, La Villa G, Pinzani M, Buzzelli G, Pampana A, Smorlesi C, Moscarella S, Birardi A (1984) Pathogenetic mechanisms in renal functional impairment in cirrhotics. Front Gastrointest Res 8: 235-245
Gentilini P, La Villa G, Laffi G, Buzzelli G, Pinzani M, Cominelli F, Moscarella S, Birardi A (1986) Sodium retention in cirrhosis: aspects of pathophysiology and treatment. Front Gastrointest Res 9: 203-218
Heyd CG (1931) Liver deaths in surgery of the gall bladder. JAMA 97: 1847-1850

Laffi G, Daskalopoulos G, Kronborg I, Hsueh W, Gentilini P, Zipser R (1986a) Effects of sulindac and ibuprofen in patients with cirrhosis and ascites. Gastroenterology 90: 182-187

Laffi G, La Villa G, Pinzani M, Ciabattoni G, Patrignani P, Mannelli M, Cominelli F, Gentilini P (1986b) Altered renal and platelet arachidonic acid metabolism in cirrhosis. Gastroenterology 90: 274-282

Lichtman SS, Sohval AR (1937) Clinical disorders with associated hepatic and renal manifestations with special reference to the so-called hepatorenal syndrome. Am J Dig Dis 4: 26-32

Perez-Ayuso RM, Arroyo V, Campo J, Rimola A, Costa J, Gaya J, Rivera F, Rodes J (1984) Renal kallikrein excretion in cirrhosis with ascites: relationship to renal haemodynamics. Hepatology 4: 247-252

Pinzani M, Daskalopoulos G, Laffi G, Gentilini P, Zipser R (1987) Altered furosemide pharmacokinetics in chronic alcoholic liver disease with ascites contributes to diuretic resistance. Gastroenterology 92: 294-298

Reznick RK, Langer B, Taylor BR, Seif S, Blendis LM (1983) Hyponatraemia and arginine vasopressin secretion in patients with refractory hepatic ascites undergoing peritoneovenous shunting. Gastroenterology 84: 713-718

Scharschmidt LA, Dunn JM (1983) Prostaglandin synthesis by rat glomerular mesangial cells in culture. J Clin Invest 71: 1756-1764

Vaamonde CA, Papper S (1979) The kidney in liver disease. In: Early LE, Gottschalk CW (eds) Strauss and Welt's Diseases of the kidney. Little Brown, Boston

Zipser RD, Meyers S, Needleman P (1980) Exaggerated prostaglandin and thromboxane synthesis in the renal vein constricted rabbit kidney: modulators of renal resistance. Circ Res 47: 231-237

Zipser RD, Radvan GH, Kronborg I, Duke R, Little TE (1983) Urinary thromboxane B2 and prostaglandin in the hepatorenal syndrome: evidence for E2 increased vasoconstrictor and decreased vasodilator factors. Gastroenterology 84: 692-703

Zipser RD, Kronborg I, Rector W, Reynolds TB, Daskalopoulos G (1984) Therapeutic trial of thromboxane synthesis inhibition in the hepatorenal syndrome. Gastroenterology 87: 1228-1232

# Pathophysiology of Cirrhotic Ascites

Giovanni Gasbarrini, Mauro Bernardi, Franco Trevisani, and Rossana de Palma
Patologia Speciale Medica I, University of Bologna, Italy

Discussing the pathophysiology of cirrhotic ascites is a hard task. We could not succeed in covering all the aspects arising from the tremendous amount of research carried out by several groups in the last few years. Rather, we will try to give basic information on the primary mechanisms leading to ascites formation.

The appearance of ascites represents a precise landmark in the course of cirrhosis and implies a poor prognosis: according to several authors, up to 50% of patients can be dead within a year from the appearance of ascites (Ratnoff and Patek 1942; Sherlock et al. 1966; Arroyo and Rodes 1975). In our experience, acquired more recently, the survival appeared to be higher, most likely because of the recent improvement in the management of major complications: 85% of our cases survived 1 year and 48% up to 3 years. In any case, ascites tells the physican that the disease is advanced.

Our knowledge of the pathophysiological mechanisms leading to ascites formation in cirrhosis has considerably improved in recent years. However, we still do not know exactly what triggers ascites formation in a previously compensated patient, or whether bleeding episodes from esophageal varices or ascitic decompensation will prevail in the natural history experienced by a cirrhotic. In contrast, we are well aware, from a clinical point of view, that several factors can precipitate ascites.

The most frequent causes of ascitic decompensation in our experience are reported in Table 1. The impact of such factors, however, is conditioned by the pathophysiological background of the individual patient, as suggested by the cases in which ascites appeared without evident precipitating cause.

Ascites is due to the interaction of several pathogenetic factors, which can be classified as "local" and "systemic."

**Table 1.** Events precipitating ascites formation in a group of 120 hospitalized cirrhotics

| Event | Percentage of patients |
|---|---|
| Gastrointestinal bleeding | 31% |
| Infection | 29% |
| Alcoholic hepatitis | 20% |
| Hepatotoxic drugs | 17% |
| Hepatocellular carcinoma | 11% |
| Surgical trauma | 11% |
| Extrahepatic cholestasis | 6% |
| Spontaneous appearance | 14% |

Assessment and Management of Hepatobiliary Disease
Eds.: L. Okolicsányi, G. Csomós, and G. Crepaldi

*Local factors.* Primary local factors are the postsinusoidal portal hypertension and the reduced plasma oncotic pressure due to hypoalbuminemia which synergically affect the equilibrium of the Starling forces (Atkinson and Losowsky 1961). Portal hypertension is able to increase hepatic lymph production linearly, as shown by Barrowman and Granger (1984) in an experimental model of cirrhosis in the rat. A boundary level of plasma colloid osmotic pressure between cirrhotics with and without ascites has been identified as about 20 mmHg by at least two groups of authors (Cerrick et al., 1960; Henriksen et al. 1980). Once the maximal flow capacity of the thoracic duct is overwhelmed, the transudate accumulates within the peritoneal cavity (Dumont and Witte 1966).

Other factors may affect the reabsorption of ascites and thus the rate of ascites accumulation, e.g., the hydrostatic pressure of the peritoneal capillaries, influenced by portal hypertension and intra-abdominal pressure, and the anatomical status of the peritoneum itself (Buhac et al. 1984). Little is known, however, about the impact of these factors on ascites pathophysiology.

*Systemic factors.* Patients with cirrhosis and ascites have long been recognized to have low renal sodium excretion. Two basic points have to be discussed: when such sodium retention appears, and which factors promote the positive sodium balance.

Cirrhotics show an increased blood volume, even before ascites formation, whether this is hemodynamically effective or not. After the complete report by Lieberman and Reynolds (1967), such a finding has been confirmed by several authors (Wernze et al. 1978; Bosch et al., 1980; Bernardi et al. 1983b). Moreover, the total exchangeable sodium pool is already expanded at this stage of the disease (Roberti et al. 1966). We believe these findings to represent strong evidence that sodium retention occurs before the appearance of ascites, and Lieberman's overflow theory of ascites formation (Lieberman et al. 1970) coincides well with them. According to this theory, blood volume expansion represents a primary pathogenetic factor which is directly responsible for ascites formation once portal hypertension and the reduction in plasma colloid osmotic pressure reach crucial levels. If we accept this concept, we also have to understand how cirrhotic patients succeed in remaining ascites-free.

There is reasonable evidence that in cirrhotics without ascites, blood volume expansion is hemodynamically effective: plasma renin activity has as a rule been found to be reduced, both by us (Bernardi et al. 1983 and by many others (Wilkinson et al. 1977a, 1979a; Wernze et al. 1978; Epstein et al. 1977; Bosch et al. 1980). We were also able to confirm this finding in a circadian study (Bernardi et al. 1986). It was evident that cirrhotics without ascites had significantly depressed levels of plasma renin activity with respect to normal controls during the whole day, with a behavior very close to that which has been described in normal subjects receiving an infusion of saline (Modlinger et al. 1976).

These patients, therefore, are able periodically to equilibrate their volume, probably through a natriuretic escape. As shown by Wilkinson et al. (1979b) and by Naccarato et al. (1981), with different experimental approaches, such a homeostatic mechanism can progressively become incomplete, and ascites can therefore appear. A reduced hepatic production of natriuretic factor may be at least in part responsible.

The second question we will try to answer is: Which factors promote renal sodium retention? There is "historic" evidence of the role of aldosterone, such as the frequent finding of increased urinary excretion or plasma levels of aldosterone in patients accumulating ascites (Luetscher and Johnson 1954; Coppage et al. 1962; Vecsei et al. 1969), the effectiveness of bilateral adrenalectomy (Giuseffi et al. 1957), and, above all, the efficacy of antimineralocorticoid drugs in antagonizing sodium retention in cirrhosis (Eggert 1970; Pérez-Ayuso et al. 1983). We have recently demonstrated in patients with cirrhosis, ascites, and unimpaired renal perfusion that the daily dose of spironolactone needed to induce a negative sodium balance is directly correlated with plasma aldosterone levels (Bernardi et al. 1985a). Moreover, in cirrhotics with sodium retention and preserved renal perfusion, this occured at both proximal and distal sites, the latter being quantitatively more important (Wilkinson et al. 1979c).

Nonetheless, doubts are cast on the role of aldosterone by two kinds of observations:

1. Reductions in plasma aldosterone, obtained by different means, were not followed by proportional increases in renal sodium excretion. In one study, aldosterone synthesis was suppressed by aminoglutethimide (Rosoff et al. 1975). Patients in that study, however, had long-standing diuretic-resistant ascites, which is generally associated with poor renal perfusion, and hence with proximal tubular sodium reabsorption. In other studies, plasma aldosterone concentration was reduced by central volume redistribution through isothermic water immersion (Epstein et al. 1977), dietary sodium load (Chonko et al. 1977), or inhibition of angiotensin I converting enzyme by captopril (Espiner and Nicholls 1982). However, it should be pointed out that the relationship between aldosterone and sodium excretion is not linear but hyperbolic, which means that patients with very elevated plasma aldosterone levels need a striking reduction in aldosterone to obtain a modest increase in renal sodium excretion. The inverse applies to patients with moderately increased or normal aldosterone. On taking this hyperbolic relationship into account, the changes in sodium excretion which followed $\beta$-blocker administration in cirrhotics with ascites were exactly as would have been predicted from the changes in urinary aldosterone (Wilkinson et al. 1977b). The same applies when plasma aldosterone concentrations are studied (Fig. 1). Finally, the decrease in tubular rejection fraction of sodium due to the change in posture by cirrhotics with ascites was inversely related to the increase in plasma aldosterone concentration (Bernardi et al. 1985b).

2. Plasma aldosterone is normal (or even reduced) in all the compensated patients and in 40%-60% of patients accumulating ascites for the first time (Wernze et al. 1978; Wilkinson et al. 1979c; Epstein et al. 1977; Bosch et al. 1980, Bernardi et al. 1983b). The possible answer to this criticism on the role of the hormone in sodium retention is that in cirrhosis there is an abnormal relationship between aldosterone and renal sodium excretion. First suggested by Wilkinson et al. (1979c), it has been confirmed by us (Bernardi et al. 1983b). Our findings also suggest that such an abnormality precedes ascites formation and worsens as the disease progresses. For any given value of plasma aldosterone, patients with ascites excreted about one-fourth and compensated about two-thirds as much sodium as controls (Fig. 2). This would seem to imply an increase in sensitivity of the renal tubules to mineralocorticoid activity or a deficiency in natriuretic factor, as previously reported. The two interpretations are not mutually exclusive. The same abnormality could explain the effectiveness of spironolactone also in ascitic patients with normal aldosteronemia (Pérez-Ayuso et al. 1983; Bernardi et al. 1985a).

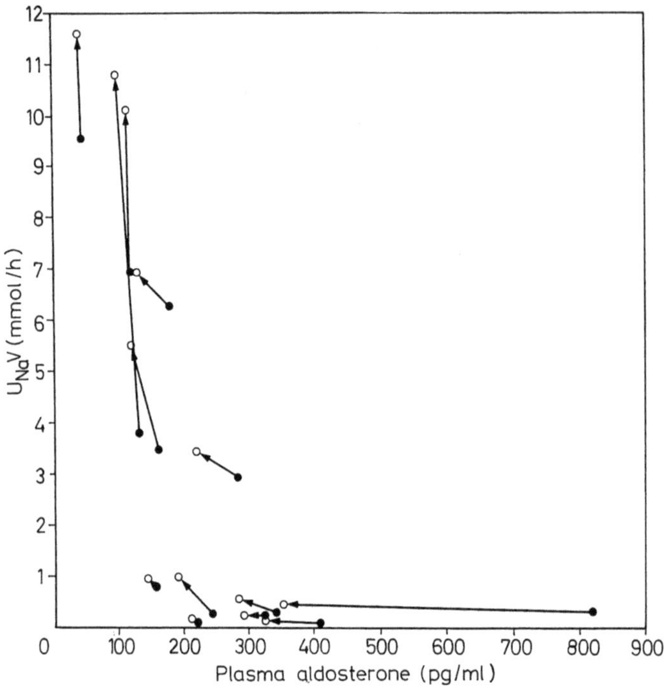


**Fig. 1.** The relationship between plasma aldosterone concentration (PAC) and renal sodium excretion (UNaV) has the form of a rectangular hyperbole. ● before, ○ after effective $\beta$-blockade induced propranolol in cirrhotics with ascites (glomerular filtration rate $\geq 55$ ml/min). *Arrows* show the direction of change. The changes in UNaV were exactly as would have been predicted based on the changes in PAC. *r* values were $-0.79$ ($p < 0.01$) before and $-0.87$ ($p < 0.01$) after $\beta$-blockade

The progression of the disease, however, is associated with profound derangements in systemic hemodynamics. Namely, peripheral resistances tend to be reduced, with a compensatory rise in cardiac output (Better and Schrier 1983). In such circumstances, a reduction in effective volemia ensues, even if total blood volume can remain above normal limits (Lieberman and Reynolds 1967; Wernze et al. 1978; Bosch et al. 1980; Bernardi et al. 1983b). The afferent stimuli mediated by different baroreceptors lead to the activation of several systems involved in volume homeostasis. In this condition a true "underfilling" status results (Epstein 1982).

The plasma levels of renin activity and aldosterone are progressively enhanced as the natural history of the disease progresses (Bernardi and Gasbarrini 1986) (Fig. 3). Parallel to this, mineralocorticoid-dependent renal sodium retention worsens. Effective hypovolemia also means hyperactivity of the sympathoadrenergic system (Bernardi et al. 1982, 1983;) Plasma norepinephrine concentration has been found to be inversely related with renal sodium excretion (Bichet et al. 1982; Bernardi et al. 1985b). The sympathetic nervous system can promote sodium retention at the proximal renal tubule, by $\alpha$-receptor-mediated stimulation, irrespective of hemodynamic effects (Bello-Reuss et al. 1976). In such patients, therefore, sodium retention may also be attributable, in part, to adrenergic hyperactivity.

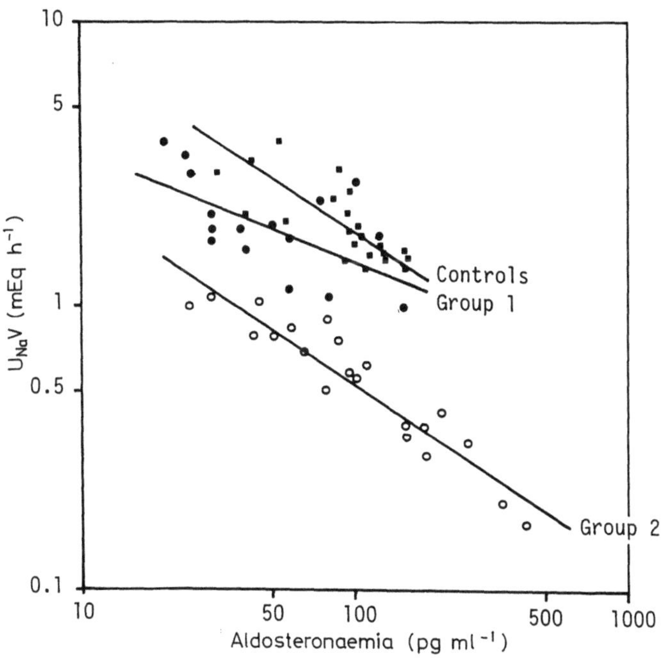


**Fig. 2.** Relationship between plasma aldosterone concentration and renal excretion of sodium (VNaV) in healthy controls [■], cirrhotics without ascites [group 1, ●], and cirrhotics with ascites [group 2, ○]. The relationship appears to be linear because log scales were used on the axes. *r* values were −0.78 ($p<0.001$), −0.59 ($p<0.05$), and −0.94 ($p<0.001$). The regression line was progressively and significantly shifted to the abscissa (group 1 vs controls $p<0.01$; group 2 vs group 1 $p<0.001$)

We feel, however, that aldosterone plays a prevalent role in promoting sodium retention also in this context. Using a chronobiological approach, we analyzed the correlation of renal sodium excretion with plasma aldosterone and urinary norepinephrine excretion in cirrhotics with ascites and preserved renal perfusion (Trevisani et al. 1984). Natriuresis was inversely related to plasma aldosterone during the whole day. In contrast, the correlation with urinary norepinephrine reached statistical significance only at night, when we found the adrenergic system to be maximally stimulated (Table 2).

The most important determinant of sodium retention in advanced cirrhosis, in addition to aldosterone, is the reduced renal perfusion. In Fig. 3 four classes of patients which may represent the natural history of cirrhosis are reported. Glomerular filtration rate and renal plasma flow progressively decrease. When renal perfusion declines, proximal sodium retention occurs (Wilkinson et al. 1975). This explains why, in such circumstances, diuretics acting more proximally than antimineralocorticoids are needed to counteract the positive sodium balance. The enhanced proximal sodium reabsorption is also the main mechanism leading to impaired free water generation capacity and hyponatremia in such patients (Schedl and Bartter 1960).

Finally, we would like to deal briefly with refractory or resistant ascites, which must

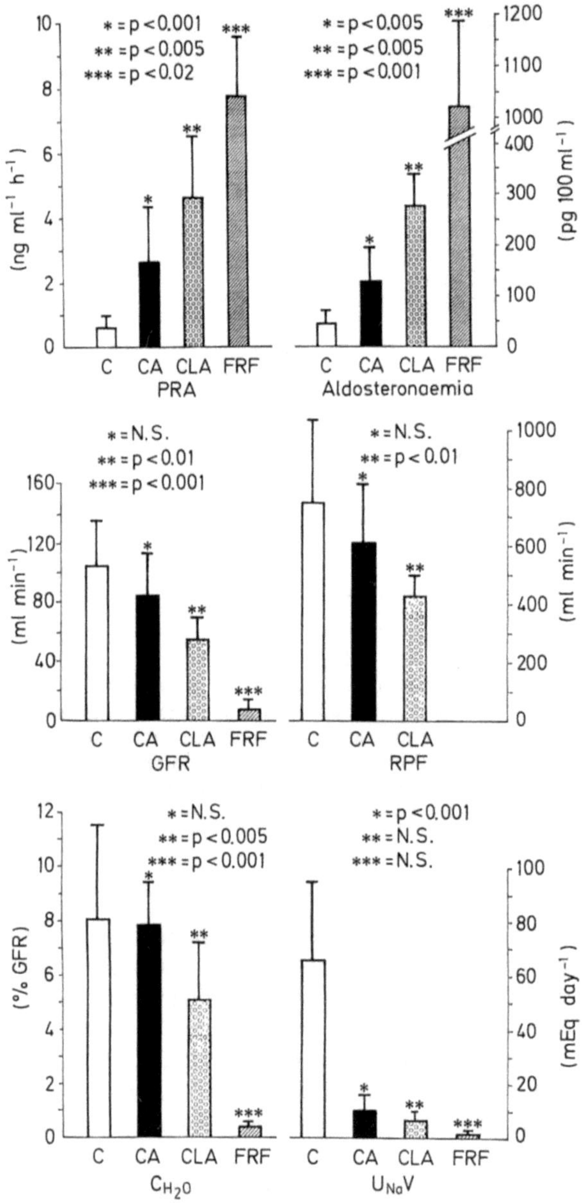


**Fig. 3.** Progressive activation of the renin-aldosterone axis, reduction of renal plasma flow *(RPF)*, glomerular filtration rate *(GFR)*, urine sodium excretion *(UNaV)*, and free water clearance ($CH_2O$) during the course of cirrhosis. *C*, cirrhosis without ascites; *CA*, cirrhosis with ascites at the first appearance; *CLA*, cirrhosis with long-standing ascites; *FRF*, cirrhosis with hepatorenal syndrome; *PRA*, plasma renin activity

* = statistical significance compared to C.

**Table 2.** Correlations between plasma aldosterone concentration (PAC), urinary excretion of norepinephrine (UneV) and renal sodium excretion (UNaV) in nine cirrhotics with ascites

| Clock time (urine collection periods) | 8-16 | 16-24 | 24-4 | 4-8 |
|---|---|---|---|---|
| PAC vs UNaV (*r* value) | −0.74* | −0.84* | −0.79* | −0.73* |
| UneV vs UNaV (*r* value) | 0.24 | −0.33 | −0.57 | −0.64* |

* $p<0.05$ or less

be readily recognized, since diuretic treatment is ineffective and alternative therapeutic approaches have to be considered (Levy et al. 1975; Epstein 1982).

Most authors refer to this condition as ascites which is not successfully reduced by energic diuretic therapy. We find such a definition confusing, not only because different diuretic regimes may have been employed, but also, and mostly, because it encompasses two distinct entities.

We use this term when the diuretic does induce a renal response, body weight declines, but ascites volume persists unmodified or even increases. In such cases localizing factors do not allow the removal of even small quantities of ascites, and diuretic-induced uremia is likely to occur.

When an adequate diuretic treatment does not reduce ascites volume because of insufficient renal response, in most cases we face pre-existing renal failure of a different nature. We prefer to define these patients as having renal failure rather than refractory ascites.

In conclusion, we believe that overflow and underfilling co-exist in the pathophysiology of cirrhotic ascites. The former appears to explain the considerable amount of data provided by experimental observation of cirrhotic patients before ascites formation and when ascites first accumulates. Once natural complications (such as bleeding, vomiting, changes in systemic hemodynamics) and/or iatrogenic complications (mainly represented by exaggerated diuretic administration) determine effective hypovolemia, the whole pattern of underfilling appears.

## References


Arroyo V, Rodes J (1975) A rational approach to the treatment of ascites. Postgrad Med J 51: 558-563

Atkinson M, Losowsky MS (1961) The mechanism of ascites formation in chronic liver disease. Q J Med 30: 153-166

Barrowman JA, Granger DN (1984) Effects of experimental cirrhosis on splanchnic microvascular fluid and solute exchange in the rat. Gastroenterology 87: 165-172

Bello-Reuss E, Trevino DL, Gottshalk C (1976) Effect of renal sympathetic nerve stimulation on proximal water and sodium reabsorption. J Clin Invest 57: 1104-1107

Bernardi M, Gasbarrini G (1986) The renin-angiotensin-aldosterone system in human hepatic cirrhosis. Isr J Med Sci 22: 70-77

Bernardi M, Trevisani F, Santini C, Ligabue A, Capelli M, Gasbarrini G (1982) Impairment of blood pressure control in patients with liver cirrhosis during tilting: study on adrenergic and renin-angiotensin systems. Digestion 25: 124-130

Bernardi M, Trevisani F, Santini C, Zoli G, Baraldini M, Ligabue A, Gasbarrini G (1983a) Plasma norepinephrine, weak neurotransmitters, and renin activity during active tilting in liver cirrhosis: relationship with cardiovascular homeostasis and renal function. Hepatology 3: 56-64

Bernardi M, Trevisani F, Santini C, de Palma R, Gasbarrini G (1983b) Aldosterone-related blood volume expansion before and during the early phases of ascites formation. Gut 24: 761-766

Bernardi M, Servadei D, Trevisani F, Rusticali AG, Gasbarrini G (1985a) Importance of plasma aldosterone concentration on the natriuretic effect of spironolactone in patients with liver cirrhosis and ascites. Digestion 31: 189-193

Bernardi M, Santini C, Trevisani F, Baraldini M, Ligabue A, Gasbarrini G (1985b) Renal function impairment induced by change in posture in patients with cirrhosis and ascites. Gut 26: 629-635

Bernardi M, de Palma R, Trevisani F, Santini C, Capani F, Baraldini M, Gasbarrini G (1986) Chronobiological study on factors affecting plasma aldosterone concentration in cirrhosis. Gastroenterology 91: 683-691

Better OS, Schrier RW (1983) Disturbed volume homeostasis in patients with cirrhosis of the liver. Kidney Int 23: 303-311

Bosch J, Arroyo V, Betriu A, Mas A, Carrilho F, Rivera F, Navarro-Lopez F, Rodes J (1980) Hepatic hemodynamics and the renin-angiotensin-aldosterone system in cirrhosis. Gastroenterology 78: 92-99

Buhac I, Flesh L, Kishore R (1984) Intraabdominal pressure and resorption of ascites in decompensated liver cirrhosis. J Lab Clin Med 104: 264-270

Cerrik GR, Kerr DNS, Read AE, Sherlock S (1960) Colloid osmotic pressure and hydrostatic pressure relationships in the formation of ascites in hepatic cirrhosis. Clin Sci 19: 361-365

Chonko AM, Bay WH, Stein JH, Ferris TF (1977) The role of renin and aldosterone in the salt retention of edema. Am J Med 63: 881-889

Coppage WS, Island DP, Cooner AE, Liddle GW (1962) The metabolism of aldosterone in normal subjects and in patients with hepatic cirrhosis. J Clin Invest 41: 1672-1680

Dumont AE, Witte MH (1966) Contrasting patterns of thoracic duct lymph formation in hepatic cirrhosis. Surg Gynaecol Obstet 122: 524-528

Eggert RC (1970) Spironolactone diuresis in patients with cirrhosis and ascites. Br Med J 4: 401-403

Epstein F (1982) Underfilling versus overflow in hepatic ascites. N Engl J Med 307: 1577-1578

Epstein M (1982) Peritoneo-venous shunt in the management of ascites and hepatorenal syndrome. Gastroenterology 82: 790-799

Epstein M, Levinson R, Sancho J, Haber E, Re R (1977) Characterization of the renin-aldosterone system in decompensated cirrhosis. Circ Res 41: 818-829

Espiner EA, Nicholls MG (1982) Hormones and fluid retention in cirrhosis (Letter). Lancet 2: 501-502

Giuseffi J, Werk EE, Larson PU, Schiff L, Elliott DW (1957) Effect of bilateral adrenalectomy in a patient with massive ascites and psotnecrotic cirrhosis. N Engl J Med 257: 796-803

Henriksen JH, Stage JG, Schlichting P, Winkler K (1980) Intraperitoneal pressure: ascitic fluid and splanchnic vascular pressures and their role in prevention and formation of ascites. Scand J Clin Lab Invest 40: 493-502

Levy VG, Opolon P, Pauleau N, Caroli J (1975) Treatment of ascites by reinfusion of concentrated peritoneal fluid - review of 318 procedures in 210 patients. Postgrad Med J 51: 564-566

Lieberman FL, Reynolds TB (1967) Plasma volume in cirrhosis of the liver: its relation to portal hypertension, ascites and renal failure. J Clin Invest 46: 1297-1308

Lieberman FL, Denison EK, Reynolds TB (1970) The relationship of plasma volume, portal hypertension, ascites and renal sodium retention in cirrhosis. The overflow theory of ascites formation. Ann NY Acad Sci 170: 202-206

Luetscher JA, Johnson BB (1954) Observations on the sodium retaining corticoid (aldosterone) in the urine of children and adults in relation to sodium balance and edema. J Clin Invest 33: 1441-1446

Modlinger RS, Sharif-Zadeh K, Ertel NH, Gutkin M (1976) The circadian rhythm of renin. J Clin Endocrinol Metab 43: 1276-1282

Naccarato R, Messa P, d'Angelo A, Fabris A, Messa M, Chiaramonte M, Gregolin C, Zanon G (1981) Renal handling of sodium and water in early chronic liver disease. Evidence for a reduced natriuretic activity of the cirrhotic urinary extracts in rats. Gastroenterology 81: 205-210

Pérez-Ayuso RM, Arroyo V, Planas R, Gaya J, Bory F, Rimola A, Rivera F, Rodes J (1983) Randomized comparative study of efficacy of furosemide versus spironolactone in non-azotemic cirrhosis with ascites. Gastroenterology 84: 961-968

Ratnoff OD, Patek AJ (1942) The natural history of Laennec's cirrhosis of the liver: an analysis of 386 cases. Medicine (Baltimore) 21: 207-268

Roberti A, Traverso H, Vesin P, Viguie R, Blanchon P (1966) Etude du Na et du K échangeables et des liquides extracellulaires dans les cirrhoses éthyliques. Sem Hop Paris 42: 1714-1718

Rosoff L, Zia P, Reynolds T, Horton R (1975) Studies of renin and aldosterone in cirrhotic patients with ascites. Gastroenterology 69: 698-705

Schedl HP, Bartter FC (1960) An explanation for and experimental correction of the abnormal water diuresis in cirrhosis. J Clin Invest 39: 248-261

Sherlock S, Senewiratne B, Scott A, Walker JG (1966) Complications of diuretic therapy in hepatic cirrhosis. Lancet 1: 1049-1053

Trevisani F, Bernardi M, Santini C, de Palma R, Baraldini M, Ligabue A, Gasbarrini G (1984) Circadian evaluation of factors affecting renal sodium handling in liver cirrhosis (abstract). Ital J Gastroenterol 16: 143

Vecsei P, Dusterdieck G, Janecke J, Lommer D, Wolff HP (1969) Secretion and turnover of aldosterone in various pathological states. Clin Sci 36: 241-256

Wernze H, Spech HJ, Muller J (1978) Study on the activity of the renin-angiotensin-aldosterone system (RAAs) in patients with cirrhosis of the liver. Klin Wochenschr 56: 389-397

Wilkinson SP, Moodie H, Alam A, Williams R (1975) Renal retention of sodium in cirrhosis and fulminant hepatic failure. Postgrad Med J 51: 527-531

Wilkinson SP, Smith IK, Clarke M, Arroyo V, Richardson J, Moodie H, Williams R (1977a) Intrarenal distribution of plasma flow in cirrhosis as measured by transit renography: relationship with plasma renin activity and sodium and water excretion. Clin Sci Mol Med 52: 469-475

Wilkinson SP, Bernardi M, Smith IK, Jowett TP, Slater JDH, Williams R (1977b) Effect of beta-adrenergic blocking drugs on the renin-aldosterone system, sodium excretion, and renal haemodynamics in cirrhosis with ascites. Gastroenterology 73: 659-663

Wilkinson SP, Smith IK, Williams R (1979a) Changes in plasma renin activity in cirrhosis: a reappraisal based on studies in 67 patients and "low renin" cirrhosis. Hypertension 1: 125-129

Wilkinson SP, Smith IK, Moodie H, Poston L, Williams R (1979b) Studies on mineralocorticoid "escape" in cirrhosis. Clin Sci 56: 401-406

Wilkinson SP, Jowett TP, Slater JDH, Arroyo V, Moodie H, Williams R (1979c) Renal sodium retention in cirrhosis: relationship to aldosterone and nephron site. Clin Sci 56: 169-177

# Treatment of Ascites

Juan Rodés and Vicente Arroyo
Liver Unit, Hospital Clinic i Provincial, Barcelona, Spain

## Bed Rest and Low-Sodium Diet

The assumption of an upright posture by patients with cirrhosis and ascites is associated with a striking activation of the renin-angiotensin system and the sympathetic nervous system, a reduction of GFR, and an enhancement of tubular sodium reabsorption [1]. Therefore, from a theoretical point of view, bed rest could be useful for the treatment of ascites, particularly in patients who do not respond satisfactorily to diuretics.

Low-sodium diet (40-60 mEq/day) is another useful measure for the treatment of cirrhotics with ascites. Approximately 20% of these patients may decrease their ascites only by reducing the sodium content in their diet. In the remaining cases, sodium restriction diminishes the diuretic requirements. An important cause of diuretic-resistant ascites is inadequate sodium restriction. This should be suspected in any patient whose ascites does not decrease despite a good natriuretic response to diuretics. Once ascites has disappeared, many cirrhotics continue to require a strict sodium diet and diuretics. Others, however, can be maintained free of ascites with moderate sodium restriction and low doses of diuretics. Finally, it is not infrequent to observe patients who spontaneously recover their ability to excrete sodium normally. Therefore, the long-term management of cirrhotics with ascites varies markedly from patient to patient, and every effort should be made to adjust sodium intake and diuretic dosage to individual requirements at each moment during the course of the disease.

## Diuretics

Loop diuretics, in particular furosemide, and distal diuretics, especially spironolactone, are the commonest drugs in the treatment of cirrhotics with ascites.

Loop diuretics exert their primary action in the ascending limb of the loop of Henle. They are the most powerful diuretics used in clinical practice today. High dosage can increase sodium excretion to 30% of the filtered sodium. This high natriuretic potency can be attributed to two features. First, between 20% and 50% of the filtered sodium is reabsorbed in the loop of Henle, representing a major substrate for the action of diuretics. Second, in the absence of hyperaldosteronism, the distal and collecting tubules, which are downstream from the loop of Henle, have a limited capacity for sodium reabsorption and are incapable of mitigating the diuresis induced by loop diuretics. These agents circulate in blood strongly bound to plasma proteins. At the proximal tubule, they are actively secreted into the tubular lumen by the organic acid transport pathway from which they are carried with the luminal fluid to the ascending limb

Assessment and Management of Hepatobiliary Disease
Eds.: L. Okolicsányi, G. Csomós, and G. Crepaldi

of the loop of Henle. Therefore, the active fraction of loop diuretics is that which reaches the tubular lumen. The natriuretic action of loop diuretics is mainly related to their inhibitory effect on a specific cotransport system, the $Na^{+}2Cl^{-}$ $K^{+}$ carrier, in the luminal membrane of the ascending limb cells. Loop diuretics increase the renal synthesis of prostaglandins, which are powerful natriuretic substances [2]. Therefore, prostaglandins may also be involved in the natriuretic effect of these drugs. In fact, prostaglandin inhibition reduces the natriuretic activity of loop diuretics [2].

Spironolactone has a much lower natriuretic potency than loop diuretics. It can increase sodium excretion to 2% of the filtered sodium. Spironolactone inhibits sodium reabsorption in the distal and collecting tubules by antagonizing the tubular effect of aldosterone and is therefore particularly effective in patients with hyperaldosteronism. The therapeutic dosage of spironolactone depends on the plasma aldosterone concentration [3]. Patients with moderately increased aldosterone levels require low doses of the drug (100–150 mg/day). However, as much as 500 mg/day may be required to antagonize the tubular effect of aldosterone in cases of marked hyperaldosteronism.

Contrary to what would be expected on the basis of their intrinsic natriuretic potency, spironolactone is more effective than loop diuretics in nonazotemic patients with cirrhosis and ascites. The administration of a loop diuretic alone is followed by a satisfactory diuretic response in only 50% of these patients [3]. In contrast, spironolactone is effective in most cirrhotics without renal failure [3, 4]. This apparently paradoxical observation could be explained by considering the site of action of these agents and the mechanism of sodium retention in cirrhosis. Cirrhotics with ascites usually present a marked hyperaldosteronism and tend to retain sodium avidly in the distal nephron. On the other hand, loop diuretics inhibit sodium reabsorption in the ascending limb of the loop of Henle but have no effect in the distal nephron. Therefore, it is possible that loop diuretics fail to increase sodium excretion in many of these patients because most of the sodium not reabsorbed in the loop of Henle by the action of these agents is subsequently taken up along the distal nephron by the action of aldosterone. In fact, in one of these studies, patients not responding to furosemide were those with higher plasma aldosterone levels [3]. The most rational treatment of cirrhotics with ascites is therefore the administration of spironolactone alone or associated with a loop diuretic. A therapeutic schedule used in many centers starts with 40 mg/day furosemide and 100 mg/day spironolactone. If there is no response, the dosage is increased stepwise to 160 mg/day furosemide and 400 mg/day spironolactone. Patients not responding to this program should be considered as having diuretic-resistant ascites.

The response to diuretics in patients with cirrhosis and ascites can be predicted on the basis of renal function [1]. Patients with normal BUN and serum creatinine concentration usually respond to standard doses of these agents. By contrast, cirrhotics with impaired GFR do not respond to diuretics or require very high doses of these drugs. This different behavior is probably related to differences in intrarenal sodium handling. In nonazotemic cirrhotics the main cause of sodium retention is increased distal sodium reabsorption, a process that can be reversed with the diuretics currently available. By contrast, the predominant mechanisms of sodium retention in patients with impaired renal hemodynamics are decreased sodium filtration and enhanced sodium reabsorption in the proximal tubule. An additional mechanism contributing to the poor response to diuretics in patients with azotemia may be impaired tubular secretion of these agents.

## Peritoneovenous Shunt

In 1974 LeVeen and associates introduced the peritovenous shunt (PVS) for the treatment of cirrhotics with refractory ascites. This device consists of a perforated intra-abdominal tube connected through a one-way pressure-sensitive valve to a silicone tube that traverses the subcutaneous tissue to empty into the superior vena cava. The aim of the shunt is to produce a sustained circulating blood volume expansion by the continuous passage of ascites from the peritoneal cavity to the general circulation.

Numerous studies have shown that peritoneovenous shunting is capable of correcting most abnormalities thought to be involved in the pathogenesis of ascites formation. The insertion of a PVS produces a striking reduction of the plasma levels of renin [5], aldosterone [5], norepinephrine (L. Blendis, personal communication), and antidiuretic hormone [6], indicating an improvement in the effective hypovolemia. This is associated with a marked increase in urine volume, sodium excretion and free water clearance and with the disappearance of ascites in most patients. In addition, in cirrhotics with functional renal failure, peritoneovenous shunting may improve renal blood flow and GFR [7]. Finally, a marked fall in the wedged-to-free hepatic venous pressure gradient has been reported to occur after the insertion of a PVS [8]. During follow-up, a significant proportion of patients treated with PVS display persisting minimal ascites despite a normal sodium diet and low diuretic dosage [9].

Unfortunately, PVS is associated with a high rate of complications [9–11]. Obstruction of the shunt occurs in more than 30% of patients. This may happen early in the postoperative period or at any time during follow-up and is usually due to fibrin deposition around the catheter or to a large clot obstructing the superior vena cava. Less frequently, obstruction is caused by fibrin deposition within the valve. Shunt obstruction is frequently, but not necessarily, followed by reaccumulation of ascites. Acute bacterial infection, generally staphylococcal, is perhaps the most frequent serious complication in these patients. The prosthesis is usually colonized and the infection cannot be eradicated unless the shunt is removed. Practically all patients treated with PVS develop laboratory changes of intravascular coagulation within the early postoperative period. The mechanism of this complication is unknown, although it has been proposed that it may be secondary to the presence in ascites of activated tissue thromboplastin and clotting factors, plasminogen activators, endotoxin, fibrin split products, and collagen. Fortunately, the incidence of symptomatic coagulopathy is low. Other complications occurring postoperatively such as gastrointestinal hemorrhage, pulmonary edema, and acute myocardial infarction, are related to the acute expansion of circulating blood volume. These complications can be prevented by reducing the ascitic fluid volume prior to the insertion of the PVS. The intra-abdominal tube may produce peritoneal fibrosis, causing intestinal obstruction. Finally, pulmonary thromboembolism and right-sided endocarditis have also been reported in these patients. Because many patients have died secondarily to these complications, PVS should be restricted to patients with medically intractable ascites.

The morbidity and survival rates of cirrhotics treated with PVS correlate with the degree of impairment of liver and renal function [12, 13], patients with severe hepatic and/or renal failure being those with a higher incidence of complications and lower survival. Therefore, the best results with this procedure should be expected to occur in those very few patients with diuretic-resistant ascites and preserved hepatic function.

## Paracentesis

Therapeutic paracentesis was abandoned after the introduction of the modern diuretics because it was generally considered to entail a great risk of inducing circulatory hypovolemia, renal failure, dilutional hyponatremia, and hepatic encephalopathy. However, at that time there was no study proving these contentions. During the last year two investigations have been published reevaluating the possible usefulness of this procedure in the management of cirrhotics with ascites. Quintero et al. [14] performed a controlled trial comparing conventional diuretic treatment with large paracentesis in 72 cirrhotics with ascites. Paracentesis of 4-6 associated with i.v. albumin infusion was performed daily until disappearance of ascites in 38 patients. The conventionally treated group of 34 randomly selected patients received spironolactone and furosemide in standard dosage. Paracentesis was effective in all 38 patients and did not induce significant changes in serum creatinine, BUN, serum sodium concentration, or serum albumin concentration. Diuretics were effective in 28 of 34 patients and produced significant increases in BUN and serum creatinine and a significant reduction in serum sodium. Mean arterial pressure decreased slightly with both therapeutic procedures. The incidence of major complications, the number of patients who died, and the duration of hospitalization were lower in the paracentesis group. The long-term survival was similar in the two groups. Kao et al. [15] performed 5-l paracentesis in 18 cirrhotic patients with tense ascites and peripheral edema, none of whom developed changes in blood pressure, plasma volume, or serum concentrations of urea, creatinine, or sodium. These two studies therefore suggest that paracentesis is a rapid, effective, and safe therapy for cirrhotics with ascites. If their findings are confirmed by further investigations, paracentesis will again become a first-choice treatment in these patients.

## References

1. Bernardi M, Santini C, Trevisani F, Baraldini M, Ligabue A, Gasbarrini G (1985) Renal function impairment induced by change in posture in patients with cirrhosis and ascites. Gut 26: 629-635
2. Olsen UB (1983) Diuretics and kidney prostaglandins. In: Dunn MJ, Patrono G, Cinotti GA (eds) Prostaglandins and the kidney. Plenum, New York, pp 205-212
3. Pérez-Ayuso RM, Arroyo V, Planas R, Gaya J, Bory F, Rimola A, Rivera F, Rodés J (1984) Randomized comparative study of efficacy of furosemide versus spironolactone in nonazotemic cirrhosis with ascites. Gastroenterology 84: 961-968
4. Campra JL, Reynolds TB (1978) Effectiveness of high-dose spironolactone therapy in patients with chronic liver disease and relatively refractory ascites. Dig Dis Sci 23: 1025-1030
5. Berkowitz DH, Mullen JL, Miller LD, Rosato EF (1978) Improved renal function and inhibition of renin aldosterone secretion following peritoneovenous (LeVeen) shunt. Surgery 84: 120-126
6. Blendis LM, Greig PD, Langer B, Baigrie RS, Ruse J, Taylor BR (1979) The renal and hemodynamic effects of the peritoneovenous shunt for intractable ascites. Gastroenterology 77: 250-257
7. Schoeder ET, Anderson GH, Smulyan H (1979) Effects of portacaval or peritoneo-venous shunt on renin in the hepatorenal syndrome. Kidney Int 15: 54-61
8. Henriksen JH, Malchom-Moller A, Ring-Larsen H, Lejerstofte Jensen J, Dietrichson O, Staehr-Johansen T, Juhl E (1983) Peritoneovenous shunt in treatment of ascites in patients with cirrhosis. A preliminary report with special reference to pathophysiology. Scand J Gastroenterol 18: 529-535

9. Smajda C, Franco D (1985) The LeVeen shunt in the elective treatment of intractable ascites in cirrhosis. A prospective study on 140 patients. Ann Surg 201: 488-493
10. Greig PD, Langer B, Blendis LM, Taylor BR, Clynn MFX (1980) Complications after peritoneovenous shunting for ascites. Am J Surg 139: 125-131
11. Epstein M (1982) Peritoneovenous shunt in the management of ascites and the hepatorenal syndrome. Gastroenterology 82: 790-799
12. Turner WW, Pate RM (1982) The Denver peritoneo-venous shunt: relationship between hepatic reserve and successful treatment od ascites. Am J Surg 144: 619-623
13. Gleysteen JJ, Klamer TW (1984) Peritoneovenous shunt: predictive factors of early treatment failure. Am J Gastroenterol 79: 654-658
14. Quintero E, Ginés P, Arroyo V, Rimola A, Bory F, Planas R, Viver J, Cabrera J, Rodés J (1985) Paracentesis versus diuretics in the treatment of cirrhotics with tense ascites. Lancet 1: 611-612
15. Kao HW, Rakow NE, Savage E, Reynolds TB (1985) The effect of large volume paracentesis on plasma volume: a cause of hypovolemia? Hepatology 5: 403-407

# Low-Sodium Diet in the Management of Ascites in the Cirrhotic Patient

Giuseppe Giusti and Michele Russo

Clinic of Infectious Diseases, 1st Medical School, University of Naples, 80135 Napoli, Italy
c/o Ospedale Gesù e Maria, Via D. Cotugno n.1, 80135 Napoli, Italy

## Introduction

Guilbert [1], in his book on medical training, suggests collecting data on the behavior that distinguishes medical efficiency from inefficiency and using these data in order to improve medical training. With this in mind, we attempted to verify family doctors' competence in prescribing dietary sodium restriction to patients suffering from liver cirrhosis with ascites. A number of cirrhotic patients with ascites hospitalized in our clinic in the last 3 years were questioned on the subject. Most had been generally advised to follow a low-sodium diet or to eat without salt. No specific information was given about avoiding such salt-rich foods as bread, canned foods, etc. Some patients had received no information at all on the necessity of a dietary sodium restriction. Virtually no diet sheets were given. Consequently, before hospitalization nearly all of the patients had a high dietary sodium intake (about 3 g daily).

The purpose of this review is to suggest how to cater for a cirrhotic patient with ascites requiring a low-sodium diet; our aim is to make such a diet both well-balanced and palatable.

## Sodium Content in the Normal Italian Diet

In Italy, average sodium intake is not less than 3 g daily, ranging from 2 to 6 g (equivalent to 5-15 g sodium chloride). This amount includes the salt used in cooking, the salt which is added at the table and the salt already contained in each single item of food.

Sodium is contained to different degrees in all foods (Table 1). Several foods are enriched with salt during commercial preparations (fresh dairy produce, sausage, canned vegetables and soups); some commercial foods contain sodium as additives (sodium propionate to cheese, sodium alginate to ice cream, sodium glutamate to soup cubes, sodium lactate to long-storage bread, and so on).

## Use and Abuse of Dietary Salt as a Consequence of Custom and Cultural Tradition

The addition of salt to dishes is not necessary, since the sodium content of food is sufficient for our requirements [2]. Up to the twentieth century the Eskimos of Godhavn, West Greenland, the Tungusis, the Chirguises, the Boscimanis and some aborigines of the Dutch East Indies were not acquainted with salt and had no word for it. Salt is still

Assessment and Management of Hepatobiliary Disease
Eds.: L. Okolicsányi, G. Csomós, and G. Crepaldi

**Table 1.** Sodium contents of some foods (mg sodium/100 g food)

| 1-10 | 20-30 | 40-50 | 50-70 | 70-100 |
|---|---|---|---|---|
| Flour, potatoes | Mushrooms | Milk | Beef | Veal |
| Pasta, rice | Lentils | Rabbit | Turkey | Chicken |
| Fresh peas | Carrots | Trout | Pork | Liver |
| Aubergines | Cabbage | Salmon | One egg (average 50 g) | Whiting |
| Courgettes | Cauliflower | Unsalted butter | | Haddock |
| Marrow | Artichokes | | | Dentex |
| Tomatoes | Melon | | | Bream |
| Onion | | | | Sole |
| Fresh fruit | | | | Turbot |
| Nuts | | | | Mascarpone (Galbani) |
| Honey | | | | Cottage cheese |
| Sugar | | | | |
| Olive oil | | | | |
| Jam | | | | |
| Barley | | | | |

1 mEq sodium corresponds to 23 mg sodium

unknown to the unacculturated Yanomamo Indians of the tropical equatorial forests of northern Brazil and southern Venezuela [3]. They do not use salt in their diet, which consists mainly of the cooking banana with irregular supplements of game, fish, insects, and wild vegetable foods. Their urinary excretion of sodium is lower than 10 mEq/day.

The habit of using salt is acquired very quickly: the acculturated monkeys of Koshima quickly learned to salt potatoes and raw cereals by wetting them in sea-water.

The use and abuse of dietary salt is due to a deep-rooted custom and represents a status symbol rising from an ancient tradition. Among nomadic peoples salt is a symbol of amity. In the Bible salt is mentioned as necessary to life (Sir 39, 26), for sacrifice (Exodus 30, 35), and for alliance (2 Chronicles 13, 14). In classic culture salt is a symbol of fraternity and amity (Demostene, Cicerone), but the Egyptians, Greeks, and Romans also sprinkled salt on their sacrificial victims. Also in Christian tradition salt was important: it was a symbol of amity and wisdom, was used in food for catechumens, was the first food for the newborn, and is a component of holy water.

## Sodium Balance in the Cirrhotic Patient with Ascites

Cirrhotic patients who accumulate ascites on an unrestricted sodium diet show low urinary sodium excretion (from 20 mEq down to less than 10 mEq daily). Extrarenal sodium loss is about 22 mEq/day, and consequently cirrhotic patients on a normal diet retain about 2 g (87 mEq) sodium daily. The retention of every gram of sodium will cause a retention of 200-300 ml of fluid. The easiest way to monitor fluid retention in patients suffering from cirrhosis is daily checking of their weight. Outpatients should make a practice of recording their own weight every day.

Sodium restriction is usually regarded as essential for managing ascites. It is known that a strict low-sodium diet (10 mEq/24 h) could lead to a mobilization of 300 ml as-

**Table 2.** An example of a diet containing 250 mg sodium (for cirrhotic patients without diabetes and without hepatic encephalopathy)

*Breakfast:* tea or coffee with 50 g milk; 5-10 g sugar or 15 g jam; two salt-free biscuits
*Dinner:* 100-150 g rice or pasta, or 75 g pasta with 50 g dried beans; 50 g beef or 85 g veal or 90 g chicken or 115 g turkey or 190 g rabbit; 100 g vegetables; 25 g olive oil; 50-100 g salt-free bread; 200 g fresh fruit
*Supper:* 250 g potatoes with onions and tomatoes; two eggs or 150 g fish (trout, haddock) or 150 g cottage cheese; 25 g olive oil or butter; 50-100 g salt-free bread; 200 g fresh fruit

Dishes can be seasoned as described in the text. If salt-free bread is not available, we suggest this recipe for home-made bread: 250 g flour, 100 g potatoes, 20-30 g olive oil, and a little brewer's yeast

cites daily. However, this degree of sodium restriction is not tolerated by all patients, and consequently caloric intake may decline. Hence, especially in outpatients, we usually prescribe a less rigorous sodium restriction (22 mEq daily, equivalent to 500 mg sodium daily), and at the same time spironolactone 50-100 mg daily is prescribed to achieve adequate diuresis and an acceptable rate of weight loss (500-800 g/day). Once the initial mobilization of ascites occurs, the sodium intake can be increased to 32 mEq/day (750 mg/day); when ascites disappears, the spironolactone dosage can be reduced and in some cases discontinued, while a moderately restrictive sodium diet (32-43 mEq/day, equivalent to 750-1000 mg/day sodium) should be maintained. The medical treatment of ascites is successful in the majority of cirrhotics if proper sodium limitation is observed.

To achieve maximal compliance, patients should receive detailed information on how salt restriction may successfully be accomplished. It is necessary to discuss with the patient the sodium content in his prescribed diet, the foods to avoid, and the dishes to choose.

A monotonous low-sodium diet aggravates anorexia and makes malnutrition worse; the patient needs to be instructed on how to prepare appetizing recipes and encouraged to experiment with cuisine, as Schaffner [4] suggests. In our experience a diet with only 250 mg sodium daily is rather unpleasant, but it is usually acceptable for the 2-3 weeks necessary to obtain a rapid mobilization of ascites. A Mediterranean diet containing about 250 mg/day of sodium is reported in Table 2. It is indispensable to use salt-free bread, as ordinary bread in our area contains 400 mg sodium/100 g bread. To prepare a diet containing 500 mg, 750 mg, or 1 g sodium, we suggest adding some supplements which will make the dishes more palatable and varied (Table 3).

Listed in Table 4 are some of the most common salt-rich foods which must be strictly avoided by the patient. The high sodium content in some tinned tomato sauces and tomato soups, tinned peas, canned vegetables, pastry, and cakes containing baking powder should be taken into account. We do not encourage the use of salt substitutes with a fair amount of sodium and a high potassium content; the latter may be harmful if the patient is taking spironolactone.

Some drugs occasionally prescribed to cirrhotic patients have a high sodium content (Table 5). The physician must check the sodium content of any drugs prescribed and warn the patient against taking any drugs on his own initiative.

**Table 3.** Amounts of food containing 250 mg sodium which can be utilized as supplements, to the diet reported in Table 2

| Food | Amount | Food | Amount |
|---|---|---|---|
| Milk | 500 g | Boiled ham | 30 g |
| Galbanino | 62 g | Mortadella | 37 g |
| Parmesan | 33 g | Tinned tunny (Cirio) | 32 g |
| Swiss cheese | 40 g | Fresh artichoke | 500 g |
| Bel Paese | 36 g | Spinach | 400 g |
| Edam | 34 g | Celery | 260 g |
| Unsalted mozzarella | 125 g | Panettone (Motta-Alemagna) | 180 g |
| or mozzarella (Galbani) | | Pandoro (Motta-Alemagna) | 150 g |

As regards commercial products, we mention only those with an unvarying sodium content. We thank Cirio, Galbani, and Motta-Alemagna for information concerning their products

**Table 4.** Foods to avoid owing to high sodium content

- Ordinary bread, baking powder, deep-frozen shortcrust or puff pastry.
- Cheese spread, cream cheese, fresh and seasoned cheeses, salted butter and margarine, mozzarella
- Mayonnaise, ketchup, bottled sauces.
- Sausages, ham, bacon, kippers, shellfish, oysters, canned fish and meat.
- Olives, capers, soup cubes, salted canned vegetables.
- Commercial biscuits, cakes, puddings, and ice cream.

It is necessary to verify the sodium content of mineral water and bottled soft drinks.

**Table 5.** Drugs not to be prescribed owing to high sodium content

| Drug | Sodium content |
|---|---|
| Alcalosio, granular[a] | 297 mg/10 g |
| Calcium Sandoz forte, effervescent tablets[b] | 282 mg/tablet |
| Ca-Sterogyl, sachets[b] | 424 mg/sachet |
| Citroepatina, granular[a] | 493 mg/10 g |
| Detoxergon, sachets | 164 mg/sachet |
| Geffer, sachets[a] | 287 mg/sachet |
| Legalon, sachets | 155 mg/sachet |
| Polase, sachets | 109 mg/sachet |
| Supradyn, effervescent tablets | 300 mg/tablet |

[a] Sodium-free antacids include Maalox, Aldrox, and Mucoxin;
[b] As preparation containing calcium and vitamin D we use Calci-Ostelin $B_{12}$ syrup

## Selection of Foods to Make a Low-Sodium Diet More Palatable

The patients should choose foods which are acceptable even if cooked without added salt. For the first course, potatoes (boiled, baked, mashed), rice, dried beans, or lentils (mashed or with pasta) can be suggested; for the main course, cottage cheese, fresh or deep-frozen fish, eggs, rabbit, or chicken. Artichokes, carrots, tomatoes, marrow, courgettes, and boiled onions are among the vegetables to which the patient should give preference. The taste of the food can be improved by seasoning it with aromatic vegetables, spices, and sauces. Sherlock [5] recommends flavoring with lemon juice, orange peel, onion, vinegar, garlic, salt-free ketchup and mayonnaise, sage, parsley, thyme, marjoram, bay leaves, cloves, pepper, or mustard. We believe that pepper and mustard should be recommended only to patients with no sign of gastritis. We advise further aromatic vegetables, seeds, and spices: basil, mint, oregano, cinnamon, truffle, almonds, pine seeds, walnuts, pistachio, nutmeg, raisins, saffron, or fennel seeds.

Sherlock [5] suggests the use of two sauces: salt-free ketchup and mayonnaise. We suggest the use of other sauces, some of which help to make salt-free foods more nourishing: bechamel[1], white sauce[1], yellow sauce[1], Dutch sauce[1], "Maitre d'Hotel" sauce[1], truffled sauce[1], green sauce[2], and tunny sauce[3].

Bechamel sauce, which is prepared with milk, flour, and butter, is easily digestible, useful for increasing protein intake, and excellent for seasoning pasta, potatoes, and many other vegetables. Food seasoned with bechamel can be baked au gratin, thus becoming more digestible owing to the damp heat when baking.

## Science in the Kitchen and the Art of Eating Well

Artusi [6] gave his book the title *La scienza in cucina e l'arte di mangiar bene*, meaning that good cooking is at the same time a science and an art.

The cirrhotic patient is frequently compelled by relatives, friends, and some incompetent physicians to abstain from eating wholesome, well-seasoned meals. Competent physicians should protect patients from this harmful advice and encourage them to prepare a diet with suitably cooked and seasoned food. Obviously, the diet needs to be adjusted to each single patient in relation to the degree of liver trouble and the presence of hepatic encephalopathy or associated diseases (diabetes, peptic ulcer, cholelithiasis). The patient without cholelithiasis should be allowed olive oil or butter in normal amounts and encouraged to add an egg yolk to pasta, rice, and mashed potatoes as desired.

As regards fish, the patient should abstain only from shellfish; he must cook river or sea fish in a savory fashion. We suggest consulting Alan Davidson's *Mediterranean Sea-Food* [7] which contains plenty of tasty recipes.

A low-sodium diet should include a main course of two eggs at least twice a week; eggs do no harm to the liver. They may be cooked in various ways (hard or soft boiled, poached, scrambled, or fried); we can also suggest omelettes, which can be made with parsley, parmesan, Swiss cheese, boiled ham, or various vegetables.

As for meat dishes, we suggest some good poultry and rabbit recipes: chicken baked with lemon; chicken salad with vegetables and salt-free mayonnaise; turkey with sage, rosemary, and garlic; stewed chicken; stewed rabbit. We also suggest some beef or veal dishes: stew; fricassee; braised beef; veal cutlet; meatballs made from yolk of egg, salt-free bread, raisins, and pine seeds. Meat can be pickled with red wine, co-

---

[1] Follow Artusi's recipe [6], excluding salt and pepper.

[2] Follow Artusi's recipe [6], excluding salt and substituting capers and anchovies with pickled gherkins.

[3] Follow Artusi's recipe [6], excluding salt, pepper, capers, and anchovies.

gnac, garlic and aromatic herbs. The addition of wine, Marsala, or cognac is not harmful, because the alcohol evaporates during cooking.

Finally, nondyspeptic patients should not omit fried food, provided it is prepared at home with olive oil. Artusi [6] lists about 60 fried recipes, many of which can be included in the diet.

Many patients with liver cirrhosis and ascites are anorexic and sometimes eat only the first course, their protein intake declining as a consequence. It is useful to suggest to them a single-course meal rich in protein, for instance gateau of potatoes with salt-free mozzarella and boiled eggs; sartù of rice with boiled eggs, meat-balls, peas and artichokes; gnocchi of semolina with egg and milk; or home-made agnolotti or cannelloni with a cottage cheese filling and a bechamel sauce, remembering always to prepare a salt-free dough.

Patients without hyperglycemia should be allowed home-made cakes, with natural ingredients and no baking powder; also pandoro and panettone (Motta-Alemagna) have a moderate sodium content (see Table 3). Patients are advised to avoid commercial cakes unless the sodium content is given and is compatible with their prescribed diet. Some home-made cakes such as sponges, Sicilian, or Neapolitan cakes containing sweetened cottage cheese are suitable for their high protein content.

## References

1. Guilbert JJ (1981) Obiettivi educativi. In: Armando A (ed) Guida pedagogica, Rome
2. Quagliariello G (1958) Importanza degli alimenti inorganici. In: Idelson (ed) Scienza dell'alimentazione.
3. Oliver WJ, Cohen EL, Neel JV (1975) Blood pressure, sodium intake, and sodium related hormones in the Yanomamo Indians, a "no-salt" culture. Circulation 52: 146-151
4. Schaffner F (1985) Management of chronic hepatitis. Semin Liver dis 5: 209-220
5. Sherlock S (1963) Control of ascites. In: Diseases of the liver and biliary system. Blackwell, Oxford
6. Artusi P (1970) La scienza in cucina e l'arte di mangiar bene. Einaudi, Torino
7. Davidson A (1981) Mediterranean seafood. Chancer, Bungay (Italian edition: Il mare in pentola. Mondadori, Milan, 1983).

# Treatment of Refractory Ascites by Concentrated Ascitic Fluid Reinfusion

A. Martin, L. Rossaro, G. C. Sturniolo, and R. Naccarato
Divisione Convenzionata di Gastroenterologia "R. Farini", Policlinico Universitario, Via Giustiniani 2, 35100 Padova, Italy

## Introduction

In most cases ascites complicating liver cirrhosis responds to diet and diuretics, but in a proportion as high as 4%-10% of patients this treatment becomes ineffective and progressively ascites becomes refractory [1]. In such cases, the increase in dosages of diuretics is of no benefit and is often dangerous, since it increases the risk of encephalopathy, prerenal azotemia and electrolyte imbalance, with a frequently rapid and fatal course [2].

Many alternative treatments have been tried, including paracentesis [3], plasma volume expanders [4], angiotensin-converting enzyme inhibitors [5], prostaglandins [6], peritoneovenous shunting [7], and reinfusion of concentrated ascites [8]. This report summarizes our clinical experience of reinfusion of concentrated ascites. The Rhodiascit apparatus allows continuous concentration of the ascitic fluid, which is infused intravenously. This procedure is based on the assumption that it allows "expansion" of plasma volume, improvement in the alterations of intrarenal hemodynamics, and salvage of the proteins contained in the ascitic fluid [9].

## Patients and Methods

From 1973 to 1986 we treated 131 ascitic patients with 182 reinfusions of concentrated ascitic fluid, using the Rhodiascit pump 1 [8]. The patients included 94 males and 37 females aged 22-74 years. Their diagnoses, based on clinical, biochemical, and morphological criteria, are presented in Table 1.

Indication for the procedure was basically lack of response to conventional treatment, i.e., bed rest and diet ($Na^+ = 20$ mEq/day) over a 7-day period, with a weight

**Table 1.** Etiology of liver disease in 131 patients treated by concentrated ascitic fluid reinfusion

| Etiology | *n* |
|---|---|
| Alcoholic cirrhosis | 63 |
| HBV-related cirrhosis | 21 |
| Cryptogenic | 41 |
| Budd-Chiari syndrome | 1 |
| Wilson's syndrome | 1 |
| Primary liver cell cancer | 4 |

Assessment and Management of Hepatobiliary Disease
Eds.: L. Okolicsányi, G. Csomós, and G. Crepaldi

loss of less than 1 kg. The procedure was also indicated when diuretic treatment had to be discontinued, due to severe hyponatremia (< 125 mEq/l) and, finally, as a preoperative procedure (before implant of peritoneovenous shunting or surgical treatment of umbilical hernia). We considered as contraindications only severe encephalopathy (grade III-IV) and infection of ascites (growth of bacteria in culture and/or presence of over 300 PMN leukocytes/$mm^3$ ascites).

In our 131 cases ascites had been present for an average of 2.2 years (range 2 months to 13 years), and 42% of patients had signs of functional renal failure with elevated (> 0.5 g/l) BUN, while 29% had also oliguria (< 500 ml/day) and 11% were severely hyponatremic. The severity of liver disease according to Pugh's classification [10] was as follows: grade A, 0%; B, 38%; C, 62%.

Blood and urine samples for the routine biochemical tests were taken before and after the procedure. In nine patients, blood samples were taken every 15 min during the first hour for determination of the plasma renin activity (PRA) and of plasma aldosterone by specific radioimmunoassay.

The length of hospital stay was recorded. Although the two groups are not fully comparable, the length of hospital stay of a group of patients treated for ascites with the conventional dietary and diuretic therapy, was also recorded.

Student's t test for paired data was used for statistical analysis of the data before and after reinfusion.

## Results

Table 2 summarizes the clinical results of treatment, while Table 3 shows the effect of the reinfusion on the clinical and biochemical parameters. Most patients tolerated the treatment well; the complications observed are presented in Table 4.

The data on PRA and plasma aldosterone, published elsewhere [11], showed a significant, steady decrease of the blood levels of these hormones during the procedure.

In 38% of our patients the procedure was repeated, from two to seven times. The average interval between the procedures was 2.5 months (range 0.5-9 months).

The duration of hospital stay was $9.4 \pm 6$ days in the patients treated by the reinfusion of ascites and $19 \pm 7$ days in those receiving the routine therapy. For a tentative assessment of costs, it may be noted that in our hospital, the cost of hospital stay is about 300000 lire (US $ 200) per day. For comparison, a LeVeen catheter costs about 1300000 lire (US $ 870).

**Table 2.** Clinical results of 182 reinfusions in 131 patients

| | Mean | Range |
|---|---|---|
| Duration of treatment (h) | 13.7 | 2.0-46 |
| Weight loss (kg) | 8.3 | 3.5-23 |
| Concentrated ascites infused (l) | 4.1 | 0.6- 7.6 |
| Ultrafiltrate (l) | 7.3 | 1.0-21 |
| Diuresis (l) | 2.1 | 0.4- 7.4 |

**Table 3.** Variations in clinical and biochemical parameters after concentrated ascitic fluid reinfusion

| | Mean difference from values before treatment | $p$ (Student's t test) |
|---|---|---|
| Weight loss (kg) | − 8.33 | 0.001 |
| Diuresis[a] (l) | 0.28 | 0.01 |
| PCV (%) | − 0.73 | 0.001 |
| BUN (g/l) | − 0.016 | n.s. |
| Serum creatinine (mg/l) | − 0.074 | n.s. |
| Serum albumin (g/dl) | + 0.19 | 0.02 |
| Serum Na (mEq/l) | + 1.17 | 0.02 |
| Serum K (mEq/l) | + 0.011 | n.s. |
| Serum Osmolality (mOsm/l) | + 2.31 | n.s. |
| Urinary Na (mEq/day) | +13.09 | 0.01 |
| Urinary K (mEq/day) | + 2.69 | n.s. |
| Urinary osmolality (mOsm/l) | +22.06 | n.s. |

[a] Mean of 5 days preceding/following the reinfusion

**Table 4.** Complications observed after 182 procedures

| | $n$ | % |
|---|---|---|
| Major: | | |
| Hepatic coma | 4 | 2.5 |
| Variceal bleeding (1 death) | 4 | 2.5 |
| Left ventricular failure | 5 | 3.0 |
| Minor: | | |
| Fever | 85 | 47.0 |
| Scrotal/local edema | 13 | 7.0 |
| Arterial hypertension | 4 | 2.5 |
| Abdominal pain | 1 | 0.5 |

## Discussion

Although we claim no scientific value for our experience with ascites reinfusion, which was intended only as a clinical tool in the relatively frequent (about 20%, in our setting), cases of "resistant" ascites, we feel that some conclusions can be drawn.

First of all, the treatment is correct from the pathophysiological point of view, since it saves the patients' own proteins, increasing plasma oncotic pressure, and expands the "effective" plasma volume. The consequent improved renal perfusion is demonstrated by the significant and rapid decrease of PRA.

Although major side effects may complicate the procedure, they are relatively infrequent. The short- and medium-term (up to 6 months) results are satisfactory. The majority of patients, in fact, do not gain weight rapidly in the weeks immediately following the procedure, and the positive effect on diuresis also tends to persist for a variable length of time. The feeling that the procedure affects the pathophysiology of the ascitic decompensation, albeit only temporarily, is also supported by the observation that in as many as 62% of patients, doses of diuretics which were ineffective before the treatment, become effective again after it.

As already stated, we have employed this treatment as a clinical tool for those patients where diuretics were no longer effective or had become contraindicated, partly because we had no better alternative. For these reasons, and because of the general satisfaction with the results of the procedure, reinfusion has become our procedure of choice for "resistant" ascites. Although difficult to assess, the low cost of the materials and the possible reduction of the hospital stay may make the procedure economically appealing.

## Summary

Although variable and difficult to estimate, as many as 10%–20% of patients with ascites are "resistant" to "conventional" treatment with diet and diuretics. In 131 such cases we employed the i.v. reinfusion of concentrated ascitic fluid. Contraindications to the procedure were infection of the ascites and encephalopathy (grade III–IV). Most patients had alcoholic (63) or HBV-related (21) cirrhosis. Forty-two percent of patients had increased (>0.5 g/l) BUN, 29% had oliguria (<500 ml/day), and 11% had hyponatremia (<125 mEq/l).

The mean duration of the 182 procedures was 13.7 h, with a mean weight loss of 8.3 kg. An average of 4.1 l concentrated ascites was infused, while 7.3 l ultrafiltrate and 2.1 l urine were eliminated. Serum albumin, plasma, and urinary Na+ significantly ($p < 0.02$) increased after treatment. Major complications consisted of: variceal bleeding (4 cases), hepatic coma (4), pulmonary edema (5). Conventionally treated patients had a mean hospital stay of 19 days compared to the 9 days of those treated with reinfusion. This, considering the cost of about US $ 160 per filter, makes the procedure economically appealing.

In conclusion, the procedure is pathophysiologically sound, relatively simple, well tolerated, and major complications are infrequent. For these reasons, the good short-term results, and the low cost, it is our procedure of choice when diuretics fail.

## References

1. Sherlock S (1975) Diseases of the liver and biliary system, 5th edn. Blackwell, Oxford, pp 122–149
2. Wilkinson SP, Williams R (1979) Ascites, electrolyte disorders and renal failure. In: Wright R, Alberti KGMM, Karran S, Millward-Sadler GH (eds) Liver and biliary disease. Saunders, Philadelphia, pp 1060–1086
3. Quintero E, Arroyo V, Bory F, Viver J, Ginés P, Rimola A, Planas R, Cabrera J, Rodés J (1985) Paracentesis versus diuretics in the treatment of cirrhotics with tense ascites. Lancet 1: 611–612
4. Vlahceviz ZR, Adham NF, Jick H, et al. (1965) Renal effects of acute expansion of plasma volume in cirrhosis. N Engl J Med 272: 387–390
5. Shepherd AN, Neligan P, Hayes PC (1983) Captopril and resistant ascites. Lancet 1: 1391–1392
6. Epstein M, Lifschitz M, Ramachandran M, et al. (1982) Characterization of renal PGE responsiveness in decompensated cirrhosis: implications of renal sodium handling. Clin Sci 63: 555–563

7. Wapnick S, Grosberg S, Kinney M, LeVeen HH (1977) LeVeen continuous peritoneal-jugular shunt. Improvement of renal function in ascitic patients. JAMA 237: 131-133
8. Wilkinson SP, Handerson J, Davidson AR, Williams R (1975) Ascites reinfusion using the Rhodiascit apparatus - clinical experience and coagulation abnormalities. Postgrad Med J 51: 583-587
9. Levy VG, Paulean N, Opolon P, Caroli J (1975) Treatment of ascites by reinfusion of concentrated peritoneal fluid - review of 318 procedures in 210 patients. Postgrad Med J 51: 564-566
10. Pugh RNH, Murray-Lyon IM, Dawson JL (1973) Transection of the oesophagus for bleeding oesophageal varices. Br J Surg 60: 646-649
11. Martin A, Sturniolo GC, Naccarato R (1980) Renin-angiotensin-aldosterone in cirrhotic ascites. Gastroenterology 78: 1123

# Concluding Remarks

N. Tygstrup

I knew that it would not be easy to comment on such rich and varied chapters as are in this section, but I would like to do so from the point of view of functional evaluation. The situation can be evaluated in two different ways, just as when you have half a bottle of whisky: you can say it is half-full or half-empty. If you say it is half-full you are an optimist, and if you say it is half-empty you are a pessimist. However, if you say it is half-full you may be satisfied with the situation, but if you say it is half-empty, then you will start to think about how to improve the situation. My pessimistic remarks should be seen in this light.

In his chapter, Dr. Blanckaert stated that functional evaluation has certainly not made great progress in hepatology for a long time. Progress has come mainly from, for instance, serology, which has little to do with liver function, from histology, and from imaging techniques like ultrasonography, endoscopy, and CT scan, which at most give very indirect information on liver functions.

This is discouraging for someone like me who considers the liver first and foremost as a biochemical factory. I feel that functional evaluation should be one of the main concerns of hepatologists. I was pleased to see that the term "liver function tests" was not used very often to refer to studies like enzyme and immune globulin levels. It could perhaps be used with some justification for one of the oldest liver tests or signs of liver disease we have, namely bilirubinemia, because it seems that some of the mysteries of bilirubin fractions may be solved by the new chromatographic techniques. Conjugation of bilirubin is a liver function, but a function one would expect not to be very important from the clinical point of view. Except for kernicterus and Crigler-Najjar syndrome, bilirubin probably has no pathogenetic significance. Only because it happens to absorb light in the visible spectrum, and thus changes the color of the skin, has it become one of the key signs in hepatology. It appears that the fraction of conjugated bilirubin is related to liver function, but it should not be accepted as a *measure* of liver function until its relationship with the capacity of the liver for conjugation of bilirubin has been proven.

The same may be said concerning bile acid metabolism, so well discussed by Dr. B. Billing. One would expect the function of the liver regarding bile acid mainly concerns its ability to produce this compound, which is only made in the liver and is important for the body. But this is not so. The capacity for synthesis of bile acid cannot at the moment be used for liver function evaluation. What we can measure is the efficacy of elimination and excretion. Again, as with bilirubin, the function we are concerned with is the formation of bile rather than the liver's metabolic capacity.

About 300 years ago one of my fellow countrymen, Bartholin, characterized the liver as a very uninteresting organ, a big, dull producer of a few drops of bile. It would be

Assessment and Management of Hepatobiliary Disease
Eds.: L. Okolicsányi, G. Csomós, and G. Crepaldi

a pity if in the future we still had to evaluate the liver by its ability to make slimy bile. The fact that attempts are being made to evaluate it more directly is encouraging. We would like to know more about and learn how to measure the functions which are important in keeping us healthy and happy, with or without bile, with or without jaundice, but so far little has been achieved in this respect.

It has been pointed out in this section that an important function of the liver may be regulation of endocrine substances. Since the number of hormones is increasing very rapidly now, with all the peptide hormones, a great deal of attention is being paid to them. I find it very difficult, however, to see how we can relate the effect of the liver on hormonal regulation to liver function as such, before we know more about the metabolism of the hormones in the liver and how this is regulated.

We have heard about the effects of drugs, toxins, and foodstuffs, and that the difference between the categories of substances which we ingest may not be great as far as the liver is concerned. One important substance, which is at the same time a drug, a food, and a toxin, is alcohol. It is well-known that alcohol has a great influence on the liver and that the liver has a great influence on the metabolism of alcohol. Again, however, it is difficult to distinguish between the different roles of alcohol and the role of liver function. It has been noted that some tests may prove valuable in deciding whether a patient is alcoholic or not. This may be an acceptable pragmatic approach, but I think it will not bring us very far until we have clarified what we mean by "alcoholic." Is it a patient who takes so much alcohol that it will damage his or her liver? This may be one level. Is it the one who drinks more than I do? If so, then it is - I hope - a slightly lower level. Or is it all those who drink alcohol occasionally, in which case it is an even lower level? I think that this should be looked at critically, and not only regarding the definition of alcoholism or alcoholic liver disease, but also regarding liver disease in general. We have heard reports of tests which reveal minimal liver disease, but what *is* minimal liver disease? Is it defined histologically or clinically? I feel that clinical definitions should always be preferred, with all the difficulties this entails.

Therefore, it is not difficult for me to include the last part of this section, i.e. that on ascites, in this point of view. What we are interested in is, after all, the effect liver function has on the organism as a whole. We know very little about the effect of liver function on the liver itself, we have to look at effects in other parts of the body - the brain, the kidneys, etc.

However, as pointed out by Dr. Galambos, we are perhaps a little too inclined to forget the liver. When we discuss complications, their relation to liver function should always be kept in mind. Encephalopathy is not just a question of branched-chain amino acids or of false neurotransmitters; it is basically a change in liver function.

What can we do, what can we expect or hope for? I think we should aim at measuring some liver functions which are important for our existence and well-being. As yet, however, we don't know which. We have heard something about quantitative liver functions, and I believe this is the area in which we may find some answers. But probably we first must find substances which are more pathogenetically relevant than aminopyrine, antipyrine, galactose, and caffeine.

The next question is how to use such tests. We have some help from outside, namely, from liver transplantation. You must forgive me, but I personally consider liver transplantation as something coming from outside, as not really pertinent to hepatology and liver function. I think you will agree that liver transplantation is not the answer to the essential problems in hepatology. It is something that may help hepatology by defining new problems, by showing us the importance of quantitating the function of the liver of a candidate for transplantation. This new development in surgical technique will thus contribute to progress in the most important area of hepatology, namely functional evaluation.

I was not present when Hans Popper first came to a meeting in Padova in 1921, but I was present 8 years ago at the meeting of the European Association for the Study of the Liver, and I think that some progress has been made in functional evaluation since then. There is a greater awareness of the problem, and I would very much like to come back 8 years from now and see that some of the current questions have been answered. One thing we can do already is to try to standardize our observations better. In his chapter Dr. Blanckaert gave us data from various centres on variation in methods, units, and reference intervals. We have had a similar experience, so I wasn't shocked, but it *is* a great problem. If we want to make quantitative evaluation of liver function, and to utilize it for communication, we have to standardize our observations - and persuade our clinical chemists to do the same.

Above all, however, there should be more meetings to discuss the problems in this field. The papers in this volume have focused on the assessment and management of hepatobiliary disease and I hope that they have contributed to raising the level in that whisky bottle of ours, labeled "Functional Evaluation of the Liver."

# Management of Liver Disease

# Liver and Aging

Hans Popper

Stratton Laboratory for the Study of Liver Diseases, Mount Sinai School of Medicine of the City University of New York, New York, NY 10029, U.S.A.

Upsurge of interest in a medical or other scientific problem is usually stimulated by discoveries, conceptual or technological. The rising concern with the medical effects of aging and also its action on the liver has been created not by such factors but rather by sociologic concerns, namely by the rapid increase of the aged segment of the population as expressed in demographic data (U.N. World Assembly 1982; Butler and Bearn 1985). In the United States, since 1983, persons over 65 years of age exceed the number of teenagers. In 2050 one-third of the population will be 55 and over, and one-fourth over 65 years of age. According to United Nations data, those over 60 years will double in number from 1985 to 2000 and in 2025 will represent one-seventh of the world population. The most rapidly growing segment of the United States' population is those aged 85 and over; in 1949 it represent 1.3% of the population, in 1982 1.9%, and is projected to rise to 2% in 2000 and to 16 million in the year 2050. This alarming problem is further complicated by the greater demand by the aged for health care, particularly drugs. Today persons over 65, 11% of the population, consume 30% of the prescription drugs, and almost all of them take several drugs. The essentially sociologic concern and increasing awareness explain the sudden emphasis on medical care of the aged - geriatrics - and on the science of aging - gerontology. The initial scientific isolation of gerontology, coupled with its rapid expansion without scientific breakthroughs, explains the often incomplete and controversial available data. Nevertheless, it stimulates a look at gerontology, attempted in this report, from the point of view of hepatology (Popper 1985, 1986). Based on the prevailing assumption of a reduction of hepatic function in aging, two questions are raised: (1) Does the liver deteriorate in aging - senesce, or wither - and to what degree is this detrimental to the organism? (2) What are the hepatologic problems in clinical management in old age?

## Theories of Biologic Aging

The four commonly listed theories of biologic aging (Dice 1985; Harman 1981; Martin 1977) may serve as introduction, though all are controversial and they are not mutually exclusive.

The first assumes that longevity and aging are programmed in development and that the number of cell divisions is genetically determined. The second claims an „error catastrophe" from increase of defects in transcription and translation, which may for instance result in an altered conformation of enzymes. The third incriminates injuries from free radicals, primarily an excess of various toxic oxygen species, and the fourth assumes damage to DNA and its repair, resulting in a reduced synthesis of protein which in view of the unchanged tissue protein concentration would postulate a re-

Assessment and Management of Hepatobiliary Disease
Eds.: L. Okolicsányi, G. Csomós, and G. Crepaldi

duced catabolism. Many observations incriminate altered ribosomal translation of RNA. Indeed, in rats the synthesis of both RNA and the polyadenylated form is reduced (Richardson and Cheung 1982). Thus, the problems of the liver and aging will be discussed under the headings of (a) morphologic and functional observations, as theoretical basis; (b) drug metabolism, for guidance in therapy; (c) the response of the liver to stimuli, important in management; and (d) age-related disease expressions, for clinical practice, in order finally (e) to address the principal question of whether the liver senesces.

## Morphologic Observations

The conventional expression of the aging of the liver at autopsy is brown atrophy; the organ appears smaller and darker. This also occurs, of course, in wasting diseases and in malnutrition. Histologically, lipofuscin accumulates around the bile canaliculi, preferentially in the perivenous zone, and focally, hepatocytes are enlarged and have dark polychromatic nuclei. Thus, morphologically the healthy aging human liver shows a reduction of weight but not of the number of acini (Tauchi and Sato 1978). But this weight loss is not uniform and thus barely usable for functional calculations, and does not occur at all in rats. The brown color comes from lipofuscin, or wear-and-tear pigment, a mainly indigestible residue of polymerized oxidation products, as also illustrated by its accumulation in many organs in vitamin E deficiency, in that case caused by toxic oxygen (Poot et al. 1986). Hepatic pigment is derived from the diet, drugs, or breakdown of organelles, which live for a much shorter time than the cells and which turn over even more rapidly in liver injury. Thus, lipofuscin reflects life experiences of the organ and of the hepatocytes. Moreover, hepatocytes, nuclei, and mitochondria all show conspicuous variations in their size. Morphometry indicates slight reductions in number and mean size. Thus, microhepatocytes and macrohepatocytes are seen (Watanabe and Tanaka 1982). However, the functional significance of all these changes is not clear.

## Functional Observations

As to the function of the aged liver, hepatic blood flow is slightly reduced, mainly on dye clearance examinations, not yet on Doppler imaging techniques. The reduction, not fully accepted, may be due to either lower liver weight or lower cardiac output. Bile flow and bile acid secretion are normal, bile acid synthesis and pool are reduced (Kitani et al. 1981), and since biliary secretion of cholesterol appears increased, cholesterol saturation of bile rises, resulting in an enhanced tendency to gallstone formation (Einarsson et al. 1985). Transcellular transport is reduced, for instance of sulfobromophthalein (BSP), but it is controversial whether transport or storage is altered. The transport of IgA from plasma to bile is decreased in rats, with reduction of the receptors, the secretory component, and this is said to account for impaired immunity of the intestinal mucosa (Schmucker et al. 1985). Thus, deficiencies of constitutive function appear to be selective, if significant at all.

Alterations of the individual hepatocytes include increase of DNA, reflected in at least focal polyploidy, and of albumin and its messenger RNA (Knook 1980), and indeed more albumin has been found in the large hepatocytes, but less BSP in cells with polyploid nuclei. Whether the mitochondria are functionally altered is not established, and one statement speaks of „less respiratory activity per liver but not per cell" (Knook and Hollander 1978). Thus the functional capacity of the enlarged hepatocytes and the functional significance of the conspicuous variations of hepatocytes and their constituents deserve clarification.

This raises the question as to the *alterations of the hepatic macromolecules,* which also might explain the excess of hepatocytic albumin and DNA. Evidence exists for a selective reduction of proetin synthesis, for instance of the rat alpha$_{\mu 2}$-globulin, vs a selective increase as reflected in increased incorporation of tagged leucine into albumin. Some catabolism, for instance of albumin, is reduced. Enzymes accumulate with either translational or post-translational changes in three-dimensional configuration, as for aldolase B and superoxide dismutase (Gershon 1979). They show a discrepancy between immunoreactive amount and reduced catalytic potency. There are repeated claims of impaired fidelity of translation, less of transcription, which may account for the variations of hepatocytes and their organelles. Possibly an inferior quality of some macromolecules, "junk" proteins, may stimulate a compensatory hyperplasia which exhausts the functional reserve and may also be related to the characteristic cellular and organelle variations.

## Regeneration and Carcinogenesis

These data are in keeping with an impaired repair of hepatocytes, more in translation than in transcription, since DNA repair in the liver is supposedly unchanged. According to several studies (Stöcker 1975), regeneration is delayed but not quantitatively reduced, i. e., less mitoses develop in a reduced periportal zone in each mitotic cycle, but this is compensated for by an increase in number of cycles.

Carcinogenesis in old age is a problem. There is no doubt about increased recognition of malignancies, which may have been initiated years or even decades before. In some experiments with chemical carcinogens, nodules appeared earlier but not more frequently, and phenobarbital also induced more nodules. However, in rats the mutagenic potency is reduced. These findings are related to the general problem as to whether the cytochrome $P_{450}$ system activates or detoxifies a specific compound. In short, it is not established whether initiation of new tumors is more or less frequent in advanced age.

## Drug Metabolism

Uncertainties apply also to many aspects of drug handling in aging (Schmucker 1985). Drug disposition appears diminished because of a questionable impairment of intestinal absorption or of albumin binding and of a better proven reduction in renal excretion. Diminished hepatic blood flow may be important in first-pass drugs, and hepatocellular drug receptors are possibly decreased. Distribution of lipid-soluble drugs may be increased, as may be target tissue sensitivity, for instance of the brain. The class I reactions, primarily the microsomal monooxygenase system, which renders lipid-soluble drugs bioactive and also generates toxic oxygen species, have, according to Schmucker (1985) and others, reduced activity in the male rat. This is accounted for by altered enzyme activity of the NADPH-dependent cytochrome C reductase and possibly by alterations of some of the multiple isoenzymes of cytochrome $P_{450}$. Such alterations also depend on changes of the phospholipid membranes in which an increased cholesterol/phospholipid ratio decreases fluidity. Moreover, some specific inducer effects were found to be reduced. However, as the important studies by Kitani (1986) show, the reduction of cytochrome $P_{450}$ activity concerns a male-specific enzyme and is thus simply a hormonal feminization. Indeed, Schmucker (Maloney et al. 1986) and others (Sutter et al. 1985) recently demonstrated an absence of age variations in both female and male subhuman primates. Thus, extrapolation from animal, particularly rodent, studies to man is hazardous.

In *humans,* we tend to presume variable tendencies: to lowered drug clearance, to effectiveness of smaller drug doses, and to increased adverse hepatic drug reactions (Popper 1985, 1986). Bioavailability of first-pass drugs, probably of propranolol, may be raised. There seems to be a great variability in response to drugs metabolized by class I reactions, possibly because of the many isoenzymes of cytochrome $P_{450}$. Class II reactions, in which conjugases and hydrases render usually biologically inert compounds water-soluble and excretable, are, mostly unchanged in aging, or even increased, as they usually are in liver injury and even in the paraneoplastic nodules produced by carcinogenic regimens. An exception is represented by some glucuronides which by precipitation may induce cholestasis, a mechanism incriminated in the adverse reactions to benoxaprofen with age-reduced metabolism. Thus it is usually stated that the metabolism of valium, librium, theophylline, and antipyrine may be lowered, but not that of Serax, Ativan, and isoniazid (Holt 1986). It is not clear whether the human response to inducing agents, including smoking, is reduced. We therefore cannot yet offer universal guidelines, and tolerance should be tested for each patient and drug. However, important are drug interactions in the frequent polypharmacy, with cimetidine often quoted. Malnutrition and diseases, including those of the liver, also influence drug metabolism in the old.

## Adaptation

Returning to less practical considerations, there appears to be reduced response to regulatory mediators, largely on the basis of extrapolations from systems other than the liver. The formation, mainly extrahepatic, of some hormones, growth factors, and cytokines is altered. Receptor action may be reduced (Konoplya et al. 1986), as for low-density lipoproteins, insulin, and glucocorticoids, Postreceptor events may be impaired, including transport, as is immune surveillance. Thus, adaptation may be disturbed, which possibly leads to susceptibility to stress. Disturbed regulation is an important function in the major abnormal hepatic reactions, for instance, hepatocellular degeneration and cholestasis. However, an assumption of increased tendency to these reactions in aging is not confirmed by clinical observations if malnutrition is absent.

## Hepatic Diseases in Aging

An increased susceptibility to experimental liver injuries is not established, nor is there a difference in the results of the routine hepatic tests. Abnormalities imply the same diseases as in the young, and only some more elaborate tests of specific metabolic processes, like the antipyrine breath test, are slightly influenced by age. There are no aging diseases of the liver, and today surgical indications are not influenced by the liver's aging. Thus, variations in incidence or severity of liver diseases in the old depend on social factors such as late-onset alcoholism or malnutrition, on delay of regeneration in hepatitis, and on immunologic disturbances, reflected in the vaccination schedule, in severity of hepatitis or occurrence of abscesses, and in the frequency of drug reactions, which might, however, also be due to use of more drugs and to interactions.

## Outlook and Conclusions

If the human liver seems to exhibit little deteriorating senescence, the question arises: Why? It enjoys a great functional reserve and regenerating potency, as we know from subtotal hepatectomy. It has an ample, indeed double blood supply, far in excess of the needs of the hepatocytes and the requirements for the liver's action on the blood. There are no functionally significant vascular diseases of the organ. Most important, however, is the very long life span of human hepatocytes. In every species the individual hepatocyte undergoes not more than two mitoses during life in the absence of injuries. In man the maximal potential life span is about 30 times longer than in rodents (Martin 1977), and this also applies to the hepatocytes. Finally, the basal metabolism, and with it the hepatic oxygen production, including that of toxic oxygen species, as well as amount of peroxidable tissue substances, are the lower the longer the life span, and usually also the greater the body's size (Parke and Ioannides 1984).

We thus come to the tentative conclusion that the impressive difference between rodents and man in life span and also in regulation, for instance by sex hormones, limits extrapolations (as is also the case for carcinogenesis). The human liver senesces less than most other organs, showing only minor constitutive defects. Regulatory deficiencies, i.e., adaptation to mainly extrahepatic factors, may reduce the functional reserve and the response to stress. Animal experiments, for instance with old dogs as donors, could indicate whether the present age limit of 45 years for donor livers in transplantation is justified. Furthermore, we can look at aging of the liver as an experiment of nature to study one factor, time, without secondary injury as seen in other organs. Finally, even if the basic theories of aging are not agreed upon, whether it is programmed death or accumulating damage, one might attempt to retard senescence of the organism by influencing liver function. This might include, besides dietary restrictions, dietary supplements to increase the antioxidative potential, to provide glutathione, and to modify phospholipid membranes. One might, by diet or medication, alter the cytochrome $P_{450}$ system or stimulate hepatic phagocytosis. Today, therefore, hepatic gerontology appears more promising than hepatic geriatrics.

## References


Butler RN, Bearn AG (eds) (1985) The aging process: therapeutic implications. Raven, New York, pp 5-9, 313-316

Dice F (1985) Cellular theories of aging as related to the liver. Hepatology 3: 508-513

Einarsson K, Nilsell K, Leijd B, Angelin B (1985) Influence of age on secretion of cholesterol and synthesis of bile acids by the liver. N Engl J Med 313: 277-282

Gershon D (1979) Current status of age-altered enzymes: alternative mechanisms. Mech Ageing Dev 9: 189-196

Harman D (1981) The aging process. Proc Natl Acad Sci USA 78: 7124-7128

Holt PR (1986) Gastrointestinal drugs in the elderly. Am J Gastroenterol 81: 403-411

Kitani K (1986) Hepatic drug metabolism in the elderly. Hepatology 2: 316-319

Kitani K, Zurcher C, van Bezooijen K (1981) The effect of aging on the hepatic metabolism of sulfobromophthalein in BN/Bi female and WAG/Rij male and female rats. Mech Ageing Dev 7: 381-393

Knook DL (1980) The isolated hepatocyte: a cellular model for aging studies. Proc Soc Exp Biol Med 165: 170-177

Knook DL, Hollander CF (1978) Embryology and aging of the rat liver. In: Newberne PM, Butler WH (eds) Rat hepatic neoplasia. MIT Press, Cambridge, pp 9-38

Konoplya EF, Luksha GL, Savateev SK, Naumov AD (1986) Steroid-receptor complexes and their interaction with the rat liver nuclei during ontogenesis. Mech Ageing Dev 35: 95-107

Maloney A, Schmucker DL, Vessey DS Wang RK (1986) The effects of aging on the hepatic microsomal mixed-function oxidase system of male and female monkeys. Hepatology 2: 282-287

Martin GM (1977) Cellular aging. I. A review. Clonal senescence. Am J Pathol 89: 484-511

Parke DV, Ioannides C (1984) Reactive intermediates and oxygen toxicity in liver injury. In: Keppler D, Popper H, Bianchi L, Reutter W (eds) Mechanisms of hepatocyte injury and death. MIT Press, Lancaster, pp 37-48

Poot M, Verkerk A, Jongkind JF (1986) Accumulation of a high molecular weight glycoprotein during in vitro ageing and contact inhibition of growth. Mech Ageing Dev 34: 219-232

Popper H (1985) Relations between liver and aging. Semin Liver Dis 5: 221-227

Popper H (1986) Aging and the liver. In: Popper H, Schaffner F (eds) Progress in liver diseases, vol 8. Grune and Stratton, Orlando, pp 659-683

Richardson A, Cheung HT (1982) The relationship between age-related changes in gene expression, protein turnover, and the responsiveness of an organism to stimuli. Life Sci 21: 605-613

Schmucker DL (1985) Aging and drug disposition: An update. Pharmacol Rev 37: 133-148

Schmucker DL, Gilbert R, Jones AL, Hradek GT, Bazin H (1985) Effect of aging on the hepatobiliary transport of dimeric immunoglobulin A in the male Fischer rat. Gastroenterology 88: 436-443

Stöcker E (1975) Zur DNS-Synthese in Zellkernen der regenerierenden Rattenleber als Funktion des Alters. In: Platt D (ed) Alternstheorien. Zellkern - Membranen. Schattauer, Stuttgart, pp 121-143

Sutter MA, Wood G, Williamson LS, Strong R, Pickham K, Richardson A (1985) Comparison of the hepatic mixed function oxidase system of young, adult, and old nonhuman primates *(Macaca nemestrina)*. Biochem Pharmacol 34: 2983-2987

Tauchi H, Sato T (1978) Hepatic cells of the aged. In: Kitani K (ed) Liver and aging. Elsevier/North Holland, Amsterdam, pp 3-19

United Nations World Assembly (1982) International plan of action. United Nations, New York

Watanabe T, Tanaka Y (1982) Age-related alterations in the size of human hepatocytes. A study of mononuclear and binuclear cells. Virchows Arch 39: 9-20

# Prognosis of Advanced Liver Disease

Niels Tygstrup
Medical Department A, Rigshospitalet, Copenhagen, Denmark

## Introduction

Advanced liver disease can be defined generally as a situation where a major part of the liver function has been destroyed by liver disease. Which functions, however, reduced to what degree? "Advanced liver disease" usually connotes liver disease with clinical manifestations recognized as indicators of bad prognosis. In acute liver disease, like fulminant hepatic failure, it is a qualitative question, – survival or not – whereas in chronic liver disease, like cirrhosis, it is a matter of duration of survival, and thus a quantitative question, which may be more difficult to handle.

## Prognostic Factors

A number of factors have been known to be associated with survival for some time. Table 1 shows 1-year survival in the presence and absence of some such factors. In a systematic search for prognostic factors the Copenhagen Study Group for Liver Diseases examined 162 variables in 488 patients with cirrhosis, and 46 of them showed an association with survival as studied by logrank analysis (Schlichting et al. 1983). Tables 2-5 list some of the variables related to prognosis and also some where such an association might be expected, but was not found.

One problem in using studies of this type to estimate prognosis is that factors appear in combination. Most patients will exhibit some manifestation indicating a bad

**Table 1.** Prognostic factors and 1-year survival (%)

| Ascites | | Jaundice | | GI bleeding | | Alcohol intake | |
|---|---|---|---|---|---|---|---|
| + | – | + | – | + | – | + | – |
| 32 | ? (1) | 26 | ? (1) | 28 | ? (1) | 74 | 72 (2) |
| 65 | ? (2) | 67 | ? (2) | 55 | ? (2) | 98 | 85 (3) |
| 62 | 88 (3) | 59 | 92 (6) | 45 | ? (5) | 82 | 80 (4) |
| 60 | 91 (6) | 60 | 82 (7) | | | 96 | 26 (5) |
| 50 | 80 (7) | | | | | | |

(1) Ratnoff and Patek (1942),
(2) Powell and Klatstein (1968),
(3) Alexander et al. (1971),
(4) Tygstrup and Juhl (1971),
(5) Borowsky et al. (1981),
(6) Orrego et al. (1983),
(7) Christensen et al. (1983)

Assessment and Management of Hepatobiliary Disease
Eds.: L. Okolicsányi, G. Csomós, and G. Crepaldi

**Table 2.** Prognostic significance of anamnestic variables

| Yes | No |
|---|---|
| Age | Alcoholic intake |
| Sex | History of jaundice |
| Duration of symptoms | History of ascites |
| History of hepatitis | History of GI bleeding |
| Working capacity | History of encephalopathy |
| | Itching |

**Table 3.** Prognostic significance of clinical signs

| Yes | No |
|---|---|
| Ascites | Palmar erythema |
| Edema | White nails |
| Nutrition | Splenomegaly |
| Spider nevi | Distended abdominal veins |
| Liver size | Skin haemorrhage |
| Muscle wasting | Liver consistency |

**Table 4.** Prognostic significance of laboratory and X-ray variables

| Yes | No |
|---|---|
| Hemoglobin | Body weight |
| Bilirubin | Sedimentation rate |
| Prothrombin | Thymol turbidity |
| Acetylcholinesterase | Aminotransferase |
| Albumin | Alkaline phosphatase |
| Gamma-globulin | Cholesterol |
| BSP | Leucocyte counts |
| ANF | LE cell |
| RAT | Antiglobulin consumption |
| Varices on X-ray | Ulcer on X-ray |

**Table 5.** Prognostic significance of histologic variables

| Yes | No |
|---|---|
| Biopsy size | Biopsy fragmentation |
| Destruction of architecture | Bile duct proliferation |
| Size of nodules | Cholestasis |
| Inflammation of connective tissue | Acidophilic bodies |
| Inflammation of parenchyma | Confluence liver cell necrosis |
| Large piecemeal necrosis | Fatty infiltrations |
| Mallory bodies | Granulomas |
| Kupffer cell proliferation | Ground-glass affearance |
| Histologic activity | Nonseptal fibrosis |
| Chronic active hepatitis | Abnormality of bile ducts |

**Table 6.** Child-Turcotte criteria. (From Child and Turcotte 1964)

| Class | A | B | C |
|---|---|---|---|
| Bilirubin | $<2$ | 2–3 | $>3$ |
| Albumin | $>3.5$ | 3–3.5 | $<3$ |
| Ascites | None | Contr. | Uncontr. |
| Neurologic disorder | None | Minimal | Coma |
| Nutrition | Excellent | Good | Poor |

**Table 7.** Variables in the combined clinical/laboratory index developed by Orrego et al. (1983)

| Clinical | Laboratory |
|---|---|
| Encephalopathy | Prothrombin |
| Collateral circulation | Hematocrit |
| Edema | Albumin |
| Ascites | Bilirubin |
| Spider nevi | Alkaline phosphatase |
| Weakness | |
| Anorexia | |

prognosis and others with the opposite effect. In view of this the classification suggested by Child and Turcotte in 1964 has gained some popularity (Table 6).

This approach, however, leaves a number of problems unsolved. Firstly, the criteria are selected on the basis of general clinical experience, and not after a systematic search. Secondly, the final classification based on the score can be defined in several ways. Thirdly, a given score can be obtained by several combinations not known to be of equal prognostic significance. And fourthly, the relation between score and survival remains open.

It is evident that the effect of combined factors cannot be studied directly by following patients with all combinations. To study five factors with two possible outcomes each, the material would have to be divided into 120 groups, most of which would be too small for analysis in any conceivable material.

## Prognostic Scores

Orrego et al. (1983) instead elaborated their combined clinical laboratory index from estimations of "relative risks" in groups with different outcomes of a series of variables. The index was based an analysis of 253 patients, of whom 51 died within 1 year, and embroces seven clinical and five laboratory variables (Table 7), but no histologic data. For intervals of the index, which may be between 1 and 25, the 1-year survival probability can be estimated.

Problems associated with this approach are: (1) it includes variables which are probably correlated, i.e., the effect of a feature expressed in several variables may be overemphasized; (2) it gives only 1-year survival probability; (3) it gives survival probability only for intervals, not for single values of the index; and (4) it does not utilize the observations fully, because censored patients, i.e., survivors followed for less than 1 year, are excluded from the evaluation.

## Regression Analysis

Multivariate regression analysis, recently used for estimation of prognostic factors in cirrhosis by Milani et al. (1985) and Mannes et al. (1986), may eliminate some of these problems. On analysis of 73 fatal cases, Milani et al. found that albumin, ascites, encephalopathy, and GI bleeding were the most powerful prognostic indicators, and bilirubin, gamma-globulin, and cholesterol contributed more modestly (Table 8). Evaluation of the prognosis from the analysis is not mentioned.

In the study carried out by Mannes et al. (1986) on 76 patients with 16 deaths in 1 year, a similar approach revealed significant prognostic information in four clinical and six laboratory observations (Table 9). It was shown that a combination of serum bile acids and number connection test has a large predictive value concerning 1-year survival. In this respect it has the same limitations as the study by Orrego et al. (1983).

In the above-mentioned study by the Copenhagen Study Group for Liver Diseases (Schlichting et al. 1983), it was found by multivariate regression analysis that among the 46 factors showing significant relation to prognosis by univariate analysis only two clinical, two laboratory, and four histologic variables had independent prognostic significance (Table 10).

## Prognostic Index

By adjusting the scores to ensure proportionality with the risk of dying, a prognostic index was made from the sum of scores and the regression coefficients of the significant variables for each patient. The index can be converted to survival probability for any given period within the range of observation or to estimated mean survival time (Schlichting et al. 1983).

Since the data came from a randomized clinical trial of steroid treatment it was also possible to estimate the prognostic influence of this therapy (Christensen et al. 1985). It turned out that four variables (Table 11) were related to the prognosis of treated patients.

It is evident that the prognosis may be estimated more precisely if changes in the variables are considered. Of two patients with the same prognostic index, one may later develop ascites or gastric hemorrhage and will probably have a shorter survival than the patient who does not. A method to account for such changes has recently been developed by the Copenhagen Study Group for Liver Diseases (Christensen et al. 1986). It is seen (Table 12) that the analysis makes is possible to include further variables. Recent observations of the variables must be available if the analysis is to be of full value.

**Table 8.** Prognostic variables listed by Milani et al. (1985)

| Variable | "Weight" |
|---|---|
| Albumin | 35.5% |
| Ascites | 17.9% |
| Encephalopathy | 13.8% |
| Varices | 13.2% |
| Bilirubin | 8.0% |
| Gamma-globulin | 7.2% |
| Cholesterol | 4.3% |

**Table 9.** Prognostic variables listed by Mannes et al. (1986)

| Clinical | Laboratory |
|---|---|
| Child-Turcotte classification | Bile acids |
| Number conn. test | Albumin |
| Ascites | Acetylcholinesterase |
| Nutrition | Bilirubin |
| Age | Prothrombin |

**Table 10.** Variables with a significant coefficient of the prognostic index in the CSL study. (From Schlichting et al. 1983)

| Variable | Score | Coefficient |
|---|---|---|
| Sex | M=1 | 0.32 |
| Age | years − 60 | 0.05 |
| Prothrombin | ln(val) − 4 | −0.49 |
| Acetylcholinesterase | ln(val*100) − 4 | −0.61 |
| Inflammation | + =1, + + =2, + + + =3 | −0.39 |
| Veins in nodules | (+)=1, + =2 | 0.26 |
| Focal necroses | + =1 | 0.31 |
| Eosinophils | (+)=1, + =2, + + =3 | 0.30 |

**Table 11.** Variables with significantly different coefficients in treated and untreated patients. (From Christensen et al. 1985)

| Variable | Score | Coefficients | |
|---|---|---|---|
| | | Prednisone | Control |
| Ascites | (+)=1, + =2 | 0.72 | 0.11 |
| Antinuclear factor | + =1, + + =2 | −0.12 | 0.31 |
| Large piecemeal necrosis | + =1 | −0.74 | 0.73 |
| Size of nodules | >lobules=1 | 0.73 | −0.61 |

**Table 12.** Variables with a significant coefficient in the time-dependent model. (From Christensen et al. 1986)

| Variable | Score | Coefficient |
|---|---|---|
| Prothrombin | ln(val) − 4 | −0.83 |
| Ascites + | 1 | 1.17 |
| GI bleeding | 1 | 1.41 |
| Age | years − 60 | 0.052 |
| Alcohol > 10 g | 3 | 0.14 |
| Alcohol > 50 g | 9 | |
| Malnutrition | 1 | 0.56 |
| Bilirubin > 70 | 1 | 0.94 |
| Albumin | ln(val) − 4 | −1.20 |
| Alkaline phosphatase | ln(val) − 4 | 0.11 |
| Inflammation | 1 | −0.56 |

**Table 13.** Variables with significant coefficient

| Variable | Score | Coefficient | variable | score | coefficient |
|---|---|---|---|---|---|
| Primary biliary cirrhosis | | | Alcoholic cirrhosis | | |
| Bilirubin | log(val) | 2.51 | Sex | M = 1 | 0.87 |
| Age | exp((years − 20)/10) | 0.007 | Age | years − 57 | 0.027 |
| Cirrhosis | + = 1 | 0.88 | Acetylcho- | | |
| Albumin | g/l | −0.05 | linesterase | log(val/2.58) | −0.49 |
| Central | + = 1 | 0.68 | Ascites | + = 1 | 0.39 |
| cholestasis | | | From Tygstrup and Juhl 1985 | | |
| Azathioprine | no = 1 | 0.52 | | | |
| From Christensen et al. 1985b | | | | | |

## Prognosis and Decision Making

The great advantage of calculating a prognostic index and then using it to estimate the survival probability for a given period or the mean survival time is that it can be applied to individual patients. It may therefore also be helpful in making therapeutic decisions. It should be noted, however, that the type of patients included in the "learning set" and the nature of the variables studied has a great influence on the prognostic index. Table 13 shows scores and coefficients of variables derived from a material consisting purely of alcoholic cirrhosis and primary biliary cirrhosis.

## Conclusion

It seems that we have now obtained much better methods to assess the prognosis of patients with cirrhosis, but there are still many problems to be solved. The relatively complicated statistical analysis is a problem, because it may be misleading unless the statistician and the clinician have a good understanding of each other's methods. Furthermore, differences in the composition of the material, the criteria used, and the variables observed may lead to very divergent and confusing results.

To my mind the most important achievement of the studies made so far has been to reveal the great significance of these most fundamental problems. Hopefully this approach will also help to solve them.

## References

Alexander JF, Lischner MW, Galambos JT (1971) Natural history of alcoholic hepatitis. II. The long-term prognosis. Am J Gastroenterol 56: 515-525

Borowsky SA, Strome S, Lott E (1981) Continued heavy drinking and survival in alcoholic cirrhosis. Gastroenterology 80: 1405-1409

Child CG, Turcotte JG (1964) Surgery and portal hypertension. In: Child CG (ed) The liver and portal hypertension. Saunders, Philadelphia

Christensen E, Schlichting P, Fauerholdt L, et al. (1983) Prognostic value of Child-Turcotte criteria in medically treated cirrhosis. Hepatology 4: 430-435

Christensen E, Neuberger J, Crowe J, et al. (1985) Beneficial effect of azathioprine and prediction of prognosis in primary biliary cirrhosis. Final results of an international trial. Gastroenterology 89: 1084-1091

Christensen E, Schlichting P, Andersen PK, et al. (1986) A therapeutic index that predicts the individual effects of prednisone in patients with cirrhosis. Gastroenterology 88: 156-165

Mannes GA, Thieme C, Stellaard F, et al. (1986) Prognostic significance of serum bile acids in cirrhosis. Hepatology 6: 50-53

Milani A, Marra L, Siciliano M, Rossi L (1985) Prognostic significance of clinical and laboratory parameters in liver cirrhosis. A multivariate statistical approach. Hepatogastroenterology 32: 270-272

Neuberger J, Altman DG, Christensen E, Tygstrup N, Williams R (1986) Use of prognostic index in evaluation of liver transplantation for primary biliary cirrhosis. Transplantation 41: 713-716)

Orrego H, Israel Y, Blake JE, Medline A (1983) Assessment of prognostic factors in alcoholic liver disease. Toward a global quantitative expression of severity. Hepatology 3: 896-905

Powell WJ Jr, Klatskin G (1968) Duration of survival in patients with Laennec's cirrhosis, influence of alcohol withdrawal, and possible effects of recent changes in general management of the disease. Am J Med 44: 406-420

Ratnoff OD, Patek AJ Jr (1942) The natural history of Laennec's cirrhosis of the liver: an analysis of 386 cases. Medicine (Baltimore) 21: 207-268

Schlichting P, Christensen E, Andersen PK, et al. (1983) Prognostic factors in cirrhosis identified by Cox's regression model. Hepatology 3: 889-895

Tygstrup N, Juhl E (1971) The treatment of alcoholic cirrhosis. The effect of continued drinking and prednisone on survival. In: Gerok W, Sickinger K, Hennekeuser HH (eds) Alcohol and the liver. Schattauer, Stuttgart

Tygstrup N, Kragh Andersen P, Riegels Thomsen BL (1986) Prognostic evaluation in alcoholic cirrhosis. Acta Med Scand [Suppl 703] 218: 149-156

# Virus and Host Factors in the Evolution of Chronic Hepatitis Type B: Choice of Treatment

G. Realdi, G. Fattovich, A. Alberti, S. Boscaro, A. Fraiese, A. M. Rigoli, and A. Ruol
Instituto di Medicina Clinica, Clinica Medica II Università degli Studi di Padova, Italy

Hepatitis B virus (HBV) infection is associated with different clinical manifestations (acute hepatitis, chronic hepatitis, liver cirrhosis, and hepatocellular carcinoma), which appear temporally linked, from longitudinal studies of patients who could be followed over time with subsequent clinical and histological evaluations (Dudley et al. 1972). However, several issues related to the natural history of HBV infection and to the associated disease remain unresolved, mainly due to the scarcity of proper studies on this topic and to the still incomplete knowledgment of all the factors which may modify the course of the disease.

Our partial understanding of the natural evolution and chronic sequelae of acute hepatitis is mainly related to the fact that the course of chronic liver disease of viral etiology is usually long, thus making it difficult to collect a consistent number of patients with an adequate follow-up for statistical evaluation. Moreover, the disease is often asymptomatic and is rarely recognized at its onset, but often becomes overt at late stages, when complications of cirrhosis have developed. Finally, the protracted course of these chronic liver diseases makes possible the intervention of other agents causing liver damage, either of viral or of chemical origin, which modify the possibly more benign history of HBV-related liver damage.

When considering the evolution of liver disease caused by HBV, it seems essential to describe separately the virus factors and the host factors that together participate in the clinical expression of the infection. As far as the virus itself is concerned HBV does not behave as a cytopathic agent and liver damage is considered the consequence of the host's immune response to viral antigens expressed in the infected cells. Recent studies based on molecular hybridization techniques have provided evidence for two distinct states of HBV-DNA in the liver, where free and integrated forms have been detected. The former pattern is associated with production of complete viral particles, while with viral integration into the host genome, complete virions are not produced and only HBsAg particles are detected in serum (Yokosuka et al. 1986). These two virological phases, that is the replicative and the nonreplicative phase, can be identified by specific markers in liver and in serum.

Serum HBeAg is the best standardized and easiest to perform marker currently available for evaluation of viral replication. However, its sensitivity is not absolute and virus replication may occur in HBeAg-negative cases (Bonino et al. 1986), as shown by detection of HBcAg in the liver by immunohistochemical methods (Alberti et al. 1983).

The most sensitive method for detection of virus replication in serum is that of spot hybridization for HBV-DNA sequences. Longitudinal studies have now demonstrated that the biology of the virus changes during the course of the infection. In fact, in individual cases the replicative phase is often confined to the early period of infection,

Assessment and Management of Hepatobiliary Disease
Eds.: L. Okolicsányi, G. Csomós, and G. Crepaldi

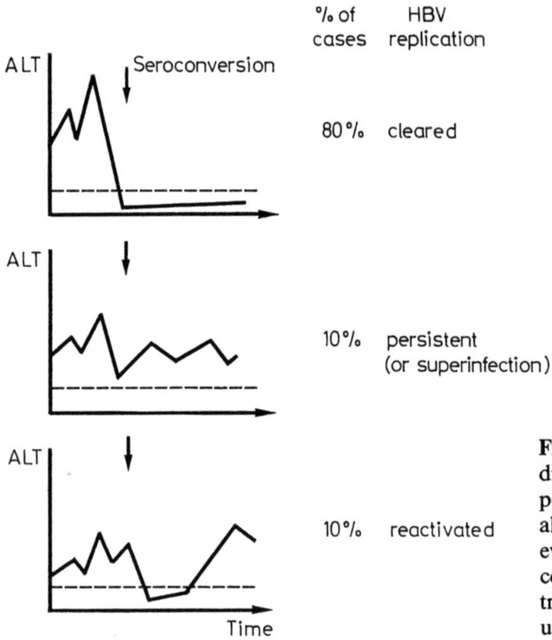


**Fig. 1.** Cumulative results of a longitudinal study of HBsAg- and HBeAg-positive chronic hepatitis (Fattovich et al. 1986a). The figure summarizes the events observed after anti-HBe seroconversion. ALT means alanine aminotransferase. Dashed line indicates the upper limit of the normal range

ranging usually from 3 to 6 years but sometimes up to 10 years or more. In the later phases of infection, viral replication ceases and HBV-DNA becomes integrated into the host genome (Shafritz et al. 1981).

These changes in the biology of the virus are associated with several important modifications of the pattern of liver disease. In fact, in our recent longitudinal study of HBsAg chronic carriers (Fattovich et al. 1986a), seroconversion to anti-HBe was associated with biochemical and histologic remission of disease activity in the majority of patients (Fig. 1). However, in about 20% of cases in our geographical area, viral replication may persist in spite of anti-HBe seroconversion, or reactivation of viral replication may be observed after apparent remission of disease activity.

As far as host factors are concerned, the most important is certainly the immune response to the viral antigens. It has been suggested that the cellular immune response, mediated by cytotoxic T-lymphocytes, is responsible for clearance of infected hepatocytes (Mondelli et al. 1982), while the humoral immune response expressed by virus-specific antibodies is relevant for neutralization and clearance of circulating virions (Alberti et al. 1984).

In the light of these considerations we have recently analyzed virus and host factors in a group of consecutive patients who, at presentation, were HBsAg-positive, had had normal alanine aminotransferase (ALT) values for at least 1 year and liver histology showing chronic active hepatitis (CAH) without cirrhosis. All patients were then followed for a minimum of 1 year after liver biopsy. Table 1 shows that after a mean follow-up period of about 6 years, three different outcomes could be observed. There was a first group of patients (34% of all cases) who developed morphological signs of cirrhosis. Another 32% of the cases showed unchanged features at subsequent liver biop-

**Table 1.** Long-term outcome of HBsAg-positive chronic active hepatitis

| Outcome | Percentage of cases | Years of follow-up (mean ± SD) |
|---|---|---|
| Evolution to cirrhosis | 34 | 5.9 ± 3.4 |
| Unchanged (persistent CAH) | 32 | 4.9 ± 2.2 |
| Improvement (histologic and biochemical remission) | 34 | 5.9 ± 2.2 |

sy, that is persistence of signs of CAH. Finally, a third group of patients had biochemical and histologic evidence of remission of inflammatory liver disease. Two examples of this last pattern of behavior are illustrated in Figs. 2, 3. The patient of Fig. 2 showed a persistent normalization of transaminases after seroconversion and clearance of replicating virions. Liver histology in 1986 (not shown in the figure) showed evidence only of portal fibrosis. Substained ALT normalization also occurred in the patient of Fig. 3 after anti-HBe seroconversion. However, liver biopsy taken by laparoscopy at the end of the follow-up was consistent with an inactive cirrhosis.

The behavior of HBV infection and of liver disease in these two cases suggests that the outcome of chronic hepatitis after anti-HBe seroconversion depends on the degree of liver damage preexisting this serologic event, that is, on the severity of the lesions that developed during the early replicative phase of infection (Realdi et al. 1987). In those cases in whom cirrhosis has not yet developed, the disease may end up with a histology typical of chronic persistent hepatitis (CPH) or slight fibrosis, or even of a normal liver (Rugge et al. 1986). By contrast, in those cases who have already developed cirrhosis, a reduction of inflammation and of disease activity may be seen, but the complications of cirrhosis, particularly portal hypertension (Realdi et al. 1987), are often seen during follow-up.

Progression to cirrhosis seems to be closely related to long persistence of viral replication. This has to be considered the essential prerequisite for progression of liver damage, although it should not be assumed by itself to be sufficient to cause evolution to cirrhosis. This is well illustrated in the patient of Fig. 4, in which progression to cirrhosis and even to hepatocellular carcinoma was seen in the presence of continuing viral replication, as shown by the permanent presence of HBV-DNA in the serum (Fig. 4).

Two additional types of evolution have also been observed after anti-HBe seroconversion, although they occurred in a minority of cases (about 20% in our experience). Liver disease in these patients persists despite anti-HBe seroconversion, as shown by elevated ALT levels, and evolution to cirrhosis may be observed (Fig. 5). In this group there is evidence of continuing virus replication with the results of serum HBV-DNA tests sometimes fluctuate over time, making serial testing necessary during follow-up (Alberti et al. 1986).

Finally, anti-HBe seroconversion may be associated with complete, but only transient ALT normalization, lasting sometimes for a few years, which is than followed by new peaks of enzyme elevation, mimicking a novel hepatitis attack. In these cases serum HBV-DNA testing is also very useful as positive results allow identification of the etiologic role of HBV in determining reactivation of liver damage, and make it unlikely

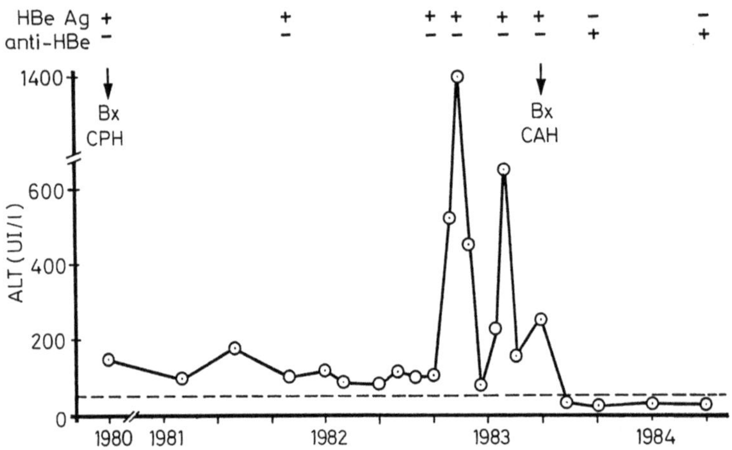


**Fig. 2.** Long-term follow-up of a patient with HBsAg- and HBeAg-positive chronic persistent hepatitis (CPH) at first biopsy. At the end of the third year of observation the patient presented two vigorous alterations of ALT during which liver histology was consistent with CAH with marked lobular inflammation. Subsequently, seroconversion to anti-HBe occurred, accompanied by persistent normalization of ALT. A third liver biopsy taken in 1986 (not shown in the figure) showed slight portal fibrosis

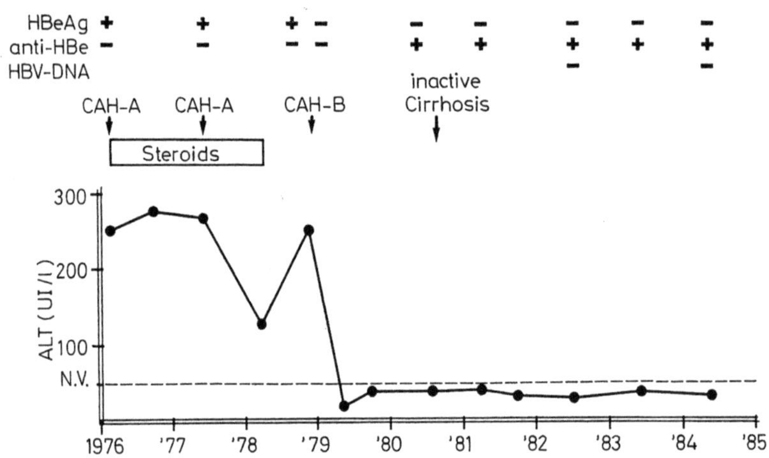


**Fig. 3.** Outcome of a patient with HBsAg- and HBeAg-positive CAH at moderate activity, who was treated with prednisone (maintenance dose of 8 mg/day) between 1976 and 1978. Withdrawal of the drug was followed by a peak of ALT with contemporary seroconversion to anti-HBe and subsequent persistent normalization of transaminases. The last liver biopsy showed a picture of inactive cirrhosis. Tests for HBV-DNA in the last 3 years were always negative

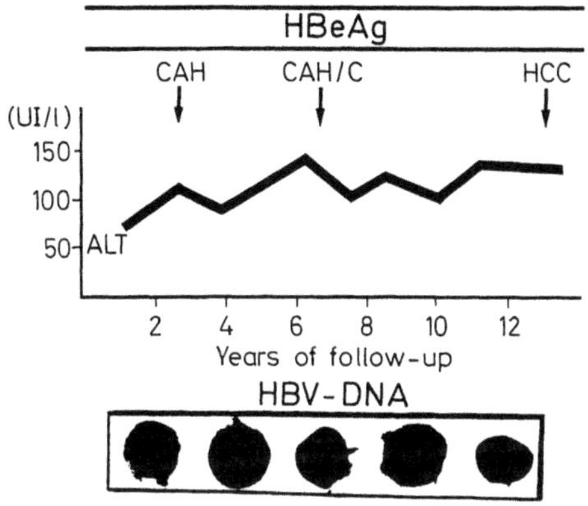


**Fig. 4.** Evolution to cirrhosis *(CAH/C)* and then to hepatocellular carcinoma *(HCC)* during a period of 13 years of observation in a patient with an initial liver biopsy of CAH and in whom there was persistence of HBV replication during the entire period of follow-up. The patient was also affected by repeated suppurations of an abdominal wound caused by an accident

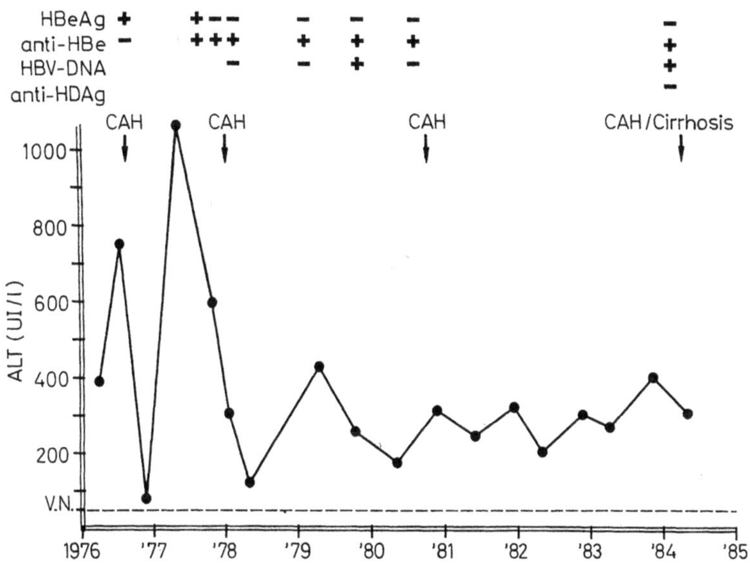


**Fig. 5.** Long-term follow-up of a drug-addict with HBsAg- and HBeAg-positive CAH at first observation. After 2 years of observation the patient had seroconversion to anti-HBc without normalization of ALT. The last biopsy showed a picture of CAH with superimposed cirrhosis. HBV-DNA tests of serum were transiently positive on some occasions

that other viral or toxic cofactors could have contributed to the liver damage (Fig. 6). These patients, who seemed not to benefit from anti-HBe seroconversion in terms of regression of liver disease, may well constitute part of the group of patients who are then seen as cases with anti-HBe-positive, HBV-DNA-positive chronic hepatitis type B. Our results further underline the clinical importance of this group that, as shown in other studies (Bonino et al. 1986), may have a severe clinical evolution. However, our results indicate that this unfavorable outcome after anti-HBe seroconversion occurs only in a minority of patients, at least in our region. These patients are then selected by the continuing inflammatory liver disease being more easily recognized among anti-HBe-positive carriers.

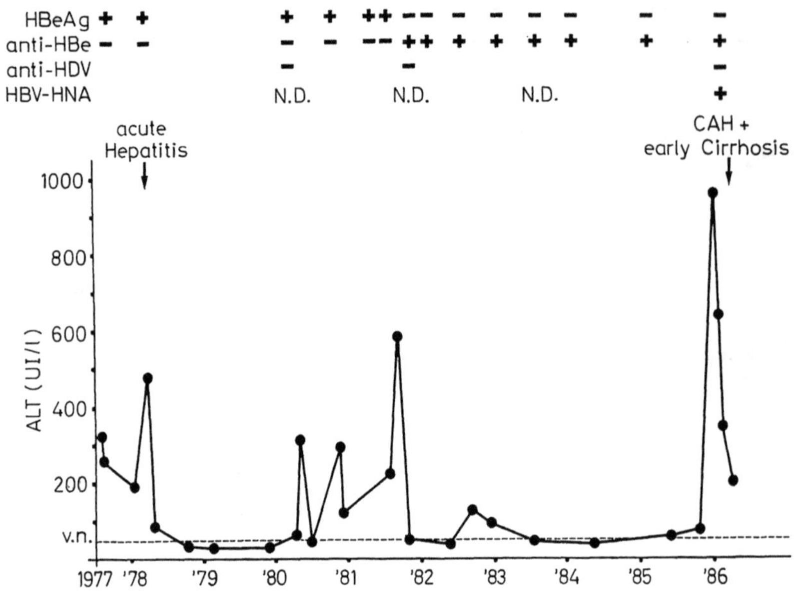


**Fig. 6.** Long-term follow-up of a health-care employee who had HBsAg- and HBeAg-positive, histologically confirmed acute hepatitis in 1977. Subsequently, ALT fluctuated over time, with periods of apparent normalization. Anti-HBe seroconversion was observed in 1982, preceded by a further ALT peak and followed by a long period of normal or quite normal ALT. In 1986 a sudden important increase of ALT was observed, resembling a new acute attack of hepatitis. Liver biopsy showed a histology of CAH with early cirrhosis. HBV-DNA tests were positive in this occasion

Thus, the following four distinct virologic and clinical outcomes can be seen after anti-HBe seroconversion:

1. Permanent ALT normalization with remission of liver disease activity and clearance of complete virus markers. The outcome may be with portal fibrosis or with a normal liver (Rugge et al. 1986). The healthy state of being a HBsAg carrier may be generated in this way (Bortolotti et al. 1987).
2. Permanent normalization of ALT with remission of inflammatory liver disease activity, associated with inactive cirrhosis (Fattovich et al. 1986a). Virus replication is absent and in some patients clearance of HBsAg may even occur, giving rise to HBsAg-negative cirrhosis, otherwise defined as cryptogenic cirrhosis (Morgan et al. 1986).
3. Continuing elevation of transaminase levels, often with significant fluctuations, and HBV-DNA remaining detectable in serum. The evolution of these forms is related to the duration of persistent virus replication.
4. Transient ALT normalization, with remission of inflammatory and necrotic activity in the liver, accompanied by transient termination of virus replication. These events are then followed by reactivation of virus replication and of liver disease. When hepatotoxic factors other than HBV are excluded, virus reactivation seems to be related to exogenous or endogenous events causing immune suppression. However superinfection with a different subtype of HBV is also a possibility.

**Table 2.** Risk factors for evolution to cirrhosis or for improvement of HBsAg-positive chronic active hepatitis

| Variable | Coefficent of regression | Risk ratio | $P^a$ |
|---|---|---|---|
| HBV replication | | | |
| Persistent | 0.32 | 5.11 | <0.001 |
| Clearance | 0.95 | 0.03 | <0.001 |
| HDV superinfection | 0.59 | 8.75 | <0.001 |
| Immunosuppressive therapy | 0.42 | 4.38 | <0.001 |
| Age over 30 years | 0.1 | 4.01 | <0.001 |

[a] Linear regression analysis

Various factors have been examined in the attempt to differentiate patients with evolution to cirrhosis from those showing improvement during follow-up (Realdi et al. 1987). When we applied multiple linear regression analysis to our data, it was possible to show that continuing virus replication, hepatitis delta virus (HDV) superinfection, previous steroid therapy, and age above 30 years, significantly correlated with evolution to cirrhosis. In contrast, the only factor found to be significantly related to improvement of liver disease was termination of virus replication with anti-HBe seroconversion and permanent clearance of HBV-DNA from serum. Regression coefficents, risk ratios and *P* values for all variables are summarized in Table 2.

From the results of our longitudinal study we can conclude that virus factors, mainly related to persistence or termination of viral replication, and host factors particularly connected with the state of the immune system, are the important determinants of the type and duration of liver disease activity. Evolution to cirrhosis or remission of the disease would depend on the interaction between these two factors, leading to different patterns of severity and duration of liver inflammation. Other factors, however, should also be considered, including superinfection by other hepatotropic agents (HDV, non-A, non-B agents, hepatitis A virus), or the presence of hepatotoxic factors, like alcohol and drugs. The importance of these factors depends mainly on the geographical distribution of the disease; ethnic and genetic factors seem to influence the outcome of the disease.

It is clear that the precise identification of these different factors is of paramount importance to predict the outcome of the disease, to further understand the pathogenesis of liver damage, and to improve future overall management strategies.

As to the choice of therapy in chronic hepatitis type B, it is clear from several previous studies that immunosuppressive drugs should be avoided. The correct therapeutic approach to chronic HBV infection is that of stimulation of the immune system, on the one hand, and eradication of the virus from the liver, on the other. As far as immunostimulation is concerned, we have recently obtained promising results with Levamisole (L-tetramisole), a rather inexpensive drug with no relevant side-effects. In a controlled study we observed that the majority of patients treated with 150 mg three times a week had an increase in ALT levels, as the expression of a potentiation of the immune response induced by the drug (Fattovich et al. 1986b). The results obtained were consistent with the conclusion that long-term treatment with levamisole is able to induce a significant trend toward normalization of ALT and termination of HBV replication, suggesting that the drug may be of real benefit in chronic hepatitis type B.

On the other hand, major efforts, are currently being devoted to the use of several antiviral agents, primarily interferon. In patients who are HBV-DNA-negative, the use of immunosuppressive therapy has been proposed, at least when autoimmune features are present. However, we did not detect autoimmune markers in these patients. Finally, patients with HDV superinfection also appear as candidates for interferon therapy and several trials are currently underway for the evaluation of the efficacy of interferon in HDV-positive chronic hepatitis.

## References

Alberti A, Tremolada F, Fattovich G, Bortolotti F, Realdi G (1983) Virus replication and liver disease in chronic hepatitis B virus infection. Dig Dis Sci 28: 962-966

Alberti A, Pontisso P, Schiavon E, Realdi G (1984) An antibody which precipitates Dane particles in acute hepatitis type B: relation to receptor sites which bind polymerized human serum albumin on virus particles. Hepatology 4: 220-226

Alberti A, Pontisso P, Fattovich G, Schiavon E, Chemello L, Bortolotti F, Tremolada F, Realdi G (1986) Changes in serum hepatitis B Virus (HBV) DNA positivity in chronic HBV infection: Results of a long-term follow-up study of 138 patients. J Infect Dis 154: 562-569

Bonino F, Rosina F, Rizzetto M, Rizzi R, Chiaberge E, Tardanico R, Callea F, Verme G (1986) Chronic hepatitis in HBsAg carrier with serum HBV-DNA and anti-HBe. Gastroenterology 90: 1268-1273

Bortolotti F, Cadrobbi P, Armigliato M, Rude L, Rugge M, Realdi G (1987) Prognosis of chronic hepatitis B transmitted from HBsAg positive mothers. Arch Dis Childhood 62: 201-203

Dudley FG, Scheuer PJ, Sherlock S (1972) Natural history of hepatitis-associated antigen-positive chronic liver disease. Lancet II: 1388-1393

Fattovich G, Rugge M, Brollo L, Pontisso P, Noventa F, Guido M, Alberti A, Realdi G (1986a) Clinical, virologic and histologic outcome following seroconversion from HBeAg to anti-HBe in chronic hepatitis type B. Hepatology 6: 167-172

Fattovich G, Brollo L, Pontisso P, Pornaro E, Rugge M, Alberti A, Realdi G (1986b) Levamisole therapy in chronic type B hepatitis: results of a double blind randomized trial. Gastroenterology 91: 692-696

Mondelli M, Mieli-Vergani G, Alberti A, Vergani D, Portmann B, Eddleston ALWF, Williams R (1982) Specificity of T lymphocytes cytotoxicity to autologous hepatocytes in chronic hepatitis B virus infection: evidence that T cells are directed against HBV core antigen expressed on hepatocytes. J Immunol 129: 2773-2778

Morgan TR, Redeker AG, Yamada S, Ashcavai M (1986) HBsAg clearance in chronic active hepatitis B. A possible cause of cryptogenic cirrhosis. Dig Dis Sci 31: 700-704

Realdi G, Fattovich G, Pontisso P, Alberti A, Bortolotti F, Noventa F (1987) Natural history of cirrhosis due to virus. In: Tygstrup N, Orlandi F (eds) Liver cirrhosis. Academic (to be published)

Rugge M, Fattovich G, Guido M, Pontisso P, Ghimenton C, Realdi G (1986) Liver histology and viral replication in chronic hepatitis type B. Front Gastrointest Res 9: 118-125

Shafritz D, Shouval D, Sherman HI, Hadziyannis SJ, Kew MC (1981) Integration of hepatitis B Virus DNA into the genome of the liver cells in chronic liver disease and hepatocellular carcinoma: studies in percutaneous liver biopsies and postmortem specimens. N Engl J Med 305: 1067-1073

Yokosuka O, Omata M, Imazeki F, Ita Y, Okuda K (1986) Hepatitis B Virus RNA transcripts and DNA in chronic liver disease. N Engl J Med 315: 1187-1192

# Antiviral Treatment of Chronic Hepatitis

Neil McIntyre

Academic Department of Medicine, Royal Free Hospital and School of Medicine, Pond Street, London NW3 2QG, United Kingdom

Viral hepatitis is a common, worldwide problem. It can to a large extent be prevented by strict hygienic measures, and the risk of transmission in certain subgroups of the population can be minimized because potentially infective material such as blood and blood products can be screened for the presence of HBsAg. Passive immunization is of value in some instances. Active immunization against hepatitis B is obviously a major preventive advance, and hopefully we will eventually have effective vaccines against hepatitis A and the other types of viral hepatitis.

Currently, however, we must care for those patients who suffer from the various types of viral hepatitis. The development of drugs which appear to be active against viral infections has led to their use in the field of viral hepatitis. Theoretically they might be of use in all the viral hepatitides, but their cost and side effects, and the difficulties of demonstrating their efficacy, limit their attraction for the treatment of hepatitis A, which is generally a benign, self-limited disease. We have no markers to confirm the diagnosis of non-A, non-B hepatitis and cannot therefore be certain that it is actually a viral infection; and at present we know relatively little about the biology of delta infection.

By contrast we now know a good deal about the hepatitis B virus (HBV) and its effects. While many patients suffer an illness similar to that of hepatitis A infection, a significant proportion tend to carry the virus in their blood for a long time and are a potential risk to others – directly or indirectly. Furthermore, many suffer serious liver disease, developing chronic hepatitis and cirrhosis and also carrying the long-term risk of primary liver cell carcinoma. Not surprisingly, there has been great interest in the possibility that antiviral drugs might be capable of eradicating HBV infection. This would reduce the infectivity of the patients to others, and minimize the risk of superimposed delta infection. One might hope that eradication of the virus would prevent further progression of chronic hepatitis and reduce the incidence of cirrhosis, and that it might also lead to a decrease in the number of patients who go on to develop primary liver cell carcinoma.

Given the very large number of patients who are currently suffering from hepatitis B infection, the first question to be asked is which patients should be treated. The treatment of acute HBV would be valuable if as a result there was a reduction in the severity and duration of the acute illness, and if it prevented progression in the small number of patients who appear to go on to acquire a chronic hepatitis. There would, of course, be formidable problems in setting up an appropriate trial; because so many of the patients run a self-limited course of variable severity, large numbers of patients would be needed to assess efficacy.

There are many patients, however, who have chronic infection with hepatitis B and

Assessment and Management of Hepatobiliary Disease
Eds.: L. Okolicsányi, G. Csomós, and G. Crepaldi

the clinical picture in these is also variable (Anderson and Murray-Lyon 1985). Some are apparently healthy carriers of hepatitis B who may have normal liver function and little evidence of abnormality in their liver biopsy (Koretz et al. 1978). While they are infective to others, and may run a small risk of progression to chronic hepatitis and cirrhosis, and to hepatocellular carcinoma, their prognosis in general appears to be very good. It is clear that such patients should not be in the vanguard of trials designed to assess the efficacy of antiviral therapy when the main benefit to be gained is the loss of their infectivity to others. Similar considerations hold with regard to the treatment of patients with either *chronic lobular hepatitis* (Liaw et al. 1982), without evidence of portal or periportal inflammation, or *chronic persistent hepatitis* (Chadwick et al. 1979; Weissberg et al. 1984; Sanchez-Tapias et al. 1984). In both cases the prognosis appears to be reasonably good, although the outlook, particularly in the latter condition, does appear to be related to the persistence of HBeAg in serum (Aldershville et al. 1982). Clearly we need further studies on the natural history of chronic lobular and chronic persistent hepatitis, and particularly on the many factors, including HBeAg/anti-HBe status, which may affect the outcome in patients with these conditions. If an effective antiviral treatment for HBV is found, then trials in these groups of patients will be necessary to show that the benefits which result outweigh the cost and complications of therapy.

The major interest in antiviral therapy for HBV infection has, understandably, been in the treatment of patients with HBV chronic active hepatitis (HBV-CAH), and there are now many studies of various agents, but unfortunately they have not as yet provided unequivocal results or a clear solution to the problem of antiviral treatment. There are many reasons for this. They arise in part because the prognosis, even in the untreated patient, is variable. The outlook, in terms of the activity of the chronic hepatitis, appears to depend on the persistence of viral replication within the liver, as evidenced by the persistence of HBV-DNA and HBeAg in serum. When they disappear, and when there is seroconversion to anti-HBe, then biochemical and histological evidence of activity is less marked and there may be a return of standard liver function tests to normal. The outlook in clinical terms is also markedly dependent on the degree of morphological change which has already been produced in the liver. Not surprisingly, the outlook is worse if cirrhosis has developed and if there is severe impairment of hepatocellular function (Hoofnagle et al. 1983; Fattovich et al. 1986).

Seroconversion to anti-HBe may occur spontaneously, and this clearly affects the interpretation of results in testing the efficacy of drugs used to treat HBV-CAH. Furthermore, the seroconversion rate varies in different groups of patients; homosexuals, for example, appear to have a lower rate than heterosexual males. The seroconversion rate seems to be increased if there is intercurrent infection with other hepatotrophic agents such as delta, non-A, non-B or hepatitis A.

Our problems are further compounded because there is as yet no complete agreement on the nature of the mechanisms underlying the continuing inflammation which takes place in HBV-CAH, a problem which is not helped by our complete lack of understanding of why some patients develop CAH and why others do not, and why, in some patients, viral replication persists even in the absence of hepatic damage. Furthermore, our knowledge of the mode of action of antiviral drugs is in its infancy, and there is little understanding of why some viruses are affected and others not, or why in vitro effects are often quite different from those in vivo. The study of antiviral agents in

HBV infection has not stemmed from any detailed knowledge of the action of these agents against HBV. It has resulted from the knowledge that some drugs appear to work in some viral infections, often due to viruses quite different from HBV itself, and the optimism that such drugs might therefore work in the treatment of hepatitis B. Finally, there are a large number of factors which may influence the course of HBV-CAH (Anderson and Murray-Lyon 1985). These may affect the natural history of the HBV infection per se, e.g. sex, ethnic origin, age at infection, mode of transmission and associated clinical conditions, or they may be factors which have a direct and deleterious effect on the liver, such as alcohol, drugs and superimposed infections.

These many influences on the course of HBV chronic hepatitis are likely to be important in determining the apparent outcome of antiviral treatment and need to be taken into account in the interpretation of the studies. They probably explain at least some of the differences found by different groups of workers; we must therefore be cautious in assuming that results obtained in one population of patients will necessarily apply to other groups, even when dealing with such apparently simple results as the HBeAg, HBV-DNA status and biochemical investigations.

Although immunosuppressive drugs are not "antiviral agents" they have been widely used in the treatment of CAH, and initially the aetiology of the CAH was not always clear. It is generally agreed that the outcome of auto-immune chronic hepatitis is favourably influenced, mortality and morbidity being reduced, by treatment with prednisolone (Cook et al. 1971), or with a combination of prednisolone and azathioprine (Soloway et al. 1972). Review of the HBV-associated cases in the early trials suggests that they responded less well than the auto-immune patients (Schalm et al. 1976). Subsequent studies have been done in patients with HBV-CAH, because of the clinical and histological similarities of the two conditions and because immune mechanisms are thought to be important in the pathogenesis of HBV-CAH (Thomas et al. 1986).

Clinical and biochemical improvement have been reported during long-term treatment with prednisolone (Weller et al. 1982), but it appears to enhance viral replication (Sagnelli et al. 1983), and in some studies mortality and morbidity have been higher in the steroid-treated group (Lam et al. 1981). Cessation of therapy has been associated with seroconversion to anti-HBe in many patients, but this may have been due to delay of spontaneous seroconversion during therapy (Realdi et al. 1980), and in some patients with advanced liver disease there has been serious exacerbation of the disease (Nowicki et al. 1984). The general feeling is that immunosuppressive therapy should not be used alone in HBeAg-positive patients; there may be a role for such treatment in patients with anti-HBe in serum, but the necessary trials have yet to be reported.

Adenine arabinoside is thought to inhibit DNA polymerase and thus to interfere with DNA synthesis, and it may have more effect on the viral than host cell mechanisms. Several groups have used it, or its less toxic monophosphate derivate ARA-AMP, in the treatment of HBV-CAH, but the trials have involved small numbers of patients for a relatively short time and have often been poorly designed. ARA-AMP appears effective in inhibiting HBV replication and there is a fall in serum HBV-DNA and HBeAg with persistent conversion to anti-HBe in some, but it is difficult to be sure that this would not have occurred spontaneously. In many patients there is reappearance of these viral markers in the serum. In a study done at the Royal Free, six of 15 patients treated with intramuscular ARA-AMP for 4 weeks lost serum HBV polymerase, DNA and HBcAg and the concentration of HBsAg fell; five developed anti-

HBe. There were no similar changes in the 14 control patients, but interpretation was rendered difficult because some patients in the treatment group suffered infection with other hepatic viruses (two delta, one HAV) which may have affected the conversion to anti-HBe. In this and in a parallel study, it was shown that while about 50% of heterosexual carriers responded to ARA-AMP, none of 24 homosexuals responded, and it was thought that this might have been due to an altered state of immunity in these patients (Novick et al. 1984).

There seems to be general agreement that ARA-AMP alone is not the answer to the treatment of HBV-CAH, and this, and concern about toxicity, has led to the withdrawal of ARA-A and ARA-AMP for this condition in Britain and the U.S.A. Some workers still believe that ARA-AMP may be useful if it is given following a short course of steroids, as increased seroconversion to anti-HBe was noted in two trials in which it was used in this way (Perrillo et al. 1985; Yokosuka et al. 1985).

Acyclovir is another drug which inhibits DNA synthesis. Its specificity against viruses, which renders it relatively non-toxic, is thought to depend on its conversion to a triphosphate derivative by a viral thymidine kinase. This enzyme is absent from HBV but acyclovir does appear to inhibit HBV replication in high doses. It has only a weak and transient effect in animal and human studies, and does not alone significantly increase the rate of seroconversion to anti-HBe. In a preliminary report it has been claimed that it may be effective in human HBV-CAH when given with interferon (Schalm et al. 1985), and in studies in the Pekin duck it appears to be effective in inhibiting duck hepatitis virus replication when given following the administration of suramin (Tsiquaye et al. 1986).

Currently the major interest in the antiviral treatment of HBV infection lies in the use of interferons (IFN). They were identified in 1957 as a group of proteins which are produced in response to viral infection and which inhibit the growth of a wide range of viruses through cellular processes involving synthesis of both RNA and protein (Taylor-Papadimitriou 1985). It is the availability of purified IFN, and the subsequent cloning and expression of the IFN genes, which has revolutionized the IFN field. Unfortunately, the large number of native IFN which have been identified and the wide range of actions of those which have been studied combine to make this a difficult area to understand, particularly in relation to their use in the treatment of human viral infections. It is clearly a major problem to test all these IFN (singly and in combination) for their possible role in the genesis of the different HBV-induced disorders and to establish their effects in treatment.

There are three basic types of IFN, alpha, beta and gamma, and these are derived from different types of cells and in response to different stimuli. Alpha-IFN, of which there are at least 13, are produced by leukocytes (probably macrophages) and by lymphoblastoid cell lines. Beta-IFN appears to be a single protein produced by solid tissues, e.g. fibroblasts and epithelial cells. Both alpha- and beta-IFN are produced by viral infection, probably by the insertion into the cell of double-stranded RNA. Gamma-IFN is produced mainly by T cells in response to antigenic stimulation, which includes that by viral antigens.

IFN appear to act in many different ways to inhibit viral infections, and the effects differ with different IFN, with the type of virus and with the animal and cell type involved. In some viral infections there seem to be effects on the attachment, penetration and uncoating of the virus, or on the eventual assembly, maturation and release of the virus. It is claimed that these effects occur with retroviruses which have some analogies with the hepadnaviridiae (Billiau 1986).

Two important effects of IFN lie in the activation of a protein kinase and of 2-5-A synthetase. The protein kinase is one which phosphorylates the eukaryotic initiation factor and so interferes with the translation of mRNA. 2-5-A synthetase causes the production of 2′,5′-linked oligonucleotides of adenosine; these activate an endogenous endonuclease which degrades both messenger and ribosomal RNA. Both these effects lead to inhibition of host cell as well as viral protein production. These mechanisms would affect viral replication directly, but IFN may also have indirect antiviral effects in that they tend to increase the surface display of the major histocompatibility antigens, and the combination of HLA 1 and viral antigen on the hepatocyte surface may enhance destruction of infected cells by cytotoxic T cells.

Pignatelli et al. (1986) at the Royal Free have shown an enhanced display of HLA I antigens in livers of patients with active HBV-CAH, and an increased display following administration of IFN. There is also an increase in serum beta$_2$-microglobulin, which appears greater in those who respond to IFN therapy. Furthermore, the IFN have effects on several parts of the immune system which may play a role in the removal of infected cells. Unfortunately, we do not yet understand how these various mechanisms interact in the effects of IFN in HBV infection, either in explaining the effects of HBV infection, or the effect of administered IFN.

There have been a number of reports on the use of interferon in HBV-CAH since the original study in 1976 by Greenberg and his colleagues, who demonstrated reduction of serum DNA-polymerase and other HBV markers in three patients given different doses of alpha-IFN for varying periods of time. In subsequent studies using the same type of IFN, together with adenine arabinoside, the Stanford group found that about 37% of patients lost HBsAg (Scullard et al. 1981). Furthermore, Scullard et al. (1982) found that serum from treated patients who had lost the viral markers was no longer infectious to chimpanzees. Because two drugs were used it was difficult to assess the effect of the IFN per se.

At a meeting in London in November, 1985, 14 groups reported their results with IFN (mainly alpha-IFN produced in lymphoblastoid cells) in chronic HBV infection. Their results were summarized in a leading article in the BMJ (Alexander and Williams 1986). Courses of alpha-IFN given 3 × week in doses of about 5 × 10 MU/m$^2$ for 3 months inhibit viral replication and appear safe. Toxicity minimizes the advantages of a larger dose. Shorter courses seem to be ineffective and larger courses confer no advantage. A hepatitis-like illness occurs in some patients during the 3rd month and tends to be followed by seroconversion from HbeAg to anti-HBe. Patients whose initial transaminase levels were high seemed more likely to seroconvert; this raises the question of whether they would have seroconverted without treatment, perhaps at a later date. Subsequently there has been a preliminary report to suggest that recombinant alpha$_2$-IFN may also be effective in some patients with chronic delta hepatitis (Rosina et al. 1986), and in those there was a rise in aminotransferase during the first week of treatment.

Howard Thomas and his group at the Royal Free have now treated about 100 patients with lymphoblastoid or recombinant alpha-IFN. About 50% of them clear HBeAg and HBV-DNA with seroconversion to anti-HBe, and in most of them there is an improvement in biochemical markers of hepatitis with return of aminotransferases to normal levels. A small number (about 5%) of those who have cleared HBeAg relapse after several months.

The probability of response to IFN, particularly in terms of clearance of HBsAg, appears to be greater if treatment is started early in the course of the infection; presumably if HBV-DNA has integrated into the host genome, continued production of HBsAg can occur. The integration of HBV-DNA may have another effect on IFN responsiveness. It has been found that there is a sequence within the HBV genome which is similar to the "consensus" sequence which is present close to the genes for proteins whose production is stimulated by IFN. If HBV-DNA integrates at these sites it may interfere with the IFN stimulus to protein synthesis. Alternatively, HBV-DNA inserted elsewhere may compete for the "messenger" molecules which would normally attach at the consensus sequences. In some in vitro studies Andrew Lever has inserted fragments of HBV-DNA into cells and shown that their presence does reduce the subsequent responsiveness of those cells to IFN.

From the studies at the Royal Free it would appear that homosexuals respond as well as heterosexual males to IFN; this is in contrast to the unresponsiveness of homosexuals to ARA-AMP. Lok et al. (1986) in Hong Kong consider that Chinese patients do not appear to respond well to IFN. This may accord with data from the Royal Free, where Thomas et al. (1986) have evidence that patients who acquired their infection from carrier mothers do not appear to respond to IFN or ARA-AMP. It is postulated that transplacental transfer of IgG anti-HBc has altered their immune response and thus interfered with the clearance of HBV-infected cells by T cells sensitized to HBc or HBe. An alternative explanation is that the transfer of viral protein to the neonate may have induced a certain degree of tolerance to the virus.

A number of interesting questions arise from the results of the studies which have so far been reported. As the IFN are natural compounds, does their effect in some patients suggest that an inadequate or insufficient IFN response plays a part in the genesis of the chronic carrier state? There is some evidence that this might be the case (Thomas et al. 1986). Some Western European carriers of HBV have a defect in the ability of their blood mononuclear cells to produce alpha-IFN in response to Sendai virus when tested in vitro. They also have evidence of suboptimal activation of hepatocytes by IFN as levels of hepatic 2-5-A synthetase are only minimally elevated, and levels of the same enzyme in peripheral mononuclear cells are low compared with those seen in acute viral infections, including hepatitis B. Consistent with this is the failure of infected hepatocytes to show increased display of HLA class I proteins; these are present in relatively low density in periportal hepatocytes in chronic HBV carriers, in contrast to the diffuse enhancement of display seen in acute hepatitis B.

But if this is so, then why does alpha-IFN take so long to work if its effect is due to a direct antiviral action? At the London meeting Omata (1986) suggested that certain types of replicative HBV-DNA (supercoiled) are relatively resistant to the effects of IFN and that this resistant DNA may form the transcribing template in those in whom viral replication continues after treatment. Alternatively, it may be that the benefits of treatment are not due to a direct antiviral action but to the effects of IFN on the immune system. If this is so, then gamma-IFN may prove more effective than alpha-IFN, as it is a more potent activator of macrophages, enhancing expression of markers such as the Fc receptor, and functions such as microbial and tumour cell killing. It also increases the display of both class I and class II MHC antigens on macrophages and other cells, while alpha-IFN appears to enhance only expression of class I antigens. That the immune system is important in the response to IFN is suggested by the recent finding of Howard Thomas and his colleagues that patients with chronic hepatitis B who are HTLV III-Ab positive do not respond to IFN.

It is hoped that the seroconversion to anti-HBe which occurs with IFN and other antiviral drugs will lead to an improvement in the outcome of the disease in these patients; the reduction in biochemical and histological activity suggests that the chronic hepatitis is ameliorated and that progression to cirrhosis will be halted. This should improve the outlook of the condition as regards the classical hepatocellular complications of chronic liver disease. What we do not yet know is whether such treatment will have a long-term effect on the development of primary liver cell carcinoma. If viral integration is the major oncogenic factor then the effect may depend on how early the drug is given. If cirrhosis and continuing hepatocyte regeneration are important in tumour production then IFN may still prove effective in reducing the incidence even after integration has occurred.

Clearly the answers to these and many other important questions may come from the many further studies on the basic mechanisms of HBV infection, on the ways in which the body responds to HBV, and on the molecular mechanisms by which antiviral drugs exert their effects. The studies done to date have been promising but they have merely scratched the surface of a very complicated area.

## References

Aldershville J, Dietrichson O, Skinhoj P, Mathiesen LR, Christoffersen P, Nielsen JO (1982) Chronic persistent hepatitis: serological classification and meaning of the hepatitis Be system. Hepatology 2: 243-246

Alexander G, Williams R (1986) Antiviral treatment in chronic infection with hepatitis B. Br Med J 292: 292-294

Anderson MG, Murray-Lyon IM (1985) Natural history of the HBsAg carrier. Gut 26: 848-860

Billiau A (1986) The mode of action of interferons in viral infections and their possible role in the control of hepatitis B. J Hepatol (in press)

Chadwick RG, Galizzi J, Heathcote J, Lyssiotis T, Cohen BJ, Scheuer PJ, Sherlock S (1979) Chronic persistent hepatitis: hepatitis B virus markers and histological follow-up. Gut 20: 372-377

Cook GC, Mulligan R, Sherlock S (1971) Controlled prospective trial of corticosteroid therapy in active chronic hepatitis. Q J Med 40: 159-185

Fattovich G, Rugge M, Brollo L, Pontisso P, Noventa F, Guido M, Alberti A, Realdi (1986) Clinical, virological and histologic outcome following seroconversion from HBeAg to Anti-HBe in chronic hepatitis type B. Hepatology 6: 167-172

Greenberg HB, Pollard RB, Lutwick LI, Gregory PB, Robinson WS, Merigan TC (1976) Effect of human leukocyte interferon on hepatitis B virus infection in patients with chronic active hepatitis. N Engl J Med 295: 517-522

Hoofnagle JH, Davis GL, Hanson RG (1983) Chronic type B hepatitis: clinical course. In: Verme G, Bonino F, Rizzetto (eds) Viral hepatitis and delta infection. Liss, New York, pp 41-53

Koretz RL, Lewin CJ, Rebhun DJ, Gitnick G (1978) Hepatitis B surface antigen carriers – to biopsy or not to biopsy. Gastroenterology 83: 860-863

Lam KC, Lai CL, Ng RP, Trepo C, Wu PC (1981) Deleterious effect of prednisolone in HBsAg positive chronic active hepatitis. N Engl J Med 304: 380-386

Liaw YF, Chu CM, Chen TJ, Lin DY, Chang-Chien CS, Wu CS (1982) Chronic lobular hepatitis: a clinicopathological and prognostic study. Hepatology 2: 256-261

Lok ASF, Lai CL, Wu PC (1986) Spontaneous and interferon induced HBe antigen to antibody

seroconversion in chronic hepatitis B virus infection in Hong Kong Chinese. J Hepatol (in press)
Novick DM, Lok ASF, Thomas HC (1984) Diminished responsiveness of homosexual men to antiviral therapy for HBsAg positive chronic liver disease. J Hepatol 1: 29-35
Nowicki MJ, Tong MJ, Nair PV, Stevenson D (1984) Detection of anti-HBc IgM following prednisolone treatment in patients with chronic active hepatitis B virus infection. Hepatology 4: 1129-1133
Omata M (1986) In vivo study on mechanism of action of interferon and ARA-A against HBV and DHBV replication in the liver. J Hepatol (in press)
Perrillo R, Regenstein F, Bodicky C, Campbell CR, Sanders GE, Sunwoo YC (1985) Comparative efficacy of adenine arabinoside 5'monophosphate and prednisolone withdrawal followed by adenine arabinoside 5'monophosphate in the treatment of chronic active hepatitis B. Gastroenterology 89: 780-786
Pignatelli M, Waters J, Brown D, Lever A, Schaff Z, Gerety R, Thomas H (1986) HLA class I antigens on the hepatocyte membrane during recovery from acute hepatitis B infection and during interferon therapy in chronic HBV infection. Hepatology (in press)
Realdi G, Alberti A, Rugge M, Bortolotti F, Rigoli AM, Tremolada F, Ruol A (1980) Seroconversion from hepatitis Be antigen to anti-HBe in chronic hepatitis B infection. Gastroenterology 79: 195-199
Rosina F, Saracco G, Actis GC, Brunetto MR, Maran E, Pintus C, Dianzani F, Verme G, Rizzetto M, Bonino F (1986) Treatment of chronic delta hepatitis with alpha-2 recombinant interferon (Abstr). Gastroenterology 90: 1762
Sagnelli E, Piccinino F, Manzillo G, Felaco FM, Filippini P, Maio G, Pasquale G, Izzo CM (1983) Effect of immunosuppressive therapy on HBsAg-positive chronic active hepatitis in relation to presence or absence of HBeAg and Anti-HBe. Hepatology 3: 690-695
Sanchez-Tapias JM, Vilar JH, Costa J, Bruguera M, Ballesta AM, Rodes J (1984) Natural history of chronic hepatitis B: relationship between hepatitis B replication and the course of the disease. J Hepatol 1: 15-27
Schalm SW, Summerskill WJH, Gitnick GL, Elveback LR (1976) Contrasting features and responses to treatment of severe chronic active liver disease with and without hepatitis Bs antigen. Gut 17: 781-786
Schalm SW, Heytink RA, Van Buuren HR, De Man RA (1985) Acyclovir enhances the antiviral effect of interferon in chronic hepatitis B. Lancet II: 358-360
Scullard GH, Pollard RB, Smith JL, Sacks SL, Gregory PB, Robinson WS, Merigan TC (1981) Antiviral treatment of chronic hepatitis B virus infection. Changes in viral markers with interferon combined adenine arabinoside. J Infect Dis 143: 772-773
Scullard GH, Greenberg HB, Smith JL, Gregory PB, Merigan TC, Robinson WS (1982) Antiviral treatment of chronic hepatitis B virus infection: infectious virus cannot be detected in patient serum after permanent responses to treatment. Hepatology 2: 39-49
Soloway RD, Summerskill WHJ, Baggenstoss AH, Geal MG, Gitnick GL, Elveback LR, Schoenfield LJ (1972) Clinical, biochemical and histological remission of severe chronic active liver disease: a controlled study of treatments and early prognosis. Gastroenterology 63: 820-833
Taylor-Papadimitriou J (ed) (1985) Interferons: their impact in biology and medicine. Oxford University Press, Oxford
Thomas HC, Lever AML, Scully LJ, Pignatelli M (1986) Approaches to the treatment of hepatitis B and delta-related liver disease. Semin Liver Dis 6: 34-41
Tsiquaye KN, Collins P, Zuckerman AJ (1986) Screening of antiviral agents for treatment of hepatitis B. J Hepatol (in press)
Weissberg JI, Andres LL, Smith CI, Weick S, Nichols JE, Garcia G, Robinson WS, Merigan TC, Gregory PB (1984) Survival in chronic hepatitis B: an analysis of 379 patients. Ann Intern Med 101: 613-616
Weller IVD, Bassendine MF, Murray AK, Craxi A, Thomas HC, Sherlock S (1982) Effects of prednisolone/azathioprine in chronic hepatitis B infection. Gut 23: 650-655
Yokosuka O, Omata M, Imazeki F, Hirota K, Mori J, Uchiumi K, Ito Y, Okuda K (1985) Combination of short-term prednisolone and adenine arabinoside in the treatment of chronic hepatitis B. Gastroenterology 89: 246-251

# Autoimmune Hepatitis: Diagnosis and Treatment

E. Pisi, F. Cassani, M. Fusconi, and F. B. Bianchi
Istituto di Patologia Medica, Cattedra di Clinica Medica II, Università di Bologna, Bologna, Italy

A chronic liver disease (CLD) is defined as autoimmune when the two following criteria are fulfilled: absence of any known cause of liver damage and presence of serum marker autoantibodies [1].

The exclusion of a number of etiological agents must be as careful as possible; in the case of non-A, non-B virus, it can be made only on the basis of clinical history, since no reliable markers of infection are yet available. Clinical features reported in the original description of the so-called lupoid hepatitis [2] such as age (young or perimenopausal) and sex (mainly females) should be carefully considered. Laboratory assessment of autoimmune involvement of other organs (thyroid, salivary glands, stomach), only rarely seen on clinical observation, should be included. The existence of the HLA DR3 phenotype would add some extra weight, but the search for it cannot be proposed for routine use. It is apparent, however, that autoimmune CLD remains largely an exclusion diagnosis. According to our experience, in Italy, where hepatitis B virus (HBV) and alcoholic liver disease (ALD) are the most frequent, about 20%-30% of CLD patients are scored as cryptogenic.

Serum non-organ-specific autoantibodies – antinuclear (ANA) and smooth muscle (SMA) – are the only positive diagnostic criteria. Both are currently regarded as heterogeneous families of antibodies recognizing a wide range of distinct antigenic targets [3, 4]. A number of studies, mainly concerning connective tissue diseases, have demonstrated the possibility of gaining more detailed diagnostic information by identifying relevant subspecificities; this point, however, does not yet seem to have been completely taken up even by recent hepatological investigators. In fact, crude ANA and/or SMA, detected by indirect immunofluorescence (IFL) on conventional tissue cryostatic sections, are still considered with no other specification except the titer, which should be "high" (usually $\geq 1:40$, but there is no well-defined consensus).

A good example of autoantibody heterogeneity is SMA. By IFL on rat kidney sections, three patterns can be detected: $SMA_V$ (positivity of vessels only), $SMA_G$ (vessels + glomeruli), and $SMA_T$ (vessels + glomeruli + peritubular structures) [5]. The introduction of cell line cultures as IFL substrates (namely human embryonic fibroblasts treated with vinblastine) disclosed the close relationship between SMA and antibodies to the cytoskeletal components: microfilaments (MF), intermediate filaments (IMF), and microtubules [4]. At a molecular level, actin has been identified as the target antigen of the SMA found in autoimmune CLD [6]. Anti-actin antibodies are detected by IFL on kidney sections as $SMA_T$ and $SMA_G$ and, far more easily, on cell cultures as anti-MF, with a variable sensitivity according to the cell line used [7]. In our hands, an optimal visualization of anti-actin antibodies was reached by IFL using cryostatic sections of liver from rats previously treated with phalloidin; due to the drug-induced ac-

Assessment and Management of Hepatobiliary Disease
Eds.: L. Okolicsányi, G. Csomós, and G. Crepaldi

**Table 1.** SMA in chronic liver disease

| | $SMA_{T\text{-}G}$ (tissue) | Anti-MF (HEp-2) | $SMA_V$ (tissue) | Anti-IMF (HEp-2) |
|---|---|---|---|---|
| Cryptogenic (82) | 16%* | 16%* | 43% | 20% |
| HBV-ALD (80) | 2% | 2% | 29% | 31% |
| Healthy controls (50) | - | - | 12% | 15% |

* Cryptogenic vs HBV-ALD: $p < 0.01$ ($chi^2$ Yates')

cumulation of filamentous actin at the biliary pole and outer cytoplasm of the hepatocytes [8], even low-titer anti-actin antibodies can be detected. The gain in sensitivity provided by an immunoenzymatic assay for antibodies to globular actin does not appear to be of clinical utility because of the even higher decrease in specificity [9]. The results of SMA characterization in a series of patients with CLD of unknown and known (HBV, ALD) etiology are reported in Table 1. Only anti-actin reactivities ($SMA_{T\text{-}G}$ on tissue sections and anti-MF on HEp-2 cells) proved to be significantly associated with cryptogenic cases (probably marking the autoimmune subgroup), whereas $SMA_V$ and anti-IMF did not discriminate among the different forms of CLD. It must be pointed out that these last reactivities are also found in the vast majority of patients with acute viral hepatitis and in a variety of other viral diseases [4].

The heterogeneity of ANA has been extensively resolved in connective tissue diseases [3], but no data are yet available about the molecular targets of CLD-associated ANA. Compared with conventional IFL, a more reliable and accurate immunomorphological characterization of ANA can again be obtained by the use of cell cultures (HEp-2) as substrate. When applied to the study of serum from liver patients, this immunological approach has allowed identification of relevant ANA patterns (like the anticentromere antibody, Cen) with the highest gain of clinical information in primary biliary cirrhosis [10]. As to autoimmune CLD, ANA giving a homogeneous (H) pattern are said to be commonly found [1]. In our experience (Table 2) both the homogeneous and speckled (S) patterns are more frequent in cryptogenic than in HBV and ALD cases, the statistical significance being higher for the former. The known candidate antigens of ANA-H are histones and double-stranded (ds) DNA; anti-dsDNA antibodies, however, are highly specific for systemic lupus erythematosus (SLE) and very rare in CLD, as assessed by IFL on *Crithidia luciliae*. One more feature differentiating CLD-associated from SLE-associated ANA is the absence of antibodies to extractable nuclear antigens (ENA); they are in fact commonly detected (by immunodiffusion or counterimmunoelectrophoresis, CIE) in SLE sera exhibiting a strong IFL ANA-S reactivity. An ENA-like precipitating system, called XR, has been recently described in autoimmune CLD [11]; the close correlation we found between XR and SMA, but not ANA, would suggest that the corresponding antigen is actually actin.

The impact of the use of the "new" instead of the "old" markers in the diagnostic assessment of our patients is summarized in Table 3. It is apparent that the diagnosis of autoimmune CLD would certainly be rarer, but probably more specific. Further studies are needed to ascertain the reliability of such a diagnostic rearrangement.

The importance of a correct diagnosis of autoimmune CLD is far from limited to more accurate nosographic classification. In fact, evidence has been produced in the

**Table 2.** ANA in chronic liver disease

| | ANA (tissue) | H (HEp-2) | S (HEp-2) | Cen (HEp-2) | dsDNA *(Crithidia)* |
|---|---|---|---|---|---|
| Cryptogenic (82) | 33%* | 27%** | 39%*** | 2% | 2% |
| HBV-ALD (80) | 15% | 6% | 16% | 2% | - |
| Healthy controls (50) | 5%-19% | 0%-3% | 8%-12% | - | - |

Anti-ENA was never detected by CIE
Cryptogenic vs HBV-ALD (chi²): $*p<0.001$ $**p<0.002$ $***p<0.01$

**Table 3.** "Old" and "new" markers in chronic liver disease

| *Old* ANA and/or SMA (IFL tissue 1:40) | | | *New* ANA-D and/or anti-MF (IFL HEp-2 1:40) | | |
|---|---|---|---|---|---|
| Cryptogenic CLD (82) | | | Cryptogenic CLD (82) | | |
| ANA | SMA | ANA+SMA | ANA-D | anti-MF | ANA-D+anti-MF |
| 11 | 25 | 16 | 17 | 8 | 5 |
| Autoimmune: 52/82 (63%) | | | Autoimmune: 30/82 (37%) | | |
| HBV-ALD (80) | | | HBV-ALD (80) | | |
| ANA | SMA | ANA+SMA | ANA-D | anti-MF | ANA-D+anti-MF |
| 8 | 21 | 4 | 5 | 2 | - |
| Total: 33/80 (41%) | | | Total: 7/80 (9%) | | |

past by several clinical trials on (mainly) autoimmune CLD patients that steroids with or without azathioprine do have an overall beneficial effect in terms of survival, evolution to cirrhosis, and biochemical parameters [12]. However, a proportion of nonresponder cases, scored as autoimmune on the basis of conventional markers, have been reported [13]. It is suggested that better selection of the patients by use of the relevant ANA and/or SMA subspecificities would possibly allow avoidance of inappropriate steroid courses (and the associated untoward side effects). It remains to be clearly assessed whether serological markers may play a role in the monitoring of therapy. The titer of granulocyte-specific ANA (found in CLD and rheumatoid arthritis) has been reported to decrease under steroid treatment [14]; this finding, however, has not been confirmed.

## References


1. Mackay IR (1983) Immunological aspects of chronic active hepatitis. Hepatology 5: 724-728
2. Mackay IR, Taft LJ, Cowling DC (1956) Lupoid hepatitis. Lancet ii: 1323-1326
3. Tan EM (1982) Autoantibodies to nuclear antigens: their immunobiology and medicine. Adv Immunol 33: 167-240
4. Toh BH (1979) Smooth muscle autoantibodies and autoantigens. Clin Exp Immunol 38: 621-628
5. Bottazzo GF, Florin-Christensen A, Fairfax A, Swana G, Doniach D, Gröschel-Stewart U (1976) Classification of smooth muscle autoantibodies detected by immunofluorescence. J Clin Path 29: 403-410
6. Lidmann K, Biberfeld G, Fagraeus A, Norberg R, Tortensson R, Utter G, Carlsson L, Luca J,

Lindberg U (1976) Anti-actin specificity of human smooth muscle antibodies in chronic active hepatitis. Clin Exp Immunol 24: 266-272
7. Zauli D, Crespi C, Bianchi FB, Pisi E (1985) Immunofluorescent detection of anti-cytoskeleton antibodies using vinblastine-treated mononuclear cells. J Immunol Methods 82: 77-82
8. Gabbiani G, Montesano R, Tuchweber B, Salas M, Orci L (1975) Phalloidin-induced hyperplasia of actin filaments in rat hepatocytes. Lab Invest 33: 562-569
9. Bretherton L, Brown C, Pedersen JS, Toh BH, Clarke FM, Mackay IR, Gust D (1983) ELISA assay for IgG autoantibody to G-actin: comparison of chronic active hepatitis and acute viral hepatitis. Clin Exp Immunol 51: 611-616
10. Cassani F, Bianchi FB, Lenzi M, Volta U, Pisi E (1985) Immunomorphological characterization of antinuclear antibodies in chronic liver disease. J Clin Path 38: 801-805
11. Bernstein RM, Neuberger JM, Bunn CC, Callender ME, Hughes GRV, Williams R (1984) Diversity of autoantibodies in primary biliary cirrhosis and chronic active hepatitis. Clin Exp Immunol 55: 553-560
12. Wright EC, Seeff LB, Berk PD, Jones EA, Plotz PH (1977) Treatment of chronic active hepatitis. An analysis of three controlled trials. Gastroenterology 73: 1422-1430
13. Lebovics E, Schaffner F, Klion FM, Simon C (1985) Autoimmune chronic active hepatitis in postmenopausal women. Dig Dis Sci 30: 824-828
14. Whittingham S, Morstyn G, Wilson TW, Mackay IR (1981) An autoantibody reactive with nuclei of polymorphonuclear neutrophils: a cell differentiation marker. Blood 58: 766-771

# Serum $\beta_2$-Microglobulin and Anti-$\beta_2$m Antibodies in Chronic Liver Disease

A. Pár[1], A. Falus[2], and T. Jávor[1]

[1] First Department of Medicine, University Medical School, Pécs, Hungary
[2] National Institute for Rheumatology and Physiotherapy, Budapest, Hungary

$\beta_2$-Microglobulin ($\beta_2$m) is a low-molecular-weight (11800-dalton) protein, free of carbohydrates, consisting of a single polypeptide chain of 100 amino acid residues. The amino acid sequence and the structure of $\beta_2$m are homologous with the chains of immunoglobulin. $\beta_2$m binds to MHC class I antigens and also to tumor-specific antigens, as "light chain", on the surface of nucleated cells. The most significant function of $\beta_2$m seems to be the intracellular transport of MHC class I antigens and the formation and maintenance of their active membrane configuration. $\beta_2$m is produced at a relatively constant rate in healthy subjects and released into the body fluids as a result of cell turnover. It is eliminated from the organism by the kidneys, where it is filtered through the glomeruli and reabsorbed and catabolised by the proximal tubular cells. Normally only trace amounts of $\beta_2$m are excreted in urine, but its excretion is markedly increased after derangements of the functional integrity of the proximal tubuli. The serum level of $\beta_2$m reflects the glomerular filtration rate more accurately than does that of serum creatinine.

Soluble $\beta_2$m as a shed membrane protein subunit of HLA antigens can be found in relatively low concentration in biological fluids of healthy persons, while increased production and high serum $\beta_2$m levels have been detected in malignant, infectious, and autoimmune diseases. There is strong evidence that lymphocytes are a major source of $\beta_2$m, and their activation is associated with an increased release of this protein. $\beta_2$m is highly cytophilic, showing preferential binding to $\beta_2$m-receptor structures of activated cells and to the Fc receptors of macrophages (Berggard and Bearn 1968; Grey et al. 1973; Peterson et al. 1974; Wibell and Karlsson 1973).

An autoantibody against $\beta_2$m may develop, and this $\beta_2$m-binding antibody (anti-$\beta_2$m) represents part of the lymphocytotoxic antibodies reacting with surface antigens. Antibodies specific to $\beta_2$m, in addition to their complement-dependent cytotoxicity, express a mitogenic effect on B and T lymphocytes and inhibit the mitogenic, allogeneic, and antigenic activation of lymphocytes (Falus 1984).

So far, only few authors have studied the serum $\beta_2$m level in liver diseases (Beorchia et al. 1982; Hallgren 1979; Rashid et al. 1981) and only Revillard et al. (1981) reported on anti-$\beta_2$m determinations in hepatitis. Although these previous findings raised the possibility that $\beta_2$m as a marker of lymphocyte activation may also reflect the hepatic mesenchymal reaction, conclusions were contradictory regarding the diagnostic value of $\beta_2$m determinations in liver diseases.

In the present study we describe the distribution of serum $\beta_2$m and anti-$\beta_2$m levels in a variety of chronic hepatitides. We wanted to determine to what extent the rise of these serum factors may be an expression of immune reactions in liver disorders. For comparison, assay were also performed in sera of patients with systemic lupus erythematosus (SLE), a well-known autoimmune disease.

Assessment and Management of Hepatobiliary Disease
Eds.: L. Okolicsányi, G. Csomós, and G. Crepaldi

## Patients and Methods

### Patients

Forty-one patients with biopsy-proven liver disease (19 males and 22 females) were examined. Fourteen suffered from chronic persistent hepatitis (CPH), 14 from chronic active hepatitis (CAH), and 13 from active cirrhosis (CH). Sixteen patients had hepatitis B virus (HBV)-related liver disease as shown by HBsAg and/or anti-HBc positivity. CPH could be considered as a completely "inactive" liver disease, on the basis of histological findings as well as on transaminase (GOT) and gamma-globulin serum levels, which hardly exceeded the normal. The GOT values of patients with CAH and with CH were, in general, more than double the upper limit of the normal value, while histologically the signs of "aggressiveness" (massive lymphoplasma cell infiltration and piecemeal necrosis) and cirrhosis were present. At the time of the examinations, the patients' disease was moderately active; some of them had previously been treated with low-dose prednisolone (10–15 mg daily). Renal function was normal in all of the patients with liver disease.

Nineteen patients with SLE were diagnosed on the basis of American Rheumatism Association criteria (Cohen et al. 1971). The majority required low-dose maintenance corticosteroid treatment. Two SLE patients had manifest renal involvement.

As normal controls, the sera of 27 healthy individuals were studied.

### Methods

Beside the liver function tests (serum bilirubin, transaminase, electrophoresis), the HBV markers (HBsAg and anti-HBc antibody) were determined by Abbott radioimmunoassay (AUSRIA-II and CORAB respectively). Antinuclear antibody (ANA) was detected by using the indirect immunofluorescence technique, and the presence of circulating immune complexes was verified by the polyethylene glycol precipitation method (Digeon et al. 1977).

Determination of the serum $\beta_2$m concentration was made with the Phadebas $\beta_2$m microtest using a competitive RIA kit according to the attached directions. Anti-$\beta_2$m antibody was measured with the ELISA technique, using staphylococcus protein A peroxidase. Details of performance are described elsewhere (Pár and Falus 1986).

## Results

The mean $\beta_2$m value was significantly higher than normal in each patient group (Table 1). In CPH pathological high $\beta_2$m values were found in one-third of the cases, with a frequency similar to those of anti-$\beta_2$m, ANA, and elevated gamma-globulin and immune complex levels (Table 2). In CAH the mean $\beta_2$m and the frequency of the pathological values were also higher than in CPH. Here, high $\beta_2$m concentration occurred in two-thirds of the cases. In CH results were obtained similar to those in CAH. The individual values are shown in Fig. 1. The differences between the three liver diseases were not statistically significant. In SLE, however, the mean $\beta_2$m level was significantly higher than in CPH. In the two SLE patients with renal involvement the $\beta_2$m serum concentration was especially high, i.e., 12.0 and 19.6 µg/ml.

**Table 1.** Mean $\beta_2$m and anti-$\beta_2$m values ($\pm$SEM) in various forms of liver disease and SLE

| Diagnosis | $n$ | $\beta_2$m (μg/ml) | $P$ | Anti-$\beta_2$m ($OD_{500}$) | $P$ |
|---|---|---|---|---|---|
| Controls | 27 | 1.40 ± 0.09 | | 0.350 ± 0.080 | |
| CPH | 14 | 2.63 ± 0.40 | 0.01 | 0.670 ± 0.055 | 0.001 |
| CAH | 14 | 3.39 ± 0.74 | 0.02 | 0.740 ± 0.056 | 0.001 |
| CH | 13 | 4.20 ± 0.90 | 0.01 | 0.600 ± 0.035 | 0.01 |
| SLE | 19 | 5.28 ± 1.00 | 0.001 | 0.825 ± 0.080 | 0.001 |

**Table 2.** Incidence of pathological immune markers and elevated transaminase (GOT) levels in different patient groups

| Diagnosis | $n$ | $\beta_2$m (>2.4 μg/ml) | Anti-$\beta_2$m (>0.750 $OD_{500}$) | ANA 1:10 | Gamma-globulin (>20 g/l) | Immune complexes (>680 μg/ml) | GOT (>50 IU) |
|---|---|---|---|---|---|---|---|
| | | Number of patients with pathological values | | | | | |
| Controls | 27 | 1 | 1 | 2 | 1 | 2 | 0 |
| CPH | 14 | 5 | 4 | 6 | 5 | 4 | 1 |
| CAH | 14 | 10 | 5 | 9 | 8 | 5 | 5 |
| CH | 13 | 11 | 1 | 8 | 7 | 4 | 4 |
| SLE | 19 | 16 | 12 | 17 | 7 | 14 | 1 |

Anti-$\beta_2$m occurred less frequently than a pathological $\beta_2$m level in patients with liver disease, but the mean anti-$\beta_2$m levels also differed from the controls. The anti-$\beta_2$m value was significantly higher in CAH than in CH ($P<0.01$). The incidence of high anti-$\beta_2$m concentration in SLE was markedly higher than in liver diseases (Fig. 2).

Analyzing the correlations between the different immunological parameters, the following was found. There was no correlation between the $\beta_2$m and anti-$\beta_2$m values in patients with liver disease, as $\beta_2$m and ANA positivity did not correlate. The mean $\beta_2$m concentration in the 13 patients with liver disease and with pathological immune complex levels was 5.04 ± 1.1 μg/ml, while in the 28 immune complex negative patients it was 2.60 ± 0.16 μg/ml ($P<0.05$). The mean $\beta_2$m level of 16 HBV-positive patients was 2.36 ± 0.25 μg/ml, that of the 25 HBV-negative cases 3.97 ± 0.60 μg/ml ($P<0.05$). The GOT values – indicating liver cell necrosis – did not correlate with the $\beta_2$m values. Neither was there any correlation between the anti-$\beta_2$m, ANA, gamma-globulin, and immune complex values.

## Discussion

The results suggested that in different forms of chronic inflammatory liver disease the serum $\beta_2$m and anti-$\beta_2$m levels varied. In CPH considered to be inactive histologically and immunologically, the serum $\beta_2$m level was more moderately and less frequently increased than in CAH and CH. On the other hand, serum $\beta_2$m increased similarly in

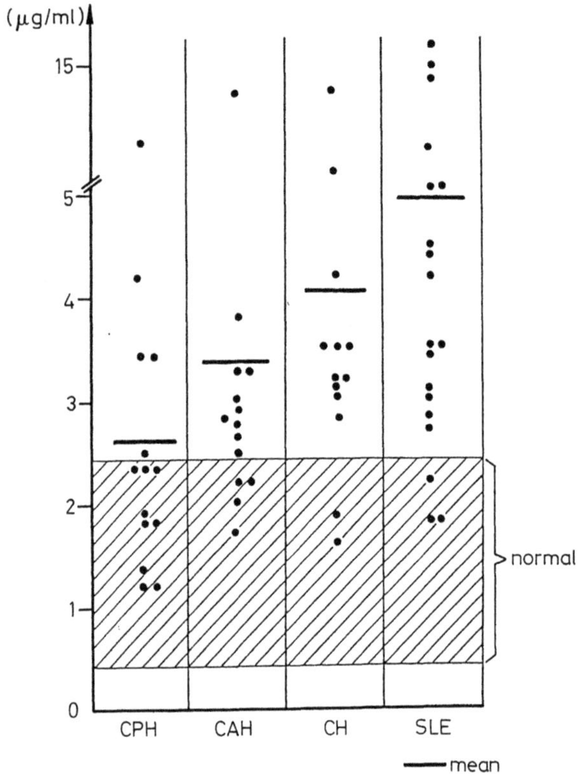


**Fig. 1.** Serum $\beta_2$m values in various types of chronic liver disease and systemic lupus erythematosus. *CPH*, chronic persistent hepatitis; *CAH*, chronic active hepatitis; *CH*, cirrhosis hepatitis; *SLE*, systemic lupus erythematosus

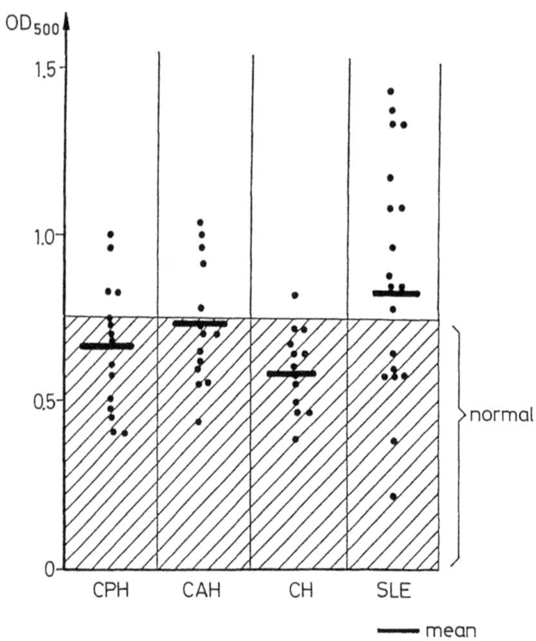


**Fig. 2.** Serum anti-$\beta_2$m values in chronic liver diseases and SLE

HBV-negative ("autoimmune") hepatitis and in cases associated with the presence of circulating immune complexes, as in SLE. These findings are in agreement with those of Beorchia et al. (1982), who assumed that autoimmune phenomena and lymphocyte activation might have a role in the elevation of the $\beta_2$m level of patients with liver disease. They noted the normalization of $\beta_2$m level in active hepatitis parallel with corticosteroid treatment, similar to the observations of Child et al. (1980) during chemotherapy of malignant lymphomas. Others, however, published contradictory results. Hallgren (1979) found that the $\beta_2$m level was not elevated in fatty liver, but was elevated in 80% of cases of alcoholic cirrhosis, while Rashid et al. (1981) observed the same in 50% of cases of chronic hepatitis and cirrhosis.

The anti-$\beta_2$m autoantibody occurred less frequently in hepatitis than in SLE. Anti-$\beta_2$m positivity was found by Revillard et al. (1981) in 50% of CAH cases. We found it in one-third of these patients, only sporadically in those with cirrhosis, and in two-thirds of SLE patients.

In conclusion, it is suggested that serum $\beta_2$m and anti-$\beta_2$m might be additional markers of inflammatory and autoimmune activities in chronic hepatitis, as in SLE. In assessing the results, it is essential to consider the well-known fact that renal impairment influences the serum $\beta_2$m concentration (Wibell and Karlsson 1973).

## Summary

Serum $\beta_2$-microglobulin concentration is increased in pathological processes associated with lymphocyte activation. $\beta_2$m and anti-$\beta_2$m autoantibody (anti-$\beta_2$m) determinations were made in the sera of 41 patients with chronic inflammatory liver diseases, in 19 with systemic lupus erythematosus (SLE), and in 27 healthy controls. High $\beta_2$m values were found in one-third of the cases of inactive persistent hepatitis and in more than two-thirds of the active hepatitis and cirrhosis cases. In SLE, high $\beta_2$m levels occurred in 16 of 19 patients. The $\beta_2$m level was elevated mainly in HBV-negative and circulating immune complex-positive patients with liver disease. Anti-$\beta_2$m occurred in one-third of chronic hepatitides, in only one of 13 cases of cirrhosis, and in 12 of 19 patients with SLE.

The results suggest that $\beta_2$m and anti-$\beta_2$m may be further laboratory indicators of immunological activity in inflammatory liver diseases, as they are already known to be in SLE.

## References

Beorchia S, Trep C, Vincent C, Revillard J-P, Brette R (1982) Intérêt pronostique et pathogénique de l'élévation de la $\beta_2$-microglobuline dans les hépatites aigues et chroniques. Gastroenterol Clin Biol 6: 679-687

Berggard I, Bearn AG (1968) Isolation and properties of a low molecular weight $\beta_2$ globulin occurring in human biological fluids. J Biol Chem 243: 4095-4103

Child JA, Spati B, Illingworth S (1980) Serum $\beta_2$-microglobulin and C-reactive protein in the monitoring of lymphomas. Cancer 45: 318-326

Cohen AS, Reynolds WE, Franklin EG, Kulka JP (1971) Preliminary criteria for the classification of systemic lupus erythematosus. Bull Rheum Dis 21: 643-648

Digeon M, Laver G, Riza J, Bach JF (1977) Detection of circulating immune complexes in human sera by simplified assay with polyethyleneglycol. J Immunol Methods 16: 165-169

Falus A (1984) Beta-2-microglobulin specific autoantibodies and complexes in autoimmune disease. Ann Immunol Hung [Suppl] 1: 371-382

Grey HM, Kubo RT, Colon S (1973) The small subunit of HLA is $\beta_2$-microglobulin. J Exp Med 138: 1608-1612

Hallgren R (1979) Serum $\beta_2$-microglobulin in liver disease. Scand J Clin Lab Invest 39: 441-447

Pár A, Falus A (1986) Serum $\beta_2$-microglobulin and anti-$\beta_2$m antibody in chronic hepatitis. Acta Med Hung (in press)

Peterson P, Rask L, Lindblom JB (1974) Highly purified papain-solubilized HLA antigens contain $\beta_2$-microglobulin. Proc Natl Acad Sci USA 71: 35-39

Rashid SA, Axon ATR, Bullen AW, Cooper EH (1981) Serum $\beta_2$-microglobulin in hepatobiliary diseases. Clin Chim Acta 114: 83-91

Revillard JP, Beorchia S, Vincent C, Trepo C (1981) Serum $\beta_2$-microglobulin levels and $\beta_2$m-binding antibodies in liver disease. Fed Proc 38: 1224-1227

Wibell L, Karlsson FA (1973) Serum $\beta_2$-microglobulin in renal disease. Nephron 10: 320-331

# Treatment of Liver Cirrhosis

J. T. Galambos, W. D. Warren, W. J. Millikan, Jr., J. M. Henderson, D. Simon, W. S. Brooks, and S. P. Riepe

Departments of Medicine and Surgery, Emory University School of Medicine, Atlanta, Georgia, 30303, U. S. A.

Morphologically, cirrhosis can be defined as an entity. However, the physiologic and clinical abnormalities produced by cirrhosis are heterogeneous. Cirrhosis cannot be used as a homogeneous entity in clinical studies without clear-cut definition of the type of patients involved and the manifestation of the severity of their disease. Neither the clinical illness nor death of cirrhotic patients is necessarily related to liver disease. For example, 40% of 4455 deaths in cirrhosis were due to causes other than hepatic or renal failure, GI bleeding, or infection. One of the best examples of the heterogeneity of the clinical manifestation of cirrhosis is provided by the data published recently by various investigators purporting to identify the key determinants which predict the prognosis for cirrhotic patients. Although the various investigators used similar statistical methods, what appeared to be prognostic in one institution was not in another, and vice versa [1-5].

The therapy of fibrosis in cirrhosis consists of dissolution of the fibrous septae or prevention of their formation, i. e., prevention of fibrogenesis or promotion of fibrolysis. Currently, there are no effective methods available to prevent collagen formation in the liver, but the use of proline and lysine analogues holds out hope for the development of effective methods of either reducing the rate of collagen synthesis or modifying collagen structure to the point that it will be easily hydrolyzable by proteolytic enzymes in the extracellular spaces [6, 7]. It must be noted that collagen is not the only rigid macromolecule in the extracellular matrix, because hydrophobic glycoproteins, laminin, and fibronectin can also be crosslinked and are insoluble. Furthermore, proteoglycans and glycosaminoglycans are also present in the extracellular matrix. Therapy in the future may also be aimed at restoring the more normal cell-to-cell and cell-to-matrix interaction disrupted by hepatic fibrogenesis leading to cirrhosis. Today, the therapy of cirrhosis is essentially the therapy of the clinical manifestations of the disease.

The most effective therapy of cirrhosis is prevention. This is available in cases of Wilson's syndrome and probably also in the treatment of precirrhotic hemochromatosis. Widespread vaccination could reduce the frequency of viral hepatitis leading to chronic active hepatitis and cirrhosis, and abstinence or at least reduction of excessive consumption of alcoholic beverages can lead to a decline of alcoholic hepatitis and cirrhosis.

The major clinical manifestations of cirrhosis – hepatic failure, chronic active hepatitis, encephalopathy, variceal hemorrhage, ascites, and renal failure – are topics for discussion at this meeting. I would like to present some recent data from our institution on two of these areas: (1) the prevention of recurrent variceal hemorrhage and (2) the treatment of ascites.

Assessment and Management of Hepatobiliary Disease
Eds.: L. Okolicsányi, G. Csomós, and G. Crepaldi

Thirty-three patients with documented variceal hemorrhage and cirrhosis were treated with endoscopic sclerotherapy and were followed for 12 months [8]. Eighteen of these 33 patients rebled and 12 of them were sclerotherapy failures. Transfusion requirements in these 12 were significantly higher (14.7 ± 8 units) than in the sclerotherapy success group (1.6 ± 3 units). Sclerotherapy failure was more common in the alcoholic (11 of 23) than non-alcoholic (1 of 10) cirrhotics. It was more common in the sickest (Child's C) patients (9 of 18) than in Child's A or B patients (3 of 15). Size of varices at the initial elective sclerotherapy session was also prognostic for rebleeding. Patients with large varices (grade 3 or 4) bled more frequently and required more blood transfusions than patients with small varices. However, this criterion alone did not adequately define the subset of patients who eventually failed sclerotherapy. Sclerotherapy in this group of patients with cirrhosis delayed recurrent hemorrhage long enough to permit clinical improvement (predominantly due to abstinence in alcoholics). The improvement was manifested by a change of at least one grade of their Child's classification in 66% of these patients followed for 1 year. Preservation of their hepatopetal portal flow was associated with quantitative improvement of hepatic functional capacity without change in their cardiac output or hepatic blood flow.

Sclerotherapy failures fell into three categories: (1) Bleeds from scleroulcers. (2) Rebleeds from esophageal varices initially controlled by sclerotherapy; the most common example was a persistent single varix. (3) Rebleeds from gastric varices; the most common example was bleeding from fundic mucosa. At times a gastric varix was seen during endoscopy but usually large gastric varices were visualized by magnetic resonance imaging and on angiography rather than by endoscopy. Early sclerotherapy failures may represent technical failures of the sclerotherapy schedule, or may be a failure of sclerotherapy per se. It is possible that a more aggressive sclerotherapy regimen could possibly have reduced the frequency of early rebleeding from esophageal varices. On the other hand, it could have produced more scleroulcers. The view that patients can always be operated if chronic sclerotherapy fails to prevent rebleeding is valid only to a point. If patients are declared sclerotherapy failures during a torrential hemorrhage when the only effective option left is emergency shunt, then surgery is performed as a life-saving maneuver. Under such conditions, it is not always possible to perform the best operation for the optimum long-term clinical course. Although urgent selective shunt can be performed in most of these sclerotherapy failures, the procedure is technically more difficult, it takes more time to perform, and, in case of the distal splenorenal shunt, it may not provide immediate total decompression of gastroesophageal varices in every patient because of renal vein hypertension [9, 10]. Elective or semi-elective surgery has a lower operative mortality and morbidity than emergency operations [10–35]. Patients who repeatedly bleed large volumes from esophageal varices and not from gastric varices or scleroulcers should be treated with more frequent sclerotherapy. For the best outcome, failure of sclerotherapy should be recognized in time to permit elective or at least semi-elective selective shunt surgery.

In a prospective randomized clinical trial, we compared selective distal splenorenal shunt (DSRS) with sclerotherapy. This trial included 71 patients with documented variceal hemorrhage requiring transfusion of two or more units. These patients were randomly assigned to DSRS [35] or sclerotherapy [36] and were followed up for a median of 26 months. None of these patients were lost to followup and all but one received the randomly allotted therapy. The two groups were well matched regarding etiology (alcoholic vs nonalcoholic), clinical stage of the disease (Child's A/B vs C), and laboratory abnormalities (conventional liver tests), as well as hemodynamic and quantitative hepatic functional parameters.

Initial evaluation included (a) clinical, biochemical, and hematologic assessment, (b) endoscopy, (c) liver biopsy, (d) angiography, and (e) measurement of liver function and hemodynamics (cardiac output, effective hepatic blood flow). Criteria for classification as Child's C were two or more of the following parameters: encephalopathy (other than that precipitated by the variceal bleed), ascites preceding or persisting after the acute bleed, serum bilirubin greater than 3 mg/dl, serum albumin less than 3 g/dl, prothrombin time more than 4 s greater than control.

DSRS was performed within a week of randomization with the exception of one patient who developed a non-A, non-B hepatitis and died of hepatic failure without surgery. Variceal sclerotherapy consisted of two initial endoscopic treatments 5-6 days apart during the first week after randomization followed by monthly sclerotherapy till the esophageal varices were obliterated at and within 3 cm of the gastroesophageal junction. Sclerosis was done with a flexible endoscope and a combination of intra- and paravariceal injections were performed using either sodium morrhuate or sodium tetradecyl sulfate. An overtube was not used on the flexible endoscope, but a proximal balloon cuff (the Brooks balloon) was fitted on the endoscope and was inflated during injection of the varix to aid in stabilization of the sclerosant in the vein after injection. The balloon was also used to control bleeding if it occurred after removal of the needle.

Reevaluations included hemodynamic studies and the quantitative tests of liver function and angiography at yearly intervals in both groups in addition to 1- to 3-monthly clinical and routine laboratory evaluations which included interval angiography in most of these patients.

Rebleeding was defined as bleeding requiring at least two units of blood transfusion. Failures of the DSRS were death or shunt thrombosis defined by direct shunt catheterization. Failure of sclerotherapy was defined as the inability to control recurrences of gastroesophageal bleeding due to portal hypertension despite repeated attempts at sclerotherapy. This decision required the concurrence of the sclerosing gastroenterologist and of a hepatologist who believed that the patient's life was threatened by withholding surgical therapy or that death due to uncontrollable recurrent bleeding with imminent. Survival and therapy failures were analyzed by the Kaplan-Meier method [36]. Comparison between groups was made by repeated measures of analysis of variance [37].

The 2-year survival of the sclerotherapy group (84%) is significantly ($p < 0.01$) better than for the DSRS group (59%). It should be noted that the 31 survivors in the sclerotherapy group include 11 patients (35.5%) who failed sclerotherapy treatment and required surgery to control recurrent variceal bleedings. The operative mortality of the DSRS group was 12%, with all four deaths occurring in Child's C patients. Eight of the ten subsequent deaths were due to hepatic failure. Four of these were Child's A/B and four were Child's C at randomization. In the sclerotherapy group one patient, Child's C died from uncontrolled bleeding. The other four deaths were due to hepatic failure. Each of these patients rebled from varices: rebleeding was controlled by further sclerotherapy in two patients, but both died of progressive hepatic failure due to the progression of their liver disease; the other two Child's C patients required emergency surgery to stop their variceal bleeding, and died 1 and 2 months post operatively.

Fifteen of 35 (42.8%) patients with DSRS were shunt failures and 13 of 36 (36%) were sclerotherapy failures. Shunt failures comprised 14 (40%) deaths and one (2.8%) shunt thrombosis who was crossed over to sclerotherapy. In the DSRS group the incidence of rebleeding was 2.8%; this patient has been successfully managed by endoscopic sclerotherapy. In the sclerotherapy group the incidence of rebleeding was 53%. Consequently, 30.6% of sclerotherapy patients were crossed over to surgery and 2.8% of DSRS to sclerotherapy. In contrast, sclerotherapy failures comprised two deaths and 11 patients who were crossed over to shunt surgery. Seven of the these 11 patients were Child's C at randomization and four were Child's A/B. Ten of the 11 failures with rebleeding were managed by surgery with a 10% operative mortality and 80% long term survival.

A single measure of hepatic function, liver volume, and hemodynamics prior to randomization did not correlate with operative or 2-year mortality in the DSRS group, or with mortality, rebleeding, or failure of sclerotherapy.

Hepatic function 1 year after randomization was significantly ($p < 0.01$) better in those patients managed by sclerotherapy than in those treated by DSRS. This difference was due to the increase of hepatic function in the sclerotherapy group (from $306 \pm 66$ to $356 \pm 82$ mg/min), which was statistically significant ($p < 0.05$); hepatic function did not change significantly in the DSRS group ($323 \pm 110$ to $287 \pm 78$, $p = 0.1$). However, hepatic function remained unchanged during the 2nd year in both groups.

Liver volume decreased significantly not only after DSRS but also in the sclerotherapy group at 1 year, but no further loss of liver volume occurred during the 2nd year in either group.

Portal perfusion was lost in 47% of DSRS patients but in only 5% of patients undergoing sclerotherapy ($p < 0.01$). Neither liver blood flow nor cardiac output changed significantly during the first year. The liver blood flow expressed as fraction of cardiac output decreased in the DSRS group, but remained unchanged in the sclerotherapy group despite reduced liver volume and improved hepatic function, suggesting an improved "efficiency" of hepatic blood flow in the sclerotherapy group. This improvement is likely to be associated with continued and probably improved portal perfusion of hepatic sinusoids.

Eight patients had a history of encephalopathy before randomization: five of these were shunted and three had sclerotherapy. Three of these five shunted patients died in the perioperative period and a fourth died later of hepatic failure. Two of the three patients with a history of spontaneous encephalopathy in the sclerotherapy group have also died within 8 months of randomization. Spontaneous encephalopathy was therefore a poor prognostic sign regardless of therapeutic assignment. The incidence of spontaneous encephalopathy during the follow-up period was not different in the two groups: 16% in the DSRS and 12% in the sclerotherapy group developed encephalopathy during a median of 26 months follow-up.

One must exercise caution in comparing the outcomes of clinical trials designed to prevent recurrent variceal bleeds or at least deaths in these patients. One should not extrapolate data from this report, containing only 61% alcoholic cirrhosis, to groups almost wholly alcoholic. Patient refusal to accept the randomly assigned therapy and losses to follow-up can compromise the validity and reliability of conclusions from clinical trials. When these trials are conducted in different institutions, the frequencies of poor- and good-risk patients enrolled are likely to vary. The severity of liver disease in study patients affects the outcome of any therapeutic or prophylactic measure used in a trial. Therefore, it should be noted that 44% of our patients were poor-risk (Child's C) cases. Our outcome compares favorably with clinical trials reported from King's College [38, 39] which represent the best available data on the efficacy of sclerotherapy. However, their cirrhotic population [38] included only 28% Child's C patients. Comparison of our results with those reported from King's indicates that sclerotherapy with surgery for the rebleeding failures has produced even better results than sclerotherapy alone in a population with a higher proportion of poor-risk (Child's C) patients. Earlier randomized studies of DSRS had achieved 70%-80% 2-year survival, but in none of these studies were more than 10% of the patients Child's C. Survival analysis of only Child's A/B DSRS patients in the present study yields a figure similar to those in earlier reports.

The only other prospective randomized study of control of variceal bleeding which has achieved better survival figures than we report here is that from Lebrec and colleagues [40]. However, they used propranolol only in Child's A patients and achieved 90% 2-year survival. However, 21% of the patients in this propranolol study were lost to follow-up, and other centers have failed to duplicate this good outcome [41].

## The Effect of Large-Volume Paracentesis

Ascites was frequently treated with repeated paracentesis until the early 1960s when a series of publications confirmed the hazards of paracentesis. It became generally accepted that the removal of more than 1 l of ascitic fluid produced a fall in cardiac output [42] and that ascitic fluid mobilization was limited, with ascites reforming at 3.5 times the maximum absorption rate after paracentesis [43]. Paracentesis has been reported to precipitate hepatic encephalopathy, renal failure, and hyponatremia, and it depletes serum albumin and can introduce infection or perforate abdominal viscera. During the last 20 years paracentesis has been used only rarely as a therapeutic measure and when it is used, the anticipated decrease of plasma volume is promptly treated with I.V. plasma or albumin. Paracentesis was considered contraindicated for the treatment of ascitic patients up to the early 1980s, but recent clinical observations have restored the therapeutic respectability of abdominal paracentesis for the treatment of ascites, particularly of tense ascites in cirrhotic patients. The pendulum is apparently beginning to swing in the opposite direction. The clinical usefulness of paracentesis is being reexamined on the basis of several recent reports [44-49] showing that removal of 5 l ascitic fluid from patients with tense ascites and peripheral edema is safe. These patients showed no changes in blood urea nitrogen concentration, hematocrit, blood pressure, or plasma volume. Indeed, repeated paracentesis of 4-6 l accompanied by the administration of intravenous albumin was thought to be as effective a way to treat cirrhotic ascites as standard diuretic therapy. Indeed, it was considered to be a more cost-effective method of managing ascites than sodium-restricted diet accompanied by diuretic therapy.

**Table 1.** Factors implicated as prognostic in one or more of five recent studies ($n = 2074$)

| One study | Two studies | Three studies |
|---|---|---|
| Alcoholic cirrhosis | Male | Albumin |
| Nutrition | Ascites | Bilirubin |
| HBsAg | Encephalopathy | Globulin |
| Cholesterol | Varices | |
| Creatinine | GI bleeding | |
| Clinical assessment | Continued alcohol consumption | |
| SGOT | Prothrombin time | |
| Serum Alkaline Phosphatase | | |
| Cholinesterase | | |
| GGTP | | |
| Liver biopsy | | |

We examined the acute (8–24 h) changes of hemodynamic, renal, and hormonal alterations produced by large – volume paracentesis in 11 patients who had cirrhosis and tense ascites. Seven of these patients had marked prolongation of their prothrombin time. All patients were hemodynamically stable at the time of study; none of them had current or recent gastrointestinal hemorrhage, and they had no evidence of bacteremia, peritonitis, pancreatitis, congestive heart failure, chronic obstructive pulmonary disease, or encephalopathy. Although renal function was not normal in these patients, their serum creatinine was 1.5 mg/dl or less. Nine of the 13 had alcoholic cirrhosis. The means and ranges of ascitic fluid protein, serum albumin, serum bilirubin concentration, prothrombin time over control, and galactose elimination capacity are described in Table 2. Before paracentesis, the patients had an equilibration period of 48 h during which diuretic therapy was discontinued. Their 2 g/day sodium diet and unrestricted fluid intake was continued. The night before the study a Swan-Ganz catheter was inserted aseptically via the right internal jugular vein, and hemodynamic monitoring began 12 h prior to paracentesis. Eight hours prior to the study, the patients were placed on a regimen of nothing by mouth and the insensible water loss was replaced by intravenous infusion of 5% galactose. The first 50 ml ascitic fluid removed was used for measurement of protein content and for routine laboratory analysis, including culture for bacteria. Ascitic fluid was removed rapidly, at first 1 l, then 2 l at a time during a 15–30-min period, following which a 60-min equilibration period was permitted. Paracentesis was discontinued once 8 l had been removed or no further fluid was obtainable. After the completion of the paracentesis and repetition of hemodynamic measurements, the patients resumed their previous diet and activities. Hemodynamics were monitored by measuring cardiac output with the thermodilution technique including three or more measurements each time until triplicate matching results were obtained. The systemic vascular resistance was calculated from the following formula: mean arterial pressure minus central venous pressure divided by cardiac output X 80. The results are given in Table 3.

In each of the patients there was a consistent increase of cardiac output after completion of an 8-l paracentesis. Twenty-four hours after the beginning of the paracentesis, i.e., the next morning, cardiac output declined toward the pre-paracentesis level but remained consistently higher, despite the fact that the patients did not receive any

**Table 2.**

| Patient | Etiology of cirrhosis | Ascitic fluid protein (g) | Bilirubin (mg/dl) | Albumin (g/dl) | Prothrombin time (s) | Galactose elimination capacity (mg/min) |
|---|---|---|---|---|---|---|
| 1 | ETOH | 2.5 | 1.8 | 3.1 | 1.6 | 224 |
| 2 | ETOH | 1.1 | 1.4 | 2.6 | 1.8 | 352 |
| 3 | ETOH | 1.29 | 10 | 2.0 | 2.1 | 472 |
| 4 | PBC | 0.62 | 5.7 | 2.5 | 1.6 | 241 |
| 5 | ETOH | 2.2 | 0.3 | 2.8 | 1.1 | 295 |
| 6 | ETOH | 1.26 | 6.9 | 3.1 | N.A. | N.D. |
| 7 | ETOH | 2.5 | 1.4 | 2.4 | 3.4 | 449 |
| 8 | ETOH | 2.3 | 0.3 | 2.5 | 1.3 | N.D. |
| 9 | ETOH | 4.3 | 0.5 | 3.3 | 3.0 | 224 |
| 10 | NANB | 1.7 | 1.9 | 3.1 | 1.5 | N.D. |
| 11 | NANB | 0.57 | 2.7 | 2.5 | 2.3 | N.D. |
| | Mean | 1.7 | 3.7 | 2.65 | 2.3 | 323 |

ETOH, alcoholic; PBC, primary biliary cirrhosis; NANB, non-A, non-B; N.D., not done; N.A., not available

**Table 3.**

| Observations | Time[a] | | |
|---|---|---|---|
| | Zero | 8 hours | 24 hours |
| Cardiac output (l/min) | 6.64 ± 0.7 | 8.81 ± 0.86 | 7.5 ± 0.79 |
| Central venous pressure (mmHg) | 9.1 ± 0.96 | 8.6 ± 0.91 | 6.8 ± 0.72 |
| Main pulmonary artery pressure (mmHg) | 19.3 ± 2.0 | 18.8 ± 1.9 | 18.2 ± 2.1 |
| Pulmonary capillary wedge pressure (mmHg) | 13.1 ± 1.4 | 11.1 ± 1.3 | 9.89 ± 1.1 |
| Pulse | 90 ± 7 | 85 ± 6.8 | 89 ± 7 |
| Mean arterial pressure (mmHg) | 92 ± 7.4 | 91 ± 7.3 | 89 ± 7.2 |
| Effective hepatic blood flow (ml/min) | 1133 ± 151 | 995 ± 132 | |
| Systemic vascular resistance (dynes·s·cm$^{-5}$) | 1283 ± 135 | 884 ± 93 | 995 ± 105 |
| A-V $O_2$ difference | 379 ± 44 | 341 ± 40 | 352 ± 64 |
| Respiration (breaths/min) | 23 ± 2 | 16.5 ± 1.4 | 16.8 ± 1.6 |
| Blood urea nitrogen (mg/dl) | 13.3 ± 1.0 | 11.7 ± 0.94 | 11.9 ± 0.95 |
| Creatinine (mg/dl) | 0.88 ± 0.07 | 0.84 ± 0.07 | 0.9 ± 0.07 |
| Serum Na (mEq/l) | 135 ± 10 | 133 ± 10 | 133 ± 10 |
| Creatinine clearance (ml/min) | 77.11 ± 10.2 | | 67.2 ± 10.3 |
| Urine osmolarity (osmol/kg) | 502 ± 40 | 396 ± 37 | 398 ± 34 |
| Urine $Na^+$ (mEq/l) | 43 ± 3.5 | 38 ± 3.6 | 27 ± 2.6 |
| Urine $K^+$ (mEq/l) | 42.5 ± 3.7 | 34.7 ± 3 | 29.8 ± 3.1 |

[a] Hours indicate time before study that diuretics were discontinued (aldactone was the only diuretic that any patient was receiving). "Zero" indicates that patient had never taken diuretics or that they were discontinued more than 5 days prior to study

I. V. colloid to expand their plasma volume. For central venous pressure measurement, the zero point was at the estimated level of the right atrium. There was a consistent, albeit small, decline, of central venous pressure at the conclusion of the paracentesis and a further decline by 24 h after the initiation of the paracentesis. There was a small random decline of mean pulmonary artery pressure. The decline of pulmonary capillary wedge pressure was more marked and again continued after the cessation of paracentesis, like central venous pressure. These changes of cardiac function were accompanied by negligible changes of mean arterial pressure and pulse. There was a marked reduction of respiratory rate which then remained stable after the completion of the paracentesis. Systemic vascular resistance declined after the completion of the paracentesis but rose overnight as cardiac output declined. The systemic arterial-venous (peripheral artery – pulmonary artery) oxygen difference declined markedly after the conclusion of the paracentesis and remained stable or rose slightly during the next day. Effective hepatic perfusion as measured by the galactose clearance technique declined 10% during the paracentesis. Blood urea nitrogen concentration decreased at the end of the paracentesis. It remained below pre-paracentesis levels for at least 48 h. Serum creatinine concentrations rose slightly during the second 24 h after paracentesis. This was accompanied by a decrease of creatinine clearances, which declined further during the second 24 h after the paracentesis. Urinary sodium and potassium concentrations declined during these periods and urine osmolality also decreased. Serum renin activity declined slightly at the conclusion of the paracentesis compared to before paracentesis, but almost doubled during the next 24 h. In contrast, serum aldosterone concentrations, which initially declined immediately after the conclusion of the paracentesis, rose subsequently only to the same level observed prior to paracentesis. Serum atrial natriuretic factor (ANF) remained stable during and after paracentesis and was not associated with changes of creatinine clearance or urinary sodium excretion.

Our observations support those of others suggesting the clinical safety of large-volume paracentesis in cirrhotic patients with tense ascites. It is interesting to note that although paracentesis resulted in a decrease of central venous pressure, it did not cause increasing azotemia. In contrast, blood urea nitrogen concentrations declined pari passu with declining central venous pressure and was accompanied by improved left ventricular function manifested by decreasing pulmonary capillary wedge pressure and increased cardiac output. However, some undesirable effects of paracentesis were also identified. There was a consistent decline of effective hepatic blood flow and creatinine clearance after paracentesis, and there was a marked rebound rise of serum renin activity. As far as renal failure is concerned, cirrhotic ascitic patients in our study had only modest declines of renal function before paracentesis was undertaken; the mean creatinine clearance was 77 ml/min and the mean serum creatinine concentration 0.88 (in malnourished patients with decreased muscle mass). Nevertheless, one can assume that these patients had already developed renal cortical ischemia. While four of the patients had normal serum bilirubins and another four had only minimal elevations, five of them were jaundiced with modest elevations of the serum bilirubin and seven had marked prolongation of their prothrombin time. The response of the jaundiced patients was not materially different from that of the anicteric ones.

## References


1. Bradbear R, Jenkins WJ, Ashby D, Sherlock S (1985) Prognostic factors in alcoholic cirrhosis. J Hepatol [Suppl] 2: S199
2. Christensen E, Schlichting P, Andersen PK, et al. (1985) Prognostic index to update prognosis in cirrhosis. J Hepatol [Suppl] 2: S213
3. Gines P, Quintero E, Arroyo V, et al. (1985) Prognostic factors in compensated cirrhosis. J Hepatol [Suppl] 2: S242
4. Milani A, Marra L, Siciliano M, Rossi L (1985) Prognostic significance of clinical and laboratory parameters in liver cirrhosis. A multivariate statistical approach. Hepatogastroenterology 32: 270-272
5. D'Amico G, Morabito A, Pagliaro L, Marubini E (1986) Survival and prognostic indicators in compensated and decompensated cirrhosis. Dig Dis Sci 31: 468-475
6. Wu GY, Wu CH (1983) Effect of 2-aminoethyl-L-cysteine on collagen accumulation in isolated hepatic granulomas. Proc Soc Exp Biol Med 174: 79-85
7. Tan EML, Ryhanen L, Uitto J (1983) Proline analogues inhibit human skin fibroblast growth and collagen production in culture. J Invest Dermatol 80: 261-276
8. Millikan WJ Jr, Henderson JM, Potts JR III, Warren WD, Galambos J, Brooks WS, Riepe S (1984) Liver function and hemodynamic status 1 year into sclerotherapy for variceal bleeding. Gastroenterology 86: 1184
9. Nordlinger BM, Nordlinger DF, Fulenwider JT, et al. (1980) Angiography in portal hypertension: clinical significance in surgery. Am J Surg 139: 132-141
10. Potts JR III, Henderson JM, Millikan WJ Jr, Warren WD (1984) Emergency distal splenorenal shunts for variceal hemorrhage refractory to non-operative control. Am J Surg 148: 813-816
11. Warren WD (1983) Control of variceal bleeding. Reassessment of rationale. Am J Surg 145: 8-16
12. Conn HO (1974) Therapeutic portacaval anastomosis: to shunt or not to shunt. Gastroenterology 67: 1065-1071
13. Editorial (1984) Bleeding esophageal varices. Lancet i: 139-141
14. Reynolds TB (1983) What to do about esophageal varices? N Engl J Med 309: 1575-1577
15. Conn HO (1983) Endoscopic sclerotherapy: an analysis of variants. Hepatology 3: 769-771
16. Terblanche J (1985) The long term management of patients after an oesophageal variceal bleed: the role of sclerotherapy. Br J Surg 72: 88-90
17. Crafoord C, Frenckner P (1939) New surgical treatment of varicose veins of the esophagus. Acta Otolaryngol (Stockh) 27: 422-429
18. Resnick RH, Chalmers TC, Ishihara AM, et al. (1969) A controlled study of the prophylactic portacaval shunt: a final report. Ann Intern Med 70: 675-688
19. Jackson FC, Perrin EB, Felix WR, Smith AG (1971) A clinical investigation of the portacaval shunt. V. Survival analysis of the therapeutic operation. Ann Surg 174: 672-701
20. Resnick RH, Iber FL, Ishihara AM, Chalmers TC, Zimmerman H (1974) A controlled study of the therapeutic portacaval shunt. Gastroenterology 67: 843-857
21. Rueff B, Prandi D, Degos F, et al. (1976) A controlled study of therapeutic portacaval shunt in alcoholic cirrhosis. Lancet i: 655-659
22. Reynolds TB, Donovan AJ, Mikkelsen WP, Redeker AG, Turrill FL, Weiner JM (1981) Results of a 12-year randomized trial of portacaval shunt in patients with alcoholic liver disease and bleeding varices. Gastroenterology 80: 1005-1011
23. Johnston GW, Rodgers HW (1973) A review of 15 years' experience in the use of sclerotherapy in the control of acute hemorrhage from esophageal varices. Br J Surg 60: 797-800
24. Macdougall BRD, Westaby D, Theodossi A, Dawson JL, Williams R (1982) Increased long-term survival in variceal hemorrhage using injection sclerotherapy. Results of a controlled trial. Lancet i: 124-127
25. Terblanche J, Northover JMA, Bornman P, et al. (1979) A prospective controlled trial of sclerotherapy in the long term management of patients after esophageal variceal bleeding. Surg Gynecol Obstet 148: 323-333
26. Paquet KJ (1982) Prophylactic endoscopic sclerosing treatment of the esophageal wall in varices – a prospective controlled randomized trial. Endoscopy 14: 4-5

27. Mitchell KJ, Macdougall BRD, Silk DBA, Williams R (1982) A prospective reappraisal of emergency endoscopy in patients with portal hypertension. Scand J Gastroenterol 17: 965-968
28. Novis BH, Duys P, Barbezat GO, Clain J, Bank S, Terblanche J (1976) Fibreoptic endoscopy and the use of the Sengstaken tube in acute gastrointestinal haemorrhage in patients with portal hypertension and varices. Gut 17: 258-263
29. Johnson AG, Simms JM, Stoddard CJ (1982) Is there a role for injection sclerotherapy in the presence of active bleeding? In: Westaby D, Macdougall BRD, Williams R (eds) Variceal bleeding. Pitman, London
30. Cello JP, Grendell JH, Crass RA, Trunkey DD, Cobb EE, Heilbron DC (1984) Endoscopic sclerotherapy versus portacaval shunt in patients with severe cirrhosis and variceal hemorrhage. N Engl J Med 311: 1589-1594
31. Terblanche J, Yakoob HI, Bornman PC, et al. (1981) Acute bleeding varices. A five-year prospective evaluation of tamponade and sclerotherapy. Ann Surg 194: 521-530
32. The Copenhagen Esophageal Varices Sclerotherapy Project (1984) Sclerotherapy after first variceal hemorrhage in cirrhosis. A randomized multicenter trial. N Engl J Med 311: 1594-1600
33. Conn HO (1985) Ideal treatment of portal hypertension in 1985. In: Benhamou J-P (ed) Clinics in gastroenterology: portal hypertension. Saunders, Philadelphia
34. Paquet KJ, Fleig WE (1981) Sclerotherapy of esophageal varices. In: Papp JP (ed) Endoscopic control of gastrointestinal hemorrhage. CRC, Boca Raton
35. Warren WD, Millikan WJ Jr, Henderson JM, et al. (1982) Ten years portal hypertensive surgery at Emory: results and new perspectives. Ann Surg 195: 530-542
36. Kaplan EL, Meier P (1958) Nonparametric estimation from incomplete observations. J Am Statist Assoc 53: 457-481
37. Winer BJ (1971) Statistical principles in experimental design, 2nd edn. McGraw-Hill, New York
38. Westaby D, Macdougall BRD, Williams R (1985) Improved survival following injection sclerotherapy for esophageal varices: final analysis of a controlled trial. Hepatology 5: 827-830
39. Westaby D, Melia WM, Macdougall BRD, Hegarty JE, Gimson AE, Williams R (1985) B1 selective adrenoreceptor blockade for the long term management of variceal bleeding. A prospective randomised trial to compare oral metoprolol with injection sclerotherapy in cirrhosis. Gut 26: 421-425
40. Lebrec D, Poynard T, Bernuau J, et al. (1984) A randomized controlled study of propranolol for prevention of recurrent gastrointestinal bleeding in patients with cirrhosis: a final report. Hepatology 4: 355-358
41. Burroughs AK, Jenkins WJ, Sherlock S, et al. (1983) Controlled trial of propranolol for the prevention of recurrent variceal hemorrhage in patients with cirrhosis. N Engl J Med 309: 1539-1542
42. Knauer CM, Lowe HM (1967) Hemodynamics in the cirrhotic patient during paracentesis. N Engl J Med 276: 491-496
43. Shear L, Ching S, Gabuzda GJ (1970) Compartmentalization of ascites and edema in patients with hepatic cirrhosis. N Engl J Med 282: 1391-1396
44. Lieberman FL, Denison EK, Reynolds TB (1970) The relationship of plasma volume, portal hypertension, ascites, and renal sodium retention in cirrhosis: the overflow theory of ascites formation. Ann NY Acad Sci 170: 202-212
45. Iwatsuki S, Reynolds TB (1973) Effect of increased intraabdominal pressure on hepatic hemodynamics in patients with chronic liver disease and portal hypertension. Gastroenterology 65: 294-299
46. Gordon ME (1960) The acute effects of abdominal paracentesis in Laennec's cirrhosis upon exchanges of electrolytes and water, renal function, and hemodynamics. Am J Gastroenterol 33: 15-37
47. Kao HW, Rakov NE, Savage E, Reynolds TB (1985) The effect of large volume paracentesis on plasma volume – a cause of hypovolemia? Hepatology 5: 403-407
48. Quintero E, Gines P, Arroyo V, et al. (1985) Paracentesis versus diuretics in the treatment of cirrhotics with tense ascites. Lancet i: 611-612
49. Carey WD, Kohne JC, Leatherman J, Paradis K (1983) Ascitic fluid removal: does it cause renal or hemodynamic decompensation? Cleve Clin Q 50: 397-400

# Drug Therapy for Alcoholic Liver Disease*

J. C. Bode
Department of Internal Medicine (Gastroenterology), Robert Bosch Hospital, Stuttgart, Federal Republic of Germany

## Introduction

Alcohol abuse affects every organ in the body and produces manifold metabolic derangements and diseases. Quantitative and/or qualitative malnutrition with varying degrees of vitamin and trace element deficiencies increases the complexity of alcohol-related illnesses. Treatment of alcoholic liver disease has to take into consideration this multitude of organ injuries and functional disturbances including behavioral and psychosocial aspects.

In this review I shall focus only on the pharmacotherapy of alcoholic liver disease. The therapy of alcohol dependence and of complications of advanced stages of alcoholic liver disease such as ascites, encephalopathy, and bleeding from esophageal varices will not be discussed here.

In order to approach the treatment of alcohol-induced liver disease rationally, the following facts have to be kept in mind:

a) Alcohol abuse may cause a wide spectrum of hepatic changes. The histological spectrum of alcoholic liver disease extends from uncomplicated fatty liver over various degrees of alcoholic hepatitis and hepatic fibrosis to, ultimately, cirrhosis [18, 39]. Correspondingly, the clinical picture varies greatly: The extreme on the one hand is the patient without complaints or symptoms in whom routine-check up reveals an enlarged liver. The other extreme is represented by the patient with decompensated cirrhosis with jaundice, ascites, and hepatic encephalopathy [17, 39]. Therefore, in order to evaluate any type of drug treatment, the stage and severity of the underlying liver disease has to be precisely defined. In addition, the natural history of the various types of alcoholic liver disease has to be considered, and, moreover, attention has to be paid to the effects of nonspecific therapy, especially cessation of alcohol consumption, on the course and prognosis of the disease.

b) Despite major advances in the understanding of the interaction of ethanol metabolism with other metabolic pathways and in the elucidation of the possible direct or indirect contributions of many of the alcohol-induced metabolic disturbances to liver injury, the pathogenesis of alcoholic liver disease in man has not been clarified [4, 18]. Proposals for any type of drug treatment for alcoholic liver disease at present are therefore based on hypothetical pathophysiological considerations and not on proven and generally accepted facts. Drug treatment of alcoholic liver disease is still at the stage of empirical forms of therapy!

* This work was supported in part by the Robert-Bosch-Stiftung (grant F 1)

Assessment and Management of Hepatobiliary Disease
Eds.: L. Okolicsányi, G. Csomós, and G. Crepaldi

c) Unfortunately, no animal model for alcoholic liver disease observed in humans is yet available. The only exception is the liver injury observed following chronic alcohol administration to baboons [31]. Most of the "hepatoprotective" drugs have been introduced in the treatment of alcoholic liver disease on the basis of certain effects of these compounds on alcohol-induced metabolic alterations in the liver of experimental animals (rats, guinea pigs, cats, and dogs). Since none of these species develop the same histological changes after acute or chronic alcohol feeding characteristic for alcoholic liver disease in humans, the assumption that such biochemical effects are relevant for alcoholic liver disease in man is mainly speculative.

## Natural History of Alcoholic Liver Disease: Effect of Abstinence

Details of the results obtained in the large number of studies on the natural history of alcoholic liver disease are beyond the scope of this brief commentary; they have been reviewed elsewhere [17, 42].

*Alcoholic fatty liver* is assumed to be a benign condition and is completely reversed when alcohol ingestion is stopped. Hepatomegaly, the main clinical finding in patients with uncomplicated fatty liver, will return to normal within a month or two following cessation of the toxin.

The term *alcoholic hepatitis* is applied to a syndrome which may be associated with a broad spectrum of morphological and clinical symptoms [4]. It is diagnosed from the presence of hepatocellular necrosis, ballooning degeneration of hepatocytes with or without Mallory bodies, and an inflammatory reaction where polymorphonuclear leukocytes usually predominate [39].

Moderately severe alcoholic hepatitis is also largely reversible by cessation of alcohol intake [5, 29], but if it coexists with increased fibrous tissue deposition and/or perivenular hyalin sclerosis these changes will persist. Many reports indicate that severe alcoholic hepatitis often proves fatal. However, the prognosis of patients with severe alcoholic hepatitis without cirrhosis seems to be remarkably better [5, 29] than that of patients in whom an acute episode of severe alcoholic hepatitis is superimposed on complete alcoholic cirrhosis [17, 42] (Table 1). This may at least partly explain the fact that in nine separate randomized studies where glucocorticoid therapy and placebo were compared in efficacy, the early mortality in the placebo groups ranged from 19% to 100% (Table 2). Other factors which are assumed to be of prognostic value for patients with alcoholic hepatitis are as follows: presence of underlying cirrhosis, presence of encephalopathy, presence of ascites, prothrombin time prolonged (>5-6 s), initial bilirubin >15 mg/dl, renal failure (creatinine clearance <50 ml/min), and severe histological changes in the liver [4, 17].

*Alcoholic cirrhosis* also tends to improve in patients who stop drinking. In several studies of the natural history of the disease the overall 5-year survival rate was statistically better in the nondrinking groups [17, 42]. In one study [48] the death rate after 5 years was almost twice as high for drinkers (56%) as for those who stopped (32%). Poor prognostic factors in these studies were ascites, hematemesis from esophageal varices, severe fibrosis, and jaundice [17, 42].

For the judgment of the results of many, if not most, of the controlled clinical trials on the efficacy of certain drugs which will be reviewed in the following sections, it

**Table 1.** Survival rates in patients with alcohol hepatitis (AH) by the presence or absence of cirrhosis

| Authors, year | Selection of patients | Presence of cirrhosis | *n* | Mortality (%) |
|---|---|---|---|---|
| Theodossi et al. 1982 [47] | Collected data from 15 studies of *severe* AH | Yes | 121 | 70 |
| | | No | 42 | 24 |
| Bode et al. 1984 [5] | *All* patients admitted because of AH | Yes | 118 | 31.4 |
| | | No | 61 | 6.6 |

**Table 2.** Effect of corticosteroid therapy on survival in severe alcoholic hepatitis

| Authors, year | Control group | | Corticosteroid group | | Statistical significance |
|---|---|---|---|---|---|
| | *n* | Mortality (%) | *n* | Mortality (%) | |
| Helman et al. 1971 [20] | 17 | 35 | 20 | 5 | $p<0.025$ |
| Porter et al. 1971 [37] | 9 | 77 | 11 | 55 | n.s. |
| Campra et al. 1973 [8] | 25 | 36 | 20 | 35 | n.s. |
| Blitzer et al. 1977 [3] | 16 | 31 | 12 | 50 | n.s. |
| Maddrey et al. 1977 [32] | 31 | 19 | 24 | 12 | n.s. |
| Shumaker et al. 1978 [44] | 15 | 47 | 12 | 50 | n.s. |
| Lesesne et al. 1978 [30] | 7 | 100 | 7 | 29 | $p<0.001$ |
| Depew et al. 1980 [12] | 13 | 54 | 15 | 53 | n.s. |
| Theodossi et al. 1982 [47] | 28 | 57 | 27 | 63 | n.s. |
| Total | 161 | 43.5 | 148 | 38 | n.s. |

should be stressed that the criteria for the selection of patients varied greatly from study to study and that in many instances the stage and severity of the disease (for example, presence or absence of cirrhosis or encephalopathy) were not exactly defined.

As might be expected in severely ill patients in whom alcohol has affected nearly all organs, death results in many cases from causes other than liver failure. In many instances it is difficult to distinguish clearly between death from liver disease or its complications (hemorrhage, hepatic renal failure, coma) and death from other causes unrelated to the liver disease.

## Glucocorticoids

Glucocorticoids have been proposed for the treatment of alcoholic hepatitis because of increasing evidence that immune mechanisms are implicated in the pathogenesis of the disease [18, 36]. In addition, glucocorticoids might be helpful because of their effect in increasing serum albumin and decreasing hyperbilirubinemia [16]. Furthermore, the partial adrenocortical insufficiency in chronic alcoholics may lead to insufficient stress-induced cortisol production in severely ill patients.

**Short-Term Treatment**

One group from the University of North Carolina has consistently found in two placebo-controlled trials that prednisolone treatment reduces mortality in severely ill patients with hepatic encephalopathy [20, 30] (Table 2). In seven other controlled, randomized clinical studies this beneficial effect of glucocorticoid therapy on the mortality in patients with severe alcolholic hepatitis was not confirmed [3, 8, 12, 32, 37, 44, 47] (Table 2). However, in one other study early mortality was less in patients treated with prednisolone and several laboratory tests (serum bilirubin, transaminases, and albumin levels) returned to normal more quickly [32]. Possible explanations for the disparity between the highly significant beneficial effects observed by the group from North Carolina and the failure to reproduce these results at other institutions in the United States [3, 8, 12, 37, 44] and in London [47] have been discussed in detail by Conn [10, 11]. A major problem in drawing definite conclusions from the results of these studies is the inhomogeneity of the patients investigated in the various trials.

As mentioned above the prognosis of alcoholic hepatitis varies distinctly with the presence or absence of underlying cirrhosis (Table 1) and/or other factors like encephalopathy. The marked differences in mortality in the placebo-treated groups, which ranges from 19% to 100% (Table 2) indicate that the groups of patients are not at all homogeneous. It shows that the results of these trials can hardly be compared with each other. Furthermore, in most, if not in all, of the studies the number of patients was too small to provide a firm conclusion. The likelihood of avoiding a B error has been calculated only in one study [47]. In this study, in which a very high dose of prednisolone (1 g/day) was given for 3 days, the chance of detecting a 20% difference in survival rates between the two groups of patients was calculated to be only 43%.

In his critical review of glucocorticoid therapy in alcoholic hepatitis, Conn [10] analyzed the data of patients with alcoholic hepatitis and encephalopathy from six studies separately. The main findings of this evaluation are summarized in Table 3. The highly significant difference in mortality in favor of the glucocorticoid-treated group supports the assumption that this drug benefits this subgroup of patients with alcoholic hepatitis. However, since the latter data were obtained by retrospective analysis of results which should not really be evaluated together, further studies in larger and more homogeneous groups of patients with alcoholic hepatitis are necessary to identify more clearly those who might benefit from treatment with glucocorticoids.

**Table 3.** Effect of corticosteroid therapy on survival in alcoholic hepatitis with encephalopathy [10]

| Authors, year | Control group | | Steroid group | | Statistical significance |
|---|---|---|---|---|---|
| | *n* | Mortality (%) | *n* | Mortality (%) | |
| Helman et al. 1971 [20] | 6 | 100 | 9 | 11 | $p<0.01$ |
| Porter et al. 1971 [37] | 8 | 88 | 8 | 75 | n.s. |
| Campra et al. 1973 [8] | 10 | 80 | 8 | 50 | n.s. |
| Shumaker et al. 1978 [44] | 2 | 50 | 3 | 67 | n.s. |
| Blitzer et al. 1977 [3] | 6 | 0 | 6 | 33 | n.s. |
| Lesesne et al. 1978 [30] | 7 | 100 | 7 | 29 | $p<0.01$ |
| Total | 39 | 74 | 41 | 41 | $p<0.001$ |

**Long-Term Treatment**

The only well-documented controlled trial on long-term treatment of patients with alcoholic hepatitis was performed on 99 patients among a consecutive group of 483 cirrhotics investigated by the Copenhagen Study Group for Liver Diseases [43]. Forty-four patients received prednisolone 40 mg/day for 4-8 weeks and a daily dose of 10-15 mg thereafter for 5-12 years. The survival rate in this group was not significantly different from the group of 45 patients receiving placebo tablets. Long-term treatment using the same dosage of prednisolone in patients with advanced alcoholic cirrhosis adversely affects the prognosis [48] and should therefore be avoided.

## Anabolic Steroids

In patients with alcohol liver disease marked changes in the metabolism of androgenic steroids have been found [50]. The formation of testosterone is decreased, leading to reduced serum levels of this hormone and an increase in the estrogens:androgens ratio which is responsible for the development of feminization in these patients. Earlier studies in animals suggested a beneficial effect of androgenic anabolic steroids on liver injury. The administration of such substances reduced or prevented experimentally induced liver injury and accelerated liver regeneration following partial hepatectomy [33]. Another reason for the use of anabolic steroids is that they stimulate the formation of coagulation factors and accelerate the removal of hepatic fat [33]. Several uncontrolled and a few controlled studies of testosterone treatment of cirrhosis have been published. In most of them a positive effect of testosterone on physical and biochemical variables was found [33]. Mortality was significantly reduced in the treated groups in two controlled studies (Table 4). However, in these earlier trials patients with different etiology of the cirrhosis were included.

More recently Mendenhall et al. [33] studied 263 patients with moderate or severe alcoholic hepatitis. The patients were randomly assigned to a treatment with oxandrolone (80 mg/day), prednisolone (60 mg initially, stepwise reduction of dose), or placebo for 30-day periods. During this time mortality in the two groups receiving steroid therapy was not significantly different from that in the placebo group. Surprisingly, oxandrolone therapy was associated with a beneficial effect on long-term survival in patients with moderate alcoholic hepatitis. Among those patients who survived 2 months after the start of the treatment the conditional 6-months death rate was 3.5% in the group receiving oxandrolone and 19%-20% after placebo. The difference between the two groups levelled off after an additional 2-4 months. The authors tried to explain the

**Table 4.** Controlled long-term studies of therapy with testosterone in patients with liver cirrhosis

| Author(s), year | Study duration (years) | Testosterone | | Placebo | |
|---|---|---|---|---|---|
| | | *n* | Mortality (%) | *n* | Mortality (%) |
| Wells 1960 [52] | 1.5 | 26 | 31 | 27 | 55 |
| Islam and Islam 1973 [24] | 4.0 | 32 | 34 | 28 | 63 |

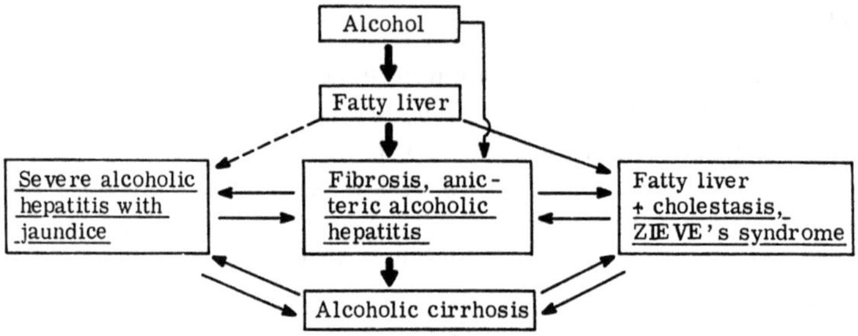


**Fig. 1.** Schematic representation of the main types of alcohol-induced liver disease

prolonged effect of the 30-day treatment by the hypothesis that oxandrolone might induce a genetic change which produces a fetal expression that results in enhanced and prolonged liver regeneration.

## Propylthiouracil

Isreal et al. [25] recently reported that chronic alcohol feeding of rats leads to a hypermetabolic state with increased rates of hepatic oxygen consumption similar to that seen in hyperthyroidism. In these animals the liver became extremly sensitive to ischemic injury. Both the hypermetabolic state and the susceptibility to ischemic injury were suppressed by thyroidectomy and prevented by administration of propylthiouracil. From these results it was suggested that hypoxia might contribute to the pathogenesis of alcoholic liver disease.

In a double-blind controlled trial in 133 patients with alcoholic liver disease the effect of short-term propylthiouracil (PTU) administration (300 mg/day) was investigated [34]. Patients with alcoholic hepatitis with and without cirrhosis showed a significantly higher rate of normalization of a composite clinical and laboratory index on PTU than on placebo. In a subgroup of 38 patients with alcoholic hepatitis without cirrhosis, those on PTU showed a greater improvement in 15 of 15 items ($p < 0.001$) of the composite clinical and laboratory index. The overall mortality was low in both groups (four in the PTU group versus six in the placeco group). Unfortunately, data for only 103 patients are shown in the report. The results have been criticized because of the lack of data and other flaws in the study design [26].

A more recent randomized double-blind controlled study [19] has failed to confirm the findings of the study mentioned above. In this trial only patients with severe alcoholic hepatitis were included. Histological examination was carried out in 63%, 30% of whom had underlying cirrhosis. Of 31 patients treated with PTU, 23% died, as compared to 19% of the 36 patients in the placebo group. The treatment produced no beneficial effect on any of the hepatic biochemical tests. The questions arising from these studies and the rationale for the use of PTU in alcoholic hepatitis have been discussed in detail by Kaplowitz [26].

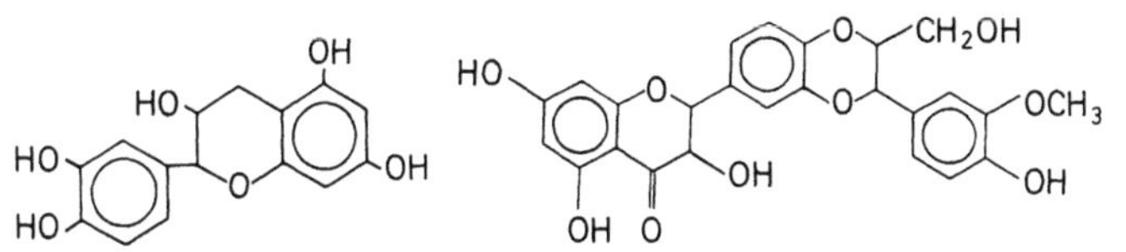


**Fig. 2.** Chemical structure of (+)-cyanidanol-3 *(left)* and silymarin *(right)*

## Flavonoids

The bioflavonoids silymarin (silibin) and (+)-cyanidanol-3 differ distinctly concerning their chemical structure (Fig. 2). Both compounds, however, have been shown to have marked hepatoprotective effects against several types of experimental liver injury, e.g., that caused by carbon tetrachloride, thioacetamide, phalloidin, and galactosamine [22, 51]. The beneficial effect of both flavonoids is observed only when they are administered before the toxins. (+)-Cyanidanol-3 acts as a potent radical scavenger and antioxidant [22, 27]. Both flavonoids change the basic properties of cytoplasmic and other cell membranes [22, 51]. Silymarin stimulated hepatic protein synthesis by increasing ribosomal RNA synthesis [45]. Because of their promising biochemical and pharmacological effects in animal experiments these flavonoids have been tried in alcoholic liver disease.

### (+)-Cyanidanol-3

The results of four randomized controlled clinical trials in patients with alcoholic liver disease are summarized in Table 5. The only investigation which gave a clearly positive result was performed by Palmas from Italy in patients with compensated cirrhosis [35]. The effect of (+)-cyanidanol-3 on symptoms and biochemical tests related to liver disease was assessed in only 30 patients with alcoholic cirrhosis (15 received (+)-cyanidanol-3 and 15 placebo). Statistically significant inprovement was reported in clinical symptoms (asthenia, anorexia, abdominal discomfort) and in a number of liver function tests (GOT, GPT, gamma-GT, prothrombin time and serum albumin). The patients obviously continued to drink, but alcohol consumption during the trial was not reported. Since patients were hospitalized during the first 1-2 months of the study a beneficial effect of reduction of alcohol intake during this period would be anticipated. However, surprisingly, no change in the mean values of the liver function tests during this early period of the study was observed. The most impressive effects of the drug were seen after 3 months therapy. Two of the other controlled trials [9, 41] also lasted for 3 months. Neither showed beneficial results. In both studies patients with alcoholic hepatitis were investigated and a smaller dose of (+)-cyanidanol-3 was given than in the group studied by Palmas [35]. In the fourth study a larger group with mild to moderate alcoholic hepatitis was treated with the same dose (3.0 g/day) of (+)-cyanidanol-3 for only 2 weeks. Improvement was seen in both groups but was attributed to abstinence; (+)-cyanidanol-3 treatment showed no significant beneficial effect.

In addition to the studies summarized in Table 5, Ugarte et al. [49] reported two studies on the effect of 2 g (+)-cyanidanol-3 daily vs placebo in two groups with alco-

**Table 5.** Effect of (+)-cyanidanol-3 therapy on alcoholic liver disease

| Author | Duration | Dosage (g/day) | *n* [(+)-cyanidanol-3/placebo] | Results |
|---|---|---|---|---|
| Colman et al. 1980 [9][a] | 3 months | 2.0 | 20/20 | No beneficial effect |
| Palmas 1981 [35][b] | 5 months | 3.0 | 20/21 | Improvement: GOT, GPT, gamma-GT, albumin, bilirubin (statistical significance) |
| Sanchez-Tapias et al. 1981 [41][a] | 3 months | 1.5 | 14/13 | No beneficial effect |
| Hennings 1981 [21][a] | 2 weeks | 3.0 | 35/35 | No beneficial effect |

[a] Alcoholic hepatitis
[b] Alcoholic cirrhosis

holic hepatitis. In one trial with 43 patients with severe alcoholic hepatitis cyanidanol had no beneficial effect, while in a smaller group of 25 patients with mild alcoholic hepatitis serum transaminases improved more rapidly in the group receiving cyanidanol. Unfortunately the period of treatment was not mentioned and too few details in study design were presented to permit meaningful evaluation of the data.

## Silymarin

Two controlled clinical studies have claimed that silymarin improves a number of laboratory parameters in patients with mild to moderate alcohol-induced liver disease [15, 40]. In one study 31 patients were treated with silymarin for 4 weeks and 35 received placebo [15]. Improvement of serum GPT in the silymarin group was the only statistically significant difference. In addition, no details of study design and histological findings were presented. Salmi and Sarna [40] studied 97 patients with mild to moderate liver disease selected on the basis of elevated serum transaminase levels. Ninety of the patients had liver biopsies. Forty-seven received silymarin (420 g/day) and 50 placebo for 4 weeks. There was a statistically significantly greater decrease of serum GPT and, less pronounced, GOT in the treated group than in the controls. The liver disease was assumed to be mainly induced by alcohol abuse; however, no details on alcohol consumption and incidence of histological findings compatible with alcoholic liver disease were given. Furthermore, the distinctly higher initial GPT than GOT values in both groups cast doubt on the assumption that mainly patients with alcoholic liver diseases were included in the trial. Moreover, there were marked differences in the incidence of signs of acute liver injury in the initial biopsy in the treated group. In summary, the two studies give no clear evidence for a beneficial effect of silymarin on alcohol-induced liver injury.

In a controlled double-blind multicenter trial from Vienna, the effect of silymarin was studied on the course and outcome of 170 patients with cirrhosis of various etiology over a period of 40–50 months. Preliminary results of this study were published by Benda et al. [2]. The most important finding was a statistically significant increase in the 4-year survival rate in the subgroup of patients with alcoholic cirrhosis. Since details of the study are presented in a separate communication by Ferenci et al. [14] in this volume, they will not be discussed here.

## Antifibrogenic Drugs

Many of the complications of alcoholic cirrhosis stem from the derangement of liver architecture that follows progressive formation of collagen in the liver. Two drugs – colchicine and D-penicillamine – which are known to inhibit collagen deposition or stimulate collagen breakdown have been proposed for treatment of patients with alcoholic liver diseases.

### Colchicine

Colchicine inhibits microtubular protein assembly in fibroblasts, and thereby collagen formation [23]. Kershenobich and associates [28] studied 43 patients with liver cirrhosis. Twenty-three received colchicine (1 mg/day, 5 days a week) and 20 placebo for 4 years. Mortality decreased from 40% with placebo to 17% in the treatment group. Because of the small number of patients, these results did not reach statistical significance. Ascites, encephalopathy, and splenomegaly improved significantly ($p<0.05$) in the group receiving colchicine. Although the results of this study are encouraging, confirmation in a larger population sample is needed.

### D-Penicillamine

D-Penicillamine is known to retard the cross-linking of collagen molecules thus rendering newly-formed fibers susceptible to collagenolytic activity [23]. As a consequence this drug has been considered a potentially useful inhibitor of fibrogenesis in the liver. Resnick et al. [38] studied the effect of D-penicillamine on the course of 40 patients with moderately severe alcoholic hepatitis without cirrhosis in a double-blind controlled trial. 19 received D-penicillamine (100 mg/day) and 21 received placebo for 8 weeks. The groups of patients were similar in demographic data and in clinical, biochemical, and histological features. No improvement in survival or in liver function tests was seen in the experimental group. Reduction in degree of hepatocellular necrosis and in the deposition of collagen, determined histologically after 8 weeks of therapy, appeared to be greater in the D-penicillamine-treated patients. The number of patients who had biopsies before and after treatment was too small to allow statistically significant conclusions.

## Insulin Plus Glucagon

In animal experiments the presence of hepatotrophic factors in portal blood has repeatedly been documented [46]. Particularly insulin and glucagon from the pancreas were shown to be potent stimuli of hepatocellular regeneration [6]. The administration of these hormones ameliorated fulminant murine hepatitis [13]. Stimulation of regeneration by infusion of these hormones might provide an useful approach to treatment of severe alcoholic hepatitis in man.

Baker et al. [1] recently conducted a randomized, double-blind controlled trial of insulin and glucagon infusion in 50 patients with alcoholic hepatitis. Twenty-five received 24 U regular insulin and 2.4 mg glucagon over 12 h daily for 3 weeks, and 25 received 200 ml dextrose solution in the same manner as placebo. Mortality (three in the treatment group, six in the placebo group) was not significantly different. However, in a subgroup of 34 patients with prothrombin times prolonged by 3 s over controls, a tendency to fewer deaths was observed in the treatment group ($p < 0.1$). In addition, total serum bilirubin and prothrombin time improved more rapidly in the insulin- and glucagon-infused group. Complications of therapy included hypoglycemia in three patients, one of whom died, superficial thrombophlebitis at the site of infusion in all treated patients, and generalized macular skin eruptions in three patients. This type of therapy seems to be a promising approach for the most severely ill patients, in whom the rate of hepatocellular regeneration might be a critical factor for survival. However, so far it should be considered experimental.

## References

1. Baker AL, Jaspan JB, Haines NW, Hatfield GE, Krager PS, Schneider JF (1981) A randomized clinical trial of insulin and glucagon infusion for treatment of alcoholic hepatitis: Progress report in 50 patients. Gastroenterology 80: 1410-1414
2. Benda H, Dittrich H, Ferenzi P, Frank H, Wewalka F (1981) Zur Wirksamkeit von Silymarin auf die Überlebensrate von Patienten mit Leberzirrhose. In: de Ritis F, Csomos G, Braatz R (eds) Der toxisch metabolische Leberschaden. Hansisches Verlagskontor, Lübeck, pp 59-68
3. Blitzer BL, Mutchnik MG, Joshi PH, Phillips MM, Fessel JM, Conn HO (1977) Adrenocorticosteroid therapy in alcoholic hepatitis. A prospective, double-blind randomized study. Am J Dig Dis 22: 477-484
4. Bode JC (1981) Die alkoholische Hepatitis, ein Krankheitsspektrum. Internist (Berlin) 22: 536-545
5. Bode JC, Kruse G, Mexas P, Martini GA (1984) Alkoholfettleber, Alkoholhepatitis und Alkoholzirrhose; Trinkverhalten und Häufigkeit klinischer, klinisch-chemischer und histologischer Befunde bei 282 Patienten. Dtsch Med Wochenschr 40: 1516-1521
6. Bucher NLR, Swaffield MN (1975) Regulation of hepatic regeneration in rats by synergistic action of insulin and glucagon. Proc Natl Acad Sci USA 72: 1157-1160
8. Campra JL, Hamlin EM, Kirschbaum RJ, Olivier M, Redeker AG, Reynolds TB (1973) Prednisone therapy of acute alcoholic hepatitis. Report of a controlled trial. Ann Intern Med 79: 625-631
9. Colman JC, Morgan MY, Scheuer PJ, Sherlock S (1980) Treatment of alcohol-related liver disease with (+)-cyanidanol-3: a randomized double-blind trial. Gut 21: 965-969
10. Conn HO (1978) Steroid treatment of alcoholic hepatitis. The yeas and the nays. Gastroenterology 74: 319-326
11. Conn HO (1985) The rational management of alcoholic liver disease. In: Hall P (ed) Alcoholic liver disease – pathobiology, epidemiology and clinical aspects. Arnold, London, pp 266-289
12. Depew W, Boyer T, Omata M, Redeker A, Reynolds T (1981) Double-blind controlled trial of prednisolone therapy in patients with severe acute alcoholic hepatitis and spontaneous encephalopathy. Gastroenterology 78: 524-529
13. Farivar M, Wands JR, Isselbacher KJ, Bucher NLR (1976) Effect of insulin and glucagon on fulminant murine hepatitis. N Engl J Med 295: 1517-1519
14. Ferenci P, Dragosics B, Dittrich H, Frank H, Lochs H, Pamperl H, Meryn S (1986) Silymarin treatment in patients with cirrhosis of the liver: a prospective study.
15. Fintelmann V, Albert A (1980) Nachweis der therapeutischen Wirksamkeit von Legalon bei toxischen Lebererkrankungen im Doppelblindversuch. Therapiewoche 30: 5589-5594

16. French SW, Burbige EJ (1979) Alcoholic hepatitis: clinical, morphologic, pathogenic and therapeutic aspects. Prog Liver Dis 6: 557-579
17. Galambos JT (1974) Alcoholic hepatitis. In: Schaffner F, Sherlock S, Leevy CM (eds) The liver and its diseases. Thieme, Stuttgart, pp 255-267
18. Hall P (1985) Pathology and pathogenesis of alcoholic liver disease. In: Hall P (ed) Alcoholic liver disease – pathobiology, epidemiology and clinical aspects. Arnold, London, pp 41-68
19. Hallé P, Pare P, Kaptein K, Kanel G, Redeker AG, Reynolds TB (1982) Double-blind, controlled trial of propylthiouracil in patients with severe acute alcoholic hepatitis. Gastroenterology 82: 925-931
20. Helman RA, Temko MH, Nye SW, Fallon HJ (1971) Alcoholic hepatitis. Natural history and evaluation of prednisolone therapy. Ann Intern Med 74: 311-321
21. Henning H (1981) Influence of (+)-cyanidanol-3 on chronic alcoholic liver injury. In: Conn HO (ed) International workshop on (+)-cyanidanol-3 in diseases of the liver. Academic, London; Grune and Stratton, New York, pp 177-179 (The Royal Society of Medicine, International congress and symposium series, no 47)
22. Hennings G (1981) Biochemical, pharmacological and toxicological evaluation of (+)-cyanidanol-3. In: Conn HO (ed) International workshop on (+)-cyanidanol-3 in diseases of the liver. Academic, London; Grune and Stratton, New York, pp 7-9 (The Royal Society of Medicine, International congress and symposium series, no 47)
23. Hirayama C (1974) Hepatic fibrosis: biochemical considerations. In: Schaffner F, Sherlock S, Leevy CM (eds) The liver and its diseases. Thieme, Stuttgart, pp 273-282
24. Islam N, Islam A (1973) Testosterone propionate in cirrhosis of the liver. Br J Clin Pract 27: 125-128
25. Isreal Y, Videla L, MacDonald A, Bernstein J (1973) Metabolic alterations produced in the liver by chronic ethanol administration: comparison between the effects produced by ethanol and by thyroid hormones. Biochem J 134: 523-539
26. Kaplowitz N (1982) Propylthiouracil treatment for alcoholic hepatitis: Should it and does it work? Gastroenterology 82: 1468-1472
27. Kappus H (1981) (+)-Cyanidanol-3 inhibition of lipid peroxidation induced by hepatotoxic chemicals in the rat. In: Conn HO (ed) International workshop on (+)-cyanidanol-3 in diseases of the liver. Academic, London; Grune and Stratton, New York, pp 17-18 (The Royal Society of Medicine, International congress and symposium series, no 47)
28. Kershenobich D, Uribe M, Suarez GI, Mata JM, Perez-Tamayo R, Rojkind M (1979) Treatment of cirrhosis with colchicine. A double-blind randomised trial. Gastroenterology 77: 532-536
29. Klatskin G (1971) Alcoholic hepatitis. In: Gerok W, Sickinger K, Hennekeuser HH (eds) Alcohol and the liver. Schattauer, Stuttgart, pp 282-287
30. Lesesne HR, Bozymski EM, Fallon HJ (1978) Treatment of alcoholic hepatitis with encephalopathy. Comparison of prednisolone with caloric supplements. Gastroenterology 74: 169-173
31. Lieber CS (1986) Alcohol and the liver. In: Arias IM, Frenkel M, Wilson JHP (eds) The liver annual 5. Elsevier, Amsterdam, pp 116-167
32. Maddrey WC, Boitnott JK, Bedine MS, Weber FL, Mezey E, White RI (1978) Corticosteroid therapy of alcoholic hepatitis. Gastroenterology 75: 193-199
33. Mendenhall CL, Anderson S, Garcia-Pont P, et al. (1984) Short-term and long-term survival in patients with alcoholic hepatitis treated with oxandrolone and prednisolone. N Engl J Med 311: 1464-1470
34. Orrego H, Kalant H, Isreal Y, Blake J, Medline A, Rankin JG, Armstrong A, Kapur B (1979) Effect of short-term therapy with propylthiouracil in patients with alcoholic liver disease. Gastroenterology 76: 105-115
35. Palmas S (1981) Treatment of alcoholic cirrhosis with (+)-cyanidanol-3. In: Conn HO (ed) International workshop on (+)-cyanidanol-3 in diseases of the liver. Academic, London; Grune and Stratton, New York, pp 167-175 (The Royal Society of Medicine, International congress and symposium series, no 47)
36. Paronetto F (1985) Ethanol and the immune system. In: Seitz HK, Kommerell B (eds) Alcohol-related diseases in gastroenterology. Springer, Berlin Heidelberg New York Tokyo, pp 269-281
37. Porter HP, Simon FR, Pope CE, Volwiler W, Fenster LF (1971) Corticosteroid therapy in severe alcoholic hepatitis. A double-blind drug trial. N Engl J Med 284: 1350-1355

38. Resnick RH, Boitnott J, Iber FL, Makopour H, Cerda JJ (1974) Preliminary observations of d-penicillamine therapy in acute alcoholic liver disease. Digestion 11: 257-265
39. Review by an international group (1981) Alcoholic liver disease: morphological manifestations. Lancet i: 707-711
40. Salmi HA, Sarna S (1981) Effect of silymarin on chemical, functional, and morphological alterations of the liver. A double-blind controlled study. Scand J Gastroenterol 17: 517-521
41. Sanchez-Tapias JM, Fiol B, Rodes J (1981) (+)-Cyanidanol-3 in mild alcoholic hepatitis. In: Conn HO (ed) International workshop on (+)-cyanidanol-3 in diseases of the liver. Academic, London; Grune and Stratton, New York, pp 173-175 (The Royal Society of Medicine, International congress and symposium series, no 47)
42. Schenker S (1984) Alcoholic liver disease: evaluation of natural history and prognostic factors. Hepatology 4: 36S-43S
43. Schlichting P, Juhl E, Poulsen H, Winkel P and the Copenhagen Study Group for Liver Diseases (1976) Alcoholic hepatitis superimposed on cirrhosis. Clinical significance and effect of long-term prednisone treatment. Scand J Gastroenterol 11: 305-312
44. Shumaker JB, Resnick RH, Galambos JT, Makopour H, Iber FL (1978) A controlled trial of 6-methylprednisolone in acute alcoholic hepatitis. Am J Gastroenterol 69: 443-449
45. Sonnenbichler J, Machicao F, Mattersberger J, Rosen H (1981) Gesteigerte Leberzellregeneration unter dem Einfluß von Silymarin. In: de Ritis F, Csomos G, Braatz R (eds) Der toxischmetabolische Leberschaden. Hansisches Verlagskontor, Lübeck, pp 28-36
46. Starzl TE, Terblanche J (1979) Hepatotrophic substances. Prog Liver Dis 6: 135-152
47. Theodossi A, Eddleston ALW, Williams R (1982) Controlled trial of methylprednisolone therapy in severe acute alcoholic hepatitis. Gut 23: 75-79
48. Tygstrup N, Juhl E and the Copenhagen Study Group for Liver Diseases (1971) The treatment of alcoholic cirrhosis. The effect of continued drinking and prednisone on survival. In: Gerok W, Sickinger K, Hennekeuser HH (eds) Alcohol and the liver. Schattauer, Stuttgart, pp 519-526
49. Ugarte G, Bunout D, Iturriaga H (1981) Effect of (+)-cyanidanol-3 on alcoholic liver disease with and without overt hepatic failure. In: Conn HO (ed) International workshop on (+)-cyanidanol-3 in diseases of the liver. Academic, London; Grune and Stratton, New York, pp 181-184 (The Royal Society of Medicine, International congress and symposium series, no 47)
50. Van Thiel DH, Lester R (1979) The effect of chronic alcohol abuse on sexual function. Clin Endocrinol Metab 8: 499-510
51. Vogel G, Trost W, Braatz R, Odenthal KP, Brüsewitz G, Antweiler H, Seeger R (1975) Untersuchungen zur Pharmakodynamik, Angriffspunkt und Wirkungsmechanismus von Silymarin, dem antihepatotoxischen Prinzip aus Silybum mar. (L.) Gaertn. 2. Besondere Untersuchungen zum Angriffspunkt und Wirkungsmechanismus (auch an anderen Organen als der Leber). Arzneimittelforsch 25: 179-188
52. Wells R (1969) Prednisolone and testosterone propionate in cirrhosis of the liver. A controlled trial. Lancet 1: 1416-1419

# Silymarin Treatment in Patients with Cirrhosis of the Liver – a Prospective Study

P. Ferenci[1], B. Dragosics[1], H. Dittrich[2], H. Frank[3], H. Lochs[1], H. Pamperl[1], and S. Meryn[1]

[1] First Department of Gastroenterology and Hepatology, University of Vienna, Austria
[2] Ambulatorium Süd der Wiener Gebietskrankenkasse, Vienna, Austria
[3] Department of Internal Medicine, Sophienspital, Vienna, Austria

## Introduction

Silymarin is the collective name for the flavolignans silibinin, silidianin and silichristin, extracted from the milk thistle *Silybum marianum* (L.) *gaertneri*. This drug was shown to protect experimental animals against various hepatotoxins, including phalloidin [1, 2], $\alpha$-amanitin [3], carbon tetrachloride [4, 5], thioacetamide [6], and galactosamine [4]. The mechanism by which silymarin exerts its "hepatoprotective" action is under intensive investigation. The antitoxic effects of silymarin against the *Amanita phalloides* toxins phalloidin and $\alpha$-amanitin are mediated by the inhibition of the binding of phalloidin to specific receptors on liver cell membranes [7] and by the antagonism to the blocking effects of $\alpha$-amanitin on RNA polymerase [8-10]. Furthermore, the hepatoprotective properties of silymarin may be related to the inhibition of lipid peroxide formation in liver cells [11] and to changes of physical properties of plasma membranes induced by silymarin, making cells more resistant to osmotic lysis and to the action of detergents [12, 13].

The role of silymarin for treatment of patients with liver disease remains to be established. Silibinin-C-2′-3-dihydrogen-succinate, the water-soluble active form of silymarin, prevents hepatocellular disease when administered intravenously to patients within the first few hours after the ingestion of *Amanita phalloides* [2]. In patients with various forms of mild alcoholic liver disease treated with silymarin, abnormal liver function tests improved much earlier than in patients receiving a placebo [14, 15]. The present prospective, double-blind randomized study was initiated to investigate whether silymarin is able to improve the outcome of patients with cirrhosis of the liver.

## Patients and Study Protocol

One hundred and seventy patients with cirrhosis of the liver were included in the study. In 70% of cases the diagnosis of cirrhosis was confirmed by liver histology. In the remaining patients no liver biopsy could be obtained due to coagulation disorders. Patients with end-stage liver failure or known malignancies were excluded from the study, as were patients on immunosuppressive treatment and patients with primary biliary cirrhosis. All potential candidates were followed for at least 3 months before they were asked to participate. By this means very sick patients and probably noncompliant patients were excluded.

At the entry into the study the severity of the underlying liver disease was classified using the Child-Turcotte criteria [16], and the etiology using clinical, biochemical, im-

Assessment and Management of Hepatobiliary Disease
Eds.: L. Okolicsányi, G. Csomós, and G. Crepaldi

munological, and histological criteria as described previously [17]. The patients were randomly assigned to a group receiving either 420 mg silymarin (140 mg t.i.d orally) or an identical-looking placebo. This dose of silymarin was calculated, based on pharmacokinetic studies, to yield a hepatic concentration of the drug similar to that effective in in vitro studies [18]. Both the drug and the placebo were kindly supplied by Madaus (Cologne, FRG). All patients were advised to abstain from alcohol completely. The degree of alcohol consumed during the study was estimated by questioning the patients and their relatives. Furthermore, serial determinations of serum gamma-glutamyl transpeptidase (SGGTP) activity in the blood were a useful parameter for detection of major alcohol abuse during the study. Any therapy for treatment of complications of liver disease or of other conditions unrelated to liver disease was recorded in the protocol. The use of steroids and of D-penicillamine was not allowed.

After randomization the patients were seen in the outpatient clinic at intervals of 3 months. At each outpatient visit the patient was examined clinically and blood was drawn to determine routine parameters of liver function (bilirubin, SGOT, SGPT, alkaline phosphatase, SGGTP, prothrombin time, albumin, pseudocholinesterase, serum electrophoresis, alpha-1-fetoprotein, HBsAg).

At the beginning of the study and at each following visit to the outpatient clinic the patients received a 3-month supply of the drug and were asked to return the containers at the next scheduled visit. The counting of the unused capsules served as a measure for compliance. Patients were withdrawn from the study and considered as "dropouts" if they failed to come to a scheduled outpatient visit within 14 days or if they had not used at least 80% of the supplied capsules. If a patient died during the study, the physician treating the final event was contacted to determine the cause of death.

Originally, the study was designed for 2 years. Later, the study committee decided to extend it as lońg as possible. Each patient who completed the 2-year study period was asked to continue the treatment. The study was terminated when the last patient entered completed the 2-year study period and the code was broken. The mean duration of treatment was 41 months (range 2–6 years).

## Statistical Analysis

The data were evaluated by computer using the life table and survival function analysis (BMDP Statistical Software, Inc., Regents of the University of California 1983). By this program the product limit estimate of survival was computed. Statistical comparison of the results was performed using a general Wilcoxon (Breslov) test and the Mantel-Cox test [19]. The Mantel-Cox test weights mortality equally during the whole study, the Wilcoxon-Breslov test is more sensitive in the early phase of survival. The $\chi^2$ test was used for comparison of demographic data and of biochemical parameters of liver function between the study groups and to compare mortality figures after 2 years.

## Results

Eighty-three patients received placebo and 87 were treated with silymarin. The two study groups were well matched regarding etiology and severita of the underlying liver disease, age, sex, and biochemical findings (Table 1).

**Table 1.** Demographic and biochemical data of patients with cirrhosis of the liver in the silymarin trial at randomization

| | Placebo | Silymarin |
|---|---|---|
| Male *(n)* | 62 | 61 |
| Female *(n)* | 21 | 26 |
| Age (years) | 58 ± 12 | 57 ± 12 |
| Etiology of liver disease | | |
| Alcoholic *(n)* | 45 | 47 |
| Nonalcoholic *(n)* | 38 | 40 |
| Child's classification | | |
| A *(n)* | 42 | 47 |
| B *(n)* | 32 | 37 |
| C *(n)* | 9 | 3 |
| Serum bilirubin (mg/dl) | 2.5 ± 2.1 | 1.6 ± 1.1 |
| SGOT (U/l) | 40 ± 38 | 36 ± 30 |
| SGPT (U/l) | 28 ± 33 | 29 ± 22 |
| SGGTP (U/l) | 150 ± 178 | 129 ± 160 |
| Serum albumin (g/l) | 35.6 ± 6.6 | 35.8 ± 6.0 |
| Prothrombin time (%) | 67 ± 22 | 69 ± 17 |
| HBsAg positive *(n)* | 12 | 9 |

Data shown as mean ± SD
SGOT, serum glutamic oxaloacetic transaminase (normal up to 12 U/l); SGPT, serum glutamic pyruvic transaminase (normal up to 12 U/l); SGGTP, serum gamma-glutamyl transpeptidase (normal up to 28 U/l). Normal range for serum albumin: 35-50 g/l; normal range for prothrombin time: 70%-130%

Silymarin treatment was well tolerated over the whole study period. Only four patients (two in the silymarin group and two in the control group) complained of nausea and epigastric discomfort. These complaints disappeared after stopping the drug treatment.

Twenty-four patients (10 in the placebo group and 14 in the silymarin group) were considered as dropouts. The reasons for dropout included drug-related complaints (see above, two in each group), intercurrent major nonhepatic disease (one in each group), and change of the treating physician due to change of home (one in control group and two in silymarin group). In the remaining 15 patients no clear reasons for dropout were apparent (= true noncompliance). Six of the dropouts had died within 2 years after randomization (two in the control group and four in the silymarin group) and seven were still alive (two in the control group and five in the silymarin group). The remaining 11 patients died 2½-6½ years after randomization.

After subtracting the dropouts, 73 patients in each group remained in the study. Of these, 105 were still alive at the end of the 2-year study period (48 in the control group and 57 in the treatment group). As 10 patients finished the 2-year study period within 3 months after the last patients entered the study, only 95 were eligible to continue the study. Forty-three were studied for 3-4 years and 29 for 4 years or more. The mean duration of treatment was 41 months. Within the 2-year study period 25 (34%) and 16 (22%) patients had died in the placebo group and the silymarin group respectively ($p = 0.06$). In two patients in the placebo group and in three patients in the silymarin group death was attributed to nonhepatic diseases. Thus, the liver-related mortality was 23 and 13 ($p < 0.05$) in the placebo group and the treatment group respectively.

**Table 2.** Causes of death among patients dying during the silymarin study

| | Placebo *(n)* | Silymarin *(n)* |
|---|---|---|
| End-stage liver failure | 21 | 11 |
| Upper GI hemorrhage | 8 | 3 |
| Hepatocellular carcinoma | 1 | – |
| Nonhepatic malignancies | 3 | 1 |
| Accident | 1 | 1 |
| Heart failure | 1 | 2 |
| Cerebral hemorrhage | 1 | – |
| Pneumonia | – | 1 |
| Meningitis | – | 1 |
| Unknown | 1 | 4 |
| Total | 37 | 24 |

Over the whole study period, an additional 12 patients in the placebo group and eight in the treatment group had died. The causes of death are listed in Table 2. Thirty-two patients (21 in the control group and 11 in the silymarin group) developed end-stage liver failure and died. Eleven patients without overt signs of end-stage liver failure died following massive upper gastrointestinal hemorrhage, nine due to rupture of esophageal varices and two to a bleeding duodenal ulcer. One patient developed a hepatocellular carcinoma 4½ years after randomization and died shortly after the diagnosis. In 12 patients the cause of death was unrelated to liver disease. In five patients the cause of death could not be determined with confidence. One of them collapsed while walking down the street and died. The four remaining patients were found dead in their apartments. Fifty-three of the 61 dead patients underwent autopsy. At the postmortem examination, in eight cases (five in the control group and three in the silymarin group) a small hepatocellular carcinoma was found which had not been suspected clinically.

After 4 years, the cumulative survival rate (±SE) was 58%±9% and 38%±9% in the treatment group and the control group respectively ($p = 0.03$). In addition, survival rates were analyzed separately according to the etiology of the liver disease (alcoholic vs nonalcoholic) and according to the severity of liver disease. In alcoholic cirrhosis the number of deaths in the control group was three times as high as in the treatment group and treatment was associated with a better outcome ($p < 0.01$). Conversely, in the nonalcoholic cirrhosis group survival rates were not significantly influenced by treatment with silymarin. In patients originally identified as Child A, the most favorable category, survival was significantly improved by treatment with silymarin ($p < 0.01$). In patients originally rated Child B or C, survival rates were not different in the two groups.

Analysis of liver function tests such as transaminases, SGGTP, bilirubin, and alkaline phosphatase revealed no difference between the two study groups. As judged by SGGTP determinations, 33 patients in the control group and 26 patients in the treatment group consumed alcohol.

## Discussion

This study demonstrates that long-term treatment with silymarin markedly reduces the mortality of patients with cirrhosis. Evaluation of the efficacy of drug treatment in patients with liver cirrhosis is difficult, as there are no reliable parameters to assess a beneficial effect of the drug on the progression of chronic liver disease. Mortality is possibly not the best parameter, but still the best one available in therapeutic trials in patients with liver cirrhosis [20]. Undoubtedly, mortality is determined not only by drug treatment but also by several other factors, which are unlikely to be influenced by any treatment. The value of serial liver biopsies or of laboratory parameters to assess the efficacy of treatment in patients with alcoholic cirrhosis has never been documented [21]. Furthermore, liver biopsies are subject to sample error and cannot be obtained safely from patients with advanced liver disease. In this study, follow-up of transaminases, serum albumin, and serum bilirubin revealed no differences between the two study groups. However, it should be noted that in the control group twice as many patients died of hepatic failure as in the treatment group. As these patients had highly abnormal laboratory findings, after their death the mean value for a certain parameter improved in the remaining patients. Thus differences between the two groups could have existed but been missed.

Whether a patient will benefit from treatment with silymarin depends on the extent of liver damage. In patients originally rated as Child A, the most favorable score, mortality was significantly reduced by treatment with silymarin, but not in patients rated Child B. This finding indicates that when the degree of liver damage is extensive, the outcome is determined by secondary complications of liver disease rather than by liver disease itself, and is therefore unlikely to be changed by medical treatment.

A drug protecting the liver cell from toxic substances could do much toward preventing hepatocellular necrosis and could thus delay or competely prevent the occurrence of hepatic failure in patients with cirrhosis. A reduction in mortality due to hepatic failure can therefore be attributed to effect of drug treatment. If silymarin treatment reduced the extent of hepatocellular damage, it could also have reduced the extent of the formation of scar tissue and of pseudolobules in the liver, thus mitigating the extent of circulatory changes in the liver and in the portal system. Therefore decreased mortality due to variceal hemorrhage may possibly be related to the effect of drug treatment.

The mechanisms of action of silymarin are uncertain. In all clinical studies performed so far the beneficial effects of silymarin were documented in alcoholic or toxin-induced liver diseases [14, 15]. In this study too, the beneficial effect of silymarin on mortality was most pronounced in the group of patients with alcoholic cirrhosis. Although all patients denied alcohol intake during the study, a complete cessation of alcohol abuse in a group of chronic alcoholic patients without any psychiatric treatment is very unlikely. As judged by serial determinations of SGGTP activity in the blood, about 60% of the patients with alcoholic cirrhosis in each group still consumed appreciable quantities of alcohol. Thus, the effect of silymarin is to prevent some metabolic or toxic effects of alcohol on the liver. Based on the results of this study, no discussion of mechanisms by which silymarin could act is possible.

In conclusion, long-term treatment with silymarin appears to be safe and effective in improving survival in patients with alcoholic cirrhosis.

## Summary

Silymarin, the active principle of the milk thistle *Silybum marianum,* protects experimental animals against various hepatotoxic substances. To determine the effect of silymarin on the outcome of patients with cirrhosis, we performed a double-blind, prospective, randomized 2-year study in 170 patients with cirrhosis. Eighty-seven patients (46 alcoholic, 41 nonalcoholic; 61 male, 26 female; 47 Child A, 37 Child B, 3 Child C; mean age 57) received 140 mg silymarin three times daily. Eighty-three patients (45 alcoholic, 38 nonalcoholic; 67 male, 21 female; 42 Child A, 32 Child B, 9 Child C; mean age 58) received a placebo. Noncompliant patients and patients who failed to come to a control were considered as dropouts and withdrawn from the study. All patients who completed the 2-year study period remained on the same treatment until the last patient entered had completed the 2 years. The mean observation period was 41 months. There were 11 dropouts in the placebo and 14 in the treatment group. In the placebo group 37 patients had died, and in 31 death was related to liver disease. In the treatment group 24 had died, and in 18 death was related to liver disease. The mean 4-year survival rate (±SE) was 58%±9% in silymarin-treated patients and 39%±9% in the placebo group ($p=0.02$). Analysis of subgroup indicated that treatment was effective in patients with alcoholic cirrhosis ($p=0.01$) and in patients initially rated Child A ($p=0.03$). No side effects of drug treatment were observed. The results of this study indicate that treatment with silymarin effectively reduces mortality in patients with cirrhosis.


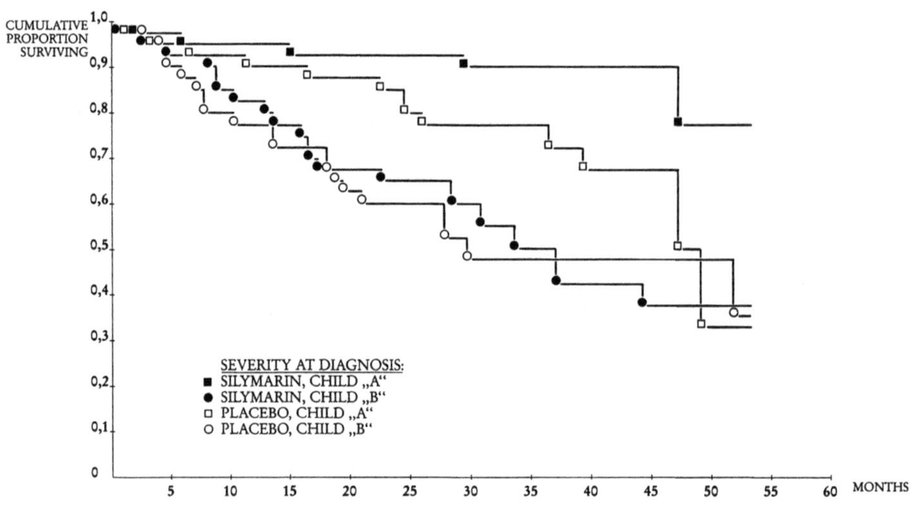


**Fig. 1.** Survival curves for 170 patients with cirrhosis of the liver treated with silymarin or placebo; data analyzed according to the severity of liver disease at randomization (placebo vs. silymarin, Child A: Wilcoxon-Breslov-test p=0.031, Mantel-Cox-test p=0.016; Child B: Wilcoxon-Breslov-test p=0.65, Mantel-Cox-test p=0.86).

## References

1. Tuchweber B, Sieck R, Trost W (1979) Prevention by silybin of phalloidin induced acute hepatotoxicity. Toxicol Appl Pharmacol 51: 265-275
2. Floersheim GL (1978) Experimentelle Grundlagen zur Therapie von Vergiftungen durch den grünen Knollenblätterpilz *(Amanita phalloides)*. Schweiz Med Wochenschr 108: 185-197
3. Hahn G, Lehmann HD, Kürten M, Uebel H, Vogel G (1968) Zur Pharmakologie und Toxikologie von Silymarin, des antiheptotoxischen Wirkprinzipes aus Silybum marianum (L.) Gaertn. Arzneimittelforsch 18: 698-704
4. Rauen HM, Schriewer H (1971) Die antihepatotoxische Wirkung von Silymarin bei experimentellen Leberschädigungen der Ratte durch Tetrachlorkohlenstoff, D-Galaktosamin und Allylalkohol. Arzneimittelforsch 21: 1194-1212
5. Rauen HM, Schriewer H (1973) Die antihepatotoxische Wirkung von parenteral verabreichtem Silymarin bei der Leberschädigung der Ratte durch $CCl_4$. Arzneimittelforsch 23: 148-149
6. Schriewer H, Badde R, Roth G, Rauen HM (1973) Die antihepatotoxische Wirkung des Silymarins bei der Leberschädigung durch Thioacetamid. Arzneimittelforsch 23: 160-161
7. Lotter HL (1984) Untersuchung der Struktur-Wirkungsbeziehung antihepatotoxischer Naturstoffe (Silybin-Antamanid) durch Röntgenstrukturanalyse. Z Naturforsch 39c: 535
8. Sonnenbichler J, Zetl I (1984) Untersuchungen zum Wirkungsmechanismus von Silibinin. V. Einfluß von Silibinin auf die Synthese ribosomaler RNA, mRNA und tRNA in Rattenlebern in vivo. Hoppe Seylers Z Physiol Chem 365: 555-560
9. Machicao F, Sonnenbichler J (1977) Mechanism of the stimulation of RNA synthesis in rat liver nuclei by silybin. Hoppe Seylers Z Physiol Chem 358: 141-147
10. Faulstich H (1979) New Aspects of *Amanita* poisoning. Klin Wochenschr 57: 1143-1152
11. Bindoli A, Cavallini L, Siliprandi N (1977) Inhibitory action of silymarin of lipid peroxide formation in rat liver mitochondria and microsomes. Biochem Pharmacol 26: 2405-2409
12. Valenzuela A, Barria T, Guerra R, Garrido A (1985) Inhibitory effect of the flavonoid silymarin on the erythrocyte hemolysis induced by phenylhydrazine. Biochem Biophys Res Commun 126: 712-715
13. Ramellini G, Meldolesi J (1974) Stabilization of isolated rat liver plasma membranes by treatment in vitro with silymarin. Arzneimittelforsch 24: 806-808
14. Salmi HA, Sarna S (1982) Effect of silymarin on chemical, functional and morphological alterations of the liver. Scand J Gastroenterol 17: 517-520
15. Fintelmann V, Albert A (1980) Nachweis der therapeutischen Wirksamkeit von Legalon® bei toxischen Lebererkrankungen im Doppelblindversuch. Therapiewoche 30: 5589
16. Child CG, Turcotte JG (1964) Surgery and portal hypertension. In: Child CG (ed) The liver and portal hypertension. Saunders, Philadelphia, pp 50-56
17. Ferenci P, Dragosics B, Marosi L, Kiss F (1984) Relative incidence of primary liver cancer in cirrhosis in Austria. Etiological considerations. Liver 4: 7-14
18. Bulles H, Bulles J, Krumbiegel G, Mennicke WH, Nitz D (1975) Untersuchungen zur Verstoffwechselung und zur Ausschcidung von Silybin bei der Ratte. Arzneimittelforsch 25: 902-905
19. Cox DR (1972) Regression models and life tables (with discussion). J R Statist Soc [B] 34: 187-220
20. Preisig R (1981) Problems in phase I and phase II trials with "hepatoprotective" drugs. In: Conn HO (ed) International workshop on (+)-cyanidanol-3 in diseases of the liver. Academic, London; Grune & Stratton, New York, pp 41-48 (The Royal Society of Medicine, International congress and symposium series, no 47)
21. Juhl E, Christensen E, Tygstrup N (1977) The epidemiology of the gastrointestinal RCT. N Engl J Med 296: 20-22

# Protein Malnutrition in Chronic Liver Disease: Corrective Measures

F. Fiaccadori, H. Graf v. Lehndorff, G. Pedretti, and P. Pizzaferri
Cattedra di Malattie Infettive, Università di Parma, Parma, Italy

Malnutrition and nutrient abnormalities are often associated with chronic liver disease, and may contribute to the development of several complications. The liver's role being central in nitrogen metabolism, hepatic damage frequently causes derangements in protein metabolism (Mezey 1978). In most patients with chronic liver disease, protein requirements for maintenance of nitrogen balance (NB) are no different from those of normal individuals. It follows that the accuracy of either oral or parenteral protein equivalent administration can play a major role in liver disease progress. Besides, one must take into consideration the fact that an increased requirement of protein, in order to repair the hepatic damage, leads to deficiencies in other organs; specifically, it causes muscle wasting, since amino acids are continuously deaminated so as to provide a source of energy (Soeters and Fischer 1976). This picture is characteristic of chronic liver disease, with a trend to: (a) an increase in plasma concentrations of amino acids normally removed by the liver, i.e., essential and nonessential aromatic and sulfurated amino acids; (b) a decrease in the amino acids preferentially taken up by extrahepatic tissues, i.e., essential branched-chain amino acids (BCAA) such as valine, leucine, and isoleucine. Therefore, the most common amino acid pattern observed in chronic liver disease consists of increases in the aromatic amino acids (AAA) tyrosine and phenylalanine, glutamic acid, methionine, and sometimes cystine, and a decrease in the BCAA valine, leucine, and isoleucine (Rosen et al. 1977). In addition, patients with chronic liver disease display a decrease in urea synthesis which results in ammonia accumulation (Rudman et al. 1973). In normal conditions the liver eliminates the nitrogen in amino acids by means of transamination with glutamic acid formation. Furthermore, ammonia produced in various tissues can be removed by amination of glutamic acid with the formation of glutamine. Since nitrogen released in the liver as ammonia is unable to enter the urea cycle, ammonia accumulates. The hepatic activities of Krebs-Henseleit urea cycle enzymes have proved to be depressed in liver cirrhosis (Khatra et al. 1974). This, however, does not necessarily account for the decrease in urea synthesis with consequent ammonia accumulation, since changes in hepatic blood flow, hepatic mass, and alternate pathways because of removal of ammonia may also be relevant in this connexion.

Amino acid pattern in derangement, hyperammonemia, and decreased urea synthesis are the qualitative signs of a quantitative dysfunction, such as the negative NB. As has already been reported (Fiaccadori et al. 1981), at the onset of hepatic encephalopathy (HE) all the patients of a studied group showed a negative NB. In the same study a high incidence of this quantitative alteration was observed even in cirrhotics who were seemingly at a clinically compensated stage.

From what has been stated above, one can infer that poor dietary protein intake is

Assessment and Management of Hepatobiliary Disease
Eds.: L. Okolicsányi, G. Csomós, and G. Crepaldi

probably the principal cause of nutritional deficiency in chronic liver disease. In addition, most cirrhotics being alcoholics, disturbances in digestion and absorption may be associated. In this case the provision of adequate nutrition is needed in order to avoid both further damage to the liver and depletion of poor protein stores.

The aims of the present study are (a) to report the nitrogen balance status in cirrhotics both with and without HE, and (b) to evaluate the effects of the measures indicated to restore the NB and, consequently, altered protein metabolism in chronic liver disease. This study deals with three groups of patients with negative NB; the nutritional measures were carried out by either the parenteral or the oral route, according to the clinical conditions.

## Patients and Methods

Nitrogen metabolism was studied in 280 cirrhotic patients consecutively admitted to our department between September 1979 and December 1985.

The diagnosis of liver cirrhosis was based on clinical and laboratory findings, and was confirmed in 253 cases (90.3%) by liver biopsy.

Nitrogen metabolism was assessed by measuring the NB, calculated as the difference between nitrogen intake and urinary (24-h pool) and fecal (3-day pool) excretion; skin losses were assumed to be 0.5 g/day. Following the method of Kopple et al. (Grodstein et al. 1980), the balance was corrected for body weight variation.

One hundred and seventeen (41.8%) of the 280 patients had negative NB and entered the study (Fig. 1). The presence of HE and its grade (evaluated by means of neuroclinical and electroencephalographic parameters) were the criteria used to assign the patients to the different protocols.

The hepatic decompensation was caused by the following factors: HE (62 cases; 52.9%), jaundice (24 cases; 20.5%), ascites (37 cases; 31.6%), gastrointestinal bleeding (12 cases; 10.2%), and hepatorenal syndrome (four cases; 3.4%) (Fig. 2).

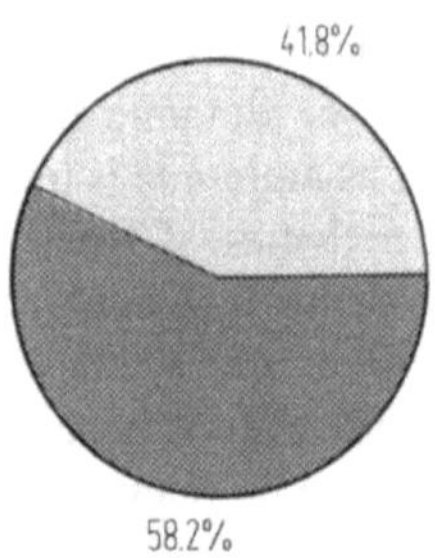


**Fig. 1.** Incidence of positive (▩) and negative (□) nitrogen balance in 280 patients evaluated from September 1979 to December 1985

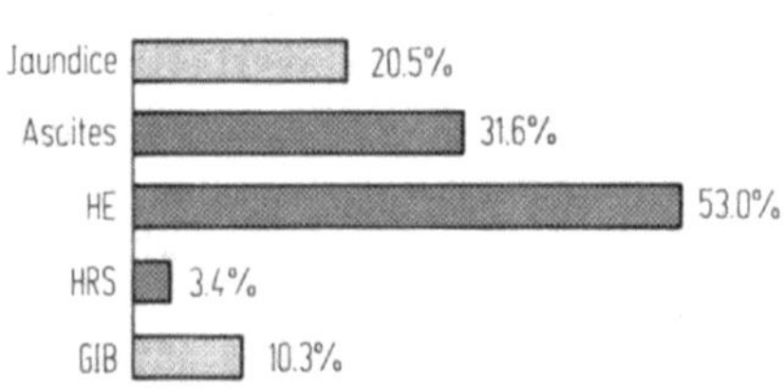


**Fig. 2.** Clinical features of hepatic decompensation in 117 patients with negative nitrogen balance. *GIB*, gastrointestinal bleeding

The caloric intake ranged between 30 and 35 kcal/kg body weight/day for all patients, independently from the protocols used. Treatment with lactulose (administered orally, through a nasogastric tube, or in enema form) in doses varying from 150 to 300 ml/day was combined with each of the therapeutic protocols. Neither steroids nor other drugs were administered during the study period.

The therepeutic protocols were as follows:

*Group A*. Seventy-one patients without HE were given a "metabolic diet" prepared in a special kitchen by trained staff according to the individual patients' tastes with foods selected on the basis of their high BCAA content (Swart et al. 1981). The protein intake was 0.8–1 g/kg BW/day.

NB was evaluated at time 0 and then on the 5th, 10th, and 15th days. During the same period blood urea and blood ammonia were measured, both by the enzymatic method.

*Group B*. In 20 of the 71 patients without previous HE, after the 15 days of treatment by metabolic diet NB was still negative and one or more episodes of recurrent HE (grade I) developed. In these patients the protein intake (see above) was then supplemented with an oral BCAA mixture equal to a protein equivalent of 0.3 g/kg BW/day. The mixture (L-valine 40%, L-leucine 40%, L-isoleucine 20%) was provided in sachets containing 5 g BCAA granular preparation. In all, the protein intake was 1.1 g/kg BW/day; the treatment period lasted 4 weeks. At the baseline time and at the end of treatment the following parameters were evaluated: EEG, number connection test (NCT) according to Conn et al. (Conn and Lieberthal 1979), ammonia, blood urea, *p*-cholinesterase, and aspartate aminotransferase, as well as some nutritional parameters, i.e., albumin and prealbumin, and anthropometric indexes, such as triceps skinfold, mid-arm circumference, and creatinine-height index [expressed as the ratio between daily urinar creatinine excretion of each patient and expected daily urinary creatinine of normal adult subjects of equal height (Bistrian and al. 1975)].

*Group C*. Forty-six patients with grade II–III or IV HE were given total parenteral nutrition (TPN), through a subclavian vein, with hypertonic glucose (30%) plus a special amino acid solution high in BCAA and low in AAA. Among them, 18 died during the observation period (four of recurrent bleedings, one of hepatorenal syndrome (HRS), 13 of HE grade II–IV). NB, blood urea, and blood ammonia were measured in 28 patients before and after 10 days of parenteral treatment. HE grade was assessed by two independent observers evaluating mental state, asterixis, and NCT (only for the patients with grade II and III of HE). EEGs were also performed.

Statistical analysis was performed using Stundent's t-test for paired data at the beginning and at the end of the study. Data were elaborated using an IBM PC/XT.

## Results

### Group A

With regard to the 71 patients who received the metabolic diet alone, 51 of them reached a positive NB after 15 days of treatment (from $-3.99 \pm 1.0$ to $+2.89 \pm 0.78$ g $N_2$/24 h) (Fig. 3).

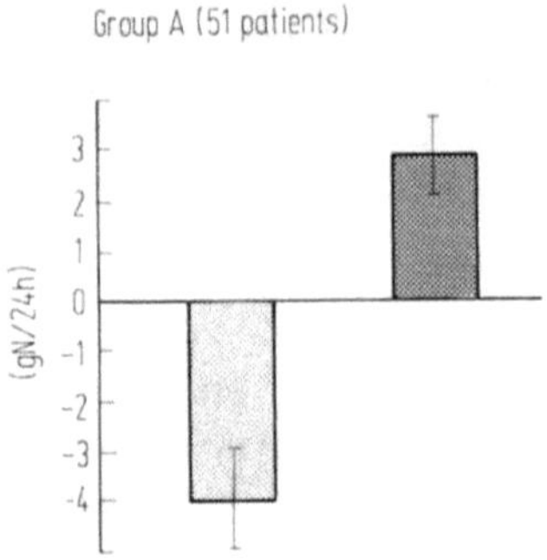


**Fig. 3.** Mean values of NB before oral diet (□) and on the 15th day of oral diet (■) in group A

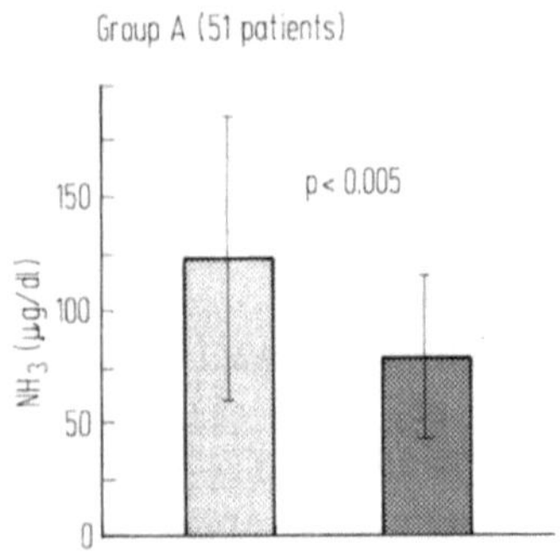


**Fig. 4.** Mean values of ammonia before oral diet (□) and on the 15th day of oral diet (■) in group A

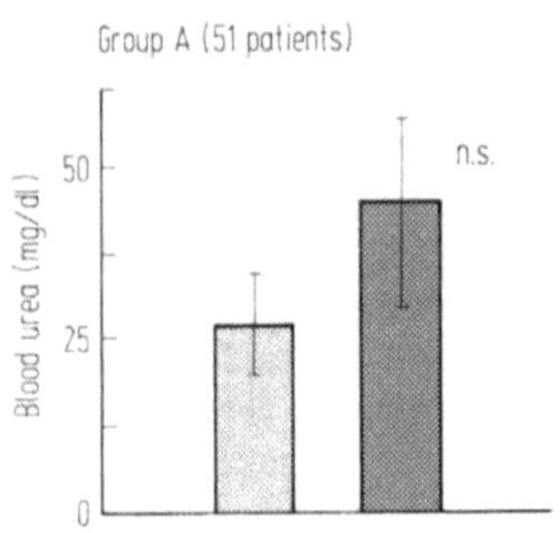


**Fig. 5.** Mean values of blood urea before oral diet (□) and on the 15th day of oral diet (■) in group A

In this group blood ammonia levels showed a statistically significant decrease (from 121.97 ± 63.4 to 76.92 ± 38.3 μg%, $p < .005$) (Fig. 4). Blood urea, however, was increased (from 26 ± 8 to 45 ± 12 mg/dl) (Fig. 5).

## Group B

During the supplementation of the diet with oral BCAA mixture, no patient developed HE. The NCT showed a positive variation in mean performance time (139.4 ± 13.7 and 101.3 ± 9.9 s respectively at the beginning and the end of the treatment, $p < .001$) (Fig. 6). None of the liver chemistry parameters studied achieved statistical significance. The difference between basal and final mean values of blood urea showed sta-

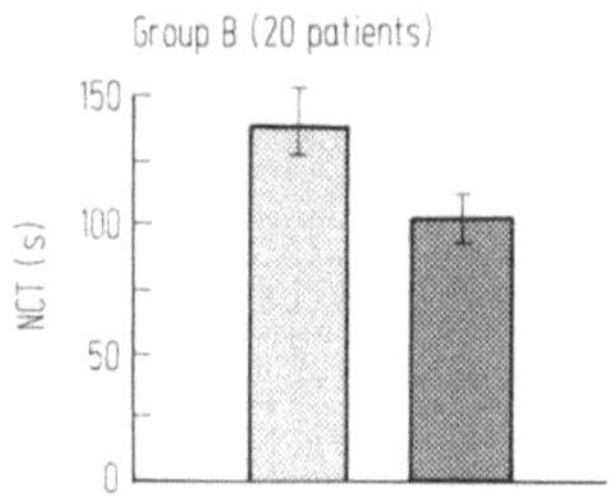


**Fig. 6.** Variations in NCT at beginning (□) and end (■) of oral BCAA supplementation in group B

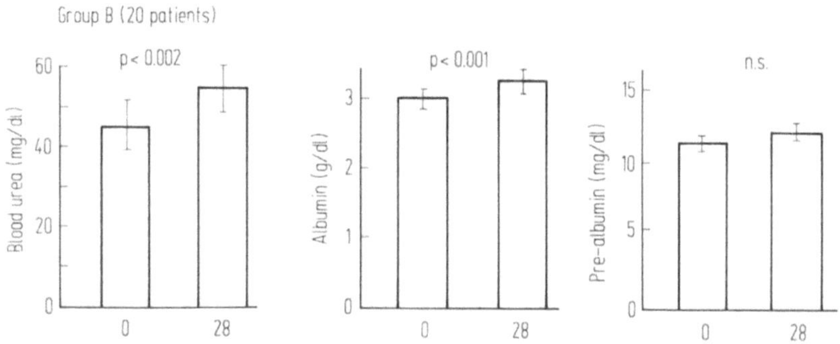


**Fig. 7.** Nutritional parameters before *(0)* and after *(28)* oral BCAA supplementation

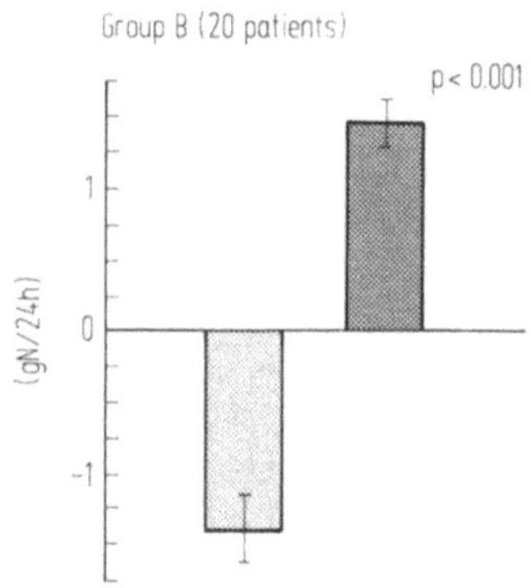


**Fig. 8.** Mean values of NB before BCAA (□) and on the 28th day of oral BCAA supplementation (■) in group B

tistical significance (from 42±4 to 52±4 mg/dl, $p<.002$), as did the albumin values (from 2.94±0.08 to 3.10±0.10 g/l, $p<.001$); prealbumin did not reach statistical significance, although the final values showed a notable increase (from 10.92±0.75 to 12.19±0.97 mg/dl) (Fig. 7). NB achieved positive values in all patients on the 7th day of treatment and the positiveness was maintained at the end of the treatment; the difference between basal and final data (−1.38±0.24 vs +1.45±0.19 g $N_2$/24 h) was highly significant ($p<.001$) (Fig. 8). Regarding the anthropometric measures, the only change to attain statistical significance was that of triceps skinfold which increased from 6.44±0.48 to 7.05±0.56 and from 6.22±0.59 to 7.09±0.64 cm respectively in the right and left arm ($p<0.003$) (Fig. 9). No correlation was found on comparing NB negative or positive values with creatinine-height index (Fig. 10).

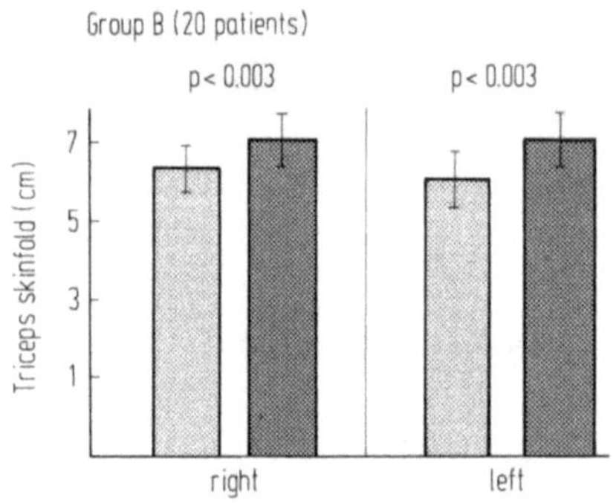


**Fig. 9.** Behavior of triceps skinfold in right and left arm before (□) and after (■) oral BCAA supplementation in group B

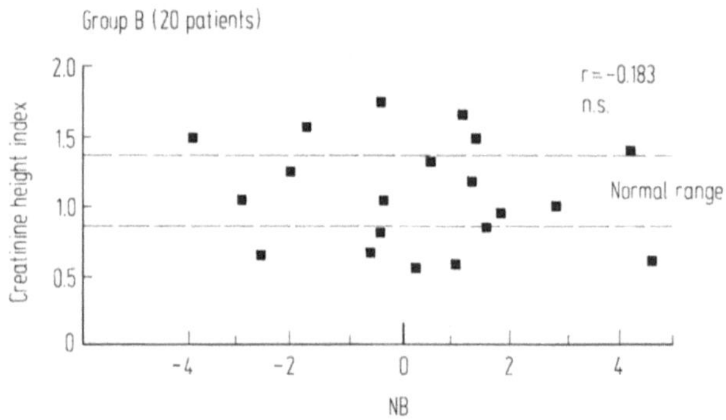


**Fig. 10.** Comparison between creatinine-height index and negative or positive NB in group B. The data show no correlation

## Group C

NB became positive on average on the 10th day of treatment in the 28 cases given TPN (from $-5.11 \pm 0.8$ to $+2.43 \pm 0.7$ g $N_2$/24 h) (Fig. 11). Blood ammonia mean values showed a statistically significant decrease (from $172.31 \pm 64.2$ to $103.60 \pm 61.32$ μg/dl, $p < 0.005$) (Fig. 12); blood urea levels showed a highly significant increase (from $20 \pm 6$ to $33 \pm 8$ mg/dl, $p < 0.001$) (Fig. 13).

## Comment and Conclusions

Attention has recently been drawn to the role played by energy metabolism in determining abnormalities related to HE. In particular, both negative NB and muscle protein breakdown have been described in chronic liver disease (Rikkers et al. 1978).

As previously reported (Fiaccadori et al. 1981), a high incidence or negative NB has been observed even in seemingly compensated cirrhotics, probably as a consequence of inadequate home diet. The lack of both adequate energy supply and suitable protein intake can enhance the catabolic state and lead to a worsening of the patient's conditions. In patients both with and without encephalopathy, nitrogen metabolism imbal-

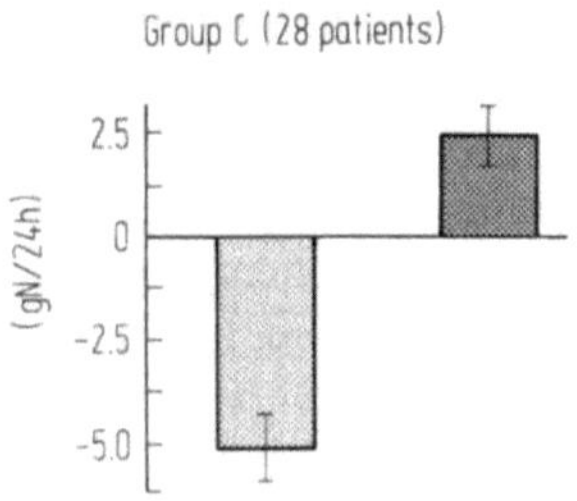


**Fig. 11.** Mean values of NB before (□) and on the 10th day of (■) TPN with BCAA-enriched mixtures in group C

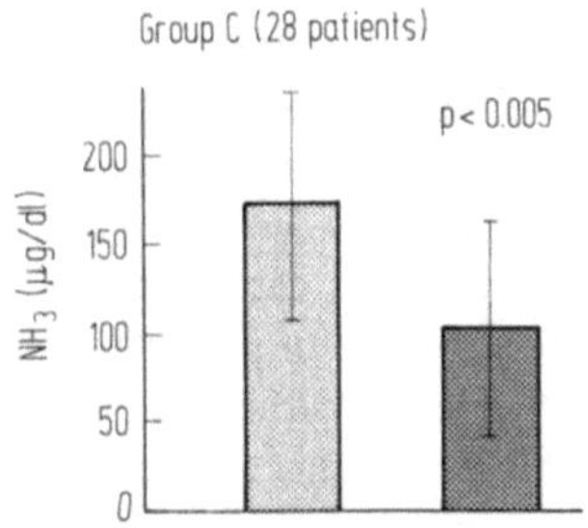


**Fig. 12.** Mean values of ammonia before (□) and on the 10th day of (■) TPN with BCAA-enriched mixtures in group C

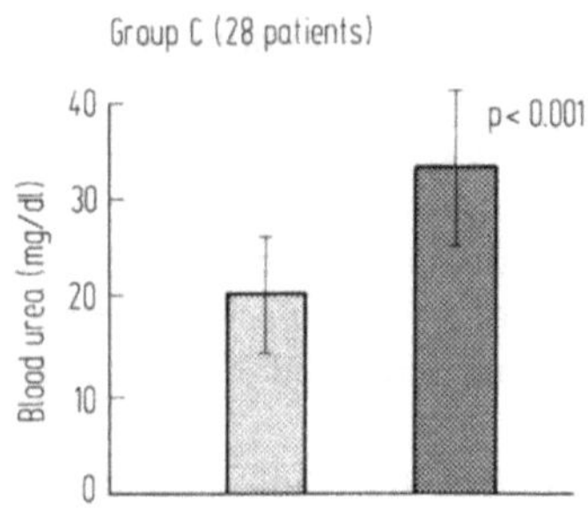


**Fig. 13.** Mean values of blood urea before (□) and on the 10th day of (■) TPN with BCAA-enriched mixtures in group C

ance is expressed by low urea levels, hyperammonemia, and altered amino acid pattern. This is a result of the utilization of endogenous body protein as a source of energy, the cirrhotic liver being unable to metabolize AAA: the consumption of BCAA by muscle, kidney, and fat is therefore increased. It follows that the administration of adequate nutritional support with an appropriate supply of proteins and calories represents a cornerstone of the treatment. Nevertheless, in patients who are both protein-intolerant and protein-depleted, the protein component of the nutritional therapy remains one of the main problems.

Theoretically, infusion or oral administration of adequate amounts of BCAA should promote positive NB, stimulate muscle protein synthesis, and decrease muscle degradation without precipitating encephalopathy (Marchesini et al. 1982).

For many years, solutions rich in BCAA and low in AAA have been suggested as a nutritional support. This therapeutic approach seems to give an adequate answer to the problem, by either correcting the altered plasma amino acid pattern or supplying a sufficient protein equivalent. The amino acid composition of the mixture utilized in this study was in agreement with Fischer's principles, i.e., was aimed at normalizing the plasma amino acid imbalance together with both reversal of encephalopathy and efficacious nutrition.

As for the HE problem, the results of some prospective randomized trials on patients with a severe clinical picture using both dextrose as a source of energy and enriched BCAA solutions, the efficacy of BCAA has been clearly established, in terms of both recovery from coma and survival, in respect to controls (Cerra et al. 1982; Fiaccadori et al. 1985; Rossi-Fanelli et al. 1982).

Moreover, achievement of a positive NB has been reported by many authors in patients given BCAA mixtures, the improvement being correlated with a trend toward normalization in plasma amino acid pattern (Fiaccadori et al. 1984a) along with the decrease in ammonia levels and reversal of clinical encephalopathy signs.

In the present study the results obbained in group C confirm that at more advanced stages of encephalopathy, TPN by BCAA-enriched mixtures influences the NB and effects clinical and neurological improvement by correcting the previous catabolic state. The clinical conditions seem not to be influenced by the different types of precipitating factors. It has already been reported (Fiaccadori et al. 1981; Holdsworth et al. 1981) that treatment with glucose only failed to improve the neurological status and to bring the patients to a positive NB, although this treatment was associated with NB less negative than before commencing therapy, probably since it prevents the use of endogenous proteins as a source of energy and acts upon the insulin/glucagon ratio (Marchesini et al. 1981).

It is worth pointing out that in the study mentioned above (Fiaccadori et al. 1984a, b), patients with grade IV HE given TPN including BCAA-enriched solutions showed a negative correlation between NB and BCAA/AAA ratio initially, but a positive correlation after 7 days of treatment, owing to the decrease of AAA. A positive correlation between the amount of BCAA given intravenously and improved NB had also been found by Freund et al. (1979, 1982).

Finally, in a study (Marchesini et al. 1982) on six cirrhotics, the venous administration of a BCAA mixture for 3 days and of the same mixture together with 250 g glucose daily for 3 more days was associated with a reduction in both AAA concentration and methylhistidine excretion, while plasma alanine levels increased. These phenomena were offered as evidence of reduced muscle catabolism.

The efficacy of the oral treatment with BCAA was shown in some anectodal series (Egberts et al. 1985; Horst et al. 1984), where NB and encephalopathic signs were carefully monitored. Horst's study clearly showed that a BCAA-supplemented diet was superior to a mixed-protein one in preventing HE in susceptible patients. Egberts et al., in a cross-over trial against placebo, demonstrated the nutritional efficacy of equimolar amounts of BCAA given with a dietary base. Besides the achievement of positive NB and a decrease in ammonia levels, possibly due to anabolic effect, the authors demonstrated an improvement of cerebral functions as measured by psychometric tests. In another study (Holm 1982), patients receiving first a standard diet and then a BCAA-supplemented diet showed, as a result of the supplementation, a high (about 100%) increase of plasma valine, leucine, and isoleucine. BCAA given orally are also known to increase protein tolerance and to induce positive NB to approximately the same degree as an equivalent amount of dietary protein without inducing encephalopathy as frequently (Fiaccadori et al. 1984b).

In contrast, no improvement was achieved by dietary BCAA supplementation in HE in a cross-over trial involving a small number of patients carried out by Eriksson and Wahren (1981). Their results have been strongly criticized by Fischer (1984), who denied that their study could be taken as an indication of an unfavorable trend. In four cirrhotics given either 50 g of a casein diet or 20 g of casein plus 30 g of protein equivalent by BCAA, no difference was demonstrated between the two treatments for NB mean values. Thus, it has been assumed that oral BCAA mixture supplementation has the same capacity of restoring negative NB as has casein. Although it leads the amino acid pattern toward normal, it does not ameliorate encephalopathy (McGhee et al. 1983).

Our study was aimed at demonstrating that a well-balanced oral diet can also improve malnutrition and/or nutrient abnormalities developing in chronic liver disease, and that in case of protein intolerance with clinical related symptoms, BCAA oral supplementation is able to correct this abnormality without the necessity of reducing protein intake.

In our patients liver function was relatively stable, so that they appeared the most suitable for demonstrating the effects of the new therapeutic approach. Besides, therapeutic alternatives would have been either protein restriction, which may have unfavorable side effects when applied for long periods, or increased lactulose doses, the side effects of which are taste and abdominal discomfort leading to poor compliance in the long term.

Fifty-one of 71 cirrhotics with negative NB of the group A reached the positivity after a dietary protein intake of 0.8–1 g/kg BW/day together with 30–35 kcal/kg/day. This indicates previous inappropriate protein and/or caloric nutrition which can be corrected by a well-balanced diet. Twenty of the 71 patients, on the same diet, developed one or more episodes of HE, which indicates protein intolerance and reveals a latent encephalopathic state. In this situation characterized by persistently negative NB, protein restriction could worsen instead of improving the clinical state. We then thought it suitable to give the patients an extra selected isonitrogenous amount of BCAA: during the observation period, these patients showed neither clinical worsening nor HE episodes. The improvement was parallel to NB positivity, meaning the protein dietary intolerance can be corrected by BCAA supplementation. The altered psychometric tests (i.e., NCT) also came down to the normal range; among anthropometric indexes triceps skinfold showed a statistically significant increase. In keeping with the results of other authors (Holm et al. 1983), some nutritional parameters, i.e., urea and albumin, also showed a statistically significant difference between basal and final mean values. No variations were observed in liver function tests.

Although the minimum protein requirement in advanced liver disease has been calculated as $0.74 \pm 0.08$ g/kg/day (Swart et al. 1981), this has not been confirmed in our selected cases. Their nitrogen balance, indeed, was negative even after 15 days of a diet with 0.8 g/kg/day protein intake: for this reason their diet was orally supplemented by an isonitrogenous amount of BCAA corresponding to 0.3 g/kg/day. Our results confirm the possibility of supplementing a basal diet of 0.8 g/kg/day in cirrhotics affected by episodic encephalopathy with a surplus of protein equivalent until a positive NB can be reached and maintained: this supplementation involves neither unfavorable neuroclinical signs nor side effects during the period of treatment.

We can conclude that supplementation by BCAA must be reserved for (a) residual cases without HE, nonresponders to the dietetic treatment alone; and (b) all cases with episodic or recurrent HE presenting both negative NB and alterations in psychometric tests after the failure of a diet with minimum protein requirement.

*Acknowledgements.* We are grateful to Prof. Sergio Tognella (Boehringer Biochemia Robin, Milan) for his help in supplying the mixtures of amino acids (BS 666-BS 692-BS702) and to T. Annese, D. Rinaldi, N. Soverini and F. Tanferri of the Dietary Service of Parma Regional Hospital for their continuous cooperation in diet controls.

## References

Bistrian BR, Blackburn GL, Sherman M, Scrimshaw NS (1975) Therapeutic index of nutritional depletion in hospitalized patients. Surg Gynecol Obstet 141: 512

Cerra FB, Cheung NK, Fischer JE (1982) A multicenter trial of branched chain enriched amino-acid infusion (F080) in hepatic encephalopathy (HE). Hepatology 2: 699

Conn HO, Lieberthal MM (1979) Assessment of mental state. In: Conn HO, Lieberthal MM (eds) The hepatic coma syndromes and lactulose. Williams and Wilkins, Baltimore, pp 169-188

Egberts EH, Schomerus H, Hamster W, Jurgens PJ (1985) Branched chain aminoacids in the treatment of latent portosystemic encephalopathy. A double blind placebo-controlled cross-over study. Gastroenterology 88: 887-895

Eriksson S, Wahren J (1981) Failure of oral branched chain aminoacids administration to improve chronic hepatic encephalopathy. In: Walser M, Williamson JR (eds) Metabolism and clinical implications of branched chain amino and ketoacids. Elsevier/North Holland, New York, pp 481-485

Fiaccadori F, Ghinelli F, Pedretti G, Pelosi G, Sacchini D, Spadini G (1981) Negative nitrogen balance in cirrhotics. A correct therapeutic approach. Ric Clin Lab 11: 259-268

Fiaccadori F, Ghinelli F, Pedretti G, Pelosi G, Sacchini D (1984a) Different nutritional approaches in liver cirrhosis. Effects on nitrogen balance, preliminary report. Front Gastrointest Res 8: 254-265

Fiaccadori F, Ghinelli F, Pedretti G, Perinotto P (1984b) Oral BCAA as nutritional supplementation in cirrhotics. In: Holm E, Kasper H (eds) Metabolism and nutrition in liver disease. MTP Press, Lancaster, pp 351-354

Fiaccadori F, Ghinelli F, Pedretti G, Pelosi G, Sacchini D, Zeneroli ML, Rocchi E, Gibertini P, Ventura E (1985) Branched chain enriched aminoacid solutions in the treatment of hepatic encephalopathy: a controlled trial. Ital J Gastroenterol 17: 5-10

Fischer JE (1984) Branched chain aminoacids in hepatic encephalopathy: results of parenteral trials. In: Holm E, Kasper H (eds) Metabolism and nutrition in liver disease. MTP Press, Lancaster, pp 259-273

Freund H, Yoshimura N, Fischer JE (1979) Chronic hepatic encephalopathy. Long term therapy with a branched chain aminoacid enriched elemental diet. JAMA 242: 347

Freund H, Dienstag J, Lehrich J, Yoshimura N, Bradford RR, Rosen H, Atamian S, Slemmer E, Holroyde J, Fischer JE (1982) Infusion of branched chain enriched aminoacid solutions in patients with hepatic encephalopathy. Ann Surg 196: 209-220

Grodstein GP, Blumenkrantz MJ, Kopple JD (1980) Nutritional and metabolic response to catabolic stress in uremia. Am J Clin Nutr 33: 1411-1416

Holdsworth JD, Clague MB, James OFW (1981) The effect of branched chain aminoacid infusion on protein synthesis and breakdown in chronic liver disease. Proceedings of 16th Meeting EASL, Lisbon

Holm E (1982) BCAA enriched diets for oral treatment of patients with liver cirrhosis: a controlled study of biochemical variables, psychometric performance and the EEG. Ajimoto Symposium, Raleigh

Holm E, Leweling H, Staedt U (1983) Metabolism and nutritional supply of aminoacids in hepatic failure. In: Kleinberger G, Deutsch E (eds) New aspects of clinical nutrition. Karger, Basel, pp 377-399

Horst D, Grace ND, Conn HO, Schiff E, Schenker S, Viteri A, Law D, Atterbury CE (1984) Comparison of dietary protein with an oral branched chain enriched aminoacid supplement in chronic portal systemic encephalopathy: A randomized controlled trial. Hepatology 4: 279-287

Khatra BS, Smith RB, Millikan WG, Sewell CW, Warren WD, Rudman D (1974) Activities of Krebs-Henseleit enzymes in normal and cirrhotic human liver. J Lab Clin Med 84: 708-715

Marchesini G, Zoli M, Angiolini A (1981) Muscle protein breakdown in liver cirrhosis and their role of altered carbohydrate metabolism. Hepatology 1: 294-299

Marchesini G, Zoli M, Dondi C, Bianchi GP, Cirulli M, Pisi E (1982) Anticatabolic effect of branched chain aminoacid enriched solutions in patients with liver cirrhosis. Hepatology 2: 420-425

McGhee A, Hendersson JM, Millikan WJ, Bleier JC, Vogel R, Kassouny M, Rudman D (1983) Comparison of the effects of hepatic-aid and a casein modular diet on encephalopathy, plasma aminoacids, and nitrogen balance in cirrhotic patients. Ann Surg 3: 288-293

Mezey E (1978) Liver disease and nutrition. Gastroenterology 74: 770-783

Rikkers L, Jenko P, Rudman D, Freides D (1978) Subclinical hepatic encephalopathy detection, prevalence and relationship to nitrogen metabolism. Gastroenterology 75: 462

Rosen HM, Yoshimura N, Hodgman JM, Fischer JE (1977) Plasma aminoacid patterns in hepatic encephalopathy of differing etiology. Gastroenterology 72: 482-487

Rossi-Fanelli F, Riggio O, Cangiano C, Cascino A, de Conciliis D, Merli M, Stortoni M, Giunchi G (1982) Branched chain aminoacids vs lactulose in the treatment of hepatic coma. A controlled study. Dig Dis Sci 27: 929-935

Rudman D, di Fulco TJ, Galambos JT (1973) Maximal rates of excretion and synthesis of urea in normal and cirrhotic subjects. J Clin Invest 52: 2241-24249

Soeters PB, Fischer JE (1976) Insulin, glucagon, aminoacid imbalance, and hepatic encephalopathy. Lancet 2: 880-882

Strata A, Giuberti T, Magnati G, Regolisti M, Sacchini D, Fiaccadori F (1984) Diete ad apporto proteico controllato e prevenzione dell'encefalopatia epatica. Minerva Dietol Gastroenterol 3: 245-250

Swart GR, Frenkel M, van den Berg IWO (1981) Minimum protein requirements in advanced liver disease; a metabolic ward study of the effects of oral branched chain aminoacids. In: Walser M, Williamson GR (eds) Metabolic and clinical implications of branched chain amino and ketoacids. Elsevier/North Holland, New York, pp 427-432

# The Management of Primary Biliary Cirrhosis

Maria Chiaramonte, Annarosa Floreani, and Remo Naccarato

Divisione Convenzionata di Gastroenterologia "R. Farini" Istituto di Medicina Interna, Policlinico Universitario, Via Giustiniani, 2, 35100-Padova, Italy

Primary biliary cirrhosis (PBC) is a chronic liver disease involving the intrahepatic bile ducts and progressing to liver failure. The etiology and pathogenic mechanisms are unknown, but there is much evidence for an autoimmune process [1]. Although the incidence in Italy is unknown, in England an incidence of 5.8 cases per million population and a prevalence of 54 cases per million are reported [2-4]. The classic signs include pruritus, jaundice, fatigability, and xanthomatosis. However, PBC includes heterogeneous groups of patients: asymptomatic, with symptoms of cholestasis and/or autoimmune conditions, and with decompensated cirrhosis.

The diagnosis in asymptomatic patients is often made after a physician investigates the cause of unexplained hepatomegaly or an elevated level of serum alkaline phosphatase found during a routine examination. The life expectancy in asymptomatic patients does not differ from that of a control population matched for age and sex [5]. Thus these patients probably do not require any treatment, especially considering that so far no one drug which may act on immunological mechanisms has been shown to be of certain benefit in this disease. In the other groups of patients, treatment can be divided into three areas: relief of symptoms and prevention of complications, specific therapy, and liver transplantation.

## Relief of Symptoms and Prevention of Complications

*Pruritus* (Table 1) is usually well alleviated by cholestyramine, which binds bile salts in the gut, preventing their enterohepatic circulation. The doses vary individually between 8 and 24 g/day preferentially before meals.

Patients with intractable itching may need high doses, but in these cases osteomalacia and hypoprothrombinemia may get worse because cholestyramine reduces fat-solu-

**Table 1.** Management of pruritus in PBC

| Treatment | Dosage |
|---|---|
| Cholestyramine | 4-24 g/day per os |
| Terfenadine | 60 mg twice daily per os |
| Chlorpheniramine maleate | 4 mg twice daily per os |
| Phenobarbital | 50 mg per os at bedtime |
| Zinc sulphate | 220 mg 2-3 times/day |
| Phototherapy | ultraviolet B irradiation for 9-12 min/day |
| Plasmapheresis | ? |

Assessment and Management of Hepatobiliary Disease
Eds.: L. Okolicsányi, G. Csomós, and G. Crepaldi

ble vitamin absorption. It has recently been suggested that terfenadine, a new specific antihistamine that is relatively free of sedative side effects, may be effective in controlling this symptom [6].

In severe cases small doses of phenobarbital at bedtime may be added [7]. Phototherapy with ultraviolet B irradiation has been proposed in intractable pruritus [8]. Serum bile acid concentrations decrease after exposure for 9–12 min a day, and temporary relief can be obtained, but pruritus recurs within 2 weeks. Thus phototherapy is ineffective in the late stages of the disease [9].

Plasmapheresis has been used in sporadic cases of intractable pruritus and neuropathy due to xanthomatosis [10]. However, the high cost and the considerable risk of side effects, such as non-A, non-B hepatitis, limit the use of this technique to selected cases.

*Steatorrhea,* usually associated with bile secretory failure or pancreatic insufficiency, can be reduced by a diet with low fat content and with medium-chain triglycerides which do not require bile salts for absorption.

*Pancreatic dysfunction,* which may be attributed to "dry gland syndrome," is common in PBC, but severe pancreatic failure is quite rare [11, 12]. These cases respond to conventional management with oral pancreatic enzyme supplements together with a histamine $H_2$-receptor blocker (cimetidine or ranitidine) as required. Fat-soluble vitamin should be administered parenterally every 4 weeks. Vitamin A may be administered orally (25000–50000 U/day for 4–12 weeks) in patients with abnormal dark adaptation or skin lesions [13]. Shepherd et al. [14] suggest that routine treatment with vitamin A is not indicated because of the hepatotoxicity of this vitamin. Vitamin A supplementation should not be given to women of childbearing age, since it is teratogenic [15]. Low serum zinc levels may be corrected by oral supplementation ($3 \times 220$ mg daily).

Very occasional in PBC is the association with *osteodystrophy.* Osteomalacia does occur infrequently but readily improves on oral or parenteral administration of vitamin D or its active metabolites [16]. Osteoporosis, characterized by a reduction in bone mineral mass without impairment of bone mineralization, is more common than osteomalacia. Oral vitamin D (25-hydroxy-vitamin $D_3$) fails to improve osteoporosis [17, 18]; more benefit seems to be gained from parenteral administration of vitamin D (100000 U i.m. every 4 weeks). Furthermore, a controlled trial in 64 postmenopausal PBC women receiving parenteral vitamin $D_2$ showed that addition of calcium gluconate and microcrystalline hydroxyapatite compound prevents bone thinning and promotes positive cortical bone balance [19].

Dislipidemia, very frequent in PBC patients, is characterized by increased serum cholesterol phospholipids, HDL cholesterol, and also lipoproteins such as LDL and $HDL_2$ [53, 54]. HDL cholesterol is statistically correlated to serum cholesterol, in contrast to familial hypercholesterolemia and other forms of cholestasis, and this might explain the relative lack of atherosclerotic lesions in PBC patients.

No specific treatment for dislipidemia is required. If dislipidemia is associated with bile secretory failure with steatorrhea, a low-fat diet is indicated.

## Treatment of Major Complications

In the late stages, management of major complications such as ascites, bleeding from oesophageal varices, and encephalopathy should be considered. In these cases treatment is the same as in other forms of end-stage liver disease. Ascites should be controlled by diet with salt restriction and aldosterone antagonists. Although esophageal bleeding is rare at the time of presentation of the disease, portal hypertension is common, even in patients with normal bilirubin and no regenerative nodules on biopsy [20]. It has been suggested that this may partially be explained by the pericellular fibrosis which surrounds sinusoidal areas, so that portal hypertension in PBC may originate at a sinusoidal rather than postsinusoidal level [21].

Esophageal varices were recognized in 20%, 50%, and 90% at 1, 3, and 9 years respectively after the onset of pruritus and/or itching in a follow-up of 24 PBC patients [22]. In another study the mean duration of survival from the time that portal hypertension was recognized was 14.9 months [20]. Endoscopic injection sclerotherapy probably produces an improvement in survival, although no controlled trials relate specifically to PBC.

The management of encephalopathy, as in other forms of chronic liver disease, includes dairy and vegetable protein diets with oral branched-chain amino acids, lactulose, and paramomicine.

## Specific Treatment

The goal of specific treatment in PBC is the improvement of (1) symptoms, (2) biochemical abnormalities, (3) histological progression and (4) survival. Unfortunately, so far no progress has been made in specific treatment. The main reason is that the pathogenic mechanism of PBC is still unknown.

Penicillamine seemed at one time to be the best such treatment, credited with copper chelation [23]. reduction in collagen synthesis [24], and immunosuppression [25]. Between 1977 and 1984, 767 patients were included in seven trials in Europe and the United States (Table 2). The oral dose varied between 250 and 1000 mg/day. After the first enthusiastic preliminary report from thc Royal Free Hospital, in which statistically significant reductions in copper concentration, AST, and immune complexes [26, 27] were demonstrated, the conclusive results of the trials failed to show any beneficial effect of D-penicillamine. All the studies report a high percentage of severe side effects (average 30%), including bone marrow suppression, proteinuria, myasthenia gravis, skin lesions, and cholestatic snydrome (see Table 2). Although a modest improvement in biochemical indexes may occur, no statistical benefit concerning survival has been reported. After these discouraging results it is clear that the cost/benefit ratio is too high to justify treatment with penicillamine in a wide number of patients [37]. There is probably little justification for any of the mechanisms of action which have been postulated in PBC. Although liver copper concentration may reach levels similar to those occurring in Wilson's disease, there is no evidence that copper plays a significant role in the pathogenesis of PBC [38]. On the other hand, immune complexes may be only an epiphenomenon, rather than an important pathogenic factor [39].

**Table 2.** Controlled trials of D-penicillamine

| Trials | No. of patients | Dose (mg/day) | Side effects | Conclusive results | | Biochemical improvement |
|---|---|---|---|---|---|---|
| | | | | Histological progression | Survival | |
| European multicenter [25] | 189 | 1200 | 36% (severe) | No benefit | No benefit | No benefit |
| Royal Free Hospital [26-29] | 98 | 600 | 33% (severe) | No benefit | No benefit | No benefit |
| Mayo Clinic [31, 32] | 310 | 1000 | 105/106 | No benefit | No benefit | ↓AST, immunoglobulins, copper |
| Boston [30] | 52 | 1000 | 31% (severe) | No benefit | No benefit | ↓AST, copper |
| Newcastle [34] | 59 | 250-1000 | 37.5% (severe) | No benefit | No benefit | ↓AST, alkaline phosphatase, immunoglobulins |
| Sheffield [35] | 35 | 875 | 1 patient withdrawn | Benefit [36] | No benefit | No benefit |
| Holland [36] | 24 | 1000 | 22% (severe) | No benefit | No benefit | ↓Immunoglobulins, copper |

Other treatments are at present under consideration, in spite of their side effects. Corticosteroids have been administered in only a small number of patients because they may induce osteoporosis [40, 41]. These sporadic reports are not valuable, but until the results of controlled trials are available, corticosteroids may be considered for a small group of symptomatic patients with autoimmune-associated disorders (systemic lupus erythematosus, rheumatoid arthritis, myasthenia gravis) and in mixed forms of PBC with chronic active hepatitis [42]. The doses should be kept (about 10 mg prednisolone daily) with calcium and vitamin D supplementation.

Cyclosporin, another interesting immunosuppressive drug, has been used in two studies. In the first [43], six patients received cyclosporin at a dose of 10 mg/kg/day for 8 weeks. A decreased helper/suppressor T lymphocyte ratio and an improvement in alkaline phosphatase were reported. Unfortunately the study had to be stopped after 8 weeks because of nephrotoxicity. In the second pilot study, ten patients received cyclosporin at a dose of 150-300 mg daily for 6 months. Biochemical improvement was modest, with relief of pruritus in five of seven patients and of the symptoms of sicca syndrome in three of three patients. The drug improved T suppressor function [44]. Further major trials with this drug are now in progress. Chlorambucil, an alkylating agent, has been administered in a single randomized trial by the National Institutes of Health in Bethesda [45]. Thirteen patients received chlorambucil (0.5-4 mg/day) and 11 received placebo. Evaluations revealed lower mean serum bilirubin at 2 years and lower mean IgM levels at 1, 2, and 3 years in treated patients. Hepatic histology demonstrated a marked decrease in inflammatory infiltrates in six of ten treated patients and in three of ten control patients. Nevertheless, chlorambucil had to be permanently discontinued in four patients because of marrow suppression (Table 3). After this trial chlorambucil has been abandoned because of the risk of acute leukemia in long-term treatment.

More encouraging, though controversial, are the data regarding azathioprine. Two

**Table 3.** PBC specific therapy: chlorambucil

| | Treated | Untreated |
|---|---|---|
| No. of patients | 13 | 11 |
| Dose | 0.5-4 mg/day | |
| Follow-up | | |
| - Biochemical improvement | ↓bilirubin at 2 years<br>↓IgM at 1, 2, 3 years | - |
| - Histological improvement | 6/10 | 3/10 |
| - Severe side effects | 4/13 | |

Hoofnagle et al. [45]

**Table 4.** Controlled trials with azathioprine in PBC

| | | Dose | Histology | Duration | Survival | Biochemical parameters |
|---|---|---|---|---|---|---|
| Royal Free Hospital 1976 [46] | 22 drug<br>23 placebo | 2 mg/kg | No improvement | 6 years | No benefit | No change |
| International group (First report, 1980) [47] | 124 drug<br>112 placebo | 300-700 mg | No improvement | 18 months | No benefit | ↑albumin, ↓IgG, ↓thyroid antibody |
| (Final report, 1985) [48] | 127 drug<br>121 placebo | 300-700 mg | No improvement | 10 years | Benefit ($p < 0.01$) | No change |

controlled trials performed by the Royal Free Hospital group and by an international group showed that azathioprine does not significantly alter the immunologic or histologic processes [46, 47]. Nevertheless, final evaluation of the latest study has shown a significant beneficial effect of azathioprine on survival [48] (Table 4). The authors suggest that the discrepancy between the results in the two previous reports and their own is due to type 2 error, because of small sample size in the Royal Free Hospital study and limited duration of follow-up in the preliminary report of the international trial. However, the results of this report do not prove that azathioprine is the best treatment in PBC [49].

## Liver Transplantation

Individual high-risk PBC patients may be candidates for liver transplantation, but identification of them is very difficult. So far the best indication is an intolerable quality of life in the preterminal stage, characterized by intractable itching, marked and prolonged alteration of serum bilirubin, and bone disease [50]. Among the major contraindications to transplantation (Table 5) is age >55 years. In fact the average age of patients at diagnosis is about 50-55 years [4], so that in the late stage many exceed this limit. Another problem may be the recurrence of PBC in transplanted patients [51]. However, graft reaction may mimic PBC and differential diagnosis is very difficult. Thus the real potential recurrence remains to be established.

Analysis of data on 540 patients from 4 centers in the United States and Western Europe demonstrates that 3-year survival in PBC patients is about 45% [52]. Survival

**Table 5.** Indications and contraindications for liver transplant in PBC patients

| |
|---|
| *Indications* |
| Intolerable quality of life. |
| Intractable itching and jaundice in preterminal stages. |
| Decompensated cirrhosis |
| *Contraindications* |
| Absolute |
| - portal vein thrombosis |
| - severe hypoxemia due to right-to-left shunts |
| - sepsis outside the hepatobiliary system |
| - primary malignant disease outside the hepatobiliary system |
| - advanced cardiopulmonary or renal disease |
| - age >55 years |
| - inability to accept the procedure or understand its nature and/or costs |
| Relative |
| - prior abdominal surgery, particularly in the right upper quadrant |

tends to be greater for patients transplanted after January 1, 1980 than before this date, and it has been suggested that this improvement may not be wholly attributable to the more recent use of cyclosporin [52]. Despite the problems this high-risk procedure seems to be the best chance for patients with late-stage decompensated disease.

## References


1. James SP, Hoofnagle JH, Strober W, Jones EA (1983) Primary biliary cirrhosis: a model of autoimmune disease. Ann Int Med 99: 500-512
2. Hamlyn AN, Maklon AM, James O (1980) Primary biliary cirrhosis (PBC): controlled study of epidemicity and symptom onset seasonality. Gut 21: A899
3. Stuart Hislop W (1980) Primary biliary cirrhosis: an epidemiological study. Br Med J 281: 1069-1070
4. Triger DR (1980) Primary biliary cirrhosis: an epidemiological study. Br Med J 281: 772-775
5. Roll J, Boyer JL, Barry D, Klatskin G (1983) The prognostic importance of clinical and histologic features in asymptomatic and symptomatic primary biliary cirrhosis. N Engl J Med 308: 1-7
6. Duncan JS, Kennedy HJ, Triger DR (1984) Treatment of pruritus due to chronic obstructive liver disease. Br Med J 289: 22
7. Sherlock S (1985) Cholestasis. In: Diseases of the liver and biliary system, 6th edn. Blackwell, Oxford
8. Perlstein SM (1981) Phototherapy for primary biliary cirrhosis. Arch Dermatol 117: 608
9. Hanid MA, Levi AJ (1980) Phototherapy for pruritus in primary biliary cirrhosis. Lancet 2: 530
10. Cohen LB, Ambinder EP, Wolke AM, Field SP, Schaffner F (1985) Role of plasmapheresis in primary biliary cirrhosis. Gut 26: 291-294
11. Klass HJ, Braganza JM, Warnes TW (1979) The pancreas in primary biliary cirrhosis. Gut 20: A443
12. Epstein O, Chapman RWG, Lake-Bakaar G, Foo AY, Rosalk SB, Sherlock S (1982) The pancreas in primary biliary cirrhosis and sclerosing cholangitis. Gastroenterology 83: 1177-1182
13. Walt RP, Kemp CM, Lyness L, Bird AC, Sherlock S (1984) Vitamin A treatment for night blindness in primary biliary cirrhosis. Br Med J 288: 1030-1031
14. Shepherd AN, Bedford GJ, Hill A, Bouchier IAD (1984) Primary biliary cirrhosis, dark adaptometry, electrooculography, and vit A state. Br Med J 289: 1484-1485

15. Hall JG (1984) Vitamin A teratogenicity. N Engl J Med 311: 797-798
16. Davies M, Mawer EB, Klass HJ, Lumb GA, Berry JL, Warnes TW (1983) Vitamin D deficiency, osteomalacia, and primary biliary cirrhosis. Response to orally administered vitamin $D_3$. Dig Dis Sci 28: 145-153
17. Herlong HF, Recker RR, Maddrey WC (1982) Bone disease in primary biliary cirrhosis: histologic features and response to 25-hydroxyvitamin D. Gastroenterology 83: 103-108
18. Matloff DS, Kaplan MM, Neer RM, Goldberg MJ, Bitman W, Wolfe HJ (1982) Osteoporosis in primary biliary cirrhosis: effects of 25-hydroxy-vitamin $D_3$ treatment. Gastroenterology 83: 97-102
19. Epstein O, Kato Y, Dick R, Sherlock S (1982) Vitamin D hydroxyapatite and calcium gluconate in treatment of cortical bone thinning in postmenopausal women with primary biliary cirrhosis. Am J Clin Nutr 36: 426-430
20. Kew MC, Varma RR, Dos Santos HA, Scheuer PJ, Sherlock S (1971) Portal hypertension in primary biliary cirrhosis. Gut 12: 830-834
21. Warnes TW, Smith A, Haboubi NY, Cope V, Vales P (1984) Portal hypertension in primary biliary corrhosis (PBC) – an early assault on the sinusoids? Hepatology 4: 751
22. Lebrec D, Sicot C, Degott C, Benhamou G-P (1976) Portal hypertension and primary biliary cirrhosis. Digestion 14: 220-226
23. Deering TB, Dickson ER, Fleming CR, Geall MG, McCall JT, Baggenstoss AH (1977) Effect of D-penicillamine on copper retention in patients with primary biliary cirrhosis. Gastroenterology 72: 1208-1212
24. Deshmukh K, Nimni ME (1969) A defect in the intramolecular and intermolecular cross linking of collagen caused by penicillamine. J Biol Chem 244: 1787-1795
25. Multicentre Trial Group (1975) Controlled trial of D-penicillamine in severe rheumatoid arthritis: double blind controlled study of a high and low dose regimen. Ann Rheum Dis 34: 416-421
26. Jaun S, Scheuer PJ, Samourian S, McGee JOD, Sherlock S (1977) A controlled trial of D-penicillamine therapy in primary biliary cirrhosis. Lancet 1: 831-834
27. Epstein O, De-Villiers D, Jain S, Potter BJ, Thomas HC, Sherlock S (1979) Reduction of immune complexes and immunoglobulins induced by D-penicillamine in primary biliary cirrhosis. N Engl J Med 300: 274-278
28. Epstein O, Jain S, Lee RG, Cook DG, Boss AM, Scheuer PJ, Sherlock S (1981) D-Penicillamine treatment improves survival in primary biliary cirrhosis. Lancet 1: 1275-1277
29. Epstein O, Cook DG, Jain S, Sherlock S (1985) D-Penicillamine in primary biliary cirrhosis – an understand (and understable?) treatment. J Hepatol 1: S49
30. Matloff DS, Alpert E, Resnick RH, Kaplan MM (1982) A prospective trial of D-penicillamine in primary biliary cirrhosis. N Engl J Med 306: 319-326
31. Dickson ER, Wiesner RH, Baldus WP, Fleming CR, Ludwig J, McCall JT, Fleming TR (1984) D-Penicillamine trial for primary biliary cirrhosis. Gastroenterology 86: 1062
32. Neuberger J, Christensen E, Portmann B, Caballeria J, Rodes J, Ranek L, Tygstrup N, Williams R (1985) Double blind controlled trial of D-penicillamine in patients with primary biliary cirrhosis. Gut 26: 114-119
33. Dickson ER, Wiesner RH, Baldus WP, Fleming CR, Ludwig JL (1982) D-Penicillamine improves survival and retards histologic progression in primary biliary cirrhosis. Gastroenterology 82: 1225
34. Bassendine MF, Maklon AF, Mulcahy R, James OFW (1982) Controlled trial of high and low dose D-penicillamine in primary biliary cirrhosis: results at three years. Gut 23: A909
35. Triger DR, Manifold IH, Cloke P, Underwood JCE (1980) D-Penicillamine in primary biliary cirrhosis: two years results of a single centre, double blind controlled trial. Gut 21: A919-A920
36. Taal BG, Schalm SW, Tenkate FW, van Berge Henegouwen GP, Brandt KH (1983) Low therapeutic values of D-penicillamine in a short term prospective trial in primary biliary cirrhosis. Liver 3: 345-352
37. James OFW (1985) D-Penicillamine for primary biliary cirrhosis. Gut 26: 109-113
38. Epstein O (1985) The pathogenesis of primary biliary cirrhosis. Mol Aspects Med 8: 293-305
39. Goldberg H, Kaplan MM, Mitamuri T, Anderson CL, Matloff DS, Pinn VW, Agnello V (1982) Evidence against an immune complex pathogenesis in primary biliary cirrhosis. Gastroenterology 83: 677-683

40. Wilson JAC, Short IA, Varley H, Howatt HT (1958) The biochemical changes induced by corticosteroids in xanthomatous biliary cirrhosis. Gastroenterologia 89: 343-345
41. Howatt HT, Ralston AL, Varley H, Wilson JA (1966) The late results of long term treatment of primary biliary cirrhosis. Rev Int Hepatol 16: 227-238
42. Warnes TW (1985) Treatment of primary biliary cirrhosis. Semin Liver Dis 5: 228-240
43. Routhier G, Epstein O, Janossy G, Thomas HC, Sherlock S (1980) The effects of cyclosporin A on suppressor and inducer T-lymphocytes in primary biliary cirrhosis. Lancet 2: 1223-1226
44. Al-Aghbar MNA, Alexander GJM, Neuberger J, Nouri-Aria KT, Eddleston ALWF, Williams R (1983) Effect of cyclosporin A on suppressor cell function in vivo and in vitro in primary biliary cirrhosis. Gut 24: A970
45. Hoofnagle JH, Davis GL, Schafer DF, Peters MG, Avigan MI, Hanson RG, Pappas SC, Minuk GY, Dusheiko GM, Jones EA, MacSween RNM (1984) Randomized trial of chlorambucil for primary biliary cirrhosis. Hepatology 4: 1062
46. Heathcote J, Ross A, Sherlock S (1976) A prospective controlled trial of azathioprine in primary biliary cirrhosis. Gastroenterology 70: 656-660
47. Crowe J, Christensen E, Smith M, Cochrane M, Ranek L, Watkinson G, Doniach D, Popper H, Tygstrup N, Williams R (1980) Azathioprine in primary biliary cirrhosis: a preliminary report of an international trial. Gastroenterology 78: 1005-1010
48. Christensen E, Neuberger J, Crowe J, Douglas G, Altman G, Popper H, Portmann B, Doniach D, Ranek L, Tygstrup N, Williams R (1985) Beneficial effect of azathioprine and prediction of prognosis in primary biliary cirrhosis. Final results of an international trial. Gastroenterology 89: 1084-1091
49. Roll J (1985) A new treatment for primary biliary cirrhosis? Gastroenterology 89: 1195-1199
50. Schenker S (1984) Medical treatment vs transplantation in liver disorders. Hepatology 4: 1025-1065
51. Neuberger J, Portmann B, MacDougall BR, Calne RY, Williams R (1982) Recurrence of primary biliary cirrhosis after liver transplantation. N Engl J Med 306: 1-4
52. Scharschmidt BF (1984) Human liver transplantation: analysis of data on 540 patients from four centres. Hepatology 4: 95S-101S
53. Floreani A, Baldo G, Chiaramonte M, Baggio G, Fellin R, Naccarato R (1984) Serum lipid levels and HDL cholesterol (HDL-C) primary biliary cirrhosis (PBC). Ital J Gastroenterol 16: 274-275
54. Baldo-Enzi G, Baiocchi MR, Grotto M, Floreani A, Chiaramonte M, Fellin R (1985) Lipoprotein pattern and lipolytic enzymes (H-TGL and LPL) in patients with primary biliary cirrhosis. In: Crepaldi G et al. (eds) Diabetes, obesity and hyperlipidemias. Elsevier, Amsterdam, pp 147-154

# Impaired Calcitonin Response to Intravenous Calcium Load in Primary Biliary Cirrhosis

F. Szalay, J. Zséli, M. Abonyi, J. Földes, and I. Holló
First Department of Medicine, Semmelweis University Medical School, Budapest, Hungary

The pathomechanism of the process leading to osteopenia in primary biliary cirrhosis (PBC) seems to be complex. Osteomalacia heals completely in response to adequate vitamin D therapy, while osteoporotic bone disease continues despite such treatment [1]. Both the pathomechanism and the treatment of osteoporosis in PBC are controversial. Calcitonin (CT) inhibits osteoclastic activity and has been considered to have a bone protective effect [2]. This is the first report on altered CT secretion in PBC.

## Patients

Fourteen women with PBC (age 47-69 years, stage II-IV) and 13 healthy control women (age 45-61 years) were investigated. The diagnosis of PBC was based on the typical clinical signs and biochemical data, antimitochondrial antibody (AMA) positivity, the absence of extrahepatic obstruction, and compatible liver histology. Decreased bone mineral content of the nondominant radius was detected by osteodensitometry (Norland-Cameron MBA 178) in seven of 14 patients with PBC, but none of the controls. The patients were treated regularly with vitamin D3, but therapy was stopped 4 weeks before the investigation.

## Methods

*Intravenous Ca loading* was carried out at 8.00 a.m. after an overnight fast. A cannula was inserted into the antecubital vein for withdrawal of blood samples. Calcium ion 3.6 mg/kg as 0.2 ml/kg 10% solution of $CaCl_2$ was given intravenously within 3 min into the contralateral vein. Blood was withdrawn for determination of serum total Ca, ionized Ca, and CT before and 5, 15, 30, 60, and 120 min after the injection. Serum samples were stored at $-25\,°C$. The daily Ca intake from the diet of each subject did not exceed 200 mg during the last 7 days before the i.v. Ca load.

Serum *Ca* was determined using the Pye-Unicam Model SP 190 atomic absorption spectrophotometer, and serum *ionic Ca* with the Orion Model SS 20 unit. Serum *CT* was measured with the INC RIA kit, and basal *parathormone* (PTH) with the Byk-Mallincrot RIA kit.

*Statistical analysis:* the significance of differences was determined by Student's *t*-test of paired and unpaired samples.

Assessment and Management of Hepatobiliary Disease
Eds.: L. Okolicsányi, G. Csomós, and G. Crepaldi

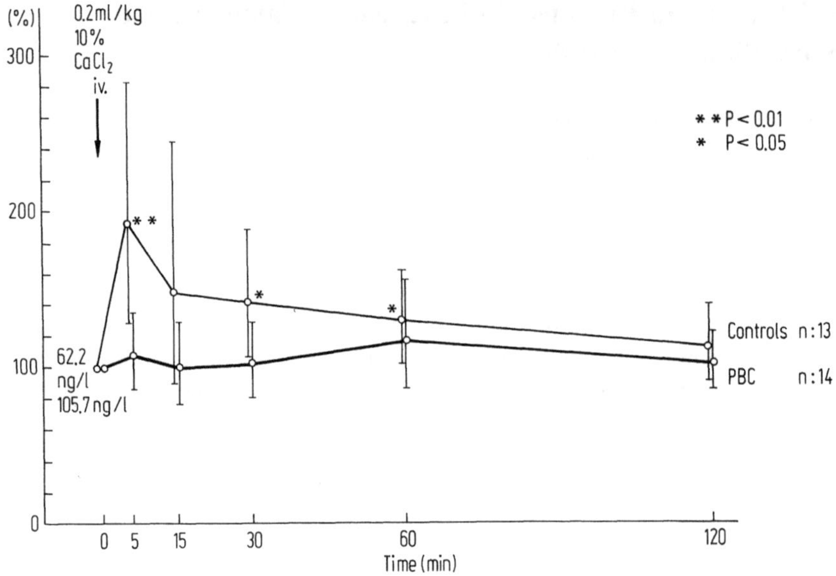


**Fig. 1.** Changes in mean serum calcitonin level and 95% confidence limits during i.v. Ca load in PBC patients and controls

## Results

The serum mean basal CT level in PBC patients was 105.7 ng/l (95% confidence limits, 85.9–130.5) and in the control subjects 62.2 ng/l (95% confidence limits, 45.0–85.9). The difference between the two groups is statistically significant ($p < 0.01$).

Different patterns of CT response to the i.v. Ca loading were found in the two groups. In the control subjects serum CT increased rapidly with a maximum at 5 min ($p < 0.01$). The 30- and 60-min values were also higher than the initial level ($p < 0.05$) (Fig. 1). In contrast, there was no significant change in the mean CT level during i.v. Ca loading in PBC patients. In some patients there was an elevation, but the peak response occurred later, at 30, 60, and, in one case, 120 min.

The serum Ca in PBC patients was $2.45 \pm 0.17$ mmol/l and in controls $2.40 \pm 0.08$ mmol/l; the ionic Ca in the PBC group was $1.13 \pm 0.04$ mmol/l and in the control subjects $1.14 \pm 0.03$ mmol/l. After the i.v. injection of Ca a highly significant elevation of serum Ca and ionic Ca ($p < 0.001$ for each) was recorded with a maximum at 5 min in both groups. There was no significant difference between the two groups in total serum Ca before and after the Ca loading. Although the ionic Ca values after i.v. Ca loading were slightly lower in the PBC patients than in the controls, neither the basal nor the 5-min peak or 15-min values differed significantly between the two groups.

In PBC patients the mean PTH level was slightly higher than that in the controls, but all the basal PTH values were within the normal range in both groups. The 25-OH D3 levels were also in the normal range, indicating adequate substitution of vitamin D.

## Discussion

Calcitonin deficiency has been observed in postmenopausal osteoporosis (POP) and has been considered to contribute to the development of this bone disease. The basal CT level was found to be lower [3, 4] and the CT reserve was considered to have diminished in response to i.v. Ca loading in POP [5, 6]. Since osteoporosis has been recognized as a common complication of PBC [7], we expected to find CT deficiency in this disease also.

Our results showed that the basal serum CT level in PBC patients was significantly higher than in healthy controls. However, there was no further increase in CT secretion to the same i.v. Ca stimulus, i.e., the CT responsiveness seems to be smaller.

The long-term deficiency in CT secretion may lead to demineralization of bones [8] per se or by augmentation of other osteopenic conditions in PBC.

## Conclusion

The alteration of CT response to calcium may perhaps be concerned in the multifactorial process leading to osteopenia in PBC.

## References

1. Matloff DS, Kaplan MM, Neer RM et al. (1982) Osteoporosis in primary biliary cirrhosis: effects of 25-hydroxyvitamin $D_3$ treatment. Gastroenterology 83: 97-102
2. Friedman J, Raisz LG (1965) Science 150: 1465-1467
3. Stevenson JC, Abeyasekera G, Hillyard CJ et al. (1981) Calcitonin and the calcium-regulating hormones in postmenopausal women: effect of oestrogens. Lancet i: 693-695
4. Chestnut CH III, et al. (1980) Basal plasma immunoreactive calcitonin in postmenopausal osteoporosis. Metabolism 29: 559-562
5. Taggart HM, Chestnut CH III, Ivey JL, Baylink DJ, Sisom K, Huber MB, Roos BA (1982) Deficient calcitonin response to calcium stimulation in postmenopausal osteoporosis? Lancet i: 475
6. Zséli J, Horváth C, Szücs J, Holló I (1982) Effect of intravenous calcium load on plasma calcitonin level in postmenopausal osteoporosis. Lancet i: 1022
7. Christensen E, Crowe J, Doniach D, Popper H, Ranek L, Rodés J, Tygstrup N, Williams R (1980) Clinical pattern and course of disease in primary biliary cirrhosis based on an analysis of 236 patients. Gastroenterology 78: 236-246
8. Talmage RV, Grubb SA, Norimatsu H, Vanderwiel CJ (1980) Evidence for an important physiological role for calcitonin. Proc Natl Acad Sci USA 77: 609-613

# Prevention of Upper Gastrointestinal Bleeding in Cirrhotic Patients

L. Pagliaro[1], G. D'Amico, L. Pasta, G. Malizia, F. Tinè, M. Traina, and G. Vizzini

[1] Clinica Medica R, Istituto di Medicina Generale e Pneumologia, Università di Palermo, Palermo, Italy

[2] Divisione di Medicina Interna, Ospedale V. Cervello, Via Trabucco, 180, 90146 Palermo, Italy

## Introduction

The prevalence of varices in patients with cirrhosis is stated to be about 50% and the risk of variceal bleeding 40% with mortality ranging from 30% to 60%. Differences may be due to patient selection and diagnostic criteria. The death risk of first bleeding seems to be higher than that of subsequent episodes (Christensen et al. 1981; D'Amico et al. 1986), indicating that the first bleeding episode causes a selection.

As a sizable proportion of patients with varices will not bleed, the first step in the prevention of bleeding is the selection of high-risk patients, especially if major surgical treatment is considered. The second step in the bleeding prevention procedure is the selection of the best available treatment in high-risk patients. Although a number of randomized controlled trials (RCTs) of prophylaxis have been reported, no treatment seems to be effective enough for use in current clinical practice.

The aims of this paper are: (1) to identify the possible indicators of bleeding risk in patients who have never bled and (2) to outline the evidence of efficacy of the different treatments so far proposed to prevent the first bleeding.

## Methods

Data on bleeding risk indicators were drawn from published reports and from our own experience dealing with a consecutive series of patients prospectively followed up for up to 4 years. Twelve RCTs of three different treatments for the prevention of first bleeding in patients with esophageal varices were reviewed (Table 1).

Methodological and statistical criteria for handling clinical information were drawn from selected references (Tygstrup et al. 1982; Sackett et al. 1985; Wulff 1981; Feinstein 1983; Collins et al. 1985; Diamond and Forrester 1983). The "pooled" risk of bleeding and of death was computed according to Collins et al. (1985).

## Identification of High-Risk Patients

*Variceal Size.* Large varices are the most reliable indicator of bleeding risk. Laplace's law, stating that the tension of the wall of a filled container is proportional to the radius, provides a theoretical basis for relating the variceal size to bleeding risk. Both retrospective and prospective studies indicate that patients with large varices do have a bleeding risk significantly higher than patients with small or medium-sized varices

Assessment and Management of Hepatobiliary Disease
Eds.: L. Okolicsányi, G. Csomós, and G. Crepaldi

**Table 1.** RCTs of treatments for the prevention of (re)bleeding in cirrhosis

| | prophylactic (p) | therapeutic (t) |
|---|---|---|
| Portacaval Shunt (PCS) vs Non-Shunt | 4* 1965–72 ⇓ | 4* 1971–81 (=) |
| Distal Splenorenal Shunt (DSRS) vs Non-Selective Shunt | – | 6* 1978–85 (=) |
| Endoscopic Variceal Sclerotherapy (EVS) vs Non-EVS | 3* 1982–86 ⇑ | 4* 1979–85 ⇧ or (=) |
| Propranolol (Prop) vs Placebo | 2* unpublished ⇧ or (=) | 2* 1981–84 (=) |

* No. of RCTs Survival in experimental groups: improved ⇧; unaffected (=); worsened ⇩

(Beppu et al. 1981; Pagliaro et al. 1980, 1984; Lebrec et al. 1980; Garcia-Tsao et al. 1985; Baker et al. 1959; Palmer and Brick 1956; Dagradi et al. 1966; Westaby et al. 1978).

*Endoscopic Features.* An overall blue appearance of varices and the presence of dilated small vessels or microtelangectasia on the variceal surface, defined as "red color sign" and including cherry-red spots, red weal marking, and hematocystic spots, have been proposed as accurate risk indicators by a retrospective Japanese study (Beppu et al. 1981). Our prospective study including 106 consecutive patients with large varices confirms these results (Fig. 1).

*Ultrasound Portal Diameter.* In a prospective study of 215 consecutive nonascitic patients we found that portal diameter above 13 mm with respiratory variations smaller than 50% in any of the portal vessels constitutes a highly sensitive (95%) indicator of the presence of large varices. Although specificity is as low as 44% (Fig. 2), about half the endoscopies can be spared if ultrasound is employed as a preliminary screening to identify patients with large varices (Cottone et al. 1986).

*Portal Pressure.* Portal pressure has been investigated as a bleeding indicator for many years, but conflicting results have been reported. Although some authors report significantly higher portal pressure in patients who have bled than in patients who have never bled (Garcia-Tsao et al. 1985; Joly et al. 1971; Viallet et al. 1975, 1980; Burcharth et al. 1980), no differences were found by other investigators (Lebrec et al. 1980; Krook 1957; Simert et al. 1978; Vinel et al. 1982; Rector and Reynolds 1985). The variability of techniques in pressure measurement and of severity of liver disease in patients without previous bleeding may be responsible for the differences in results. Further studies are needed to assess the relationship between the degree of portal hypertension and the risk of hemorrhage from esophageal varices.

*Variceal Pressure.* It has recently been reported that the incidence of rebleeding is higher in patients with variceal pressure above 20 cm $H_2O$ as assessed by a "noninvasive"

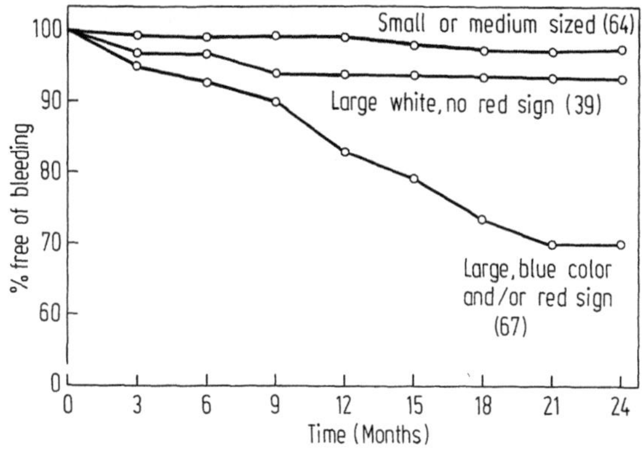


**Fig. 1.** Percentage of patients without bleeding after inclusion in the study, according to the endoscopic features of varices. The figures in *parentheses* are the numbers of patients in each group

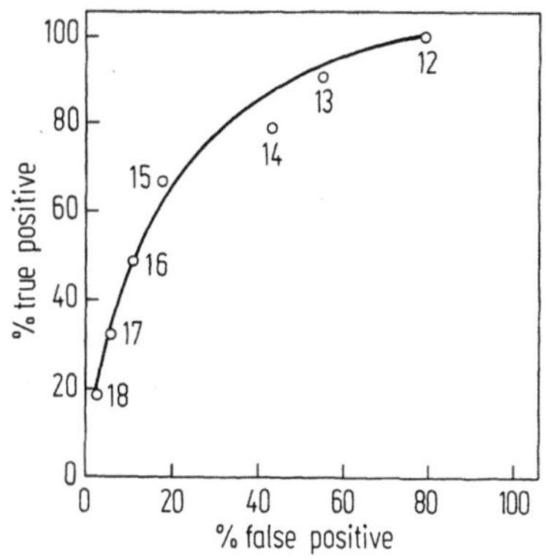


**Fig. 2.** Receiver operating characteristic curve of the ultrasound portal diameter (respiratory variation in any of the portal vessels <50%) in the screening of patients with large varices

procedure (Gertsh et al. 1982). Preliminary results from another study suggest that intravariceal pressure (direct puncture procedure) is significantly higher in patients who have recently bled than in patients without previous bleeding (Staritz 1986). If these findings are confirmed, direct variceal pressure measurement could improve the accuracy of selection of high-risk patients.

## What Is the Best Treatment?

### Portocaval Shunt Vs Nonshunt

Four RCTs published between 1965 and 1972 (Jackson et al. 1968; Resnick et al. 1969; Conn and Lindenmuth 1965; Conn et al. 1972) unanimously showed that prophylactic portocaval shunt (P-PCS) was effective in preventing upper gastrointestinal bleeding ($\Delta_{c-t}$ 3%–35%), and operative mortality was 5%–13%. Five-year survival, however, was shortened, because deaths from liver failure outnumbered the prevented deaths from bleeding. Moreover, about 20% of shunted patients were disabled by chronic and/or severe portosystemic encephalopathy (PSE) (Mutchnick et al. 1974). These results led to virtual abandonment of P-PCS.

However, in these four RCTs the size of the patients' varices was not indicated, and a number of patients with small or medium-sized varices at relatively low risk of bleeding could have been included. This could explain the relatively low incidence of bleeding and deaths from bleeding in control patients (range 19%- 39% and 10%-22% respectively). Clearly, no benefit can be expected in such patients from prophylactic procedures, while adverse effects can be anticipated from a major and nonphysiological operation such as PCS.

**Prophylactic Endoscopic Variceal Sclerotherapy**

Three RCTs have been fully published (Paquet 1982; Witzel et al. 1985; Kock et al. 1986) and preliminary data from two others have been reported (Sauerbruch et al. 1986; Fleig et al. 1986). All of these studies were performed in Germany. The first two fully reported RCTs (Paquet 1982; Witzel et al. 1985) showed significant reduction of bleeding rate and improvement of survival in treated patients. However, bleeding rate in the controls was higher than in other published series: this was particularly surprising in the study by Witzel et al. (1985) whose patients were not selected for high risk of bleeding. For both studies it has been also pointed out that the control patients were not given the best available treatment for acute hemorrhage when this occurred (Terblanche 1986). The third published RCT (Koch et al. 1986) included few patients (30 per group): no differences were observed in bleeding rate or survival, but the authors claimed a benefit from prophylactic endoscopic variceal sclerotherapy (P-EVS) if patients dying from "diffuse bleeding in terminal liver failure" were excluded from analysis.

Among the incompletely reported studies, the first (Sauerbruch et al. 1986), including 103 patients with large varices in Child class A or B failed to show any benefit from P-EVS after a mean follow-up period of 17 months. Data from the second (Fleig et al. 1986) are too preliminary to allow any confident analysis.

In conclusion, the available data on P-EVS provide no definite evidence of benefit: further RCTs are needed.

**Propranolol**

A large multicenter RCT of prophylactic propranolol vs placebo (vitamin K), in which our own group participated, was performed in Italy. Admissions were stopped in January 1984, by which time 174 patients with large varices had been included. After a mean follow-up period of 22 months, nonascitic patients given propranolol had a significantly lower bleeding incidence without improvement in survival. No benefit was found in patients with ascites. Follow-up is still in progress and definitive analysis has not yet been carried out.

A preliminary report from another RCT (Cales and Pascal 1986) including 190 patients followed up for 1 year shows that propranolol was effective in preventing bleeding and improving survival in all patients. Due to the low incidence of events in patients with less advanced disease (Child-Pugh < 9), statistical significance was reached only in those with more severe cirrhosis (Child-Pugh 9-13). These results are partly in disagreement with ours. Hemodynamic data showing that propranolol is not active or is less active on portal pressure in patients with ascites provide indirect support for our own results.

## Conclusions

On the basis of the available data it can be concluded that prevention of first variceal bleeding in patients with cirrhosis is not justified other than in controlled clinical trials. Future controlled trials should include only patients at high risk of bleeding. Analysis of published RCTs shows bleeding rates in controls ranging from 19% to 88%, and it is not surprising that the higher the bleeding rate in controls the more likely is a positive effect of the treatment. Prevention of bleeding in patients who have not yet bled should be a two-step procedure:
*Step 1:* accurate assessment of bleeding risk
*Step 2:* RCTs of treatments in patients at high risk of bleeding stratified according to their functional hepatic reserve

## Summary

Prevention of upper gastrointestinal bleeding in cirrhotics who have never bled is a two-step procedure. The aim of step 1 is the identification of high-risk patients. Large varices and "alarm features" such as blue color and/or red color sign assessed by endoscopy are the most reliable indicators. Ultrasound of portal veins can be used to screen patients for endoscopy. The role of portal pressure measurement remains to be clarified, whereas direct measurement of variceal pressure seems to be promising as a bleeding risk indicator.

Step 2 deals with prophylactic treatments in high-risk patients:

a) Cumulative evidence from four randomized controlled trials (RCTs) of portocaval shunt showed decreased survival, although bleeding was substantially reduced. However, the criteria of selection would now be considered obsolete, since the size and endoscopic features of the varices were not taken into account.
b) Cumulative evidence from three RCTs of endoscopic sclerotherapy seems to show benefit in both prevention of bleeding and survival. However, an unusually high incidence of bleeding in controls and methodological inadequacies limit the value of these results.
c) Propranolol, as evaluated in two RCTs not fully published, has hitherto shown conflicting results. Significant protection from bleeding was obtained in nonascitic patients in the first RCT, but in ascitic patients in the second.

In conclusion, data available from RCTs do not allow clear-cut guidelines for the prevention of first bleeding in cirrhosis. A better definition of high risk of bleeding is needed for the patients included in further RCTs.

## References

Baker LA, Smith C, Lieberman G (1959) The natural history of esophageal varices. Am J Med 26: 228-236

Beppu K, Inokuchi K, Koyanagi N, et al. (1981) Prediction of variceal hemorrhage by esophageal endoscopy. Gastrointest Endosc 27: 213-218

Burcharth F, Sørensen TIA, Andersen B (1980) Findings in percutaneous transhepatic portography and variceal bleeding in cirrhosis. Surg Gynecol Obstet 150: 887-890

Cales P, Pascal GP (1986) Prophylaxis of first variceal bleeding in cirrhotic patients by propranolol: final report of a multicenter randomized study (Abstr 780) USA Digestive Disease Week, San Francisco, May 18-21, pp A195

Christensen E, Fanerholdt L, Schlichting P et al. (1981) Aspect of the natural history of gastrointestinal bleeding in cirrhosis and the effect of prednisone. Gastroenterology 81: 944-952

Collins R, Yusuf S, Peto R (1985) Overview of randomized trials of diuretics in pregnancy. Br Med J 290: 17-23

Conn HO, Lindenmuth WW (1965) Prophylactic portacaval anastomosis in cirrhotic patients with esophageal varices. N Engl J Med 272: 1255

Conn HO, Lindenmuth WW, May CJ, Ramsby GR (1972) Prophylactic portacaval anastomosis. A tale of two studies. Medicine (Baltimore) 51: 27-40

Cottone M, D'Amico G, Maringhini A et al. (1986) Predictive value of ultrasonography in the screening of non-ascitic cirrhotic patients with large varices. J Ultrasound Med 5: 189-192

Dagradi AE, Stempien SI, Owens LK (1966) Bleeding esophagogastric varices. Arch Surg 92: 944-947

D'Amico G, Morabito A, Pagliaro L et al. (1986) Six week prognostic indicators in upper gastrointestinal haemorrhage in cirrhosis. In: Gentilini (ed) Liver cirrhosis II. Karger, Basel (Frontiers of gastrointestinal research, vol 23) (in press)

Diamond GA, Forrester JS (1983) Clinical trials and statistical verdicts: probable grounds for appeal. Ann Intern Med 98: 385-394

Feinstein AR (1983) Ann additional basic science for clinical medicine. II. The limitation of randomized trials. Ann Intern Med 99: 544-550

Fleig WE, Stange EF, Wordehoff D, Rainer K, Ditshuneit H (1986) Endoscopic sclerotherapy for the primary prophylaxis of variceal bleeding in cirrhotic patients. Preliminary results of a randomized, controlled trial (Abstr). International Symposium on Prophylaxis of Variceal Bleeding, Munich, Jan 24-25

Garcia-Tsao G, Croszmann RJ, Fisher RL, Conn HO, Atterbury CE, Glickman M (1985) Portal pressure, presence of gastroesophageal varices and variceal bleeding. Hepatology 5: 419-424

Gertsh PH, Loup P, Diserens H, Mosimann R (1982) Endoscopic noninvasive manometry of oesophageal varices: prognostic significance. Am J Surg 144: 528-530

Jackson FC, Perrin EB, Smith AG, Dagradi AE, Nadal HM (1968) A clinical investigation of the portocaval shunt. Survival analysis of the prophylactic operation. Am J Surg 115: 22-42

Joly JG, Marleau D, Legare A et al. (1971) Bleeding from esophageal varices in cirrhosis of the liver. Can Med Assoc J 104: 576-580

Kock H, Henning H, Grimm H, Soehendra N (1986) Prophylactic sclerosing of esophageal varices. Results of a prospective controlled study. Endoscopy 18: 40-43

Krook H (1957) Circulatory studies in liver cirrhosis. Acta Med Scand [Suppl 318] 156: 55-65

Lebrec D, deFleury P, Rueff B et al. (1980) Portal hypertension, size of esophageal varices and risk of gastrointestinal bleeding in cirrhosis. Gastroenterology 79: 1139-1144

Mutchnick MG, Lerner E, Conn HO (1974) Portal-systemic encephalopathy and portacaval anastomosis: A prospective, controlled investigation. Gastroenterology 66: 1005-1019

Pagliaro L, D'Amico G, Maringhini A et al. (1980) History of nonalcoholic cirrhosis. In: Medical and surgical problems of portal hypertension, Orloff HJ, Stipa S, Ziparo U, eds Academic, London

Pagliaro L, Pasta L, Filippazzo G et al. (1984) Emorragie digestive dei cirrotici: trattamento e prevenzione. In Progressi nella epatologia Italiana. Chianciano Terme, Siena

Palmer ED, Brick IB (1956) Correlation between the severity of esophageal varices in portal cirrhosis and their propensity towards hemorrhage. Gastroenterology 30: 85-90

Paquet KJ (1982) Prophylactic endoscopic sclerosing treatment of the esophageal wall in varices. A prospective controlled randomized trial. Endoscopy 14: 4-5
Rector WG Jr, Reynolds TB (1985) Risk factors for haemorrhage from oesophageal varices and acute gastric erosion. Clin Gastroenterol 14: 139-153
Resnick RH, Chalmers TC, Ishihara AM et al. (1969) A controlled study of the prophylactic portacaval shunt. A final report. Ann Intern Med 70: 675-688
Sackett DL, Haynes RB, Tugwell P (1985) Clinical epidemiology. A basic science for clinical medicine. Little, Brown, Boston
Sauerbruch T, Wotzka R, Köpcke W et al. (1986) Endoscopic sclerotherapy for prophylaxis of variceal bleeding in liver cirrhosis (Abstr). International Symposium on Prophylaxis of Variceal Bleeding, Munich, Jan 24-25
Simert G, Lunderquist A, Tylén U, Vang J (1978) Correlation between percutaneous transhepatic portography and clinical findings in 56 patients with portal hypertension. Acta Chir Scand 144: 27-34
Staritz M (1986) Role of variceal pressure in oesophageal hemorrhage (Abstr) International Symposium on Prophylaxis of Variceal Bleeding, Munich, Jan 24-25
Terblanche J (1986) Sclerotherapy for prophylaxis of variceal bleeding. Lancet 1: 961-963
Tygstrup N, Lachin JM, Juhl E (1982) The randomized clinical trial and therapeutic decisions. Dekker, New York
Viallet A, Marleau D, Huet PM et al. (1975) Relationship between portal hypertension and bleeding from ruptured varices in alcoholic cirrhosis patients. Gastroenterology 69: 1297-1300
Viallet A, Marleau D, Huet PM et al. (1980) Relationship between portal hypertension bleeding from ruptured varices. Gastroenterology 79: 1129
Vinel JP, Cassigneul J, Louis A (1982) Clinical and prognostic significance of portohepatic gradients in patients with cirrhosis. Surg Gynecol Obstet 155: 347-352
Westaby S, Wilkinson SP, Warren R, Williams R (1978) Spleen size and portal hypertension in cirrhosis. Digestion 17: 63-68
Witzel L, Wolbergs E, Merki H (1985) Prophylactic endoscopic sclerotherapy of oesophageal varices. Lancet 1: 773-775
Wulff HR (1981) Rational diagnosis and treatment, 2nd edn. Blackwell, Oxford

# Prophylactic Treatment of First Variceal Bleeding in Cirrhotics with Nadolol or Ranitidine: A Prospective Randomized Study*

G. Idéo[1], E. Fesce[1], R. Fesce[2], D. Grimoldi[1], and G. Bellati[1]

[1]Department A of Internal Medicine, St. Anna's Hospital, Como, Italy
[2]Institute of Pharmacology, University of Milan, Italy

Propranolol has been demonstrated to decrease portal hypertension and to reduce the incidence of rebleeding from ruptured esophageal varices in patients with well-compensated alcoholic cirrhosis [1, 2].

Variceal bleeding is a threatening event with a high mortality rate, from 28% to 80% [3-7]. To clarify the efficacy of $\beta$-blocker in preventing the first hemorrhage, we started a prospective randomized trial comparing nadolol, ranitidine, and placebo. Nadolol was chosen because it is not cardioselective, does not require extensive hepatic metabolism, does not interfere with renal flow, and extensively reduces portal hypertension [8-10]. Ranitidine was tested because of claims that peptic reflux may play some role in the rupture of esophageal varices [11-15] and because it inhibits gastric acid secretion and increases lower esophageal sphincter pressure [16].

## Material and Methods

From September 1982 to August 1985, 104 patients suffering from liver cirrhosis with varices which had never bled were considered for this study. The criteria for patient selection were: presence of large varices at the endoscopy (bleeding risk superior to 40% according to Beppu et al. [17]), no contraindication to $\beta$-blockers, absence of cardiopulmonary disease, erosive gastroduodenitis or peptic ulcer, hepatocellular carcinoma, and other neoplasia or intractable ascites. Seventy patients fulfilled these criteria. Reasons for ineligibility were: cardiopulmonary diseases (8), gastroduodenitis or peptic ulcer (11), neoplasia (7), intractable ascites (5), other conditions (6).

Clinical evaluation and liver function tests were performed prior to treatment and every 3 months afterwards. Endoscopy was performed at admission and 2 and 12 months later.

One group of 22 patients received nadolol once a day at oral doses that reduced the resting heart rate by approximately 25% (40-120 mg%). A second group of 23 patients received ranitidine (300 mg/day), and a third group of 25 received one tablet of placebo once a day.

End point of the study was gastrointestinal hemorrhage or death. Five patients (two in the nadolol, one in the ranitidine and two in the placebo group) were lost to follow-up and were not considered in the results.

* This paper was presented at the autumn meeting of the Italian Association for Study of the Liver, Erice, November 1985 and published in abstract form.

Assessment and Management of Hepatobiliary Disease
Eds.: L. Okolicsányi, G. Csomós, and G. Crepaldi

**Table 1.** Clinical data of the study group

| | All | Nadolol | Ranitidine | Placebo |
|---|---|---|---|---|
| No. of patients | 65 | 20 | 22 | 23 |
| Age | | | | |
| Mean | 55.6 | 55.3 | 57 | 53.5 |
| Range | 27 -74 | 42 -69 | 47-74 | 27 -72 |
| Alcoholism | 36 | 9 | 11 | 16 |
| Ascites | 24 | 8 | 6 | 10 |
| Encephalopathy | 5 | 2 | 1 | 2 |
| Severity of liver disease | | | | |
| Grade A or B | 51 | 15 | 17 | 19 |
| Grade C | 14 | 5 | 5 | 4 |
| Bleeding risk | | | | |
| >60% | 34 | 11 | 13 | 10 |
| <60% | 31 | 9 | 9 | 13 |
| Period of follow-up (months) | | | | |
| Mean | 19.7 | 21 | 21 | 17 |
| Range | 6 -41 | 12 -41 | 12-37 | 7 -36 |

The groups did not differ in age, sex, cause of cirrhosis, presence of ascites or encephalopathy, bleeding risk (over or under 60%), period of follow-up, or severity of liver damage graded on admission by a modification of Child's [18] classification [19] (Table 1).

Statistical analysis was performed by the chi square test, and the percentages of patients free of bleeding during the period after inclusion were calculated according to the Kaplan-Meier method and compared by means of the log-rank test [20].

## Results

Table 2 summarizes the overall results. Ten of 65 patients bled (15.4%). Seven of these cases occurred in the placebo group (30.4%) and three in the ranitidine group (13.6%). No bleeding was observed in the nadolol group. The Fisher-Yates test showed a significant statistical difference between nadolol and placebo treatment, while differences between placebo and ranitidine treatment were not significant. The clinical data of patients in which bleeding occurred are reported in Table 3. No significant difference was seen between alcoholics and nonalcoholics (7 of 36 vs 3 of 29), but bleeding occurred more frequently in ascitic than in nonascitic patients (7 of 24 vs 3 of 41; $p<0.05$). The percentages of patients free of rebleeding 1 and 2 years after inclusion were respectively 100% and 100% in the nadolol group and 78.3% and 69.6% in the placebo group; the difference between the two groups was significant ($p<0.05$; Fig. 1).

Finally, no patients had to stop taking nadolol because of side effects.

## Discussion

In this study we have demonstrated that the use of a $\beta$-blocking drug, nadolol, significantly reduces the probability of the first bleeding from esophageal varices in patients with liver cirrhosis.

**Table 2.** Results

| | All (65) | Nadolol (20) | Ranitidine (22) | Placebo (23) |
|---|---|---|---|---|
| Bleeding | 10 (15.4%) | 0* | 3 (13.6%) | 7 (30.4%) |
| Deaths due to bleeding | 4 | 0 | 1 | 3 |
| Total mortality | 12 (18%) | 3 (15%) | 3 (13.6%) | 6 (26%) |

* $p < 0.05$ in respect to placebo

**Table 3.** Clinical data of patients in which bleeding occurred

| Treatment | P | P | P | P | P | P | P | R | R | R |
|---|---|---|---|---|---|---|---|---|---|---|
| Sex | M | M | M | M | F | M | M | M | M | M |
| Age | 58 | 31 | 48 | 52 | 27 | 64 | 48 | 47 | 53 | 61 |
| Follow-up from entry to bleeding (months) | 1 | 2 | 11 | 11 | 20 | 10 | 23 | 11 | 11 | 1 |
| Alcoholism | + | + | + | + | + | – | – | + | + | – |
| Ascites | + | + | + | – | – | + | + | + | – | + |
| Child's A | | | | | | | | | | |
| Child's B | | • | • | • | • | • | • | | • | |
| Child's C | • | | | | | | | • | | • |
| Death due to bleeding | + | – | – | – | – | + | + | – | – | + |

P, placebo; R, ranitidine

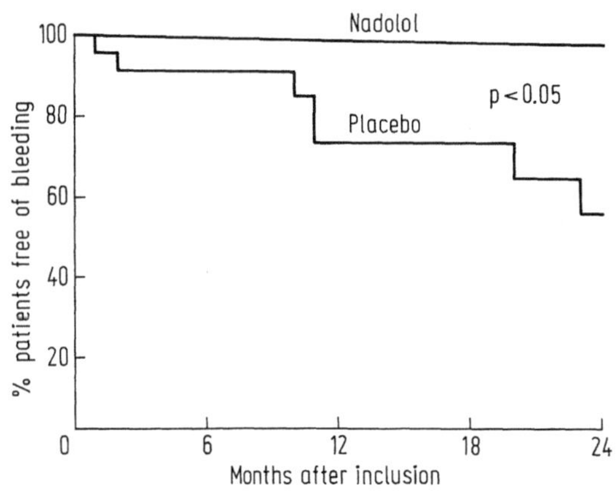


**Fig. 1.** Percentage of patients free of rebleeding as function of time after inclusion in nadolol and placebo groups

Pagliaro et al. [21] recently observed that propranolol can prevent initial bleeding from variceal bleeding in compensated cirrhosis. However, it was necessary to stop using this $\beta$-blocker because of side effects in about 30% of patients. The authors concluded that its usefulness is somewhat limited and that it should not be employed at present.

Our results are not in agreement with those of Pagliaro et al. Although our case material also contained subjects with ascites or classified as grade C (Child's classification), no patients had to stop the treatment owing to side effects.

The higher incidence of bad tolerance observed by Pagliaro et al. could be related to the different $\beta$-blocker used. The metabolization of propranolol, which takes place mainly in the liver, could be reduced in patients with liver failure, causing higher blood levels of the drug with consequent side effects. Nadolol, on the other hand, is not metabolized by the liver and is thus not affected by altered liver function. Moreover, while propranolol in some circumstances reduces renal perfusion [8], nadolol has been demonstrated to induce a significant dose-related increase in renal blood flow [8]. This interpretation might also explain the increased mortality from causes other than esophageal varices observed in cirrhotics treated with $\beta$-blocking agents, while with nadolol this mortality was similar to that of the placebo group.

As far as the effect of ranitidine is concerned, we observed a trend in favor of this drug in respect to placebo, without reaching a statistically significant difference.

In a small group of 16 cirrhotics Mac Dougall and Williams [15] showed that the frequency with which bleeding recurred in the cimetidine and placebo groups was not significantly different. Therefore it seems unlikely that $H_2$-antagonists can prevent episodes of bleeding, although we cannot exclude the possibility that with more case material we might have reached a positive, even statistically significant result with ranitidine. However, considering the efficacy of nadolol without side effects, we can conclude that this $\beta$-blocking agent is the drug of choice for the prevention of variceal bleeding in cirrhotics. Other studies should evaluate whether a combination of nadolol and ranitidine could be even more useful.

## References

1. Lebrec D, Poynard T, Hillon P, Benhamou JP (1981) Propranolol for prevention of recurrent gastrointestinal bleeding in patients with cirrhosis. A controlled study. N Engl J Med 305: 1371-1374
2. Lebrec D, Poynard T, Bernau J, Bercoff E, Nouel O, Capron JP, Poupon R, Bouvry M, Rueff B, Benhamou JP (1984) A randomized controlled study of propranolol for prevention of recurrent gastrointestinal bleeding in patients with cirrhosis: a final report. Hepatology 4: 355-358
3. Baker LA, Smith C, Lieberman G (1959) The natural history of esophageal varices. A study of 115 cirrhotic patients in whom varices were diagnosed prior to bleeding. Am J Med 26: 228-237
4. Conn HO, Lindenmuth WW, May CI, Ramsby GR (1972) Prophylactic portacaval anastomosis. A tale of two studies. Medicine 51: 27-40
5. Graham DJ, Smith JL (1981) The course of patients after variceal hemorrhage. Gastroenterology 80: 800-809
6. Paquet KJ (1982) Prophylactic endoscopic sclerosing treatment of the esophageal wall in varices. A prospective controlled randomized trial. Endoscopy 14: 4-5
7. Witzel L, Wolbergs E, Merki H (1985) Prophylactic endoscopic sclerotherapy oesophageal varices. A prospective controlled study. Lancet I: 773-775
8. Hollenberg NK, Adams DF, McKinstry DN, Williams GH, Borlucki LJ, Sullivan JM (1979) Beta-adrenoceptor blocking agents and the kidney: effect of nadolol and propranolol on the renal circulation. Br J Clin Pharmacol 7 [Suppl 2]: 219-225
9. Textor SC, Fouad FM, Bravo EL, Tarali RC, Viat DG, Gifford RW Jr (1982) Redistribution of cardiac output to the kidneys during oral nadolol administration. N Engl J Med 307: 601-605
10. Gatta A, Sacerdoti D, Merkel C, Milani L, Battaglia G, Zuin R (1984) Effects of nadolol treatment on renal and hepatic hemodynamics and function in cirrhotic patients with portal hypertension. Am Heart J 108: 1167-1172

11. Wagenknecht TW, Noble JF, Baronofsky JD (1953) Nature of bleeding in esophageal varices. Surgery 33: 869-874
12. Chiles NH, Baggenstoss AH, Olsen AM (1953) Esophageal varices: comparative incidence of ulceration and spontaneous rupture as a cause of mortal hemorrhage. Gastroenterology 25: 565-573
13. Polish E, Sullivan BG (1961) Esophagitis associated with hemorrhage from esophageal varices. Ann Intern Med 54: 900-911
14. Palmer ED (1957) Portal hypertension and esophageal varices. Clinical gastroenterology. Hoeber, New York
15. MacDougall BRD, Williams R (1983) A controlled clinical trial of cimetidine in the recurrence of variceal hemorrhage: implications about the pathogenesis of hemorrhage. Hepatology: 69-73
16. Bertaccini G, Molina E, Bobbo P, Foggi E (1981) Ranitidine increases lower oesophageal sphincter pressure in man. Ital J Gastroent 13 [Suppl]: 149-159
17. Beppu K, Inokuchi K, Koyanagi N, Nakayama S, Sakata H, Kitano S, Kobayashi M (1981) Prediction of variceal hemorrhage by esophageal endoscopy. Gastrointest Endosc 27: 213-218
18. Pugh RNH, Murray-Lyon IM, Dawson JL, Pietroni MC, Williams R (1973) Transection of the oesophagus for bleeding oesophageal varices. Br J Surg 60: 646-649
19. Child CG (1964) The liver and portal hypertension. Saunders, Philadelphia
20. Peto R, Pitie MC, Armitage P et al. (1977) Design and analysis of randomized clinical trials requiring prolonged observation of each patient II. Analysis and examples. Br J Cancer 35: 1-39
21. Pagliaro L, Pasta L, D'Amico G, Filippazzo MG, Tinè F, Morabito A, Ferrari A, Marenco G, De Pretis G (1986) A randomized clinical trial of propranolol for the prevention of initial bleeding in cirrhosis with potal hypertension. N Engl J Med 314: 244

# Hemodynamic and Clinical Evaluation of Nadolol in the Treatment of Portal Hypertension in Patients with Cirrhosis

A. Gatta, C. Merkel, D. Sacerdoti, M. Bolognesi, P. Angeli, and A. Ruol
Department of Clinical Medicine, University of Padua, Italy

## Introduction

Beta-blockers have been used in recent years for the treatment of portal hypertension in cirrhosis, following Lebrec et al.'s demonstration that propranolol lowers portal pressure (Lebrec et al. 1980) and decreases the risk of recurrent gastrointestinal bleeding (Lebrec et al. 1984). However, potentially harmful side effects of propranolol in patients with cirrhosis have recently been stressed, including decrease in liver function and occurrence of hepatic encephalopathy, central nervous system effects, and risk of overdose (Tarver et al. 1983; Arthur et al. 1985). Nadolol, another noncardioselective beta-blocker like propranolol, has pharmacological characteristics that can overcome most of these problems (Heel et al. 1980). It crosses the blood-brain barrier to a lesser degree than propranolol, and does not undergo significant hepatic metabolism, unlike propranolol. We report the results of a pathophysiological study aimed at investigating the effects of nadolol on hepatic and renal hemodynamics and function and of a controlled clinical trial aimed at verifying the clinical value of the drug in the prevention of rebleeding in patients with cirrhosis.

## Patients and Methods

### Pathophysiological Study

20 patients with biopsy-proven cirrhosis (14 with alcoholic cirrhosis, two with posthepatitic cirrhosis, four with cryptogenic cirrhosis) were studied before and after 1 month of treatment with nadolol at a dose reducing resting heart rate by approximately 25% (40-160 mg/day). All patients had esophageal varices, four had mild ascites, and eight had had previous upper gastrointestinal bleeding which occurred at least 1 month before the study. None had arterial hypertension, cardiac disease, organic renal disease, or asthma. All patients were kept on a 90 mEq/day sodium intake.

In all subjects the following were measured: mean arterial pressure (MAP), expressed as diastolic + ⅓ pulse pressure; cardiac output (CO), by means of thermal dilution; hepatic venous pressure gradient (HVPG), as occluded – free hepatic venous pressure; and hepatic blood flow (HBF) using the indocyanine green constant infusion method. To evaluate the effect of nadolol on liver function, we measured galactose - eliminating capacity (GEC) after intravenous load and aminopyrine metabolic capacity using the breath test. Esophageal varices were evaluated by endoscopy; the results were classified according to Dagradi (1973). To investigate possible effects on renal he-

Assessment and Management of Hepatobiliary Disease
Eds.: L. Okolicsányi, G. Csomós, and G. Crepaldi

modynamics and function, renal blood flow was determined by PAH clearance and glomerular filtration rate by inulin clearance. Details of the techniques employed were given in previous papers (Gatta et al. 1984; Merkel et al. 1986).

## Clinical Trial

Patients with biopsy-proven cirrhosis of different etiologies who survived an episode of variceal bleeding were entered into a prospective randomized clinical trial. Bleeding site was defined endoscopically as proven or probable. Endoscopy was always performed within 36 h from the beginning of bleeding. Trial inclusion and exclusion criteria were as follows:

*Inclusion*
- Biopsy-proven cirrhosis
- Previous digestive hemorrhage from ruptured esophageal varices diagnosed according to one of the following criteria:
  a) visualization of bleeding site
  b) visualization of a fibrin clot on a varix
  c) presence of varices in the absence of gastroduodenal lesions and of any assumption of drugs affecting gastric mucosa

*Exclusion*
- Child's C
- Massive ascites
- Renal failure persisting after compensating hemodynamic conditions (serum creatinine > 1.5 mg/dl)
- Age < 18 or > 70
- Tumors
- Contraindications to beta-blocking agents (asthma, first degree A-V block, heart failure, clinically evident diabetes)

Of 54 cirrhotic patients eligible for the study admitted to the Department of Clinical Medicine of the University of Padua from January 15th 1983 to May 15th 1984, 24 were found to fulfill admission criteria. They were randomized to receive either placebo (one tablet/day in the morning) or nadolol at a dose reducing heart rate by approximately 25% in a single daily administration in the morning (40–160 mg/day). Twelve patients received placebo, 12 nadolol. Patients were included in the trial 15–40 days after bleeding and were followed as outpatients monthly during the first 3 months, then every 3 months. In addition to the clinical examination, common liver function tests were performed and serum creatinine was measured. Follow-up lasted up to 145 weeks (mean $71 \pm 45$ weeks). End-points of the study were considered the onset of side effects necessitating withdrawal of treatment, the occurrence of digestive hemorrhage from ruptured esophageal varices, and death. Patients withdrawn from the study were offered variceal sclerosis or surgery, accepted by two and three patients respectively. The results were evaluated using life-table analysis according to the Kaplan-Meier method and the log-rank test (Peto et al. 1977). Hemorrhage from varices and death were the events for which statistical computation was carried out. Two patients in the nadolol group and three in the placebo group were lost to follow-up after 44 and 50 weeks and 13, 27, and 62 weeks respectively.

## Results

### Pathophysiological Study

After 1 month of nadolol treatment, CO, HVPG, and HBF showed significant decrease, while MAP remained steady (Fig. 1). Also esophageal varices degree was reduced in 11 patients and unchanged in the remainders. A significant correlation was found between decrease in CO and in HVPG ($p < 0.01$) (Fig. 2).

As for the effects of nadolol treatment on hepatic and renal function and on renal blood flow, all investigated parameters were unchanged after 1 month of treatment. The results are illustrated in Fig. 1.

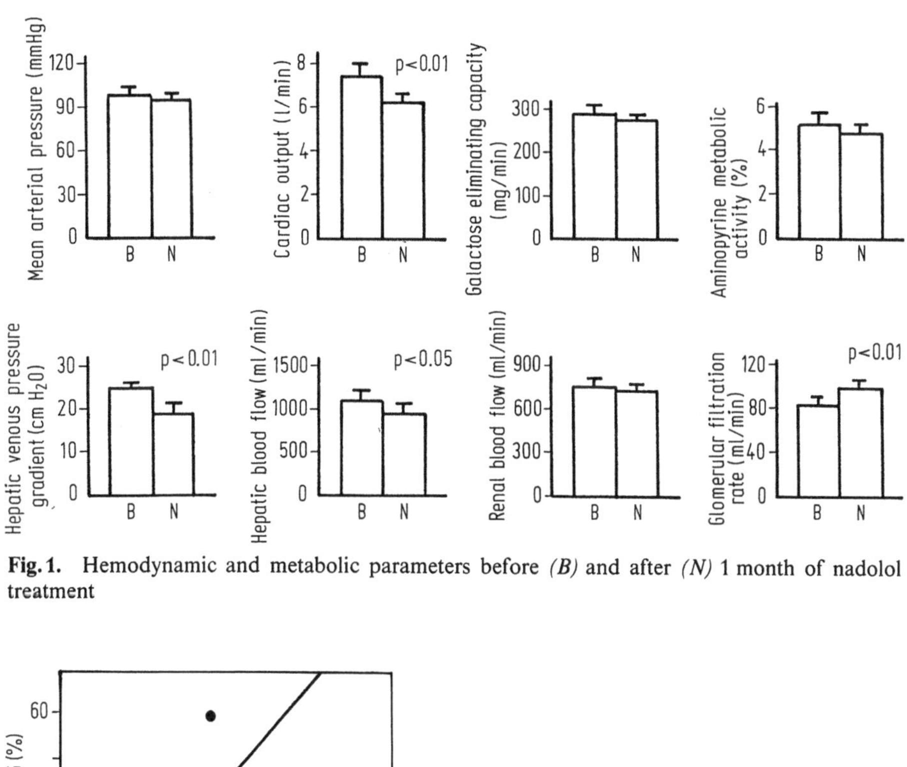


**Fig. 1.** Hemodynamic and metabolic parameters before *(B)* and after *(N)* 1 month of nadolol treatment

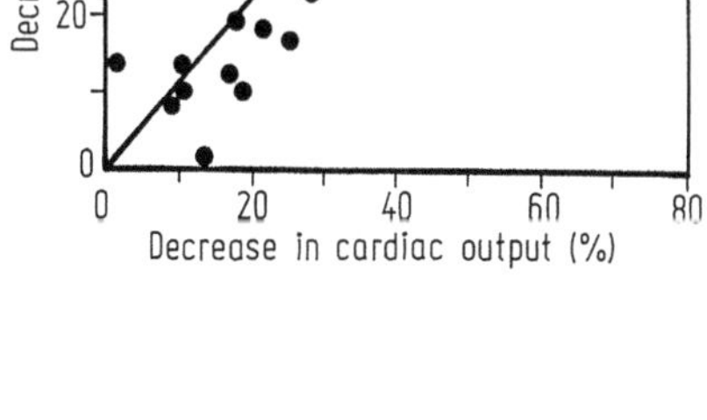


**Fig. 2.** Correlation between decrease in cardiac output and decrease in hepatic venous pressure gradient after 1 month of nadolol treatment

*Table 1.* Clinical characteristics and laboratory values of the placebo and nadolol groups

| | Nadolol | P | Placebo |
|---|---|---|---|
| Age | 49 ±13 | n.s. | 47 ±12 |
| Sex (M/F) | 9/3 | n.s. | 8/4 |
| Bilirubin (mg/dl) | 1.2 ± 0.6 | n.s. | 1.8 ± 1.1 |
| PT (%) | 57 ±15 | n.s. | 67 ±18 |
| Albumin (g/dl) | 3.50 ± 0.46 | n.s. | 3.71 ± 0.72 |
| Serum creatinine (mg/dl) | 0.9 ± 0.3 | n.s. | 1.0 ± 0.3 |
| Child (A/B) | 4/8 | n.s. | 6/6 |
| Etiology (A/NA) | 9/3 | n.s. | 9/3 |
| Severity of varices (1+2/3+4)[a] | 2/10 | n.s. | 5/7 |
| HVPG (cm $H_2O$) | 24 ± 6 | n.s. | 26 ± 5 |
| Ascites | 4 | n.s. | 2 |
| More than one previous hemorrhage | 5 | n.s. | 4 |

PT, prothrombin time; A/NA, alcoholic/nonalcoholic
[a] Dagradi's classification

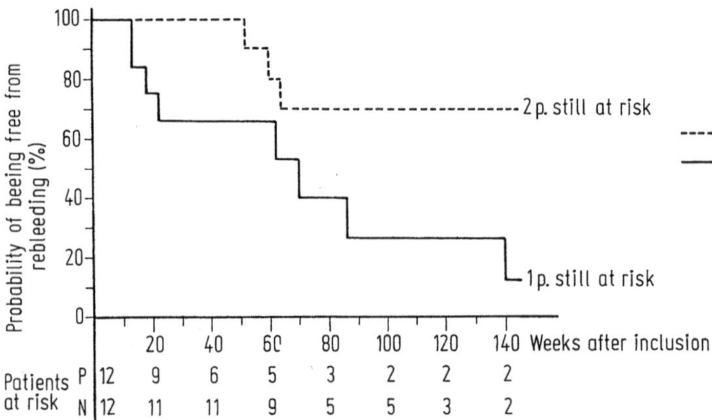


**Fig. 3.** Probability of being free of rebleeding according to the Kaplan-Meier method

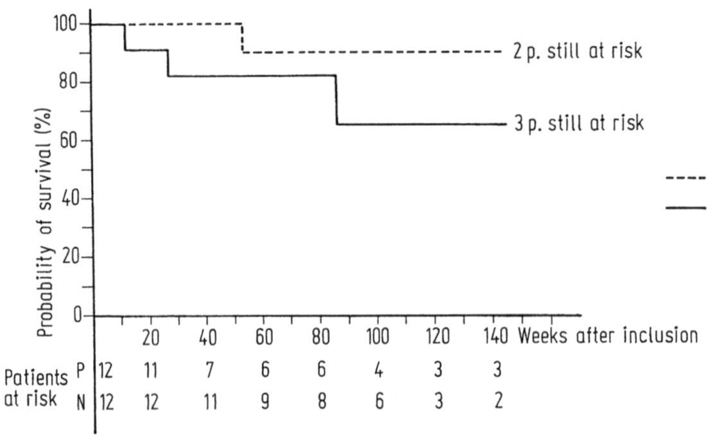


**Fig. 4.** Probability of survival according to the Kaplan-Meier method

### Clinical Trial

The two groups of patients were similar regarding sex, age, severity of liver disease and of portal hypertension, etiology of cirrhosis, number of patients with more than one previous hemorrhage, and serum creatinine, as reported in Table 1. As for the side effects of nadolol treatment, only one patient had to be withdrawn from therapy, because of asthma after 26 weeks of treatment. No other relevant side effect was found.

During the follow-up period, eight patients in the placebo group and three in the nadolol group had hemorrhage from esophageal varices. In Fig. 3 the probability of being free from rebleeding is reported for both groups according to the Kaplan-Meier method. It was found to be significantly higher in the nadolol group than in the placebo group (log-rank test: $\chi^2 = 4.32$; $p < 0.05$). Figure 4 illustrates survival in the nadolol group compared to that in the placebo group. The probability of survival was not statistically different ($\chi^2 = 1.43$), although the ratio observed/expected deaths was 0.46 in the nadolol group and 1.66 in the placebo group.

## Discussion

### Pathophysiological Study

This study aimed at verifying the effects of 1 month of nadolol treatment on systemic and regional hemodynamics and on liver and kidney function in patients with cirrhosis. In our patients with cirrhosis 1 month of nadolol treatment induced a significant decrease in portal pressure and in 11 of 20 patients also a decrease in the severity of esophageal varices. These results are concordant with those obtained with other beta-blockers (Lebrec et al. 1982; Hillon et al. 1982; Westaby et al. 1984). Percent reduction in HVPG was similar to that in CO and a significant correlation was found between them. Therefore reduction in splanchnic blood flow tributary to the portal vein seems to be mainly due to decrease in CO. However, since the splanchnic vascular system has beta-adrenergic receptors (Granger et al. 1980), it is possible that nadolol also provoked a splanchnic vasoconstriction because of unopposed alpha-adrenergic activity.

No relationship was found between decrease in HVPG and decrease in severity in esophageal varices. This is not surprising, since others (Bosch et al. 1984; Cales et al. 1985) also found a difference in the effect of propranolol on portal pressure and on collateral blood flow, as estimated by the azygous blood flow. This is a clue that beta-blockers may also have some direct effects on the portocollateral circulation, as shown by Kroeger and Grosszmann (1985) in experimental animals.

Despite decrease in HBF, liver function as estimated by quantitative techniques such as GEC and aminopyrine metabolic capacity were not affected by the treatment. This can be interpreted as showing that such a decrease in blood flow is not able to depress liver function, and/or the drug by itself does not impair liver function. It is unlikely that the onset of hepatic encephalopathy, occasionally reported after propranolol administration, is the consequence of decrease in liver blood flow, as hypothesized by some authors (Tarver et al. 1983), since nadolol, which has the same effects on liver blood flow, does not depress liver function. The effect of propranolol on liver function is in fact controversial, some reports indicating a decrease in liver microsomal activity (Greenblatt et al. 1978; Bax et al. 1981; Parker et al. 1984) and others no effect (Larrey et al. 1983). Nevertheless, propranolol has been shown to interfere with brain serotonin metabolism (Jeppson et al. 1984), and therefore a direct central nervous system effect could be the cause of encephalopathy in patients receiving propranolol.

As for the renal effects of nadolol, renal blood flow and glomerular filtration rate were unimpaired after treatment, but, since cardiac output was lowered by nadolol, an increase of the percentage of CO distributed to kidneys resulted. As a significant increase in filtration fraction was found, redistribution of intrarenal vascular resistance is to be supposed. Since renal blood flow was unchanged, simultaneous preglomerular vasodilation and postglomerular vasoconstriction can be hypothesized. It is not easy to define the mechanisms through which nadolol causes these intrarenal hemodynamic effects. Decrease of plasma renine activity and intrarenal beta$_2$-adrenergic blockade might be involved. No matter how these favorable renal effects are obtained, they may be of value in cirrhotics, because of the reduction in renal blood flow frequently found in these patients (Epstein et al. 1970; Ruol et al. 1979).

### Clinical Trial

Our clinical trial performed in patients with uncomplicated cirrhosis, whose etiology was alcoholic in most cases, shows a significantly lower rate of rebleeding in patients on nadolol than in those on placebo. In the nadolol group the probability of being free from rebleeding was 100% at 6 months, 90% at 1 year, and 70% at 2 years. In the placebo group it was 67%, 67%, and 26% respectively. The probability of rebleeding in our control group is very close to that reported in other series (Burroughs et al. 1983; Lebrec et al. 1984). This is important, since from it the statistical significance of the efficacy of treatment is derived. Our data confirm results obtained by Lebrec et al. (1984) in a similar series, in which mainly patients with alcoholic cirrhosis in otherwise good condition were included.

As for the side effects we found, only one patient had to stop treatment because of asthma, and no other relevant side effect was found: in particular, no patient had worsening of hepatic or renal function, ascites, or encephalopathy. As for the effect on survival, three patients in the placebo group and one in the nadolol group died (two and one respectively of hemorrhage). At the end of the trial the probability of survival was 90% in treated patients and 75% in placebo. This difference is not significant, although the ratio observed/expected deaths was 0.46 in the nadolol group and 1.66 in the placebo group.

In conclusion, nadolol treatment in patients with cirrhosis in otherwise good condition is both effective in reducing the risk of rebleeding and safe, particularly regarding hepatic and renal function, where no relevant side effects were observed.

### Summary

Beta-blockers such as propranolol have been used for the prevention of variceal rebleeding in patients with cirrhosis. However, side effects may follow propranolol administration in patients with liver disease, including impairment or liver and kidney function, encephalopathy, and central nervous system abnormalities. Nadolol, another nonselective beta-blocker, has some properties which could be useful in such patients, namely low hepatic metabolism, absence of central nervous system effects, and maintenance of renal blood flow.

In 20 patients with cirrhosis we evaluated systemic, portohepatic, and renal hemodynamics and liver and renal function before and after 1 month of nadolol treatment. Nadolol decreased cardiac output, portal pressure, and hepatic blood flow, while mean arterial pressure, galactose-eliminating capacity, aminopyrine breath test, and PAH and inulin clearances were all unchanged.

In another series of patients with cirrhosis who survived a documented episode of variceal hemorrhage, a prospective, controlled, randomized clinical trial was performed. Twelve patients received nadolol, 12 placebo. After a follow-up of up to 145 weeks, nine patients in the nadolol group and four in the placebo group survived free from rebleeding (log-rank test: $\chi^2=4.35$; $p<0.05$). Survival was not statistically different in the two groups (one death in the nadolol group, three in the placebo group), although the ratio observed/expected deaths was 0.46 in the nadolol group and 1.66 in the placebo group. No relevant side effect was registered, particularly on hepatic and renal function, except one case of asthma.

In conclusion, nadolol appears to represent an effective therapy for prevention of variceal rebleeding in cirrhotic patients.

## References

Arthur MJP, Tanner AR, Patel C, Wright R, Renwick AC, George CF (1985) Pharmacology of propranolol in patients with cirrhosis and portal hypertension. Gut 26: 14-19

Bax NDS, Lennard MS, Turker GT (1981) Inhibition of antipyrine metabolism by beta-adrenoreceptor antagonist. Br J Clin Pharmacol 12: 779-784

Bosch J, Hasti R, Kravetz D, Bruix J, Goya J, Rigan J, Rodes J (1984) Effects of propranolol on azygos venous blood flow and hepatic and splenic hemodynamics in cirrhosis. Hepatology 4: 1200-1205

Burroughs AK, Jenkins WJ, Sherlock S, Dunk A, Walt RP, Osuaford TOK, Mackie S, Dick R (1983) Controlled trial of propranolol for the prevention of recurrent variceal hemorrhage in patients with cirrhosis. N Engl J Med 309:1539-1542

Cales P, Braillon A, Jiron MJ, Lebrec D (1985) Superior portosystemic collateral circulation estimated by azygos blood flow in patients with cirrhosis. Lack of correlation with esophageal varices and gastrointestinal bleeding. Effect of propranolol. J Hepatol 1: 37-46

Dagradi AE (1973) Esophageal varices, splenic pulp pressure and „directional“ flow patterns in alcoholic liver cirrhosis. Am J Gastroenterol 56: 15

Epstein M, Berk DP, Hollenberg NK, Adams DF, Chalmers TC, Abrams HL, Merril JP (1970) Renal failure in the patients with cirrhosis. The role of active vasoconstriction. Am J Med 49: 175-185

Gatta A, Sacerdoti D, Merkel C, Battaglia G, Zuin R (1984) Effects of nadolol treatment on renal and hepatic hemodynamics and function in cirrhotic patients with portal hypertension. Am Heart J 108: 1167-1172

Granger DN, Richardson PDI, Kvietys PR, Mortillaro NA (1980) Intestinal blood flow. Gastroenterology 78: 887

Greenblatt DJ, Franke K, Huffman DH (1978) Impairment of antipyrine clearance in human by propranolol. Circulation 57: 1161-1164

Heel RC, Brogden RN, Pakes CE, Speight TM, Avery CS (1980) Nadolol: a review of its pharmacological properties and therapeutic efficacy in hypertension and angina pectoris. Drugs 20: 1-23

Hillon P, Lebrec D, Munoz C, Jurgens M, Goldfarb G, Benhamou JP (1982) Comparison of the effects of a cardioselective and a nonselective beta-blocker on portal hypertension in patients with cirrhosis. Hepatology 2: 528-531

Jeppson B, Bengisson F, Nobin A (1984) Effects of propranolol on brain serotonin levels after porto-caval shunt in rats. 5th International Symposium on Ammonia, Semmering

Kroeger R, Grosszman RJ (1985) Increased portal venous resistance hinders portal pressure reduction during the administration of beta-adrenergic blocking agents in a portal hypertensive model. Hepatology 5: 97-101

Larrey D, Lebrec D, Bercoff E, Pessayre D (1983) Propranolol does not further decrease the clearance of antipyrine in patients with alcoholic cirrhosis. Clin Sci 65: 203-205

Lebrec D, Nouel O, Corbic M, Benhamou JP (1980) Propranolol is a medical treatment for portal hypertension? Lancet 2: 180-182

Lebrec D, Hillon P, Munoz C, Goldfarb G, Nouel O, Benhamou JP (1982) The effect of propranolol on portal hypertension in patients with cirrhosis: a hemodynamic study. Hepatology 2: 523-527

Lebrec D, Poynard T, Bernauau J, Bercoff E, Nouel O, Capron JP, Poupon R, Bouvry M, Rueff B, Benhamou JP (1984) A randomized controlled study of propranolol for prevention of recurrent gastrointestinal bleeding in patients with cirrhosis: a final report. Hepatology 4: 355-358

Merkel C, Sacerdoti D, Finucci GF, Zuin R, Bazzerla G, Bolognesi M, Gatta A (1986) Effect of nadolol on liver haemodynamics and function in patients with cirrhosis. Br J Clin Pharmacol 21: 713-719

Parker G, Daneshmend TK, Roberts CJC (1984) Do beta-blocker differ in their effects on hepatic microsomal enzymes and liver blood flow? J Clin Pharmacol 24: 493-499

Peto R, Pike MC, Armitage P, Breslow NE, Cox DR, Howard SV, Mantel N, McPherson K, Peto J, Smith PG (1977) Design and analysis of randomized clinical trials requiring prolonged observation of each patients. II. Analysis and examples. Br J Cancer 35: 1-39

Ruol A, Gatta A, Zuin R (1979) Renal haemodynamics in liver chronic disease: clinical aspects. In: Bartoli E, Chiandussi L (eds) Hepato-renal syndrome. Piccin, Padova, pp 173-199

Tarver D, Walt RP, Dunk AA, Jenkins WJ, Sherlock S (1983) Precipitation of hepatic encephalopathy by propranolol in cirrhosis. Br Med J 287: 585

Westaby D, Bihari DJ, Gimson AES, Crossley IR, Williams R (1984) Selective and non selective beta receptor blockade in the reduction of portal hypertension. Gut 25: 121-124

# The GABA Hypothesis of the Pathogenesis of Hepatic Encephalopathy: Current Status

Peter Ferenci

First Department of Gastroenterology and Hepatology, University of Vienna, Vienna, Austria

In 1982, Schafer and Jones [1] formulated an exciting new hypothesis of the pathogenesis of hepatic encephalopathy implicating changes of GABAergic neurotransmission as cause of the neural inhibition of hepatic encephalopathy. This hypothesis is based on the following observations:

1. Sera from rabbits with galactosamine-induced liver failure inhibit the specific binding of GABA to its postsynaptic receptor. Inhibition of specific GABA binding by GABA is frequently used for the determination of GABA concentration in biological fluids. The inhibition of specific GABA binding by sera from rabbits with acute liver failure [2] and of patients with hepatic encephalopathy [3] was attributed to GABA itself. However, as the possibility that substances other than GABA may interact with the GABA receptor could not be excluded, the term GABA-like activity has been used. The increase of serum GABA (or of GABA-like activity) was explained by impaired hepatic catabolism of GABA synthesized by gut bacteria and absorbed from the gut.

2. The second important finding was the observation of an increase in the number of binding sites for GABA on postsynaptic membranes prepared from the brains of rabbits [2] or rats [4] with galactosamine-induced liver failure. It was suggested that the increase of specific GABA binding might be induced by blood GABA entering the brain through a permeable blood-brain barrier [5]. An alternative explanation for the increase in the number of GABA receptors was given by Zeneroli et al. [6], who observed in rats with galactosamine-induced liver failure that the changes of GABA receptors varied with the severity of hepatic encephalopathy. In mild-stage hepatic encephalopathy they found an increased numbers of low- and high-affinity GABA receptors, whereas in the severe stage there was complete loss of low-affinity GABA receptors. Furthermore, the activity of the enzyme catalyzing the formation of GABA from glutamate in presynaptic neurons, glutamate decarboxylase, was decreased in the brains of rats with hepatic encephalopathy [6]. Zeneroli et al. concluded that degeneration of presynaptic GABAergic terminals occurs during the course of acute liver failure and may lead to decreased production of GABA. The low GABA concentration in the synaptic cleft may induce an upregulation of postsynaptic GABA receptors. Later on, further degeneration results also in the loss of postsynaptic GABA binding sites.

The most important limitation of the GABA hypothesis of the pathogenesis of hepatic encephalopathy is that most of the experimental findings were obtained from a single model of acute hepatic failure, namely galactosamine-induced acute liver failure in rats or rabbits. There are only few data available in humans. Furthermore, the data on blood GABA concentrations in liver failure are controversial.

Assessment and Management of Hepatobiliary Disease
Eds.: L. Okolicsányi, G. Csomós, and G. Crepaldi

## Is Blood GABA Increased in Hepatic Encephalopathy?

GABA has been measured by a variety of methods in the serum of experimental animals or of patients with hepatic encephalopathy with controversial results (Table 1). By the radioreceptor assay an up to tenfold and by an ion exchange chromatography method with fluorometric detection an up to threefold increase of GABA (or of GABA-like activity) was observed [2, 3, 7]. Conversely, by gas chromatography-mass spectrometry [6] or by an enzymatic method [8] no changes in GABA concentrations were found. In the later study, however, only three patients with hepatic coma were examined, one of them with a twofold increase of serum GABA. While many methods have been used for the measurements of serum GABA, none of them really seems perfect. Surprisingly, the normal range of GABA measured by the enzymatic method or by the gas chromatography-mass spectrometry method is five to ten times that revealed by the two other methods. The basic problem of GABA determination in serum is its separation from other amino acids which are present in much higher concentration.

The radioreceptor assay for the determination of GABA was thought to be specific and very sensitive [9]. The sensitivity of the assay is about 5 pmol GABA/ml. A high specificity of the GABA receptor assay was assumed, as the postsynaptic GABA receptor has been extensively studied over the past 10 years. Only few of the thousands of different substances which have been tested for their potency to inhibit or to increase specific GABA binding actually interfered with GABA binding.

The concentration of the tested compounds, however, were limited to a range relevant for brain function and rarely exceeded 0.1 m*M*. The normal serum concentration of amino acids is between 0.1 and 0.5 m*M*. Recently, it was shown in our laboratory that several amino acids, including glutamine, glutamate, proline, and hydroxyproline, inhibit specific GABA binding with $IC_{50}$ values within their physiologic blood concentrations [10]. As the amount of inhibition of specific GABA binding is a measure for GABA concentration, interference of amino acids with specific GABA binding will result in falsely high GABA concentration readings. Furthermore, in acute liver failure the serum concentration of several amino acids is markedly increased (up to tenfold). Therefore, the radioreceptor assay for measurement of serum GABA is of limited value in acute liver failure.

**Table 1.** Blood GABA in hepatic encephalopathy

| Reference | Method | Model | Result (x controls) | Mean blood GABA concentrations in controls (n*M*) |
|---|---|---|---|---|
| Schafer et al. [2] | Radioreceptor assay | Galactosamine hepatitis (rabbits) | – 10 | 200 |
| Ferenci et al (1983) | Radioreceptor assay | Patients with hepatic encephalopathy | – 30 | 200 |
| Goetcheus and Webster [8] | Enzymatic | Patients with hepatic encephalopathy | 1–2 | 1500 |
| Zeneroli et al. [6] | GC-MS | Galactosamine hepatitis (rats) | 1 | 900 |
| Minuk et al. [7] | Ion exchange chromatography | Patients with hepatic encephalopathy | – 3 | 400 |

An estimate of the magnitude of increase of serum GABA in liver failure can be derived from studies of hepatic catabolism of GABA. In in vivo studies in galactosamine-treated rabbits, a decrease of the plasma clearance of $^3$H-GABA was observed [11]. The data were further evaluated by computer-assisted modeling analysis and a nonparametric model of GABA metabolism was developed [12]. The results of this analysis indicated that a defect in hepatic tissue extraction of GABA was sufficient to account for only 60% of the tenfold increase in serum GABA levels that occurs in acute liver failure. Liver perfusion experiments designed to study hepatic GABA catabolism in more detail revealed that a very efficient GABA uptake system is present in the liver with a $K_m$ of 38 $\mu M$ [13]. Furthermore, it was shown that once GABA is taken up by the liver it is completely catabolized. In livers of rats with $CCl_4$-induced liver failure, hepatic GABA uptake and GABA catabolism was only impaired when very high GABA concentrations were used in the perfusate. Thus, decreased plasma clearance of $^3$H-GABA in acute liver failure can be attributed only to circulatory changes in the liver secondary to liver disease.

These findings indicate that the concept that gut-derived GABA contributes to changes of GABAergic neurotransmission must be revised. More accurate methods are needed for the measurement of serum GABA, but it is very unlikely that a more than twofold increase of serum GABA occurs in liver failure.

## Cerebral GABA Receptors

As mentioned earlier, data on the status of GABA receptors in hepatic encephalopathy are derived from a single model of liver failure, namely galactosamine-induced liver failure. Few data are available in chronic encephalopathy. Table 2 summarizes the results of different studies in various models of hepatic encephalopathy. In acute hepatic encephalopathy, an increase of GABA receptors was observed only in galactosamine-induced liver failure. However, the experimental models used have to be carefully evaluated as to whether they are suitable models of hepatic encephalopathy. In thioacetamide-induced liver failure, about 50% of the animals were hypoglycemic and all had marked impairment of renal function [14]. In chronic encephalopathy in portocaval-

**Table 2.** Status of cortical GABA receptors in hepatic encephalopathy

| | Model | Animal | Result |
|---|---|---|---|
| A) Models of acute hepatic encephalopathy | | | |
| Schafer et al. (1980) | Galactosamine | Rabbit | Increased |
| Pappas et al. (1984) | Galactosamine | Rabbit | |
| Zeneroli et al. [6] | Galactosamine | Rat | Increased in mild stage |
| Ferenci et al. (1986) | Thioacetamide | Rat | Unchanged |
| Pappas et al. (1986) | Frog virus | Mouse | Decreased |
| Ferenci and Zieve (1986) | Hepatic artery ligation | Rat | Unchanged |
| B) Models of chronic hepatic encephalopathy | | | |
| Baraldi et al. (1984) | Portocaval shunt, dimethylnitrosamine | Dog | Increased |
| Pappas et al. (1986) | $CCl_4$ | Rat | Increased |
| Zanchin et al. [17] | Portocaval shunt | Rat | Unchanged |

shunted dogs, the number of GABA receptors was increased [15]. Similar preliminary observations were made in rats with $CCl_4$-induced cirrhosis [16]. In rats with portocaval shunt, no changes in GABA receptors occurred; however, these animals were clearly not encephalopathic [17].

## Data in Humans

Very few data are available in human hepatic encephalopathy. GABA-like activity is increased in the serum of patients with hepatic encephalopathy due to acute or chronic liver disease [3]. In a preliminary study the status of brain GABA receptors in patients dying from hepatic encephalopathy (all having cirrhosis) was not consistent [18].

## Summary

Based on some recent findings the GABA hypothesis of the pathogenesis of hepatic encephalopathy has to be reformulated. The importance of gut-derived GABA as source for an increase in cerebral GABA concentration has been overestimated. Furthermore, data on specific GABA binding in animal models of hepatic encephalopathy other than galactosamine-induced liver failure are not consistent with changes in GABAergic neurotransmission. However, in contrast to other experimental models, galactosamine-induced liver failure is a well-documented model of hepatic encephalopathy which is in some aspects similar to the human disease [19]. In spite of some controversial findings, there is still very good evidence that changes in GABAergic neurotransmission are involved in the pathogenesis of hepatic encephalopathy. In particular, rabbits with galactosamine-induced liver failure were found to be more sensitive to GABAergic agonists and antagonists than control animals [20, 21]. Moreover, the pattern of visual evoked responses in animals with hepatic encephalopathy is similar to those obtained by GABAergic stimulation [22]. Furthermore, the first clinical results using a specific benzodiazepine antagonist for the treatment of human hepatic encephalopathy are very encouraging. The GABA receptor is a supramolecular complex consisting of six different proteins surrounding a Cl channel. Two of these proteins have specific receptors for benzodiazepines. As predicted by the increase in GABA receptors, the number of benzodiazepine binding sites was also increased in galactosamine-treated animals [2]. Studies in galactosamine-treated rats indicated that hepatic coma can be reversed by the administration of a specific benzodiazepine antagonist [23]. Similarly, in a few patients with hepatic coma, the intravenous administration of the benzodiazepine antagonist RO 151788 induced a marked improvement of hepatic encephalopathy within a short time [24]. These data must still be validated by careful prospective studies; however, they provide good evidence that hepatic encephalopathy is associated with marked changes in GABAergic neurotransmission.

## References


1. Schafer DF, Jones EA (1982) Hepatic encephalopathy and $\gamma$-aminobutyric acid neurotransmitter system. Lancet ii: 18-20
2. Schafer DF, Fowler JM, Munson PJ (1983) Gamma-aminobutyric acid and benzodiazepine receptors in an animal model of fulminant hepatic failure. J Lab Clin Med 102: 870-880
3. Ferenci P, Kleinberger G, Schafer DF, Hoofnagle JH (1983) Serum levels of gamma-aminobutyric-acid-like activity in acute and chronic hepatocellular disease. Lancet ii: 811-814
4. Baraldi M, Zeneroli ML (1982) Experimental hepatic encephalopathy: changes in $\gamma$-aminobutyric acid. Science 216: 427-431
5. Horowitz ME, Schafer DF, Molnar P (1983) Increased blood brain transfer in a rabbit model of acute liver failure. Gastroenterology 84: 1003-1011
6. Zeneroli ML, Iuliano E, Racagni G, Baraldi M (1982) Metabolism and brain uptake of $\gamma$-aminobutyric acid in galactosamine-induced hepatic encephalopathy. J Neurochem 38: 1219-1222
7. Minuk GY, Winder A, Burgess ED, Sarjeant EJ (1985) Serum gamma-aminobutyric acid (GABA) levels in patients with hepatic encephalopathy. Hepatogastroenterology 32: 171-174
8. Goetcheus JS, Webster LT (1965) $\gamma$-Aminobutyrate and hepatic coma. J Lab Clin Med 65: 257-267
9. Ferkany JW, Smith LA, Seifert WE, Caprioli RM, Enna SJ (1978) Measurement of gamma-aminobutyric acid (GABA) in blood. Life Sci 22: 2121-2128
10. Ferenci P, Ebner J, Zimmermann CH, Kikuta CH, Schmid R, Häussinger D (1987) Overestimation of serum concentrations of gamma-aminobutyric acid (GABA) in patients with hepatic encephalopathy by the GABA-radioreceptor assay. Hepatology 7 (in press)
11. Ferenci P, Covell D, Schafer DF (1983) Metabolism of the inhibitory neurotransmitter $\gamma$-aminobutyric acid in a rabbit model of fulminant hepatic failure. Hepatology 4: 507-512
12. Covell DG, Ferenci P, Schafer DF, Jones EA (1985) A nonlinear kinetic model of $\gamma$-aminobutyric acid metabolism in a rabbit model of acute liver failure. Math Biosci 75: 121-138
13. Ferenci P, Häussinger D, Meryn S (1985) Production of gamma-aminobutyric acid (GABA) by rat liver. Hepatology 5: 974
14. Ferenci P, Zimmermann CH, Ebner J (1986) Thioacetamide-induced acute liver failure in the rat - a suitable model for hepatic encephalopathy (Abstr)? J Hepatol
15. Baraldi M, Zeneroli ML, Ventura E, Pinelli G, Ricci P, Santi M, Racagni G, Iuliano E, Casciarri I, Germini M, Cavalletti E, Tofanetti G (1984) Portalsystemic encephalopathy in dogs: changes in brain GABA receptors and neurochemical correlates. In: Kleinberger G, Ferenci P, Riederer P, Thaler H (eds) Advances in hepatic encephalopathy and urea cycle diseases. Karger, Basel, pp 353-359
16. Pappas SC (1986) Personal communication
17. Zanchin G, Maggioni F, Salassa D, Vassanelli P (1984) GABA and dopamine receptors after chronic porta-caval shunt in the rat. In: Kleinberger G, Ferenci P, Riederer P, Thaler H (eds) Advances in hepatic encephalopathy and urea cycle disease. Karger, Basel, pp 360-367
18. Ferenci P, Riederer P, Dellinger K, Schafer DF, Jones EA (1983) Changes in $\gamma$-aminobutyric acid receptors in patients with hepatic encephalopathy. Gastroenterology 84: 1371
19. Blitzer BL, Waggoner JG, Jones EA (1978) A model of fulminant hepatic failure in the rabbit. Gastroenterology 74: 664-671
20. Bassett ML, Mullen KD, Skolnik P, Jones EA (1985) GABA and benzodiazepine receptor antagonists ameliorate hepatic encephalopathy in a rabbit model of fulminant hepatic failure. Hepatology 5: 1032
21. Rzepczynski D, Zieve L, Lindblad S, LaFontaine D (1986) In vivo studies of GABAergic effects in experimental hepatic encephalopathy. Hepatology
22. Schafer DF, Pappas SC, Brody LE (1984) Visual evoked potentials in a rabbit model of hepatic encephalopathy. 1. Sequential changes and comparison with drug-induced comas. Gastroenterology 86: 540-545
23. Baraldi M, Zeneroli ML, Ventura E (1984) Supersensitivity of benzodiazepine receptors in hepatic encephalopathy due to fulminant hepatic failure in rat - reversal by a benzodiazepine antagonist. Clin Sci 67: 167-175
24. Bansky G, Meier PJ, Ziegler WH (1985) Reversal of hepatic coma by benzodiazepine antagonists (RO 15-1788). Lancet i: 1324-1325

# Lactitol in the Prevention of Recurrent Hepatic Encephalopathy in Shunted Cirrhotic Patients. Preliminary Results of a Controlled Trial

O. Riggio[1], G. Balducci[2], F. Ariosto[3], M. Varriale[3], M. Merli[3], F. Tremiterra[2], V. Ziparo[2], and L. Capocaccia[3]

[1] Department of Internal Medicine, University of L'Aquila, L'Aquila, Italy
[2] I Department of Surgery, University of Rome, Rome, Italy
[3] II Department of Gastroenterology, University of Rome, Rome, Italy

Since 1966 [1], lactulose has been the main treatment for episodes of hepatic encephalopathy (HE). The rationale for the use of lactulose in treating this condition was initially based on the acidification of the intestinal tract content following oral administration of the drug. Low colonic pH leads to the creation of a pH gradient between the intestinal lumen and the extracellular fluid which favors the trapping of ammonia and other "toxins." Additional beneficial properties of lactulose may include its favoring of the incorporation of ammonia in the bacterial proteins, its cathartic effect, and its antiendotoxic effect [2]. Even if its precise mode of action is uncertain, lactulose has been reported effective in the treatment of HE in a number of controlled and uncontrolled clinical investigations [2]. Moreover, lactulose is now accepted as the drug of choice for the management of recurrent or chronic HE. These two conditions are characterized by neurological and psychiatric alterations which occur spontaneously or after minimal precipitating events in patients with advanced cirrhosis and portal-systemic shunting.

Recurrent HE frequently occurs in patients with surgical portacaval anastomosis and represents one of the main problems in the management of these patients. The prevalence of HE in patients submitted to surgical portal-systemic shunt has been reported to vary in relation to the type of surgical portal-systemic anastomosis, but it is generally higher than in nonshunted cirrhotic patients [3]. As lactulose has greatly modified both the prevalence and the severity of post-shunt HE, it is widely used in this kind of patient.

Although lactulose is, in general, a very safe drug, it may occasionally produce diarrhea and dehydration. Moreover, lactulose is available as a syrup containing only about 65% of the disaccharide and has a very sweet taste that may prove unacceptable to a number of patients. Finally, some gastrointestinal side effects such as nausea and meteorism are usually experienced by the majority of patients [2].

Recently, lactitol - a nonabsorbable disaccaride analogous to lactulose - has been proposed as an alternative to lactulose in the treatment of HE [4]. Lactitol ($\beta$-galactoside-sorbitol) is produced from lactose in a chemically pure crystalline form, can be dispensed as a powder, is soluble in water, and is not so sweet as lactulose. Once taken, per os, lactitol is neither hydrolyzed nor absorbed in the small intestine. In the colon, lactitol is metabolized by the intestinal flora and produces organic acids such as lactate and acetate. This leads to acidification of the colonic content and favors the growth of lactobacilli and other acidophilic, fermentative bacteria and the suppression of acidophobic proteolytic bacteria. Moreover, lactitol induces osmotic diarrhea. All the abovementioned effects may reduce the production or the absorption of ammonia and other toxins by the intestine and may be beneficial in the treatment of HE.

Assessment and Management of Hepatobiliary Disease
Eds.: L. Okolicsányi, G. Csomós, and G. Crepaldi

In 1982, lactitol was first used by Bircher to treat a 61-year-old patient with alcoholic cirrhosis and portacaval anastomosis affected by chronic HE. During a 1-year administration period, lactitol was found as good as lactulose in controlling the encephalopathy but produced no taste aversion or nausea [4].

More recently, Lanthier and Morgan reported a crossover randomized controlled study in which the effect of lactitol on the symptoms related to HE was compared to that of lactulose [5]. The authors administered lactulose or lactitol to five patients with chronic HE for 3-month periods. The patients were monitored clinically, psychometrically, and electroencephalographically and the degree of HE was assessed each month. Lactitol was as effective as lactulose in the treatment of their encephalopathy. In addition, three patients considered lactitol to be as effective as lactulose in determining bowel movements, while two patients considered it superior. All the patients felt the lactitol treatment was more acceptable because the cathartic effect was more predictable and they preferred its less sweet taste.

In summary, from the above clinical study [5] lactitol can be considered a possible successor to lactulose in the treatment of HE.

## Aim of the Study

The apparent advantage of lactitol over lactulose, in terms of tolerability, may be particularly useful in patients with surgical portal-systemic anastomosis who are usually under long-term lactulose treatment.

Our aim was to verify the efficacy of lactitol in the prevention of episodes of HE in cirrhotic patients with portacaval anastomosis. For this purpose, 30 patients were included in a randomized controlled study.

## Patients and Methods

All the patients had a surgical portal-systemic anastomosis and had been included in a post-surgery follow-up for several months. They had all been on a controlled diet containing 1 g/kg/day proteins and had been taking lactulose until their inclusion in the study. About 40% of the patients had had one or more episodes of HE in the 12 months prior to the study, confirming that this kind of patient is at risk of HE. This paper refers to the first 3 months of the study.

The patients were randomly allocated to receive either lactulose or lactitol. The dosages of lactulose, given as a syrup, and of lactitol, in powder form, were regulated in the individual patient to induce two bowel movements a day. The starting dose of lactitol was 0.5/kg body weight.

The patients and their relatives were instructed to contact the medical staff immediately in the event of even minimal alteration in the patient's mental state. This allowed us to record and evaluate all the episodes of HE which occurred during the study. At the beginning of the study and every 3 months, a clinical examination and a number of biochemical analyses, including plasma ammonemia and amino acids, were performed. Conn's index was used for a quantitative evaluation of the neurological status. This index is obtained by giving a score from 1 to 4 for five different parameters: mental state, asterixis, Raitan test, electroencephalograph, and ammonia.

## Results

Tables 1 and 2 show the clinical and biochemical parameters of the patients included in the study. The two groups were similar for the majority of the parameters. However, in the patients in the lactitol group, the age was higher and the previous follow-up longer. Moreover, in this group, the basal Conn's index was slightly worse, although not significantly so.

After 3 months of lactulose treatment, Conn's index was reduced in six patients, increased in six, and stable in three. The mean values after 3 months did not show any statistical differences compared to the basal values (0.19 ± 0.12 vs 0.20 ± 0.12). In the group treated with lactitol, the mean Conn's index was slightly increased with no statistical significance (0.25 ± 0.15 vs 0.27 ± 0.11).

None of the biochemical parameters evaluated showed significant variations during the study (including blood ammonia and the BCAA/AAA plasma molar ratio).

The efficacy in inducing bowel movements was similar in the two groups. This effect was achieved with 36.4 ± 7 g lactitol and 48 ± 25 ml lactulose syrup. The palatability of lactitol was greater than that of lactulose, and meteorism and flatulence were noted only with lactulose. However, one patient in the lactitol group had to suspend treatment due to epigastric pain.

In conclusion, these preliminary data would seem to indicate that lactitol is as effective as lactulose in the treatment of HE in shunted patients. At the end of the study

**Table 1.** Clinical data of the two groups of patients

| | Lactulose | Lactitol |
|---|---|---|
| No. of patients | 15 | 15 |
| Age (years) | 49 ± 13 | 59 ± 6 |
| Sex | M 11; F 4 | M 10; F 5 |
| Child's | | |
| A | 13 | 13 |
| B | 1 | 1 |
| C | 1 | 1 |
| Portacaval shunt | 11 | 11 |
| Mesentericocaval shunt | 4 | 4 |
| Follow-up (months) | 46 ± 11 | 56 ± 12 |
| Previous HE | 7 | 5 |
| Conn's index | 0.19 ± 0.12 | 0.25 ± 0.15 |

**Table 2.** Liver function tests in the two groups of patients (mean ± SD)

| | Lactulose ($n = 15$) | Lactitol ($n = 15$) |
|---|---|---|
| Albumin (g/dl) | 3.7 ± 0.6 | 3.7 ± 0.7 |
| Bilirubin (mg/dl) | 1.7 ± 0.8 | 1.7 ± 0.9 |
| Alkaline phosphatase (mU/ml) | 56 ± 71 | 52 ± 67 |
| Glucose (mg/dl) | 100 ± 27 | 168 ± 107 |
| Alanine transferase (mU/ml) | 23 ± 12 | 30 + 23 |
| Ammonia (μg/ml) | 110 ± 53 | 113 ± 35 |

we hope to be able to state whether lactitol can be considered an alternative to lactulose in the management of this kind of patient.

## References

1. Bircher J, Muller J, Guggenheim P, Haemmerli VP (1966) Treatment of chronic portal-systemic encephalopathy with lactulose. Lancet i: 890–893
2. Conn HO, Lieberthal MM (1979) The hepatic coma syndrome and lactulose. Williams and Wilkins, Baltimore
3. Mutchnick MG, Lerner E, Conn HO (1974) Portal-systemic encephalopathy and portal anastomosis: a prospective, controlled investigation. Gastroenterology 66: 1005–1019
4. Bircher J, Buhrer M, Franz K, van Velthuijsen JA (1982) First use of lactitol in the treatment of portal-systemic encephalopathy. Schweiz Med Wochenschr 112: 1306–1307
5. Lanthier PL, Morgan MY (1985) Lactitol in the treatment of chronic hepatic encephalopathy: an open comparison with lactulose. GUT 26: 415–420

# Concluding Remarks

J. Galambos

The chapters in this book are truly good and informative and one can learn a great deal. The first section is devoted to basic science. We learn about hepatic transport mechanisms in general, and about mechanisms of cholestasis in particular. There are two types of cholestatic mechanism, the mechanical one and the metabolic one. Cholestasis of the intrahepatic variety is due either to inhibition of (a) sodium, potassium ATPase, (b) bile acid/sodium cotransport, (c) the canalicular bile acid carrier, i.e., intracellular transport, or (d) to a leaky paracellular pathway. There are probably problems in canalicular motility which are morphologically manifested by aggregation of microfilaments around the canaliculi. Calcium homeostasis in the cell is also disturbed. This mechanisms, in part, may be explained by lithocolate binding calcium. What is not explained is why the canaliculus is dilated instead of collapsed in intrahepatic cholestasis.

We are told that the vesicular transport of fluid is an alternate explanation for bulk fluid transport which is usually explained by the paracellular pathway. I am impressed by the calculated magnitude of volume transport through the vesicular transport mechanisms; that up to 20% of the hepatocyte volume can be transported per hour, and that five times the plasma membrane surface area can enter into the vesicular transport mechanism per hour. The role of the paracellular pathways and of the tight junction will, I am sure, be the subject of future investigations as well as to what degree the failure of the vesicular transport mechanism is responsible for intrahepatic cholestasis.

We also learn about transport of organic anions by an uphill flow against an electrochemical gradient. I am impressed by the fact that the liver recognizes sex, or at least gender, that organic anions like bromsulfalcin have a much higher $K_m$ in females than in males, although the $V_{max}$ is identical in both genders. It is new to me that taurocholine transport can be inhibited without altering alanine (amino-acid) transport which uses the same mechanism; that there is structural specificity of these inhibitors; and that $K_m$ is affected by competitive inhibition and the $V_{max}$ by noncompetitive inhibition. The structural specificity of the inhibitor depends the hydroxyl group in C6 and C7, which provides the structural requirement for competitive inhibition.

Being a clinician rather than a basic scientist, I found useful a very intriguing test that can be used for measuring bile acid composition; i.e., a string test in the intestine to identify the presence of compounds like sulfated bile acids. Patients who have idiopathic recurrent cholestasis may have a rise of cholestatic bile acids, such as sulfated glycholithocholate secretion before there is clinical evidence of recurrent jaundice. If this is detected in time one may prevent it by using cholestyramine as treatment. It might work because it seems that it abolishes the postprandial rise of sulfated glycholithocholate.

Assessment and Management of Hepatobiliary Disease
Eds.: L. Okolicsányi, G. Csomós, and G. Crepaldi

We also learn about the idiopathic cholestasis of pregnancy. These patients may be helped by the use of S-adenosylmethionine if adequate doses are given. But the mechanism of action has not been dissected. It seems that it improves not only bile saturation index and bile flow, but also clinical parameters like bilirubin, serum glutamic oxaloacetic transaminase (SGOT), and bile acid concentrations in the serum.

From the presentation of epidemiological data on the prevalence of gallstones, it is interesting that the data from a limited study done in Sirmione are very similar to those in a study from the GREPCO Project. We are looking forward to a larger study investigating gallstone prevalence in different parts of Italy. But we have already learned that the frequency of symptoms among gallstone patients is much higher among women than among men. My clinical impression was that cholecystectomies were much more frequent in women. Generally, women have more abdominal operations.

The formation of a gallstone requires two conditions: one is a supersaturated solution of a solute and the second is a stimulus (nucleating factor) to produce precipitation. Interestingly, we learn that this is true not only for cholesterol stones, but also for pigment stones. It the case of cholesterol stones, the problem is the well-known supersaturation of bile with cholesterol. Here, my problem is not why people with lithogenic bile have gallstones, but why people don't have stones when cholesterol is supersaturated in the bile. I am also puzzled as to why the nucleating factor in the gallbladder is so inactive. So many of the cholesterol stones are single stones. Why do they not always form a lot more stones? Although, of course, some of them do.

There is also a supersaturation problem with pigment stones. We learn that calcium carbonate in hepatic bile is present in supersaturated solution. If the pH of bile decreases in the gallbladder, bicarbonate forms and the supersaturation ceases: it is no longer supersaturated for calcium carbonate. There are at least three kinds of pigment stone: black stones, salt and pepper stones, and the brown, greasy stones. The brown, greasy stones have a higher lipid content. Calcium bilirubinate or black stones are common in the east, but much less common in western countries. A new type of therapy, laser lithotripsy, is described. This may pulverize some stones and permit their excretion.

Then the conventional evaluation of patients with liver disease is discussed. A very disturbing ripple went through my thinking when I learned that when using even the most common type of testing, such as alkaline phosphatase or aminotransferases, the values obtained in different laboratories can vary widely. The results obtained in one hospital or in one laboratory may not be comparable with those obtained in another when different techniques are used. But even when the same technique is used, there is a large coefficient of variation among the different laboratories. Hopefully, the methods can be standardized so we can interpret each other's results. To do this, it will be necessary for the clinical chemists to use a common standard together with an unknown and express the unknown in terms of the recognized accepted standard. We also learn that there are several isoenzymes of the commonly used liver tests. It may well be that alcoholism and alcoholic disease or just excessive drinking may be recognizable by a change of the ratio of mitochondrial aspartate aminotransferase (mAST) and cytoplasmic or soluble AST (sAST). Measurements of serum bile acid concentrations are sensitive measures for liver injury, but not much more useful than conventional liver tests. We also learn that looking at conjugated bilirubin in the serum (by more sophisticated techniques than the routinely used direct and indirect bilirubin tests) and deter-

# Concluding Remarks

J. Galambos

The chapters in this book are truly good and informative and one can learn a great deal. The first section is devoted to basic science. We learn about hepatic transport mechanisms in general, and about mechanisms of cholestasis in particular. There are two types of cholestatic mechanism, the mechanical one and the metabolic one. Cholestasis of the intrahepatic variety is due either to inhibition of (a) sodium, potassium ATPase, (b) bile acid/sodium cotransport, (c) the canalicular bile acid carrier, i.e., intracellular transport, or (d) to a leaky paracellular pathway. There are probably problems in canalicular motility which are morphologically manifested by aggregation of microfilaments around the canaliculi. Calcium homeostasis in the cell is also disturbed. This mechanisms, in part, may be explained by lithocolate binding calcium. What is not explained is why the canaliculus is dilated instead of collapsed in intrahepatic cholestasis.

We are told that the vesicular transport of fluid is an alternate explanation for bulk fluid transport which is usually explained by the paracellular pathway. I am impressed by the calculated magnitude of volume transport through the vesicular transport mechanisms; that up to 20% of the hepatocyte volume can be transported per hour, and that five times the plasma membrane surface area can enter into the vesicular transport mechanism per hour. The role of the paracellular pathways and of the tight junction will, I am sure, be the subject of future investigations as well as to what degree the failure of the vesicular transport mechanism is responsible for intrahepatic cholestasis.

We also learn about transport of organic anions by an uphill flow against an electrochemical gradient. I am impressed by the fact that the liver recognizes sex, or at least gender, that organic anions like bromsulfalein have a much higher $K_m$ in females than in males, although the $V_{max}$ is identical in both genders. It is new to me that taurocholine transport can be inhibited without altering alanine (amino-acid) transport which uses the same mechanism; that there is structural specificity of these inhibitors; and that $K_m$ is affected by competitive inhibition and the $V_{max}$ by noncompetitive inhibition. The structural specificity of the inhibitor depends the hydroxyl group in C6 and C7, which provides the structural requirement for competitive inhibition.

Being a clinician rather than a basic scientist, I found useful a very intriguing test that can be used for measuring bile acid composition; i.e., a string test in the intestine to identify the presence of compounds like sulfated bile acids. Patients who have idiopathic recurrent cholestasis may have a rise of cholestatic bile acids, such as sulfated glycolithocholate secretion before there is clinical evidence of recurrent jaundice. If this is detected in time one may prevent it by using cholestyramine as treatment. It might work because it seems that it abolishes the postprandial rise of sulfated glycholithocholate.

Assessment and Management of Hepatobiliary Disease
Eds.: L. Okolicsányi, G. Csomós, and G. Crepaldi

Hepatic drug metabolism and ascites is also discussed. A complete review of these would be extremely long, but suffice it to say that the treatment of ascites has made a full circle. Nevertheless, I think we are making some progress. When I started my medical career, paracentesis was a popular therapy and as a medical student I did many paracenteses in the outpatient department. Often fluid was collected in open containers. Then, as effective diuretics became generally available, I learned that I had done a terrible disservice to these patients and with zeal I joined the chorus of condemners of paracentesis as a treatment of ascites. Now, it seems that paracentesis may become a useful clinical tool again. Maybe we can do better the second time around and define a proper role for paracentesis. To correct the predictable decrease of plasma volume one can infuse 5% albumin or plasma, can reinfuse ascitic fluid itself, or be sophisticated and use ascitic fluid after ultrafiltration. It is important to realize that paracentesis will always decrease the volume of ascites, while oral diuretics may not do so each time, yet both can lead to deterioration of renal (and hepatic) function.

The method of treatment of ascites should depend on the stage of the natural history of the disease, i.e., according to the pathophysiology of the process in the patient. We are told that there is an overflow and an underfill theory, i.e., the forward or the backward failure theory. True, when the patient is in the early stage of the natural history of ascites, excessive sodium retention is the major pathophysiologic mechanism and this is what one must treat. But later in the course of the disease when the patient's hemodynamics alter (the vasculature is underfilled and the circulating blood volume becomes increasingly "ineffective"), then one has to be very cautious in using potent diuretics. One can remove fluid from the plasma if one gives enough diuretic. But, that is not the point. The difficulty is not getting water out of plasma, but getting ascitic fluid into the plasma compartment when diuresing the patient. Will diuretic therapy improve or harm the disease process? The point is that one wants to improve the patient and ensure that he or she maintains reasonable hepatic and renal function. This is an area which is not understood very well.

Another area which I feel has not been addressed adequately by clinical investigators, is what is going on in the liver of cirrhotic patient with functional renal failure. It is not the lack of kidney function which kills these patients; it's the hepatic disease. When these patients develop hepatorenal syndrome, they die *with* but not *because* of renal failure. The current state of the art of hepatorenal syndrome has been well discussed in this book, and we need to pay more attention to it.

The last section is also fascinating. I thought that asymptomatic chronic active hepatitis was a mild, benign disease, at least among the patients I and apparently Hans Popper have seen. Not all that benign, as we learn here. Patients with a smoldering non-A, non-B hepatitis develop cirrhosis with increasing frequency; the longer the follow-up, the higher the frequency of cirrhosis. Even in the asymptomatic patients more and more cirrhosis is detected.

What then are the strategies that we need to follow? I have been persuaded that hepatitis type A is an acute disease and that it does not cause chronic hepatitis. However, I have difficulty in explaining this to some of my patients who have had anti-hepatitis type A (anti-HA) IgM for well over a year and still have evidence of active liver disease. Others have also seen patients whose acute hepatitis A (anti-HA IgM) persists for well over 6 months. One of my patients had cirrhosis. Whether these are cirrhotic patients who acquire hepatitis type A and just happen to have difficulty in converting from IgM to IgG anti-HA I don't know, but I would like to call your attention to the fact that hepatitis type A may not be a short-term disease in everybody. It may have a chronic course even if it does not become a "chronic active" hepatitis.

The problem of managing viral infections is beautifully discussed. What the best antiviral treatment modalities are, we still do not know. And what really disturbs me more than not knowing how to treat active hepatitis B viral infection is not knowing what the outcome of such treatment is on the liver disease. We know the frequency of seroconversion after $\alpha$-interferon or adenine arabinoside (ara-A) therapy, but do not know if serocenversion alters the activity and course of chronic hepatitis B. What do we tell a patient who has replicating HBV-DNA in the hepatocyte nuclei before we give a combination of prednisone and ara-A or $\alpha$-interferon therapy? We are sure the patient will have side-effects: aching muscles, a flu-like syndrome. The patient will want to know what he or she will gain in return. We may eliminate viremia and infectivity, but we cannot be sure that the disease is going to improve and disappear. We don't even know whether we have improved or worsened the chances of late complications. So, at the moment we can measure hepatitis B virus markers and viral DNA, but we have to put it into proper perspective as regards the long-term effect if the therapy induced HBeAg to anti-HBe conversion, as opposed to patients who spontaneously converted from E to anti-E. The chances of having progressive disease are much less in those with anti-HBe serology and without replicating HBV-DNA than with the HBeAg serology and replicating HBV-DNA. It does not necessarily mean that eliminating viral DNA from the circulation by interferon or ara-A is permanent or that it will improve the course of the liver disease in all such patients.

# Subject Index

MIX
Papier aus verantwortungsvollen Quellen
Paper from responsible sources
FSC® C105338

If you have any concerns about our products,
you can contact us on
**ProductSafety@springernature.com**

In case Publisher is established outside the EU,
the EU authorized representative is:
**Springer Nature Customer Service Center GmbH**
**Europaplatz 3, 69115 Heidelberg, Germany**

Printed by Libri Plureos GmbH
in Hamburg, Germany